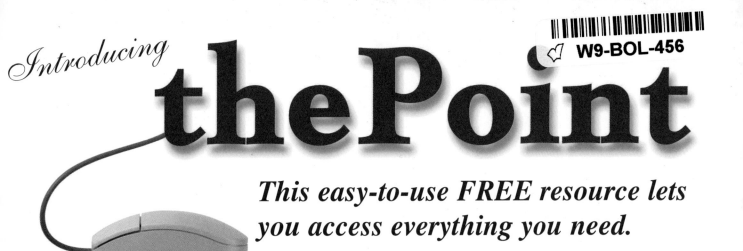
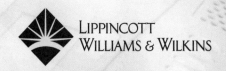

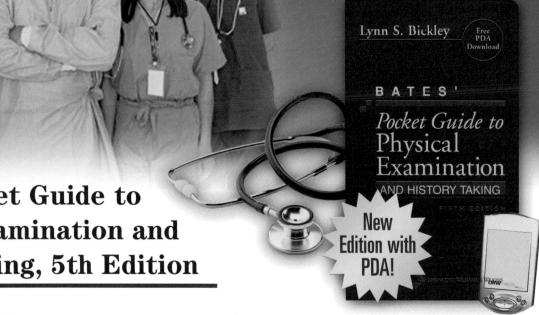
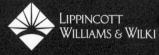

BATES'

Guide to Physical Examination

AND HISTORY TAKING

Chapter 2: Interviewing and the Health History

Elizabeth H. Naumburg, MD

Associate Dean, Advising
Professor, Department of Family Medicine
University of Rochester School of Medicine and Dentistry
Rochester, New York

Chapter 19: The Pregnant Woman
Previous edition contributions by

Joyce E. Thompson, RN, CNM, DrPH, FAAN, FACNM

Lacey Professor of Community Health Nursing
Bronson School of Nursing
Western Michigan University
Kalamazoo, Michigan

BATES'

Guide to Physical Examination

AND HISTORY TAKING

NINTH EDITION

Lynn S. Bickley, MD
Professor of Internal Medicine and Neuropsychiatry
Texas Tech Health Sciences Center
Lubbock, Texas

Peter G. Szilagyi, MD, MPH
Professor of Pediatrics
Chief, Division of General Pediatrics
University of Rochester School of Medicine and Dentistry
Rochester, New York

LIPPINCOTT WILLIAMS & WILKINS
A **Wolters Kluwer** Company
Philadelphia · Baltimore · New York · London
Buenos Aires · Hong Kong · Sydney · Tokyo

Senior Acquisitions Editor: Elizabeth Nieginski
Senior Developmental Editor: Renee Gagliardi
Senior Production Editor: Sandra Cherrey Scheinin
Senior Production Manager: Helen Ewan
Managing Editor/Production: Erika Kors
Art Director: Joan Wendt
Art Director, Illustrations: Brett MacNaughton
Interior Illustrator: Ann Rains
Manufacturing Manager: William Alberti
Indexer: Alexandra Nickerson
Compositor: Circle Graphics
Printer: R. R. Donnelley—Willard

9th Edition

9 8 7 6 5 4 3 2 1

Library of Congress Cataloging-in-Publication Data
Bickley, Lynn S.
    Bates' guide to physical examination and history taking.—9th ed. / Lynn S. Bickley,
Peter G. Szilagyi.
        p. ; cm.
    Includes bibliographical references and index.
    ISBN 0-7817-6718-0 (alk. paper)
    1. Physical diagnosis. 2. Medical history taking. I. Szilagyi, Peter
G. II. Bates, Barbara, 1928–2001. III. Title. IV. Title: Guide to physical examination
and history taking.
    [DNLM: 1. Physical Examination—methods. 2. Medical History Taking—methods. WB 205
B583b 2007]
    RC76.B38 2007
    616.07'54—dc22

2005023366

Care has been taken to confirm the accuracy of the information presented and to describe generally accepted practices. However, the authors, editors, and publisher are not responsible for errors or omissions or for any consequences from application of the information in this book and make no warranty, express or implied, with respect to the content of the publication.

The authors, editors, and publisher have exerted every effort to ensure that drug selection and dosage set forth in this text are in accordance with the current recommendations and practice at the time of publication. However, in view of ongoing research, changes in government regulations, and the constant flow of information relating to drug therapy and drug reactions, the reader is urged to check the package insert for each drug for any change in indications and dosage and for added warnings and precautions This is particularly important when the recommended agent is a new or infrequently employed drug.

Some drugs and medical devices presented in this publication have Food and Drug Administration (FDA) clearance for limited use in restricted research settings. It is the responsibility of the health care provider to ascertain the FDA status of each drug or device planned for use in his or her clinical practice.

To Gerald W. Murphy, Renaissance teacher and master clinician,
whose empathy and acumen have inspired so many.

Acknowledgments

For his thoughtful reorganization of *Chapter 18, Assessing Children: Infancy Through Adolescence,* we acknowledge the important contribution of Peter Szilagyi, MD, our pediatrics editor, to this ninth edition of *Bates' Guide to Physical Examination and History Taking.* For her expertise and careful review of *Chapter 20, The Older Adult,* we extend special thanks to Marie Bernard, MD, Professor and Chair, Reynolds Department of Geriatrics at the University of Oklahoma School of Medicine. We also extend our appreciation to Elizabeth Naumburg at the University of Rochester School of Medicine and Dentistry for *Chapter 2, Interviewing and the Health History* and to her colleagues Laurie Donohue, Valerie Gilchrest, Carl Hoffman, Brenda Lee, Anne Nofziger, Steven Lurie, and Nancy Shafer-Clark. We are grateful for the helpful suggestions of Suzanne Cox, MD from the University of Texas Southwestern; of Steven Berk, MD, Jennifer Peterson, MD, Michael Phy, DO, Fiona Prabhu, MD, Randolph Schiffer, MD, and Gary Sutkin, MD, from Texas Tech University Health Sciences Center School of Medicine; and of Susan Stangl, MD, from UCLA. Chloe Alexson, MD, Jeffrey Kaczorowski, MD, and Cheryl Kodjo, MD, MPH, from the University of Rochester School of Medicine and Dentistry have again made valued contributions to illuminating the assessment of children and adolescents.

It has been a pleasure to work with the talented and hard-working acquisitions, editorial, and production teams at Lippincott Williams & Wilkins. Elizabeth Nieginski, Senior Acquisitions Editor, has handled technical matters with unfailing patience and courtesy. Renee Gagliardi, Senior Developmental Editor, has masterminded content and schedules not only for the ninth edition, but also for its growing list of accompanying products, particularly *Bates' Pocket Guide to Physical Examination and History Taking,* 5th edition and the 18-module series *Bates' Visual Guide to Physical Diagnosis and History Taking,* 4th edition. Renee worked with Ancillary Editors Claudia Vaughn and Doris Wray to coordinate the Case Book and the Web site containing the instructor's manual, the test bank of questions, and the new on-line course in physical diagnosis. Sandra Cherry Scheinin, Senior Production Editor, is again distinguished by her meticulous care in incorporating additions and changes in both substance and format. Brett MacNaughton, Illustration Art Director, has deftly handled coordination of both photographs and illustrations with layout and text. We remain grateful to these editors, as well as to the many other members of Lippincott Williams & Wilkins who have contributed so much to this edition.

For the many small and large tasks that accompany manuscript preparation and submission, we commend Alissia Rollison and Britton Lui, and for invaluable computer expertise, Victor Gonzales.

Contents

CHAPTER 3

Clinical Reasoning, Assessment, and Plan   65

UNIT II

Regional Examinations   87

CHAPTER 4

Beginning the Physical Examination: General Survey and Vital Signs   89

CHAPTER 5

The Skin, Hair, and Nails   121

List of Tables

Introduction

Bates' Guide to Physical Examination and History Taking is designed for students of health care who are learning to talk with patients, to perform their physical examinations, and to apply clinical reasoning to understanding and assessing their problems. The ninth edition has several new features. The book is now divided into three units to facilitate learning: *Foundations of Physical Examination and History Taking, Regional Examinations,* and *Life Span Examinations.* The unit on *Life Span Examinations* includes the new chapter, *The Older Adult.* Citations in each chapter closely align content with evidence from the health care literature.

■ In Unit 1, *Foundations of Physical Examination and History Taking,* readers will find in Chapter 1 an overview of the patient interview and physical examination and an example of how these essential components of patient assessment might appear in the written record. *Chapter 2, Interviewing and the Health History,* guides students through the techniques of skilled interviewing, with a special focus on empathic interviewing, cultural competence, and ethics. *Chapter 3, Clinical Reasoning, Assessment, and Plan* completes the cycle of patient assessment. This chapter discusses the steps of clinical reasoning, illustrated by the assessment and plan of an actual case from Chapter 1. It also provides guidelines for evaluating clinical data and preparing a succinct and well-organized patient record.

■ Unit 2, *Regional Examinations,* Chapters 4 through 17, begins with the important general survey of the patient and techniques for accurate measurement of the vital signs. Subsequent chapters are devoted to the techniques of examination for each body system. These chapters are arranged in a "head-to-toe" sequence, just as you would examine the patient. Each of these regional examination chapters begins with a review of relevant anatomy and physiology, followed by pertinent health history and information useful for health promotion and counseling. The discussions then continue with the techniques of examination and examples of the written record for the physical examination of that system. Each chapter closes with tables to help students recognize selected abnormalities.

■ In Unit 3, *Life Span Examinations,* Chapters 18 through 20, students will find chapters relating to special stages in the life cycle: infancy through adolescence, pregnancy, and aging. The chapter on pediatric assessment elucidates the variations in history taking and examination pertinent to infants through adolescents. The final chapter, *The Older Adult,* details techniques for promoting the special goals of geriatrics: maintaining health and social well-being and optimal levels of function.

We assume that our student readers have had basic courses in human anatomy and physiology. Our sections on these subjects in the *Regional Examinations* chapters are intended to help students apply this knowledge to interpreting symptoms, examining the patient, and understanding physical findings.

Throughout the book, we have emphasized common or important problems rather than the rare and esoteric. Occasionally, a physical sign of a rare disorder has been included when it occupies a solid niche in classic physical diagnosis, or when recognizing the disorder is especially important for the health or even the life of the patient.

Most students learn their examination skills first by practicing on each other. Much of the anatomy and physiology and many of the techniques of examination and abnormal findings are common to both adults and children. Dr. Szilagyi's Chapter 18 helps students adapt their assessment to the remarkable developmental changes spanning infancy through adolescence. The new Chapter 20 casts a similar focus on the unique goals for assessing our growing older population.

THE NINTH EDITION

The ninth edition takes several new departures in *Bates' Guide to Physical Examination and History Taking.* As with previous editions, the changes spring from two sources: the queries of teachers and students, and the goal of making the book easier to read and more efficient to use. The three new units of the book, *Foundations of Physical Examination and History Taking, Regional Examinations,* and *Life Span Examinations,* are designed to bring a more coherent and helpful organization to students learning clinical assessment.

Readers will find both new and substantially revised chapters in the ninth edition:

- *Chapter 20, The Older Adult,* is an entirely new chapter that addresses the demographic imperative to increase not just the life span, but also the "health span" of our older population. It provides students with assessment techniques that will help older patients sustain successful aging to the end of life, enjoying rich and active lives in their homes and communities.
- *Chapter 18, Assessing Children: Infancy Through Adolescence,* has been revised substantially by Peter Szilagyi, MD, our editor for pediatrics. The content now clusters techniques of examination according to the child's developmental stage, whether it be newborn, infancy, early childhood, middle-to-late childhood, or adolescence. The chapter includes a summary of normal child development (e.g., what an infant can do); tips on how to examine children; and many new figures, tables, and boxes of clinical pearls to help you in your examination of children and adolescents.
- As requested by readers, many new tables and photographs have been added to *Chapter 5, The Skin, Hair, and Nails,* to assist beginning examiners with identification of rashes and moles.
- To help students locate the mental status examination, the Nervous System is now divided into *Chapter 16, The Nervous System: Mental Status and Behavior,* and *Chapter 17, The Nervous System: Cranial Nerves, Motor System, Sensory System, and Reflexes.*

All the chapters contain updated information relating to health promotion and counseling. Beginning with this edition, each chapter explicitly reflects an *evidence-based perspective,* listing key citations and references at the close of each chapter. For the first time, all tables are vertical so readers can page through the chapters more easily without turning the book to its side.

As in the eighth edition, each of the regional examination chapters contains sections on Anatomy and Physiology, The Health History, Health Promotion and Counseling, and Techniques of Examination. In this edition, however, Recording Your Findings, which contains samples of the write-up, is more logically placed *after* Techniques of Examination, just before the Tables of Abnormalities. Health history information about symptoms is again incorporated into the regional examination chapter most relevant to those particular symptoms. For example, symptoms and tables pertaining to headache, earache, sinusitis, and difficulty swallowing are found in the Health History and Tables of Abnormalities sections of *Chapter 6, The Head and Neck;* symptoms and a Table of Abnormalities about diarrhea appear in *Chapter 10, The Abdomen.* Throughout the book the sections on Health Promotion and Counseling have been revised and expanded according to new information and guidelines, such as for obesity, cholesterol screening, classification of hypertension, and childhood immunizations.

Chapter 4, Beginning the Physical Examination: General Survey and Vital Signs, is especially useful for students conducting the initial assessment of the patient, particularly nutritional status, measurements of height and weight using body mass index to determine excess weight and obesity, and accurate evaluation of the vital signs. This chapter also contains tables to help clinicians with nutritional assessment, dietary recommendations, and recognition of low-weight conditions such as anorexia nervosa and bulimia.

Color again demarcates chapter sections and tables more clearly, and leads students more easily to insets of key material and special tips for challenging aspects of examination such as taking the blood pressure, assessing the jugular venous pressure, and keeping the patient comfortable during the examination of the pelvis. More than 200 new and revised photographs and drawings have been added to better illustrate key points in the accompanying text.

Even with these changes, readers will recognize the basic core organization of the text. Students may study or review the Anatomy and Physiology sections according to their individual needs. They can study Techniques of Examination to learn how to do the relevant examination, then practice it under faculty guidance, and review it again afterward. Students and faculty also will benefit from identifying common abnormal findings, which appear in two places. The right-hand column of the Techniques of Examination sections presents possible abnormal findings. These are highlighted in red and linked to the adjacent text. Distinguishing these findings from the normal improves learners' observations and clinical acumen. For further information on abnormalities, readers also can turn to the Tables of Abnormalities at the end of each of the regional examination chapters. These tables display or describe various abnormal conditions in a convenient format that allows students to compare and contrast related abnormalities in a single table.

SUGGESTIONS FOR USING THE BOOK

Although the health history and the physical examination are both essential for patient assessment and care, students often learn them separately, sometimes even from different faculty members. Students learning interviewing are advised to return to *Chapter 2, Interviewing and the Health History,* as they gain experience talking with patients of different temperaments and ages. As they begin developing a smooth sequence of examination, students may wish to review the sequence of examination outlined in *Chapter 4, Beginning the Physical Examination: General Survey and Vital Signs.*

Nevertheless, students must learn to integrate the patient's story and the patient's physical findings. We suggest that students study the relevant portions of the Health History as they learn successive parts of the examination. In a few areas, symptoms may lead to examination of more than one body system. For example, chest pain prompts evaluation of both the thorax and lungs and the cardiovascular system. The symptoms of the urinary tract are relevant to the chapters on the abdomen, the prostate, and male and female genitalia.

As students progress through the body systems and regions, they should study the write-ups of the sample patient, Mrs. N, found in Chapter 1 and Chapter 3, and make frequent reference to the sections on Recording Your Findings that display samples of the patient record. This cross-checking will help students learn how to describe and organize information from the interview and physical examination into an understandable written format. Further, studying *Chapter 3, Clinical Reasoning, Assessment, and Plan,* will help students to select and analyze the data they are learning to collect.

Skimming the Tables of Abnormalities makes students more familiar with what they should be looking for and why they are asking certain questions. They should not, however, try to memorize all the detail that is presented. The best time to learn about abnormalities and diseases is when a patient, real or described, appears with a problem. Students should then use this book to try to analyze the concern or finding, and make use of other clinical texts or journals to pursue the patient's problems in as much depth as necessary. Students can refer to the Citations and Additional References at the end of each chapter for additional relevant sources.

RELATED LEARNING MATERIAL

With the ninth edition, we continue the accompanying Case Book, also revised and updated, to help students test their knowledge of symptoms and physical findings by applying principles of clinical reasoning and assessment to a series of common clinical vignettes. Faculty and teachers can again turn to resources available on Lippincott's Connection Web site, including an instructor's manual and a testbank of questions, and a new on-line course covering the basic principles of Physical Examination and History Taking.

In addition, *Bates' Pocket Guide to Physical Examination and History Taking,* 5th edition, 2005 by Lynn Bickley and Peter Szilagyi is an updated, abbreviated version of this text, designed for portability, review, and convenience. The pocket guide does not stand alone; reference to the text and illustrations of *Bates' Guide to Physical Examination and History Taking* is needed for a more comprehensive study and understanding of these subjects.

Bates' Video Guide to Physical Examination, 4th edition, is a completely revised, comprehensive, highly informative series of 18 videotapes keyed to this text. Individual and sets of modules in VHS, DVD, and streaming formats are available from Lippincott Williams and Wilkins. The accompanying front-of-book CD-ROM includes footage from these series, focusing on "Head-to-Toe Examination" and "Approach to the Patient."

EQUIPMENT

Equipment necessary for a physical examination includes the following:

An ophthalmoscope and an otoscope. If the otoscope is to be used to examine children, it should allow for pneumatic otoscopy.

A flashlight or penlight

Tongue depressors

A ruler and flexible tape measure, preferably marked in centimeters

A thermometer

A watch with a second hand

A sphygmomanometer

A stethoscope with the following characteristics:

- Ear tips that fit snugly and painlessly. To get this fit, choose ear tips of the proper size, align the ear pieces with the angle of your ear canals, and adjust the spring of the connecting metal band to a comfortable tightness.
- Thick-walled tubing as short as feasible to maximize the transmission of sound: about 30 cm (12 inches), if possible, and no longer than 38 cm (15 inches)
- A bell and a diaphragm with a good changeover mechanism

Gloves and lubricant for vaginal, rectal, and possibly oral examinations

Vaginal specula and equipment for cytological and perhaps bacteriological study

A reflex hammer

Tuning forks, ideally one of 128 Hz and one of 512 Hz

Safety pins or other disposable objects for testing two-point discrimination

Cotton for testing the sense of light touch

Two test tubes (optional) for testing temperature sensation

Paper and pen or pencil

Foundations of Physical Examination and History Taking

Overview of Physical Examination and History Taking

The techniques of physical examination and history taking that you are about to learn embody time-honored skills of healing and patient care. Your ability to gather a sensitive and nuanced history and to perform a thorough and accurate examination deepens your relationships with patients, focuses your assessment, and sets the direction of your clinical thinking. The quality of your history and physical examination governs your next steps with the patient and guides your choices from among the initially bewildering array of secondary testing and technology. Over the course of becoming an accomplished clinician, you will polish these important relational and clinical skills for a lifetime.

As you enter the realm of patient assessment, you begin integrating the essential elements of clinical care: empathic listening; the ability to interview patients of all ages, moods, and backgrounds; the techniques for examining the different body systems; and, finally, the process of clinical reasoning. Your experience with history taking and physical examination will grow and expand, and will trigger the steps of clinical reasoning from the first moments of the patient encounter: identifying problem symptoms and abnormal findings; linking findings to an underlying process of pathophysiology or psychopathology; and establishing and testing a set of explanatory hypotheses. Working through these steps will reveal the multifaceted profile of the patient before you. Paradoxically, the very skills that allow you to assess all patients also shape the image of the unique human being entrusted to your care.

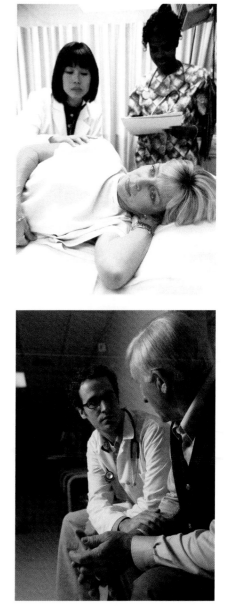

This chapter provides a road map to clinical proficiency in three critical areas: the health history, the physical examination, and the written record, or "write-up." It describes the components of the health history and how to organize the patient's story; it gives an approach and overview to the physical examination and suggests a sequence for ensuring patient comfort; and, finally, it provides an example of the written record, showing documentation of findings from a sample patient history and physical examination. By studying the subsequent chapters and perfecting the skills of examination and history taking described, you will cross into the world of patient assessment—gradually at first, but then with growing satisfaction and expertise.

After you study this chapter and chart the tasks ahead, subsequent chapters will guide your journey to clinical competence.

■ *Chapter 2, Interviewing and The Health History*, expands on the techniques and skills of good interviewing.

■ *Chapter 3, Clinical Reasoning, Assessment, and Plan*, explores the clinical reasoning process and how to document your evaluation, diagnoses, and plan for patient care.

■ *Chapters 4 to 17* detail the anatomy and physiology, health history, guidelines for health promotion and counseling, techniques of examination, and examples of the written record relevant to specific body systems and regions.

■ *Chapters 18 to 20* extend and adapt the elements of the adult history and physical examination to special populations: newborns, infants, children, and adolescents; pregnant women; and older adults.

From mastery of these skills and the mutual trust and respect of caring relationships with your patients emerge the timeless rewards of the clinical professions.

THE HEALTH HISTORY

As you read about successful interviewing, you will first learn the elements of the **Comprehensive Adult Health History.** The comprehensive history includes *Identifying Data* and *Source of the History, Chief Complaint(s), Present Illness, Past History, Family History, Personal and Social History,* and *Review of Systems.* As you talk with the patient, you must learn to elicit and organize all these elements of the patient's health. Bear in mind that during the interview this information will not spring forth in this order! However, you will quickly learn to identify where to fit in the different aspects of the patient's story.

STRUCTURE AND PURPOSES

The Comprehensive vs. Focused Health History. As you gain experience assessing patients in different settings, you will find that new patients in the office or in the hospital merit a *comprehensive health history;* however, in many situations, a more flexible *focused,* or *problem-oriented, interview* may be appropriate. Like a tailor fitting a special garment, you will adapt the scope of the health history to several factors: the patient's concerns and problems; your goals for assessment; the clinical setting (inpatient or outpatient; specialty or primary care); and the time available. Knowing the content and relevance of all components of the comprehensive health history allows you to choose those elements that will be most helpful for addressing patient concerns in different contexts.

These components of the comprehensive adult health history are more fully described in the next few pages. The *comprehensive pediatric health history* appears in Chapter 18. These sample adult and pediatric health histories follow standard formats for written documentation, which you will need to learn. As you review these histories, you will encounter several technical terms for symptoms. Definitions of terms, together with ways to ask about symptoms, can be found in each of the regional examination chapters.

■ Components of the Adult Health History

Identifying Data	■ *Identifying data*—such as age, gender, occupation, marital status
	■ *Source of the history*—usually the patient, but can be family member, friend, letter of referral, or the medical record
	■ If appropriate, establish *source of referral* because a written report may be needed.
Reliability	Varies according to the patient's memory, trust, and mood
Chief Complaint(s)	The one or more symptoms or concerns causing the patient to seek care
Present Illness	■ Amplifies the *Chief Complaint;* describes how each symptom developed
	■ Includes patient's thoughts and feelings about the illness
	■ Pulls in relevant portions of the *Review of Systems* (see below)
	■ May include *medications, allergies,* habits of *smoking* and *alcohol,* which are frequently pertinent to the present illness
Past History	■ Lists childhood illnesses
	■ Lists adult illnesses with dates for at least four categories: medical; surgical; obstetric/gynecologic; and psychiatric
	■ Includes health maintenance practices such as immunizations, screening tests, lifestyle issues, and home safety
Family History	■ Outlines or diagrams age and health, or age and cause of death, of siblings, parents, and grandparents
	■ Documents presence or absence of specific illnesses in family, such as hypertension, coronary artery disease, etc.
Personal and Social History	Describes educational level, family of origin, current household, personal interests, and lifestyle
Review of Systems	Documents presence or absence of common symptoms related to each major body system

---

The components of the comprehensive health history structure the patient's story and the format of your written record, but the order shown should not dictate the sequence of the interview. Usually the interview will be more fluid and will follow the patient's leads and cues, as described in Chapter 2.

Subjective vs. Objective Data. As you acquire the techniques of the history taking and physical examination, remember the important differences between **subjective information** and **objective information,** as summarized in the accompanying table. Knowing these differences helps you apply clinical reasoning and cluster patient information. These distinctions are equally important for organizing written and oral presentations about the patient.

■ Differences Between Subjective and Objective Data

Subjective Data	Objective Data
What the patient tells you	What you detect during the examination
The history, from Chief Complaint through Review of Systems	All physical examination findings
Example: Mrs. G is a 54-year-old hairdresser who reports pressure over her left chest "like an elephant sitting there," which goes into her left neck and arm.	*Example:* Mrs. G is an older, overweight white female, who is pleasant and cooperative. BP 160/80, HR 96 and regular, respiratory rate 24, afebrile.

THE COMPREHENSIVE ADULT HEALTH HISTORY

Initial Information

Date and Time of History.   The date is always important. You are strongly advised to routinely document the time you evaluate the patient, especially in urgent, emergent, or hospital settings.

Identifying Data.   These include age, gender, marital status, and occupation. The *source of history* or *referral* can be the patient, a family member or friend, an officer, a consultant, or the medical record. Patients requesting evaluations for schools, agencies, or insurance companies may have special priorities compared with patients seeking care on their own initiative. Designating the *source of referral* helps you to assess the type of information provided and any possible biases.

Reliability.   This information should be documented if relevant. For example, "The patient is vague when describing symptoms and cannot specify details." This judgment reflects the quality of the information provided by the patient and is usually made at the end of the interview.

Chief Complaint(s).   *Make every attempt to quote the patient's own words.*
For example, "My stomach hurts and I feel awful." Sometimes patients have no overt complaints, in which case you should report their goals instead. For example, "I have come for my regular check-up"; or "I've been admitted for a thorough evaluation of my heart."

Present Illness.   This section of the history is a complete, clear, and
chronologic account of the problems prompting the patient to seek care. The narrative should include the onset of the problem, the setting in which it has

developed, its manifestations, and any treatments. The principal symptoms should be well-characterized, with descriptions of (1) location; (2) quality; (3) quantity or severity; (4) timing, including onset, duration, and frequency; (5) the setting in which they occur; (6) factors that have aggravated or relieved the symptoms; and (7) associated manifestations. These **seven attributes** are invaluable for understanding all patient symptoms (see p. 32). It is also important to include "pertinent positives" and "pertinent negatives" from sections of the *Review of Systems* related to the *Chief Complaint(s)*. These designate the presence or absence of symptoms relevant to the *differential diagnosis,* which refers to the most likely diagnoses explaining the patient's condition. Other information is frequently relevant, such as risk factors for coronary artery disease in patients with chest pain, or current medications in patients with syncope. The *Present Illness* should reveal the patient's responses to his or her symptoms and what effect the illness has had on the patient's life. Always remember, *the data flow spontaneously from the patient, but the task of organization is yours.*

Patients often have more than one complaint or concern. Each merits its own paragraph and a full description.

Medications should be noted, including name, dose, route, and frequency of use. Also list home remedies, nonprescription drugs, vitamins, mineral or herbal supplements, oral contraceptives, and medicines borrowed from family members or friends. It is a good idea to ask patients to bring in all of their medications so you can see exactly what they take. **Allergies,** including *specific reactions* to each medication, such as rash or nausea, must be recorded, as well as allergies to foods, insects, or environmental factors. Note **tobacco** use, including the type used. Cigarettes are often reported in pack-years (a person who has smoked 1½ packs a day for 12 years has an 18-pack-year history). If someone has quit, note for how long. **Alcohol and drug use** should always be investigated (see pp. 50–51 for suggested questions). (Note that *tobacco, alcohol,* and *drugs* may also be included in the *Personal and Social History;* however, many clinicians find these habits pertinent to the *Present Illness.*)

Past History. **Childhood illnesses,** such as measles, rubella, mumps, whooping cough, chickenpox, rheumatic fever, scarlet fever, and polio, are included in the *Past History.* Also included are any chronic childhood illnesses.

You should provide information relative to **Adult Illnesses** in each of four areas:

- *Medical:* Illnesses such as diabetes, hypertension, hepatitis, asthma, and HIV; hospitalizations; number and gender of sexual partners; and risky sexual practices

- *Surgical:* Dates, indications, and types of operations

- *Obstetric/Gynecologic:* Obstetric history, menstrual history, methods of contraception, and sexual function

- *Psychiatric:* Illness and time frame, diagnoses, hospitalizations, and treatments

Also cover selected aspects of *Health Maintenance,* especially immunizations and screening tests. For *immunizations,* find out whether the patient has received vaccines for tetanus, pertussis, diphtheria, polio, measles, rubella, mumps, influenza, varicella, hepatitis B, *Haemophilus influenza* type B, and pneumococci. For *screening tests,* review tuberculin tests, Pap smears, mammograms, stool tests for occult blood, and cholesterol tests, together with results and when they were last performed. If the patient does not know this information, written permission may be needed to obtain old medical records.

Family History.   Under *Family History,* outline or diagram the age and health, or age and cause of death, of each immediate relative, including parents, grandparents, siblings, children, and grandchildren. Review each of the following conditions and record whether they are present or absent in the family: hypertension, coronary artery disease, elevated cholesterol levels, stroke, diabetes, thyroid or renal disease, cancer (specify type), arthritis, tuberculosis, asthma or lung disease, headache, seizure disorder, mental illness, suicide, alcohol or drug addiction, and allergies, as well as symptoms reported by the patient.

Personal and Social History.   The *Personal and Social History* captures the patient's personality and interests, sources of support, coping style, strengths, and fears. It should include occupation and the last year of schooling; home situation and significant others; sources of stress, both recent and long-term; important life experiences, such as military service, job history, financial situation, and retirement; leisure activities; religious affiliation and spiritual beliefs; and activities of daily living (ADLs). Baseline level of function is particularly important in older or disabled patients (see p. 852 for the ADLs frequently assessed in older patients). The *Personal and Social History* also conveys lifestyle habits that promote health or create risk such as *exercise and diet,* including frequency of exercise; usual daily food intake; dietary supplements or restrictions; use of coffee, tea, and other caffeine-containing beverages; and *safety measures,* including use of seat belts, bicycle helmets, sunblock, smoke detectors, and other devices related to specific hazards. You may want to include any *alternative health care* practices.

You will come to thread personal and social questions throughout the interview to make the patient feel more at ease.

Review of Systems.   Understanding and using *Review of Systems* questions is often challenging for beginning students. Think about asking series of questions going from "head to toe." It is helpful to prepare the patient for the questions to come by saying, "The next part of the history may feel like a million questions, but they are important and I want to be thorough." Most *Review of Systems* questions pertain to *symptoms,* but on occasion some clinicians also include diseases like pneumonia or tuberculosis.

If the patient remembers important illnesses as you ask questions within the *Review of Systems, record or present such illnesses as part of the Present Illness or Past History.*

Start with a fairly general question as you address each of the different systems. This focuses the patient's attention and allows you to shift to more specific questions about systems that may be of concern. Examples of starting questions are: "How are your ears and hearing?" "How about your lungs and breathing?" "Any trouble with your heart?" "How is your digestion?" "How about your bowels?" Note that you will vary the need for additional questions depending on the patient's age, complaints, and general state of health and your clinical judgment.

The *Review of Systems* questions may uncover problems that the patient has overlooked, particularly in areas unrelated to the *present illness*. Significant health events, such as a major prior illness or a parent's death, require full exploration. Remember that *major health events should be moved to the Present Illness or Past History in your write-up.* Keep your technique flexible. Interviewing the patient yields a variety of information that you organize into formal written format only after the interview and examination are completed.

Some clinicians do the *Review of Systems* during the physical examination, asking about the ears, for example, as they examine them. If the patient has only a few symptoms, this combination can be efficient. However, if there are multiple symptoms, the flow of both the history and the examination can be disrupted, and necessary note-taking becomes awkward. Listed below is a standard series of review-of-system questions. As you gain experience, the "yes or no" questions, placed at the end of the interview, will take no more than several minutes.

General: Usual weight, recent weight change, any clothes that fit more tightly or loosely than before. Weakness, fatigue, or fever.

Skin: Rashes, lumps, sores, itching, dryness, changes in color; changes in hair or nails; changes in size or color of moles.

Head, Eyes, Ears, Nose, Throat (HEENT): *Head:* Headache, head injury, dizziness, lightheadedness. *Eyes:* Vision, glasses or contact lenses, last examination, pain, redness, excessive tearing, double or blurred vision, spots, specks, flashing lights, glaucoma, cataracts. *Ears:* Hearing, tinnitus, vertigo, earaches, infection, discharge. If hearing is decreased, use or nonuse of hearing aids. *Nose and sinuses:* Frequent colds; nasal stuffiness, discharge, or itching; hay fever; nosebleeds; sinus trouble. *Throat (or mouth and pharynx):* Condition of teeth and gums; bleeding gums; dentures, if any, and how they fit; last dental examination; sore tongue; dry mouth; frequent sore throats; hoarseness.

Neck: "Swollen glands"; goiter; lumps, pain, or stiffness in the neck.

Breasts: Lumps, pain, or discomfort; nipple discharge; self-examination practices.

Respiratory: Cough, sputum (color, quantity), hemoptysis, dyspnea, wheezing, pleurisy, last chest x-ray. You may wish to include asthma, bronchitis, emphysema, pneumonia, and tuberculosis.

Cardiovascular: Heart trouble, high blood pressure, rheumatic fever, heart murmurs; chest pain or discomfort; palpitations, dyspnea, orthopnea, paroxysmal nocturnal dyspnea, edema; results of past electrocardiograms or other cardiovascular tests.

Gastrointestinal: Trouble swallowing, heartburn, appetite, nausea. Bowel movements, stool color and size, change in bowel habits, pain with defecation, rectal bleeding or black or tarry stools, hemorrhoids, constipation, diarrhea. Abdominal pain, food intolerance, excessive belching or passing of gas. Jaundice, liver, or gallbladder trouble; hepatitis.

Urinary: Frequency of urination, polyuria, nocturia, urgency, burning or pain during urination, hematuria, urinary infections, kidney or flank pain, kidney stones, ureteral colic, suprapubic pain, incontinence; in males, reduced caliber or force of the urinary stream, hesitancy, dribbling.

Genital: *Male:* Hernias, discharge from or sores on the penis, testicular pain or masses, scrotal pain or swelling, history of sexually transmitted diseases and their treatments. Sexual habits, interest, function, satisfaction, birth control methods, condom use, and problems. Exposure to HIV infection. *Female:* Age at menarche; regularity, frequency, and duration of periods; amount of bleeding; bleeding between periods or after intercourse; last menstrual period; dysmenorrhea; premenstrual tension. Age at menopause, menopausal symptoms, postmenopausal bleeding. If the patient was born before 1971, exposure to diethylstilbestrol (DES) from maternal use during pregnancy (linked to cervical carcinoma). Vaginal discharge, itching, sores, lumps, sexually transmitted diseases and treatments. Number of pregnancies, number and type of deliveries, number of abortions (spontaneous and induced), complications of pregnancy, birth control methods. Sexual preference, interest, function, satisfaction, any problems, including dyspareunia. Exposure to HIV infection.

Peripheral vascular: Intermittent claudication; leg cramps; varicose veins; past clots in the veins; swelling in calves, legs, or feet; color change in fingertips or toes during cold weather; swelling with redness or tenderness.

Musculoskeletal: Muscle or joint pain, stiffness, arthritis, gout, and backache. If present, describe location of affected joints or muscles, any swelling, redness, pain, tenderness, stiffness, weakness, or limitation of motion or activity; include timing of symptoms (e.g., morning or evening), duration, and any history of trauma. Neck or low back pain. Joint pain with systemic features such as fever, chills, rash, anorexia, weight loss, or weakness.

Psychiatric: Nervousness; tension; mood, including depression, memory change, suicide attempts, if relevant.

Neurologic: Changes in mood, attention, or speech; changes in orientation, memory, insight, or judgment; headache, dizziness, vertigo; fainting, blackouts, seizures, weakness, paralysis, numbness or loss of sensation, tingling or "pins and needles," tremors or other involuntary movements; seizures.

Hematologic: Anemia, easy bruising or bleeding, past transfusions, transfusion reactions.

Endocrine: Thyroid trouble, heat or cold intolerance, excessive sweating, excessive thirst or hunger, polyuria, change in glove or shoe size.

THE PHYSICAL EXAMINATION

APPROACH AND OVERVIEW

In this section, we outline the *comprehensive physical examination* and provide an *overview* of all its components. You will conduct a comprehensive physical examination on most new patients or patients being admitted to the hospital. For more *problem-oriented,* or *focused, assessments,* the presenting complaints will dictate what segments of the examination you elect to perform. You will find a more extended discussion of the approach to the examination, its scope (comprehensive or focused), and a table summarizing the examination sequence in Chapter 4, Beginning the Physical Examination: General Survey and Vital Signs. Information about anatomy and physiology, interview questions, techniques of examination, and important abnormalities are detailed in Chapters 4 through 17 for each of the segments of the physical examination described below.

For an overview of the physical examination, study the following description of the sequence of examination now. *Note that clinicians vary in where they place different segments of the examination, especially the examinations of the musculoskeletal system and the nervous system.* Some of these options are indicated below.

As you develop your own sequence of examination, *an important goal is to minimize how often you ask the patient to change position* from supine to sitting, or from standing to lying supine. Some suggestions for patient positioning during the different segments of the examination are indicated in the right-hand column in *red.*

THE COMPREHENSIVE ADULT PHYSICAL EXAMINATION

General Survey. Observe the patient's general state of health, height, build, and sexual development. Obtain the patient's weight. Note posture,

The survey continues throughout the history and examination.

motor activity, and gait; dress, grooming, and personal hygiene; and any odors of the body or breath. Watch the patient's facial expressions and note manner, affect, and reactions to persons and things in the environment. Listen to the patient's manner of speaking and note the state of awareness or level of consciousness.

Vital Signs. Measure the blood pressure. Count the pulse and respiratory rate. If indicated, measure the body temperature.

The **patient is sitting** on the edge of the bed or examining table, unless this position is contraindicated. You should be standing in front of the patient, moving to either side as needed.

Skin. Observe the skin of the face and its characteristics. Identify any lesions, noting their location, distribution, arrangement, type, and color. Inspect and palpate the hair and nails. Study the patient's hands. Continue your assessment of the skin as you examine the other body regions.

Head, Eyes, Ears, Nose, Throat (HEENT). *Head:* Examine the hair, scalp, skull, and face. *Eyes:* Check visual acuity and screen the visual fields. Note the position and alignment of the eyes. Observe the eyelids and inspect the sclera and conjunctiva of each eye. With oblique lighting, inspect each cornea, iris, and lens. Compare the pupils, and test their reactions to light. Assess the extraocular movements. With an ophthalmoscope, inspect the ocular fundi. *Ears:* Inspect the auricles, canals, and drums. Check auditory acuity. If acuity is diminished, check lateralization (Weber test) and compare air and bone conduction (Rinne test). *Nose and sinuses:* Examine the external nose; using a light and a nasal speculum, inspect the nasal mucosa, septum, and turbinates. Palpate for tenderness of the frontal and maxillary sinuses. *Throat (or mouth and pharynx):* Inspect the lips, oral mucosa, gums, teeth, tongue, palate, tonsils, and pharynx. *(You may wish to assess the cranial nerves during this portion of the examination.)*

The room should be darkened for the ophthalmoscopic examination. This promotes pupillary dilation and visibility of the fundi.

Neck. Inspect and palpate the cervical lymph nodes. Note any masses or unusual pulsations in the neck. Feel for any deviation of the trachea. Observe sound and effort of the patient's breathing. Inspect and palpate the thyroid gland.

Move behind the sitting patient to feel the thyroid gland and to examine the back, posterior thorax, and the lungs.

Back. Inspect and palpate the spine and muscles of the back.

Posterior Thorax and Lungs. Inspect and palpate the spine and muscles of the *upper* back. Inspect, palpate, and percuss the chest. Identify the level of diaphragmatic dullness on each side. Listen to the breath sounds; identify any adventitious (or added) sounds, and, if indicated, listen to the transmitted voice sounds (see p. 260).

Breasts, Axillae, and Epitrochlear Nodes. In a woman, inspect the breasts with her arms relaxed, then elevated, and then with her hands pressed on her hips. In either sex, inspect the axillae and feel for the axillary nodes. Feel for the epitrochlear nodes.

The patient is **still sitting.** Move to the front again.

A Note on the Musculoskeletal System: By this time, you have made some preliminary observations of the musculoskeletal system. You have inspected the hands, surveyed the upper back, and at least in women, made a fair estimate of the shoulders' range of motion. Use these and subsequent observations to decide whether a full musculoskeletal examination is warranted. If indicated, *with the patient still sitting,* examine the hands, arms, shoulders, neck, and temporomandibular joints. Inspect and palpate the joints and check their range of motion. (*You may choose to examine upper extremity muscle bulk, tone, strength, and reflexes at this time, or you may decide to wait until later.*)

Palpate the breasts, while at the same time continuing your inspection.

The patient position is supine. Ask the patient to lie down. You should stand at the *right side* of the patient's bed.

Anterior Thorax and Lungs. Inspect, palpate, and percuss the chest. Listen to the breath sounds, any adventitious sounds, and, if indicated, transmitted voice sounds.

Cardiovascular System. Observe the jugular venous pulsations and measure the jugular venous pressure in relation to the sternal angle. Inspect and palpate the carotid pulsations. Listen for carotid bruits.

Elevate the head of the bed to about 30° for the cardiovascular examination, adjusting as necessary to see the jugular venous pulsations.

Inspect and palpate the precordium. Note the location, diameter, amplitude, and duration of the apical impulse. Listen at the apex and the lower sternal border with the bell of a stethoscope. Listen at each auscultatory area with the diaphragm. Listen for the first and second heart sounds and for physiologic splitting of the second heart sound. Listen for any abnormal heart sounds or murmurs.

Ask the patient to roll partly onto the left side while you listen at the apex. Then have the patient roll back to the supine position while you listen to the rest of the heart. The patient should sit, lean forward, and exhale while you listen for the murmur of aortic regurgitation.

Abdomen. Inspect, auscultate, and percuss the abdomen. Palpate lightly, then deeply. Assess the liver and spleen by percussion and then palpation. Try to feel the kidneys, and palpate the aorta and its pulsations. If you suspect kidney infection, percuss posteriorly over the costovertebral angles.

Lower the head of the bed to the flat position. **The patient should be supine.**

Lower Extremities. Examine the legs, assessing three systems while the patient is still supine. Each of these three systems can be further assessed when the patient stands.

The patient is **supine.**

With the Patient Supine

- *Peripheral Vascular System.* Palpate the femoral pulses and, if indicated, the popliteal pulses. Palpate the inguinal lymph nodes. Inspect for lower extremity edema, discoloration, or ulcers. Palpate for pitting edema.

- *Musculoskeletal System.* Note any deformities or enlarged joints. If indicated, palpate the joints, check their range of motion, and perform any necessary maneuvers.

- *Nervous System.* Assess lower extremity muscle bulk, tone, and strength; also assess sensation and reflexes. Observe any abnormal movements.

With the Patient Standing

The patient is **standing**. You should sit on a chair or stool.

■ *Peripheral Vascular System.* Inspect for varicose veins.

■ *Musculoskeletal System.* Examine the alignment of the spine and its range of motion, the alignment of the legs, and the feet.

■ *Genitalia and Hernias in Men.* Examine the penis and scrotal contents and check for hernias.

■ *Nervous System.* Observe the patient's gait and ability to walk heel-to-toe, walk on the toes, walk on the heels, hop in place, and do shallow knee bends. Do a Romberg test and check for pronator drift.

Nervous System.   The complete examination of the nervous system can also be done at the end of the examination. It consists of the five segments described below: *mental status, cranial nerves* (including funduscopic examination), *motor system, sensory system,* and *reflexes.*

The patient is **sitting or supine**.

Mental Status.   If indicated and not done during the interview, assess the patient's orientation, mood, thought process, thought content, abnormal perceptions, insight and judgment, memory and attention, information and vocabulary, calculating abilities, abstract thinking, and constructional ability.

Cranial Nerves.   If not already examined, check sense of smell, strength of the temporal and masseter muscles, corneal reflexes, facial movements, gag reflex, and strength of the trapezia and sternomastoid muscles.

Motor System.   Muscle bulk, tone, and strength of major muscle groups. *Cerebellar function:* rapid alternating movements (RAMs), point-to-point movements, such as finger-to-nose (F → N) and heel-to-shin (H → S); gait.

Sensory System.   Pain, temperature, light touch, vibration, and discrimination. Compare right with left sides and distal with proximal areas on the limbs.

Reflexes.   Including biceps, triceps, brachioradialis, patellar, Achilles deep tendon reflexes; also plantar reflexes or Babinski reflex (see pp. 633–639).

Additional Examinations.   The *rectal* and *genital* examinations are often performed at the end of the physical examination. Patient positioning is as indicated.

Rectal Examination in Men.   Inspect the sacrococcygeal and perianal areas. Palpate the anal canal, rectum, and prostate. If the patient cannot stand, examine the genitalia before doing the rectal examination.

The patient is **lying on his left side** for the rectal examination.

Genital and Rectal Examination in Women. Examine the external genitalia, vagina, and cervix. Obtain a Pap smear. Palpate the uterus and adnexa. Do a rectovaginal and rectal examination.

The patient is **supine in the lithotomy position**. You should be seated during examination with the speculum, then standing during bimanual examination of the uterus, adnexa, and rectum.

RECORDING YOUR FINDINGS

Now you are ready to review an actual written record documenting a patient's history and physical findings. The history and physical examination form the database for your subsequent *assessment(s)* of the patient and your *plan(s)* with the patient for management and next steps. Your written record organizes the information from the history and physical examination and should clearly communicate the patient's clinical issues to all members of the health care team. You will find that following a standardized format is the most efficient and helpful way to transfer this information. See "Recording the History and Physical Examination: The Case of Mrs. N," for an example.

Your written record should also facilitate clinical reasoning and communicate essential information to the many health professionals involved in your patient's care. Chapter 3, Clinical Reasoning, Assessment, and Plan, will provide more comprehensive information for formulating the *assessment* and *plan* and additional guidelines for documentation.

If you are a beginner, organizing the *Present Illness* may be especially challenging, but do not get discouraged. Considerable knowledge is needed to cluster related symptoms and physical signs. If you are unfamiliar with hyperthyroidism, for example, it may not be apparent that muscular weakness, heat intolerance, excessive sweating, diarrhea, and weight loss all represent a *Present Illness*. Until your knowledge and judgment grow, the patient's story and the seven key attributes of a symptom (see p. 32) are helpful and necessary guides to what to include in this portion of the record.

TIPS FOR A CLEAR AND ACCURATE WRITE-UP

You should write the record as soon as possible, before the data fade from your memory. At first, you will probably prefer to take notes when talking with the patient. As you gain experience, however, work toward recording the *Present Illness*, the *Past History*, the *Family History*, the *Personal and Social History*, and the *Review of Systems* in final form during the interview. Leave spaces for filling in details later. During the *physical examination*, make note immediately of specific measurements, such as blood pressure and heart rate. On the other hand, recording multiple items interrupts the

(continued)

TIPS FOR A CLEAR AND ACCURATE WRITE-UP (Continued)

flow of the examination, and you will soon learn to remember your findings and record them after you have finished.

Several key features distinguish a clear and well-organized written record. Pay special attention to the *order* and the *degree of detail* as you review the record below and later when you construct your own write-ups. Remember that if handwritten, a good record is always legible!

Order of the Write-Up

The order should be consistent and obvious so that future readers, including you, can easily find specific points of information. Keep subjective items of history in the history, for example, and do not let them stray into the physical examination. Offset your headings and make them clear by using indentations and spacing to accent your organization. Create emphasis by using asterisks and underlines for important points. Arrange the *present illness* in chronologic order, starting with the current episode and then filling in the relevant background information. If a patient with long-standing diabetes is hospitalized in a coma, for example, begin with the events leading up to the coma and then summarize the past history of the patient's diabetes.

Degree of Detail

The *degree of detail* is also a challenge. It should be pertinent to the subject or problem but not redundant. Review the record of Mrs. N, then turn to the checklist in Chapter 3 on pp. 81–83. Decide if you think the order and detail included meet the standards of a good medical record.

Recording the History and Physical Examination: The Case of Mrs. N

8/30/05 11:00 AM
Mrs. N is a pleasant, 54-year-old widowed saleswoman residing in
  Amarillo, Texas.
Referral. None
Source and Reliability. Self-referred; seems reliable.

Chief Complaint: "My head aches."

Present Illness: For about 3 months, Mrs. N has had increasing problems with frontal headaches. These are usually bifrontal, throbbing, and mild to moderately severe. She has missed work on several occasions because of associated nausea and vomiting. Headaches now average once a week, usually related to stress, and last 4 to 6 hours. They are relieved by sleep and putting a damp towel over the forehead. There is little relief from aspirin. No associated visual changes, motor-sensory deficits, or paresthesias.

"Sick headaches" with nausea and vomiting began at age 15, recurred throughout her mid-20s, then decreased to one every 2 or 3 months and almost disappeared.

The patient reports increased pressure at work from a new and demanding boss; she is also worried about her daughter (see *Personal and*

(continued)

Social History). Thinks her headaches may be like those in the past, but wants to be sure because her mother died of a stroke. She is concerned that they interfere with her work and make her irritable with her family. She eats three meals a day and drinks three cups of coffee per day; cola at night.

> *Medications.* Aspirin, 1 to 2 tablets every 4 to 6 hours as needed. "Water pill" in the past for ankle swelling, none recently.
>
> **Allergies.* Ampicillin causes rash.
>
> *Tobacco.* About 1 pack of cigarettes per day since age 18 (36 pack-years).
>
> *Alcohol/drugs.* Wine on rare occasions. No illicit drugs.

Past History

Childhood Illnesses. Measles, chickenpox. No scarlet fever or rheumatic fever.

Adult Illnesses. **Medical:** Pyelonephritis, 1982, with fever and right flank pain; treated with ampicillin; develop generalized rash with itching several days later. Reports kidney x-rays were normal; no recurrence of infection. **Surgical:** Tonsillectomy, age 6; appendectomy, age 13. Sutures for laceration, 1991, after stepping on glass. **Ob/Gyn:** G3P3, with normal vaginal deliveries. 3 living children. Menarche age 12. Last menses 6 months ago. Little interest in sex, and not sexually active. No concerns about HIV infection. **Psychiatric:** None.

Health Maintenance. **Immunizations:** Oral polio vaccine, year uncertain; tetanus shots × 2, 1991, followed with booster 1 year later; flu vaccine, 2000, no reaction. **Screening tests:** Last Pap smear, 1998, normal. No mammograms to date.

Family History

The Family History: Can record as a diagram or a narrative. The diagram format is more helpful than the narrative for tracing genetic disorders. The negatives from the family history should follow either format.

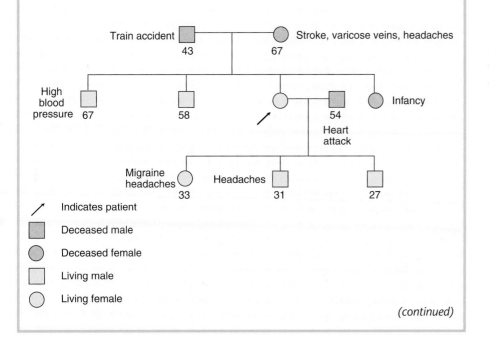

Train accident 43 — Stroke, varicose veins, headaches 67

High blood pressure 67 · 58 · 54 Heart attack · Infancy

Migraine headaches 33 · Headaches 31 · 27

/ Indicates patient

■ Deceased male

● Deceased female

□ Living male

○ Living female

(continued)

---

*Add an asterisk or underline important points.

or

Father died at age 43 in train accident. Mother died at age 67 of stroke; had varicose veins, headaches

One brother, 61, with hypertension, otherwise well; one brother, 58, well except for mild arthritis; one sister, died in infancy of unknown cause

Husband died at age 54 of heart attack

Daughter, 33, with migraine headaches, otherwise well; son, 31, with headaches; son, 27, well

No family history of diabetes, tuberculosis, heart or kidney disease, cancer, anemia, epilepsy, or mental illness.

Personal and Social History: Born and raised in Lake City, finished high school, married at age 19. Worked as sales clerk for 2 years, then moved with husband to Amarillo, had 3 children. Returned to work 15 years ago because of financial pressures. Children all married. Four years ago Mr. N died suddenly of a heart attack, leaving little savings. Mrs. N has moved to small apartment to be near daughter, Dorothy. Dorothy's husband, Arthur, has an alcohol problem. Mrs. N's apartment now a haven for Dorothy and her 2 children, Kevin, 6 years, and Linda, 3 years. Mrs. N feels responsible for helping them; feels tense and nervous but denies depression. She has friends but rarely discusses family problems: "I'd rather keep them to myself. I don't like gossip." No church or other organizational support. She is typically up at 7:00 A.M., works 9:00 to 5:30, eats dinner alone.

Exercise and diet. Gets little exercise. Diet high in carbohydrates.

Safety measures. Uses seat belt regularly. Uses sunblock. Medications kept in an unlocked medicine cabinet. Cleaning solutions in unlocked cabinet below sink. Mr. N's shotgun and box of shells in unlocked closet upstairs.

Review of Systems

General. Has *gained* about 10 lb in the past 4 years.

Skin. No rashes or other changes.

Head, Eyes, Ears, Nose, Throat (HEENT). See *Present Illness.* No history of head injury. *Eyes:* Reading glasses for 5 years, last checked 1 year ago. No symptoms. *Ears:* Hearing good. No tinnitus, vertigo, infections. *Nose, sinuses:* Occasional mild cold. No hay fever, sinus trouble. *Throat (or *mouth and pharynx):* Some bleeding of gums recently. Last dental visit 2 years ago. Occasional canker sore.

Neck. No lumps, goiter, pain. No swollen glands.

Breasts. No lumps, pain, discharge. Does breast self-exam sporadically.

Respiratory. No cough, wheezing, shortness of breath. Last chest x-ray, 1986, St. Mary's Hospital; unremarkable.

Cardiovascular. No known heart disease or high blood pressure; last blood pressure taken in 1998. No dyspnea, orthopnea, chest pain, palpitations. Has never had an electrocardiogram (ECG).

Gastrointestinal. Appetite good; no nausea, vomiting, indigestion. Bowel movement about once daily, though sometimes has hard stools for 2 to 3 days when especially tense; no diarrhea or bleeding. No pain, jaundice, gallbladder or liver problems.

(continued)

Urinary.   No frequency, dysuria, hematuria, or recent flank pain; nocturia × 1, large volume. Occasionally loses some urine when coughs hard.

Genital.   No vaginal or pelvic infections. No dyspareunia.

Peripheral Vascular.   Varicose veins appeared in both legs during first pregnancy. For 10 years, has had swollen ankles after prolonged standing; wears light elastic pantyhose; tried "water pill" 5 months ago, but it didn't help much; no history of phlebitis or leg pain.

Musculoskeletal.   Mild, aching, low-back pain, often after a long day's work; no radiation down the legs; used to do back exercises but not now. No other joint pain.

Psychiatric.   No history of depression or treatment for psychiatric disorders. See also *Present Illness* and *Personal and Social History.*

Neurologic.   No fainting, seizures, motor or sensory loss. Memory good.

Hematologic.   Except for bleeding gums, no easy bleeding. No anemia.

Endocrine.   No known thyroid trouble, temperature intolerance. Sweating average. No symptoms or history of diabetes.

Physical Examination: Mrs. N is a short, overweight, middle-aged woman, who is animated and responds quickly to questions. She is somewhat tense, with moist, cold hands. Her hair is fixed neatly and her clothes are immaculate. Her color is good, and she lies flat without discomfort.

Vital Signs.   Ht (without shoes) 157 cm (5'2"). Wt (dressed) 65 kg (143 lb). BMI 26. BP 164/98 right arm, supine; 160/96 left arm, supine; 152/88 right arm, supine with wide cuff. Heart rate (HR) 88 and regular. Respiratory rate (RR) 18. Temperature (oral) 98.6°F.

Skin.   Palms cold and moist, but color good. Scattered cherry angiomas over upper trunk. Nails without clubbing, cyanosis.

Head, Eyes, Ears, Nose, Throat (HEENT).   *Head:* Hair of average texture. Scalp without lesions, normocephalic/atraumatic (NC/AT). *Eyes:* Vision 20/30 in each eye. Visual fields full by confrontation. Conjunctiva pink; sclera white. Pupils 4 mm constricting to 2 mm, round, regular, equally reactive to light. Extraocular movements intact. Disc margins sharp, without hemorrhages, exudates. No arteriolar narrowing or A-V nicking. *Ears:* Wax partially obscures right tympanic membrane (TM); left canal clear, TM with good cone of light. Acuity good to whispered voice. Weber midline. AC > BC. *Nose:* Mucosa pink, septum midline. No sinus tenderness. *Mouth:* Oral mucosa pink. Several interdental papillae red, slightly swollen. Dentition good. Tongue midline, with 3 × 4 mm shallow white ulcer on red base on undersurface near tip; tender but not indurated. Tonsils absent. Pharynx without exudates.

Neck.   Neck supple. Trachea midline. Thyroid isthmus barely palpable, lobes not felt.

Lymph Nodes.   Small (<1 cm), soft, nontender, and mobile tonsillar and posterior cervical nodes bilaterally. No axillary or epitrochlear nodes. Several small inguinal nodes bilaterally, soft and nontender.

Thorax and Lungs.   Thorax symmetric with good excursion. Lungs resonant. Breath sounds vesicular with no added sounds. Diaphragms descend 4 cm bilaterally.

(continued)

Cardiovascular. Jugular venous pressure 1 cm above the sternal angle, with head of examining table raised to 30°. Carotid upstrokes brisk, without bruits. Apical impulse discrete and tapping, barely palpable in the 5th left interspace, 8 cm lateral to the midsternal line. Good S_1, S_2; no S_3 or S_4. A II/VI medium-pitched midsystolic murmur at the 2nd right interspace; does not radiate to the neck. No diastolic murmurs.

Breasts. Pendulous, symmetric. No masses; nipples without discharge.

Abdomen. Protuberant. Well-healed scar, right lower quadrant. Bowel sounds active. No tenderness or masses. Liver span 7 cm in right midclavicular line; edge smooth, palpable 1 cm below right costal margin (RCM). Spleen and kidneys not felt. No costovertebral angle tenderness (CVAT).

Genitalia. External genitalia without lesions. Mild cystocele at introitus on straining. Vaginal mucosa pink. Cervix pink, parous, and without discharge. Uterus anterior, midline, smooth, not enlarged. Adnexa not palpated due to obesity and poor relaxation. No cervical or adnexal tenderness. Pap smear taken. Rectovaginal wall intact.

Rectal. Rectal vault without masses. Stool brown, negative for occult blood.

Extremities. Warm and without edema. Calves supple, nontender.

Peripheral Vascular. Trace edema at both ankles. Moderate varicosities of saphenous veins both lower extremities. No stasis pigmentation or ulcers. Pulses (2 + = brisk, or normal):

	Radial	Femoral	Popliteal	Dorsalis Pedis	Posterior Tibial
RT	2+	2+	2+	2+	2+
LT	2+	2+	2+	Absent	2+

Musculoskeletal. No joint deformities. Good range of motion in hands, wrists, elbows, shoulders, spine, hips, knees, ankles.

Neurologic. *Mental Status:* Tense but alert and cooperative. Thought coherent. Oriented to person, place, and time. *Cranial Nerves:* II–XII intact. *Motor:* Good muscle bulk and tone. Strength 5/5 throughout (see p. 619 for grading system). *Cerebellar:* Rapid alternating movements (RAMs), point-to-point movements intact. Gait stable, fluid. *Sensory:* Pinprick, light touch, position sense, vibration, and stereognosis intact. Romberg negative. *Reflexes:*

	Biceps	Triceps	Brachio-radialis	Patellar	Achilles	Plantar
RT	2+	2+	2+	2+	1+	↓
LT	2+	2+	2+	2+/2+	1+	↓

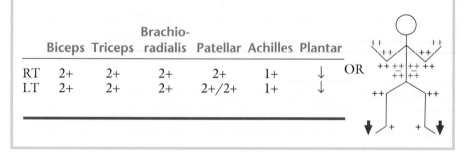

OR

Two methods of recording may be used, depending upon personal preference: a tabular form or a stick picture diagram, as shown below and at right. 2+ = brisk, or normal; see p. 633 for grading system.

Bibliography

Anatomy and Physiology

Agur AMR, Dalley AF, Grant JC, Boileau JC. Grant's Atlas of Anatomy, 11th ed. Philadelphia, Lippincott Williams & Wilkins, 2005.

Berne RM. Physiology, 5th ed. St. Louis, Mosby, 2004.

Buja LM, Krueger GRF, Netter FH. Netter's Illustrated Human Pathology. Teterboro, NJ, Icon Learning Systems, 2005.

Gray H, Standring S, Ellis, H, Berkovitz BKB. Gray's Anatomy: The Anatomical Basis of Clinical Practice, 39th ed. New York, Elsevier–Churchill Livingstone, 2005.

Guyton AC, Hall JE. Textbook of Medical Physiology, 11th ed. Philadelphia, WB Saunders, 2005.

Moore KL, Dalley AF, Agur AMR. Clinically Oriented Anatomy, 5th ed. Baltimore, Lippincott Williams & Wilkins, 2006.

Medicine, Surgery, and Geriatrics

Bailey H, Clain A (eds). Hamilton Bailey's Demonstrations of Physical Signs in Clinical Surgery, 17th ed. Bristol, UK, Wright, 1986.

Barker LR, Burton JR, Zieve PD (eds). Principles of Ambulatory Medicine, 6th ed. Philadelphia, Lippincott Williams & Wilkins, 2003.

Brunicardi FC, Schwartz SI (eds). Schwartz's Principles of Surgery, 8th ed. New York, McGraw-Hill Medical, 2005.

Cassel C, Leipzig RM, Cohen HJ, Larson EB, Meier DE. Geriatric Medicine: An Evidence-based Approach, 4th ed. New York, Springer, 2003.

Cecil RL, Goldman L, Ausiello DA. Cecil Textbook of Medicine, 22nd ed. Philadelphia, WB Saunders, 2004.

Hazzard WR. Principles of Geriatric Medicine and Gerontology, 5th ed. New York, McGraw-Hill Professional, 2003.

Kasper DL, Harrison TR (eds). Harrison's Principles of Internal Medicine, 16th ed. New York, McGraw-Hill, 2005

Mandell GL. Essential Atlas of Infectious Diseases, 3rd ed. Philadelphia, Current Medicine, 2004.

Mandell GL, Gordon R, Bennett JE, Dolin R (eds). Mandell, Douglas, and Bennett's Principles and Practice of Infectious Diseases, 6th ed. Philadelphia, Elsevier–Churchill Livingstone, 2005.

Mandell GL, Mildvan D. Atlas of AIDS, 3rd ed. Philadelphia, Current Medicine, 2001.

Orient JM, Sapira JD (eds). Sapira's Art & Science of Bedside Diagnosis, 3rd ed. Philadelphia, Lippincott Williams & Wilkins, 2005.

Townsend CM, Sabiston DC (eds). Sabiston Textbook of Surgery: The Biological Basis of Modern Surgical Practice, 17th ed. Philadelphia, Elsevier–WB Saunders, 2004.

Youngkin EQ, Davis MS. Women's Health: A Primary Care Clinical Guide, 3rd ed. Upper Saddle River, NJ, Pearson/Prentice Hall, 2004.

Health Promotion and Counseling

Agency for Healthcare Research and Quality. Clinician's Handbook of Preventive Services: Put Prevention Into Practice, 2nd ed. Available at: http://www.ahcpr.gov/clinic/ppiphand.htm. Accessed May 15, 2005.

American Public Health Association. Public Health Links (for public health professionals). Available at: http://www.apha.org/public_health. Accessed May 16, 2005.

Bluestein D. Preventive services: immunization and chemoprevention. Geriatrics 60:35–39, 2005.

National Guideline Clearinghouse. Agency for Healthcare Research and Quality (AHRQ). Available at: http://www.ahrq.gov/clinic/cps3dix.htm. Accessed May 15, 2005.

National Quality Measures Clearinghouse. Agency for Healthcare Research and Quality (AHRQ). Available at: http://www.qualitymeasures.ahrq.gov. Accessed May 15, 2005.

U.S. Preventive Services Task Force. Guide to Clinical Preventive Services, 3rd ed. Available at: http://www.ahrq.gov/clinic/cps3dix.htm. Accessed May 15, 2005.

Zimmerman RK; American Academy of Family Physicians; Advisory Committee on Immunization Practices, American College of Obstetricians and Gynecologists. The 2004 recommended adult immunization schedule. Am Fam Physician 68:2453–2456, 2003.

Interviewing and the Health History

The health history interview is a conversation with a purpose. As you learn to elicit the patient's history, you will draw on many of the interpersonal skills that you use every day, but with unique and important differences. Unlike social conversation, in which you can freely express your own needs and interests and are responsible only for yourself, the primary goal of the clinician–patient interview is to improve the well-being of the patient. At its most basic level, the purpose of conversation with a patient is threefold: to establish a trusting and supportive relationship, to gather information, and to offer information.[1–3]

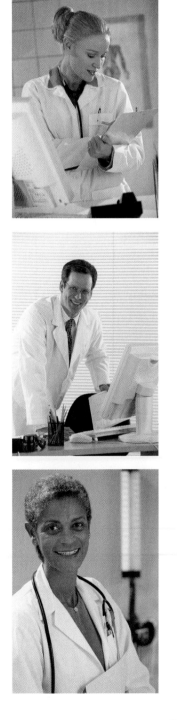

Relating effectively with patients is among the most valued skills of clinical care. As a beginning clinician, you will focus your energies on gathering information. At the same time, by using techniques that promote trust and convey respect, you will allow the patient's story to unfold in its most full and detailed form. Establishing a supportive interaction helps the patient feel more at ease when sharing information and itself becomes the foundation for therapeutic clinician–patient relationships.[4] Because illness can make patients feel discouraged and isolated, "A feeling of connectedness with the doctor, of being deeply heard and understood, reduces this feeling of isolation and despair. This feeling is the very heart of healing."[5]

This chapter introduces you to the essentials of interviewing. It emphasizes the approach to gathering the health history, but covers all the fundamental habits that you will continually use and refine in your conversations with patients. You will learn the guiding principles for skilled interviewing and how to forge trusting patient relationships. You will read about preparing for the interview, the sequence of the interviewing process, important interviewing techniques, and strategies for addressing various challenges that may arise in patient encounters. To help you navigate this journey, look over the Interviewing Milestones, on the next page, that mark the complex tasks of a skilled interview.

As a clinician facilitating the patient's story, you will come to generate a series of hypotheses about the nature of the patient's concerns. You will then test these various hypotheses by asking for more detailed information. You will also explore the patient's feelings and beliefs about his or her problem. Eventually, as your clinical experience grows, you will respond with your

Getting Ready: The Approach to the Interview

Taking time for self-reflection. Reviewing the chart. Reviewing your clinical behavior and appearance. Adjusting the environment. Taking notes.

Learning About the Patient: The Sequence of the Interview

Greeting the patient and establishing rapport. Inviting the patient's story. Setting the agenda for the interview. Expanding and clarifying the patient's story. Creating a shared understanding of the patient's concerns. Negotiating a plan. Following up and closing the interview.

Building the Relationship: The Techniques of Skilled Interviewing

Active listening. Guided questioning. Nonverbal communication. Empathic responses. Validation. Reassurance. Partnering. Summarization. Transitions. Empowering the patient.

Adapting Your Interview to Specific Situations

The silent patient. The confusing patient. The patient with impaired capacity. The talkative patient. The angry or disruptive patient. Interviewing across a language barrier. The patient with low literacy. The deaf or hard-of-hearing patient. The blind patient. The patient with limited intelligence. The patient seeking personal advice.

Sensitive Topics that Call for Special Skills

The sexual history. Mental health. Alcohol and drug use. Family violence. Death and dying.

Societal Aspects of Interviewing

Achieving cultural competence. Sexuality in the clinician–patient relationship. Ethical considerations.

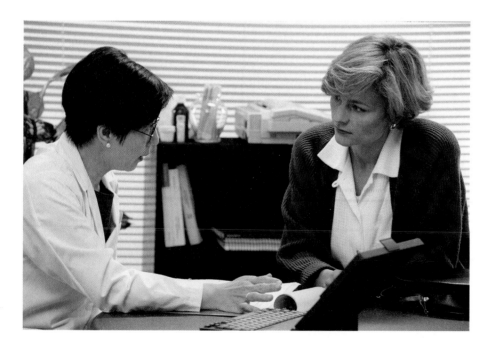

understanding of the patient's concerns. Even if you discover that little can be done, encouraging the patient to discuss the *experience of illness* is itself therapeutic, as shown by the words below from a patient with long-standing and severe arthritis:

> The patient had never talked about what the symptoms meant to her. She had never said: "This means that I can't go to the bathroom by myself, put my clothes on, even get out of bed without calling for help."

> When we finished the physical examination I said something like: "Rheumatoid arthritis really has not been nice to you." She burst into tears, and her daughter did also, and I sat there, very close to losing it myself.

> She said: "You know, no one has ever talked about it as a personal thing before. No one's ever talked to me as if this were a thing that mattered, a personal event."

> That was the significant thing about the encounter. I didn't really have much else to offer. . . . But something really significant had happened between us, something that she valued and would carry away with her.[6]

As you can see from this story, the *process* of interviewing patients requires a highly refined sensitivity to the patient's feelings and behavioral cues and is much more than just asking a series of questions. This process differs significantly from the *format* for the health history presented in Chapter 1 (p. 5). Both are fundamental to your work with patients but serve different purposes:

■ The *health history format* is a structured framework for organizing patient information in *written or verbal form* for other health care providers; it focuses the clinician's attention on specific kinds of information that must be obtained from the patient.

■ The *interviewing process* that actually generates these pieces of information is much more fluid and demands effective communication and relational skills. It requires not only knowledge of the data that you need to obtain but also the ability to elicit accurate information and the interpersonal skills that allow you to respond to the patient's feelings and concerns.

Underlying the new interviewing skills that you will learn is a mindset that allows you to collaborate with the patient and build a healing relationship.

Different Kinds of Health Histories. As you learned in Chapter 1, the kinds of information you seek varies according to several factors. The scope and degree of detail depend on the patient's needs and concerns, the clinician's goals for the encounter, and the clinical setting (e.g., inpatient or outpatient, amount of time available, primary care or subspecialty).

■ For new patients, regardless of setting, you will do a *comprehensive health history* described for adults in Chapter 1.

■ For other patients who seek care for specific complaints (e.g., cough, painful urination), a more limited interview tailored to that specific problem may be indicated, sometimes known as a *problem-oriented history.*

In a primary care setting, clinicians frequently choose to address issues of health promotion, such as tobacco cessation or reduction of high-risk sexual behaviors. A subspecialist may do an in-depth history to evaluate one problem that incorporates a wide range of areas of inquiry. Knowing the content and relevance of all the components of a comprehensive health history enables you to select the kinds of information most helpful for meeting both clinician and patient goals. Be assured that you will fully gain the knowledge of what types of information to pursue, and when to pursue them, as you deepen your clinical experience.

GETTING READY: THE APPROACH TO THE INTERVIEW

Interviewing patients requires planning. You are undoubtedly eager to begin your relationship with the patient, but first consider several steps that are crucial to success: taking time for self-reflection, reviewing the chart, setting goals for the interview, reviewing your behavior and appearance, adjusting the environment, and being ready to take brief notes.

Taking Time for Self-Reflection. As clinicians, we encounter a wide variety of individuals, each one unique. Establishing relationships with people from a broad spectrum of age, social class, race, ethnicity, and states of *health or illness* is an uncommon opportunity and privilege. Being consistently respectful and open to individual differences is one of the clinician's challenges. Because we bring our own values, assumptions, and biases to every encounter, we must look inward to clarify how our own expectations and reactions may affect what we hear and how we behave. *Self-reflection is a continual part of professional development in clinical work. It brings a deepening personal awareness to our work with patients, which is one of the most rewarding aspects of patient care.*

Reviewing the Chart. Before seeing the patient, review the medical record or chart. Doing so helps you gather information and plan what areas you need to explore with the patient. Look closely at identifying data such as age, gender, address, and health insurance, and peruse the problem list, the medication list, and details such as the documentation of allergies. The chart often provides valuable information about past diagnoses and treatments, but do not let the chart prevent you from developing new approaches or ideas. Remember that information in the chart comes from different observers and that standardized forms reflect different institutional norms. Moreover, the chart is not designed to capture the essence of the unique individual you are about to meet. Data may be incomplete, or even disagree with what you learn from the patient—understanding such discrepancies may prove helpful to the patient's care.

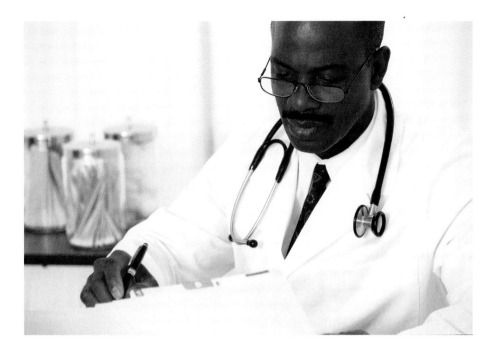

Setting Goals for the Interview.   Before you begin talking with the patient, it is important to clarify your goals for the interview. As a student, your goal may be to obtain a complete health history so that you can submit a write-up to your teacher. As a clinician, your goals range from completing forms needed by health care institutions to following up on health care issues to testing hypotheses generated by your review of the chart. *A clinician must balance these provider-centered goals with patient-centered goals.* There can be tension between the needs of the provider, the institution, and the patient and family. Part of the clinician's task is to consider these multiple agendas. By taking a few minutes to think through your goals ahead of time, you will find it easier to strike a healthy balance among the various purposes of the interview to come.

Reviewing Your Clinical Behavior and Appearance.   Just as you carefully observe the patient throughout the interview, the patient will be watching you. Consciously or not, you send messages through both your words and your behavior. Be sensitive to those messages and manage them as well as you can. Posture, gestures, eye contact, and tone of voice all convey the extent of your interest, attention, acceptance, and understanding. The skilled interviewer seems calm and unhurried, even when time is limited. Reactions that betray disapproval, embarrassment, impatience, or boredom block communication, as do any behaviors that condescend, stereotype, criticize, or belittle the patient. Although these types of negative feelings are at times unavoidable, as a health care professional, you must take pains not to express them. Guard against these feelings not only when talking to patients but also when discussing patients with your colleagues.

Your personal appearance also affects your clinical relationships. Patients find cleanliness, neatness, conservative dress, and a name tag reassuring. Remember to keep *the patient's perspective* in mind if you want to build the patient's trust.

Adjusting the Environment.   Try to make the interview setting as private and comfortable as possible. Although you may have to talk with the patient under difficult circumstances, such as in a two-bed room or the corridor of a busy emergency department, a proper environment improves communication. If there are privacy curtains, ask permission to pull them shut. Suggest moving to an empty room instead of talking in a waiting area. *As the clinician, it is part of your job to make adjustments to the location and seating that make the patient and you more comfortable.* These efforts are always worth the time.

Taking Notes.   As a novice, you will need to write down much of what you learn during the interview. Even though experienced clinicians recall much of the interview without taking notes, no one can remember all the details of a comprehensive history. Jot down short phrases, specific dates, or words rather than trying to put them into a final format, but do not let note-taking or written forms distract you from the patient. Maintain good eye contact, and whenever the patient is talking about sensitive or disturbing material, put down your pen. Most patients are accustomed to note-taking, but for those who find it uncomfortable, explore their concerns and explain your need to make an accurate record.

LEARNING ABOUT THE PATIENT: THE SEQUENCE OF THE INTERVIEW

Once you have devoted time and thought to preparing for the interview, you are fully ready to listen to the patient, elicit the patient's concerns, and learn about the patient's health. In general, an interview moves through several stages. *Throughout this sequence you, as the clinician, must always be attuned to the patient's feelings, help the patient express them, respond to their content, and validate their significance.* A typical sequence follows.

The Sequence of the Interview

- Greeting the patient and establishing rapport
- Inviting the patient's story
- Establishing the agenda for the interview
- Expanding and clarifying the patient's story
- Generating and testing diagnostic hypotheses
- Creating a shared understanding of the problem
- Negotiating a plan (includes further evaluation, treatment, and patient education)
- Planning for follow-up and closing the interview

As a student, you will concentrate primarily on gathering the patient's story and creating a shared understanding of the problem. As you become a practicing clinician, reaching agreement on a plan for further evaluation and treatment becomes more important. Whether the interview is comprehensive or focused, you should move through this sequence with close attention to the patient's feelings and affect, always working on strengthening the relationship.

Greeting the Patient and Establishing Rapport. The initial moments of your encounter with the patient lay the foundation for your ongoing relationship. How you greet the patient and other visitors in the room, provide for the patient's comfort, and arrange the physical setting all shape the patient's first impressions.

As you begin, *greet the patient* by name and introduce yourself, giving your own name. If possible, shake hands with the patient. If this is the first contact, explain your role, including your status as a student and how you will be involved in the patient's care. Repeat this part of the introduction on subsequent meetings until you are confident that the patient knows who you are: "Good Morning, Mr. Peters. I am Susannah Martinez, a third-year medical student. You may remember me. I was here yesterday talking with you about your heart problems. I am part of the medical team taking care of you."

Using a formal title to address the patient (e.g., Mr. O'Neil, Ms. Washington) is always best.[7,8] Except with children or adolescents, avoid first names unless you have specific permission from the patient or family. Addressing an unfamiliar adult as "granny" or "dear" can depersonalize and demean. If you are unsure how to pronounce the patient's name, don't be afraid to ask. You can say: "I am afraid of mispronouncing your name. Could you say it for me?" Then repeat it to make sure that you heard it correctly.

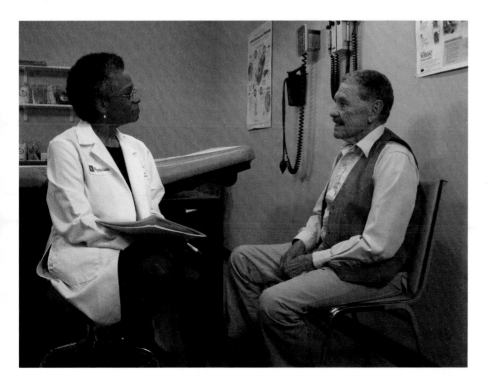

When visitors are in the room, be sure to acknowledge and greet each one in turn, inquiring about each person's name and relationship to the patient. Whenever visitors are present, *you are obligated to maintain the patient's confidentiality*. Let the patient decide if visitors or family members should remain in the room, and ask for the patient's permission before conducting the interview in front of them. For example, "I am comfortable with having your sister stay for the interview, Mrs. Jones, but I want to make sure that this is also what you want" or "Would you prefer if I spoke to you alone or with your sister present?"

Always be attuned to the patient's comfort. In the office or clinic, help the patient find a suitable place for coats and belongings. In the hospital, after greeting the patient, ask how the patient is feeling and if you are coming at a convenient time. Arranging the bed to make the patient more comfortable or allowing a few minutes for the patient to say goodbye to visitors or finish using the bedpan demonstrates your awareness of the patient's needs. In any setting, look for signs of discomfort, such as shifting position or facial expressions showing pain or anxiety. You must attend to pain or anxiety first, both to encourage the patient's trust and to allow enough ease for the interview to proceed.

Consider the best way to *arrange the room* and how far you should be from the patient. Remember that cultural background and individual taste influence preferences about interpersonal space. Choose a distance that facilitates conversation and allows good eye contact. You should probably be within several feet, close enough to be intimate but not intrusive. Pull up a chair and, if possible, sit at eye level with the patient. Move any physical barriers, like desks or bedside tables, out of the way. In an outpatient setting, sitting on a rolling stool, for example, allows you to change distances in response to patient cues. Avoid arrangements that connote disrespect or inequality of power, such as interviewing a woman already positioned for a pelvic examination. Such arrangements are unacceptable. Lighting also makes a difference. If you sit between a patient and a bright light or window, although your view might be good, the patient may have to squint uncomfortably to see you, making the interaction more like an interrogation than a supportive interview.

As you begin the interview, give the patient your undivided attention. Spend enough time on small talk to put the patient at ease, and avoid looking down to take notes or reading the chart.

Inviting the Patient's Story. Now that you have established rapport, you are ready to pursue the patient's reason for seeking health care, designated the *chief complaint*. Begin with **open-ended questions** that allow full freedom of response: "What concerns bring you here today?" or "How can I help you?" Helpful open-ended questions are "Was there a specific health concern that prompted you to schedule this appointment?" and "What made you decide to come in to see us today?" Note that these questions encourage the patient to express any possible concerns and do not restrict the patient to a minimally informative "yes" or "no" answer. Sometimes patients do not have a specific complaint or problem—they may want only a blood pressure check or a routine examination. Others may say they just want a physical examination but feel uncomfortable bringing up an underlying concern. In all these situations, *it is still important to start with the patient's story.*[9]

Train yourself to *follow the patient's leads.* Good interviewing technique includes using verbal and nonverbal cues that prompt patients to recount their stories spontaneously. If you intervene too early or ask specific questions prematurely, you risk trampling on the very information you are seeking. You should listen actively and make use of *continuers* (see p. 38), especially at the outset. These include nodding your head and phrases such as "uh huh," "go on," or "I see." Using additional guided questioning (see p. 36) helps you avoid missing any of the patient's concerns.

Listen to the patient's answer *without interrupting.* Studies show that clinicians interrupt patients during office visits after only 18 seconds![10] If patients are allowed to tell their stories, most will finish within 2 minutes. After you have given the patient the opportunity to respond fully, inquire again or even several times, "What else?," "Tell me more," or "Any further concerns?" You may need to lead patients back several times to elicit additional concerns or issues they may want to tell you about.

Establishing an Agenda. The clinician often approaches the interview with specific goals in mind. The patient also has specific questions and concerns. It is important to identify all these issues at the beginning of the encounter. This allows you to use the time available most effectively and ensures that you hear all the patient's issues. As a student, you often have enough time to cover the breadth of both your concerns and those of the patient in one visit. For a clinician, however, time is almost always constrained. As a clinician, you may need to focus the interview by asking the patient which problem is most pressing. For example, "You have told me about several different problems that are important for us to discuss. I also wanted to review your blood pressure medication. We need to decide which problems to address today. Can you tell me which one you are most concerned about?" Once you have agreed on a manageable list, let the patient know that the other problems are also important and will be addressed during a future visit—this reinforces the patient's confidence in your ongoing collaboration. Then proceed with questions such as, "Tell me more about that first problem that you mentioned."

Expanding and Clarifying the Patient's Story. You then guide the patient into elaborating areas of the health history that seem most significant. As a clinician, each symptom has attributes that you must clarify, including context, associations, and chronology. For pain and many other symptoms, understanding these essential characteristics, summarized below as the seven key attributes of a symptom, is critical.

Always pursue the seven attributes. Two mnemonics may help: **OLD CARTS** (**O**nset, **L**ocation, **D**uration, **C**haracter, **A**ggravating/**A**lleviating Factors, **Ra**diation, and **T**iming) and **OPQRST** (**O**nset, **P**alliating/**P**rovoking Factors, **Q**uality, **R**adiation, **S**ite, and **T**iming).

THE SEVEN ATTRIBUTES OF A SYMPTOM

1. *Location.* Where is it? Does it radiate?
2. *Quality.* What is it like?
3. *Quantity or severity.* How bad is it? (For pain, ask for a rating on a scale of 1 to 10.)
4. *Timing.* When did (does) it start? How long does it last? How often does it come?
5. *Setting in which it occurs.* Include environmental factors, personal activities, emotional reactions, or other circumstances that may have contributed to the illness.
6. *Remitting or exacerbating factors.* Is there anything that makes it better or worse?
7. *Associated manifestations.* Have you noticed anything else that accompanies it?

As you explore these attributes, be sure that you *use language that is understandable and appropriate* to the patient. Although you might ask a trained health professional about dyspnea, the customary term for patients is "shortness of breath." It is easy to slip into using medical language, but beware. Technical language confuses the patient and often blocks communication. Whenever possible, *use the patient's words,* making sure you clarify their meaning.

It is important to establish *the sequence and time course* of each of the patient's symptoms if you are to arrive at accurate assessments. You can encourage a chronologic account by asking such questions as "What then?" or "What happened next?" or "Please start at the beginning, or the last time you felt well, and go step by step." To fill in specific details, guide the patient's story by using different types of questions and the techniques of skilled interviewing described on pp. 35–41. You will need to use some focused questions to elicit specific information that the patient has not already offered (see p. 37). *In general, an interview moves back and forth from open-ended questions to increasingly focused questions and then on to another open-ended question.*

Generating and Testing Diagnostic Hypotheses. Eventually, as you gain experience listening to patient concerns, you will develop the skills of "clinical reasoning." You will *generate and test diagnostic hypotheses* about what disease process might be present. Identifying the various attributes of the patient's symptoms and pursuing specific details are fundamental to recognizing patterns of disease and to generating the differential diagnosis. As you learn more about diagnostic patterns and epidemiology, knowing what data you are listening for and asking about specific details become more automatic. For additional data that contribute to your analysis, use items from relevant sections of the review of systems. (In your oral presentations and written record, add the information gathered from your responses to review of systems questions to the latter paragraphs of the History of Present Illness—this information now constitutes "pertinent positives" and "pertinent negatives"—see Chapter 1, p. 7).

Appropriate questions about symptoms are also suggested in each of the chapters on the regional physical examinations. This is one way that you build evidence for and against various diagnostic possibilities. This kind of clinical thinking is illustrated by the tables on symptoms found in the regional examination chapters and further discussed in Chapter 3, Clinical Reasoning, Assessment, and Plan. The challenge is to not let this kind of inquiry dominate the interview and displace learning about the patient's perspective, conveying concern for the patient's well-being and building the relationship.[5]

Creating a Shared Understanding of the Problem. Recent literature makes it clear that delivering effective health care requires exploring the deeper meanings patients attach to their symptoms. Although the "seven attributes of a symptom" add important details to the patient's history, the **disease/illness distinction model** helps you understand the full range of what every good interview needs to cover.[11] This model acknowledges the very different yet complementary perspectives of the clinician and the patient. *Disease* is the explanation that the *clinician* brings to the symptoms. It is the way that the clinician organizes what he or she learns from the patient that leads to a clinical diagnosis. *Illness* can be defined as how the *patient* experiences symptoms. Many factors may shape this experience, including prior personal or family health, the effect of symptoms on everyday life, individual outlook and style of coping, and expectations about medical care. The melding of these perspectives forms the basis for planning evaluation and treatment. *The clinical interview needs to take into account both of these views of reality.*

Even a chief complaint as straightforward as sore throat can illustrate these divergent views. The patient may be most concerned about pain and difficulty swallowing, missing time from work, or a cousin who was hospitalized with tonsillitis. The clinician, however, may focus on specific points in the history that differentiate streptococcal pharyngitis from other etiologies, or on a questionable history of allergy to penicillin. To understand the patient's expectations, the clinician needs to go beyond just the attributes of a symptom. Learning about the patient's perception of illness means asking patient-centered questions in the six domains listed below. This information is crucial to patient satisfaction, effective health care, and patient follow-through.[12,13]

EXPLORING THE PATIENT'S PERSPECTIVE

- The patient's thoughts about the nature and the cause of the problem
- The patient's feelings, especially fears, about the problem
- The patient's expectations of the clinician and health care
- The effect of the problem on the patient's life
- Prior personal or family experiences that are similar
- Therapeutic approaches the patient has already tried

The clinician should explore the patient's thoughts about the cause of the problem by saying, for example, "Why do you think you have this stomachache?" To uncover the patient's feelings you might ask, "What concerns you most about the pain?" A patient may worry that the pain is a symptom of serious disease and want reassurance. Alternatively, the patient may be less concerned about the cause of the pain and just want relief. You need to find out what the patient expects from you, the clinician, or from health care in general . . . "I am glad that the pain is almost gone, how specifically can I help you now?" Even if the stomach pain is almost gone, the patient may need a work excuse to take to an employer.

It may be helpful to ask the patient about prior experiences, what has been tried so far, and any related changes in daily activities.

> Clinician: "Has anything like this happened to you or your family before?"

> Patient: "I was worried that I might have appendicitis. My Uncle Charlie died of a ruptured appendix."

Explore what the patient has done so far to take care of the problem. Most patients will have tried over-the-counter medications, traditional remedies, or advice from friends or family.

Ask how the illness has affected the patient's lifestyle and level of activity. This question is especially important for patients with chronic illness. "What can't you do now that you could do before? How has your backache (shortness of breath, etc.) affected your ability to work? . . . Your life at home? . . . Your social activities? . . . Your role as a parent? . . . Your function in intimate relationships? . . . The way you feel about yourself as a person?"

Negotiating a Plan. Learning about the disease and conceptualizing the illness give you and the patient the opportunity to create a complete and congruent picture of the problem. This multifaceted picture then forms the basis for planning further evaluation (e.g., physical examination, laboratory tests, consultations) and negotiating a treatment plan. It also plays an important role in building rapport with your patient. More specific techniques for negotiating a plan can be found in Chapter 3. Advanced skills, such as steps for motivating change and the therapeutic use of the clinician–patient relationship, are beyond the scope of this book.

Planning for Follow-Up and Closing. You may find that ending the interview is difficult. Patients often have many questions, and if you have done your job well, they are engaged and affirmed as they talk with you. Let the patient know that the end of the interview is approaching to allow time for the patient to ask any final questions. Make sure the patient understands the mutual plans you have developed. For example, before gathering your papers or standing to leave the room, you can say, "We need to stop now. Do you have any questions about what we've covered?" As you close, reviewing future evaluation, treatments, and follow-up is helpful. "So, you will take the medicine as we discussed, get the blood test before you leave today, and make a follow-up appointment for 4 weeks. Do you have any questions about this?" Address any related concerns or questions that the patient raises.

The patient should have a chance to ask any final questions; however, the last few minutes are not the time to bring up new topics. If that happens (and the concern is not life-threatening), simply assure the patient of your interest and make plans to address the problem at a future time. "That knee pain sounds concerning. Why don't you make an appointment for next week so we can discuss it?" Reconfirming your continued commitment to improving the patient's health is always appreciated.

BUILDING A THERAPEUTIC RELATIONSHIP: THE TECHNIQUES OF SKILLED INTERVIEWING

Building the Relationship.   You probably had many reasons to become a health care professional, but one of them was undoubtedly the desire to serve others. To succeed in fulfilling this laudable goal, you must sustain this motivation throughout your rigorous training and transform this goal into a set of behavioral approaches to your patients.

The paradigm that embeds your relationship with the patient into the therapeutic process itself now has many names and models, including the biopsychosocial model and patient-centered care, among others.[5,12,14,15] Comparing these various models reveals common elements that include interest in the patient as a whole person, an empowering approach to the patient role, and involvement of the clinician's self on an emotional and reflective level.[16] There is now robust literature demonstrating that an approach to patient care anchored in these principles is not only more satisfying for the patient and the clinician but also more effective in achieving good health care outcomes.[17]

This section describes the skills that form the basic tools of interviewing. Some of these habits are purely techniques that you can readily put into practice. Some are constructs that will inform your interviewing behaviors. You will employ these interviewing skills to achieve the tasks described earlier in the Sequence of the Interview (see p. 28) more effectively. You need to practice using these tools and find ways to be observed or recorded so that you can receive feedback on your progress. A number of these fundamental skills are listed below and then described in more detail. Pick one or two of them to incorporate into your next patient interview. Then refer back to this chapter to build your repertoire of skills.

The Techniques of Skilled Interviewing

- Active listening
- Guided questioning
- Nonverbal communication
- Empathic responses
- Validation
- Reassurance
- Partnering
- Summarization
- Transitions
- Empowering the patient

Active Listening.   Underlying all the various techniques is the habit of *active listening.* Active listening is the process of really attending to what the patient is communicating, being aware of the patient's emotional state, and using verbal and nonverbal skills to encourage the speaker to continue and expand. This takes practice. It is easy to drift into thinking about your next question or the differential diagnosis when you and the patient are best served by your concentration on listening.

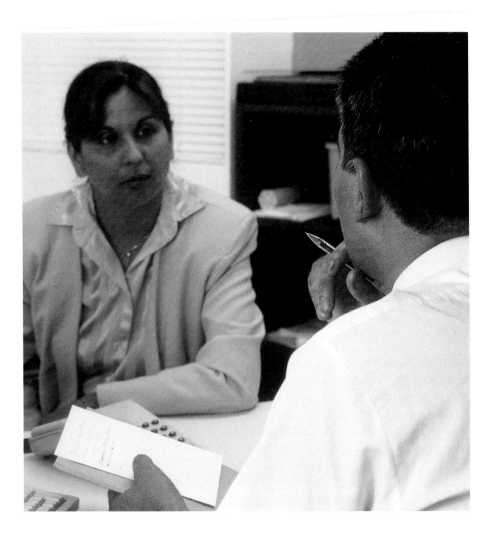

Guided Questioning: Options for Expanding and Clarifying the Patient's Story.   There are several ways you can ask for more information from the patient without interfering with the flow of the patient's story. Your goal is to facilitate the patient's fullest communication. Learning the following specific techniques will allow you to guide patients' disclosures, while minimizing the risk for distorting their ideas or missing significant details. This is how you avoid asking a series of specific questions, which takes more time and makes the patient feel more passive.

Guided Questioning: Options for Expanding and Clarifying the Patient's Story
■ Moving from open-ended to focused questions
■ Using questioning that elicits a graded response
■ Asking a series of questions, one at a time
■ Offering multiple choices for answers
■ Clarifying what the patient means
■ Offering continuers
■ Using echoing

Moving from Open-Ended to Focused Questions.   Your questioning should proceed from general to specific. Start with a truly open-ended question that does not inadvertently include an answer. A possible sequence might be:

"Tell me about your chest pain." (Pause)

"What else?" (Pause)

"Where did you feel it?" (Pause) "Show me."

"Anywhere else?" (Pause) "Did it travel anywhere?" (Pause) "To which arm?"

You should avoid *leading questions* that call for a "yes" or "no" answer. If a patient answers yes to a question such as "Is your pain pressure like . . . ?", you run the risk of turning your words into the patient's words. A better phrasing is "Please describe your pain."

Questioning that Elicits a Graded Response.   If necessary, ask questions that require *a graded response* rather than a single answer. "How many steps can you climb before you get short of breath?" is better than "Do you get short of breath climbing stairs?"

Asking a Series of Questions, One at a Time.   Be sure to *ask one question at a time*. "Any tuberculosis, pleurisy, asthma, bronchitis, pneumonia?" may lead to a negative answer out of sheer confusion. Try "Do you have any of the following problems?" Be sure to pause and establish eye contact as you list each problem.

Offering Multiple Choices for Answers.   Sometimes patients seem quite unable to describe their symptoms without help. To minimize bias, *offer multiple-choice answers:* "Which of the following words best describes your pain: aching, sharp, pressing, burning, shooting, or something else?" Almost any specific question can provide at least two possible answers. "Do you bring up any phlegm with your cough, or is it dry?"

Clarifying What the Patient Means.   At times, patients use words that are ambiguous or have unclear associations. To understand their meaning, you need to *request clarification*, as in "Tell me exactly what you meant by 'the flu' " or "You said you were behaving just like your mother. What did you mean?"

Continuers. Without specifying content, you can use posture, gestures, or words to encourage the patient to say more. Pausing with a nod of the head or remaining silent, yet attentive and relaxed, is a *cue for the patient to continue.* Leaning forward, making eye contact, and using phrases like "Mm-hmm," or "Go on," or "I'm listening" all maintain the flow of the patient's story.

Echoing. A simple repetition of the patient's last words, or *echoing,* encourages the patient to express both factual details and feelings, as in the following example:

Patient: "The pain got worse and began to spread." (Pause)

Response: "Spread?" (Pause)

Patient: "Yes, it went to my shoulder and down my left arm to the fingers. It was so bad that I thought I was going to die." (Pause)

Response: "Going to die?"

Patient: "Yes, it was just like the pain my father had when he had his heart attack, and I was afraid the same thing was happening to me."

This reflective technique has helped to reveal not only the location and severity of the pain but also its meaning to the patient. It did not bias the story or interrupt the patient's train of thought.

Nonverbal Communication. Communication that does not involve speech occurs continuously and provides important clues to feelings and emotions. Becoming more sensitive to nonverbal messages allows you to both "read the patient" more effectively and send messages of your own. Pay close attention to eye contact, facial expression, posture, head position and movement such as shaking or nodding, interpersonal distance, and placement of the arms or legs—crossed, neutral, or open. Be aware that nonverbal language is culturally bound.

Just as mirroring your position can signify the patient's increasing sense of connectedness, matching your position to the patient's can signify increased rapport. You can also mirror the patient's *paralanguage,* or qualities of speech, such as pacing, tone, and volume, to increase rapport. Moving closer or physical contact like placing your hand on the patient's arm can convey empathy or help the patient gain control of difficult feelings. Bringing nonverbal communication to the conscious level is the first step to using this crucial form of patient interaction.

Empathic Responses. Conveying empathy greatly strengthens patient rapport. As patients talk with you they may express—with or without words—feelings they may or may not have consciously acknowledged.

These feelings are crucial to understanding their illnesses and to establishing a trusting relationship. *To empathize with your patient, you must first identify the patient's feelings.* This requires a willingness and even interest on your part in hearing about and eliciting emotional content. At first, this may seem unfamiliar or uncomfortable. When you sense important but unexpressed feelings from the patient's face, voice, words, or behavior, inquire about them rather than assuming that you know how the patient feels. You may simply ask, "How did you feel about that?" Unless you let patients know that you are interested in feelings as well as facts, you may miss important insights.

Once you have identified the feelings, respond with understanding and acceptance. Responses may be as simple as "I understand," "That sounds upsetting," or "You seem sad." Empathy may also be nonverbal—for example, offering a tissue to a crying patient or gently placing your hand on the patient's arm to show understanding. When you give an empathic response, be sure that you are responding correctly to what the patient is feeling. If your response acknowledges how upset a patient must have been at the death of a parent, when in fact the death relieved the patient of a long-standing financial and emotional burden, you have misunderstood the situation. Instead of making assumptions, you can ask directly about the patient's emotional response. "I am sorry about the death of your father. What has that been like for you?"

Validation.   Another important way to make a patient feel accepted is to legitimize or validate his or her emotional experience. A patient who has been in a car accident but has no physical injury may still be experiencing significant distress. Stating something like, "Being in that accident must have been very scary. Car accidents are always unsettling because they remind us of our vulnerability and mortality. That could explain why you still feel upset," reassures the patient. It helps the patient feel that such emotions are legitimate and understandable.

Reassurance.   When you are talking with patients who are anxious or upset, it is tempting to reassure them. You may find yourself saying, "Don't worry. Everything is going to be all right." Although this may be appropriate in nonprofessional relationships, in your role as a clinician, such comments are usually counterproductive. You may fall into reassuring the patient about the wrong thing. Moreover, premature reassurance may block further disclosures, especially if the patient feels that exposing anxiety is a weakness. Such admissions require encouragement, not a cover-up.

The first step to effective reassurance is simply identifying and acknowledging the patient's feelings. This promotes a feeling of connection. The actual reassurance comes much later after you have completed the interview, the physical examination, and perhaps some laboratory studies. At that point, you can interpret for the patient what you think is happening and deal openly with expressed concerns. The reassurance comes from conveying information in a competent manner, making the patient feel confident that problems have been fully understood and will be addressed.

Partnering.   When building your relationships with patients, one of the most useful steps is to make explicit your desire to work with them in an on-going way. When you discuss a diagnosis or express uncertainty about how to explain their symptoms, it is reassuring to state that regardless of what happens with their disease, as their provider, you are committed to a continuing partnership. Even in your role as student, especially in a hospital setting, this support can make a big difference.

Summarization.   Giving a capsule summary of the patient's story during the course of the interview can serve several different functions. It indicates to the patient that you have been listening carefully. It can also identify what you know and what you don't know. "Now, let me make sure that I have the full story. You said you've had a cough for 3 days, that it's especially bad at night, and that you have started to bring up yellow phlegm. You have not had a fever or felt short of breath, but you do feel congested with difficulty breathing through your nose." Following with an attentive pause or stating "Anything else?" lets the patient add other information and confirms that you have heard the story correctly.

You can use summarization at different points in the interview to structure the visit, especially at times of transition (see below). This technique also allows you, the clinician, to organize your clinical reasoning and to convey your thinking to the patient, which makes the relationship more collaborative. *It is also a useful technique for learners to use when they draw a blank on what to ask the patient next.*

Transitions.   Patients have many reasons to feel vulnerable during a health care visit. To put them more at ease, tell them when you are changing directions during the interview. This gives patients a greater sense of control. As you move from one part of the history to another and on to the physical examination, orient the patient with brief transitional phrases like "Now I'd like to ask some questions about your past health." Make clear what the patient should expect or do next. "Before we move on to reviewing all your medications, was there anything else about past health problems?" "Now I would like to examine you. I will step out for a few minutes. Please get completely undressed and put on this gown." Specifying that the gown should open in the back may earn the patient's gratitude and save you some time.

Empowering the Patient.   The clinician–patient relationship is inherently unequal. Your sense of inexperience as a student will predictably and appropriately transition over time to a sense of confidence in your knowledge and skills and power in your role as clinician. But patients have many reasons to feel vulnerable. They may be in pain or worried about a symptom. They may be overwhelmed with the health care system or just unfamiliar with the process that you will come to take for granted. Differences of gender, ethnicity, race, or class may also create power differentials. However, ultimately, patients must be empowered to take care of themselves. They must make lifestyle changes or take the medications you recommend. They must feel confident in their ability to follow through on your advice. Listed next are principles that will help you to share power with your patients. Although many of them have been discussed in other parts of this chapter, the need to empower patients is so fundamental that it is worth summarizing them here. Keep them in mind.

EMPOWERING THE PATIENT:
PRINCIPLES OF SHARING POWER

- Inquire about the patient's perspective.
- Express interest in the person, not just the problem.
- Follow the patient's lead.
- Elicit emotional content.
- Share information with the patient (e.g., transitions).
- Make clinical reasoning transparent to the patient.
- Reveal the limits of your knowledge.

ADAPTING YOUR INTERVIEW TO SPECIFIC SITUATIONS

Interviewing patients may precipitate several behaviors and situations that seem perplexing or even vexing. Your ability to handle these situations will evolve throughout your career. *Always remember the importance of listening to the patient and clarifying the patient's concerns.*

The Silent Patient.   Novice interviewers are often uncomfortable with periods of silence and feel obligated to keep the conversation going. Silence has many meanings and many purposes. Patients frequently fall silent for short periods to collect thoughts, remember details, or decide whether you can be trusted with certain information. The period of silence usually feels much longer to the clinician than it does to the patient. The clinician should appear attentive and give brief encouragement to continue when appropriate. During periods of silence, watch the patient closely for nonverbal cues, such as difficulty controlling emotions.

Patients with depression or dementia may lose their usual spontaneity of expression, give short answers to questions, and then fall silent. If you have already tried guiding them through recent events or a typical day, try shifting your inquiry to the symptoms of depression or begin an exploratory mental status examination (see Chapter 16, pp. 573–593).

At times, silence may be the patient's response to how you are asking questions. Are you asking too many short-answer questions in rapid succession? Have you offended the patient in any way by signs of disapproval or criticism? Have you failed to recognize an overwhelming symptom such as pain, nausea, or dyspnea? If so, you may need to ask the patient directly, "You seem very quiet. Have I done something to upset you?"

The Confusing Patient.   Some patients present a confusing array of *multiple symptoms*. They seem to have every symptom that you ask about, or "a positive review of systems." With these patients, focus on the meaning or function of the symptom, emphasizing the patient's perspective (see p. 32), and guide the interview into a psychosocial assessment. There is little profit to exploring each symptom in detail. Although the patient may have several illnesses, a somatization disorder may be in play.

At other times, you may feel baffled, frustrated, and confused because you cannot make sense out of the patient's story. The history is vague and difficult to understand, ideas are poorly connected, and language is hard to follow. Even though you word your questions carefully, you cannot seem to get clear answers. The patient's manner of relating to you may also seem peculiar, distant, aloof, or inappropriate. Symptoms may be described in bizarre terms: "My fingernails feel too heavy" or "My stomach knots up like a snake." Perhaps there is a mental status change like psychosis or delirium, a mental illness such as schizophrenia, or a neurologic disorder (see Chapter 17). Consider delirium in acutely ill or intoxicated patients and dementia in the elderly. Such patients give histories that are inconsistent and cannot provide a clear chronology about what has happened. Some may even confabulate to fill in the gaps in their memories.

When you suspect a psychiatric or neurologic disorder, do not spend too much time gathering a detailed history. You will only tire and frustrate both the patient and yourself. Shift to the mental status examination, focusing on level of consciousness, orientation, memory, and capacity to understand. You can work in the initial questions smoothly by asking, "When was your last appointment at the clinic? Let's see . . . that was about how long ago?" "Your address now is. . .? . . . and your phone number?" You can check these responses against the chart or seek permission to speak with family members or friends and then obtain their perspectives.

The Patient With Altered Capacity. Some patients cannot provide their own histories because of delirium from illness, dementia, or other health or mental health conditions. Others are unable to relate certain parts of the history, such as events related to a febrile illness or a seizure. Under these circumstances, you need to determine whether the patient has "*decision-making capacity*," or the ability to understand information related to health, to make medical choices based on reason and a consistent set of values, and to declare preferences about treatments. The term *capacity* is preferable to the term "*competence*," which is a legal term. You do not need to consult psychiatry to assess capacity unless mental illness impairs decision making. For many patients with psychiatric conditions or even cognitive impairments, their ability to make decisions remains intact.

For patients with capacity, obtain their consent before talking about their health with others. Even if patients can communicate only with facial expressions or gestures, you must maintain confidentiality and elicit their input. Assure patients that any shared history will be kept confidential, and clarify what you can discuss with others. Your knowledge about the patient can be quite comprehensive, yet others may offer surprising and important information. A spouse, for example, may report significant family strains, depressive symptoms, or drinking habits that the patient has denied. Consider dividing the interview into two segments—one with the patient and the other with both the patient and a second informant. Each interview has its own value. Information from other sources often gives you helpful ideas for planning the patient's care, but remains confidential. Also learn the tenets of the *Health Insurance Portability and Accountability Act (HIPAA)* passed by Congress in 1996, which sets strict standards for disclosure for both institutions and providers when sharing patient information. These can be found at http://www.cms. hhs.gov/hipaa/.

For patients with impaired capacity, you will often need to find a *surrogate informant or decision maker* to assist with the history. Check whether the patient has a *durable power of attorney for health care* or a *health care proxy*. If not, in many cases, a spouse or family member who can represent the patient's wishes can fill this role.

Apply the basic principles of interviewing to your conversations with patients' relatives or friends. Find a private place to talk. Introduce yourself, state your purpose, inquire how they are feeling under the circumstances, and recognize and acknowledge their concerns. As you listen to their versions of the history, assess the quality of their relationship with the patient because it may color their credibility. Establish how they know the patient. For example, when a child is brought in for health care, the accompanying adult may not be the primary or even frequent caregiver, just the most available ride. Always seek the best-informed source. Occasionally, a relative or friend insists on being with the patient during your evaluation. Try to find out why, and assess the patient's wishes.

The Talkative Patient.   The garrulous rambling patient may be just as difficult as the silent or confused patient. Faced with limited time and the need to "get the whole story," you may grow impatient, even exasperated. Although this problem has no perfect solution, several techniques are helpful. Give the patient free rein for the first 5 or 10 minutes, listening closely to the conversation. Perhaps the patient simply needs a good listener and is expressing pent-up concerns. Maybe the patient's style is to tell stories. Does the patient seem obsessively detailed? Is the patient unduly anxious or apprehensive? Is there a flight of ideas or disorganized thought process that suggests a thought disorder? What about confabulation?

Try to focus on what seems most important to the patient. Show your interest by asking questions in those areas. Interrupt only if necessary, but be courteous. Learn how to be directive and to set limits when needed. Remember that part of your task is structuring the interview to gain important information about the patient's health. A brief summary may help you change the subject yet validate any concerns (see p. 40). "Let me make sure that I understand. You have described many concerns. In particular I heard about two different kinds of pain, one on your left side that goes into your groin and is fairly new, and one in your upper abdomen after you eat that you have had for months. Let's focus just on the side pain first. Can you tell me what it feels like?"

Finally, do not show your impatience. If time runs out, explain the need for a second meeting. Setting a time limit for the next appointment may be helpful. "I know we have much more to talk about. Can you come again next week? We will have a full hour then."

The Crying Patient. Crying signals strong emotions, ranging from sadness to anger or frustration. If the patient is on the verge of tears, pausing, gentle probing, or responding with empathy gives the patient permission to cry. Usually crying is therapeutic, as is your quiet acceptance of the patient's distress or pain. Offer a tissue and wait for the patient to recover. Make a supportive remark like "I am glad that you got that out." Most patients will soon compose themselves and resume their story. Aside from an acute grief or loss, it is unusual for crying to escalate and become uncontrollable.

Crying makes many people uncomfortable. If this is true for you, you will need to learn how to accept displays of emotion so that as a clinician you can support patients at these significant times.

The Angry or Disruptive Patient. Many patients have reasons to be angry: they are ill, they have suffered a loss, they lack their accustomed control over their own lives, and they feel relatively powerless in the health care system. They may direct this anger toward you. It is possible that this hostility toward you is justified . . . were you late for your appointment, inconsiderate, insensitive, or angry yourself? If so, acknowledge the fact and try to make amends. More often, however, patients displace their anger onto the clinician as a reflection of their frustration or pain.

Accept angry feelings from patients. Allow them to express such emotions without getting angry in return. Avoid joining such patients in their hostility toward another provider, the clinic, or the hospital, even when privately you may feel sympathetic. You can validate their feelings without agreeing with their reasons. "I understand that you felt very frustrated by the long wait and answering the same questions over and over. Our complex health care system can seem very unsupportive when you are not feeling well." After the patient has calmed down, help find steps that will avert such situations in the future. Rational solutions to emotional problems are not always possible, however, and people need time to express and work through their angry feelings.

Some angry patients become overtly disruptive. Few people can disturb the clinic or emergency department more quickly than patients who are angry, belligerent, or out of control. Before approaching such patients, alert the security staff—as a clinician, maintaining a safe environment is one of your responsibilities. Stay calm, appear accepting, and avoid being confrontational in return. Keep your posture relaxed and nonthreatening and your hands loosely open. At first do not try to make disruptive patients lower their voices or stop if they are haranguing you or the staff. Listen carefully. Try to understand what they are saying. Once you have established rapport, gently suggest moving to a different location that is more private (and will cause less disruption).

The Interview Across a Language Barrier. Nothing will convince you more of the importance of the history than having to do without one.

If your patient speaks a different language, make every effort to find an interpreter. A few broken words and gestures are no substitute for the full story. The ideal interpreter is a neutral person who is familiar with both languages and cultures. Recruiting family members or friends to serve as interpreters can be hazardous—confidentiality may be violated, meanings may be distorted, and transmitted information may be incomplete. Untrained interpreters may try to speed up the interview by telescoping lengthy replies into a few words, losing much of what may be significant detail.

As you begin working with the interpreter, establish rapport and review what information would be most useful. Explain that you need the interpreter to translate everything, not to condense or summarize. *Make your questions clear, short, and simple.* You can also help the interpreter by outlining your goals for each segment of the history. After going over your plans, arrange the room so that you have easy eye contact and nonverbal communication with the patient. Then speak directly to the patient . . . "How long have you been sick?" rather than "How long has the patient been sick?" Having the interpreter close by the patient keeps you from moving your head back and forth as though you were watching a tennis match.

When available, bilingual written questionnaires are invaluable, especially for the review of systems. First, however, be sure that patients can read in their language; otherwise, ask for help from the interpreter. In some clinical settings, there are speakerphone translators; use them if there are no better options.

GUIDELINES FOR WORKING WITH AN INTERPRETER

- Choose a trained interpreter in preference to a hospital worker, volunteer, or family member.
- Use the interpreter as a resource for cultural information.
- Orient the interpreter to the components you plan to cover in the interview; include reminders to translate everything the patient says.
- Arrange the room so that you and the patient have eye contact and can read each other's nonverbal cues. Seat the interpreter next to the patient.
- Allow the interpreter and the patient to establish rapport.
- Address the patient directly. Reinforce your questions with nonverbal behaviors.
- Keep sentences *short* and *simple.* Focus on the most important concepts to communicate.
- Verify mutual understanding by asking the patient to repeat back what he or she has heard.
- Be patient. The interview will take more time and may provide less information.

The Patient With Low Literacy. Before giving written instructions, assess the patient's ability to read. Literacy levels are highly variable, and marginal reading skills are more prevalent than commonly believed. Explore the many reasons people do not read: language barriers, learning disorders, poor vision, or lack of education. Some people may try to hide their inability to read. Asking about educational level may be helpful, but can be misleading. "I understand that this may be difficult to discuss, but do you have any trouble with reading?" Ask the patient to read whatever instructions you have written. (This will also address any difficulty with your handwriting.) One rapid screen is to hand the patient a written text upside down—most patients who read will turn the page around immediately. Literacy skills may be the reason the patient has not followed through on taking medications or adhered to recommended treatments. Respond sensitively, and remember that illiteracy and lack of intelligence are not synonymous.

The Patient With Impaired Hearing. Communicating with the deaf presents many of the same challenges as communicating with patients who speak a different language. Even people with partial hearing may define themselves as deaf, a distinct cultural group. Find out the patient's preferred method of communicating. Patients may use American Sign Language, a unique language with its own syntax, or various other combinations of signs and speech. Thus, communication is often truly crosscultural. Ask when hearing loss occurred relative to the development of speech and other language skills. Query about the kinds of schools the patient has attended. These questions help you determine whether the patient identifies with the Deaf culture or the Hearing culture. Written questionnaires are also useful. If the patient prefers sign language, find an interpreter and use the principles identified earlier. Time-consuming handwritten questions and answers may be the only solution, although literacy skills may also be an issue.

Hearing deficits vary. If the patient has a hearing aid, find out if the patient is using it. Make sure it is working. For patients with unilateral hearing loss, sit on the hearing side. A person who is *hard of hearing* may not be aware of the problem, a situation you will have to tactfully address. Eliminate background noise such as television or hallway conversation as much as possible. For patients who have partial hearing or can read lips, face them directly, in good light. Patients should wear their glasses to better pick up visual cues that help them understand you.

Speak at a normal volume and rate and do not let your voice trail off at the ends of sentences. Avoid covering your mouth or looking down at papers while speaking. Remember that even the best lip readers comprehend only a percentage of what is said, so having patients repeat what you have said is important. When closing, write out any oral instructions.

The Patient With Impaired Vision. When meeting with a blind patient, shake hands to establish contact and explain who you are and why you are there. If the room is unfamiliar, orient the patient to the surroundings and report if anyone else is present. It still may be helpful to adjust the light. Encourage visually impaired patients to wear glasses whenever possible. Remember to use words because postures and gestures are unseen.

The Patient With Limited Intelligence. Patients of moderately limited intelligence can usually give adequate histories. In fact, you may even be able to omit their disability from their evaluations. If you suspect problems, however, pay special attention to the patient's schooling and ability to function independently. How far have such patients gone in school? If they didn't finish, why not? What kinds of courses have they taken? How did they do? Have they had any testing done? Are they living alone? Do they need assistance with activities such as transportation or shopping? The sexual history is equally important and often overlooked. Find out if the patient is sexually active and provide information that may be needed about pregnancy or sexually transmitted diseases.

If you are unsure about the patient's level of intelligence, make a smooth transition to the mental status examination and assess simple calculations, vocabulary, memory, and abstract thinking (see Chapter 16, The Nervous System: Mental Status and Behavior).

For patients with severe mental retardation, you will have to turn to the family or caregivers to elicit the history. Identify the person who accompanies the patient, but always show interest in the patient first. Establish rapport, make eye contact, and engage in simple conversation. As with children, avoid "talking down" or using affectations of speech or condescending behavior. The patient, family members, caretakers, or friends will notice and appreciate your respect.

The Patient With Personal Problems.   Patients may ask you for advice about personal problems that fall outside the range of your clinical expertise. Should the patient quit a stressful job, for example, or move out of state? Instead of responding, explore the different approaches the patient has considered and related pros and cons, whom else they have discussed the problem with, and what supports are available for different choices. Letting the patient talk through the problem with you is usually much more valuable and therapeutic than any answer you could give.

■ SENSITIVE TOPICS THAT CALL FOR SPECIFIC APPROACHES

Clinicians talk with patients about various subjects that are emotionally charged or sensitive. These discussions can be particularly difficult for inexperienced clinicians or during evaluations of patients you do not know well. Even seasoned clinicians have some discomfort with certain topics: abuse of alcohol or drugs, sexual practices, death and dying, financial concerns, racial and ethnic experiences, family interactions, domestic violence, psychiatric illnesses, physical deformities, bowel function, and others. These areas are difficult to explore in part because of societal taboos. We all know, for example, that talking about bowel habits is not "polite table talk." Many of these topics evoke strong cultural, societal, and personal values. Mental illness, drug use, and same-sex practices are three obvious examples of issues that can touch on our biases and pose barriers during the interview. This section explores challenges to the clinician in these and other important and sometimes sensitive areas, including domestic violence and the dying patient.

Several basic principles can help guide your response to sensitive topics:

GUIDELINES FOR BROACHING SENSITIVE TOPICS

- *The single most important rule is to be nonjudgmental.* The clinician's role is to learn about the patient and help the patient achieve better health. Disapproval of behaviors or elements in the health history will only interfere with this goal.
- *Explain why you need to know certain information.* This makes patients less apprehensive. For example, say to patients, "Because sexual practices put people at risk for certain diseases, I ask all of my patients the following questions."
- Find opening questions for sensitive topics and learn the specific kinds of data needed for your assessments.
- Finally, consciously acknowledge whatever discomfort you are feeling. Denying your discomfort may lead you to avoid the topic altogether.

Look into other strategies for becoming more comfortable with sensitive areas. Examples include general reading about these topics in medical and lay literature; talking to selected colleagues and teachers openly about your concerns; taking special courses that help you explore your own feelings and reactions; and ultimately, reflecting on your own life experience. Take advantage of all these resources. Whenever possible, listen to experienced clinicians, then practice similar discussions with your own patients. The range of topics that you can explore with comfort will widen progressively.

The Sexual History. Asking questions about sexual behavior can be lifesaving. Sexual behaviors determine risks for pregnancy, sexually transmitted diseases (STDs), and AIDS—good interviewing helps prevent or reduce these risks. Sexual practices may be directly related to the patient's symptoms and integral to both diagnosis and treatment. Many patients have questions or concerns about sexuality that they would discuss more freely if you ask about sexual health. Finally, sexual dysfunction may result from use of medication or from misinformation that, if recognized, can be readily addressed.

You can introduce questions about sexual behavior at multiple points in an interview. If the chief complaint involves genitourinary symptoms, include questions about sexual health as part of "expanding and clarifying" the patient's story. For women, you can ask these questions as part of the Obstetric/Gynecologic section of the Past Medical History. You can bring them into discussions about Health Maintenance, along with diet, exercise, and screening tests, or as part of the lifestyle issues or important relationships covered in the Personal and Social History. Or, in a comprehensive history, you can ask about sexual practices during the Review of Systems. Do not forget this area of inquiry just because the patient is elderly or has a disability or chronic illness.

An orienting sentence or two is often helpful. "To assess your risk for various diseases, I need to ask you some questions about your sexual health and practices" or "I routinely ask all patients about their sexual function." For more specific complaints you might state, "To figure out why you have this discharge and what we should do about it, I need to ask some questions about your sexual activity." Try to be "matter-of-fact" in your style; the patient will be likely to follow your lead. You should *use specific language*. Refer to genitalia with explicit words such as penis or vagina and avoid phrases like "private parts." Choose words that the patient understands or explain what you mean. "By intercourse, I mean when a man inserts his penis into a woman's vagina."

In general, ask about both specific sexual behaviors and satisfaction with sexual function. Specific questions are included in Chapters 11, Male Genitalia and Hernias (pp. 413–415), and Chapter 12, Female Genitalia (pp. 432–435). Here are examples of questions that help guide patients to reveal their concerns in these discussions:

- "When was the last time you had intimate physical contact with someone?" Did that contact include sexual intercourse?" Using the term "sexually active" can be ambiguous. Patients have been known to reply, "No, I just lie there."

- "Do you have sex with men, women, or both?" Individuals may have sex with persons of the same gender, yet not consider themselves gay, lesbian, or bisexual. Some gay and lesbian patients have had sex with the opposite gender. Your questions should always be about the behaviors.

- "How many sexual partners have you had in the last 6 months? In the last 5 years? In your lifetime?" Again, these questions give the patient an easy opportunity to acknowledge multiple partners. Ask also about routine use of condoms. "Do you *always* use condoms?"

- It is important to ask all patients, "Do you have any concerns about HIV infection or AIDS?" even if no explicit risk factors are evident.

Note that these questions make no assumptions about marital status, sexual preference, or attitudes toward pregnancy or contraception. Listen to each of the patient's responses, and ask additional questions as indicated. To get information about sexual behaviors, you will need to ask more specific and focused questions than in other parts of the interview.

The Mental Health History.   Cultural constructs of mental and physical illness vary widely, causing marked differences in acceptance and attitudes. Think how easy it is for patients to talk about diabetes and taking insulin compared with discussing schizophrenia and using psychotropic medications. Ask open-ended questions initially. "Have you ever had any problem with emotional or mental illnesses?" Then move to more specific questions such as "Have you ever visited a counselor or psychotherapist?" "Have you ever been prescribed medication for emotional issues?" "Have you or has anyone in your family ever been hospitalized for an emotional or mental health problem?"

For patients with depression or thought disorders such as schizophrenia, a careful history of their illness is in order. Depression is common worldwide but still remains underdiagnosed and undertreated. Be sensitive to reports of mood changes or symptoms such as fatigue, unusual tearfulness, appetite or weight changes, insomnia, and vague somatic complaints. Two opening screening questions are: "Over the past 2 weeks, have you felt down, depressed, or hopeless?" and "Over the past 2 weeks, have you felt little interest or pleasure in doing things?"[18] If the patient seems depressed, also ask about thoughts of suicide . . . "Have you ever thought about hurting yourself or ending your life?" As with chest pain, you must evaluate severity—both depression and angina are potentially lethal. For further approaches, turn to Chapter 16, The Nervous System: Mental Status and Behavior.

Many patients with schizophrenia or other psychotic disorders can function in the community and tell you about their diagnoses, symptoms, hospitalizations, and current medications. You should investigate their symptoms and assess any effects on mood or daily activities.

Alcohol and Illicit Drugs.   Many clinicians hesitate to ask patients about use of alcohol and drugs, whether prescribed or illegal. Misuse of alcohol or drugs often directly contributes to symptoms and the need for care and treatment. Despite the high lifetime prevalence of substance abuse disorders—more than 13% for alcohol and 4% for illegal drugs in the United States—they remain underdiagnosed.[19]

Avoid letting personal feelings interfere with your role as a clinician. It is your job to gather data, assess the effects on the patient's health, and plan a therapeutic response. Clinicians should routinely ask about current and past use of alcohol or drugs, patterns of use, and family history. Make sure to include adolescents and older adults in your questioning.

Alcohol.   Questions about alcohol and other drugs follow naturally after questions about caffeine and cigarettes. "What do you like to drink?" or "Tell me about your use of alcohol" are good opening questions that avoid the easy yes or no response. Remember to assess what the patient considers alcohol—some patients do not use this term for wine or beer. To detect problem drinking, use several well-validated short screening tools that do not take much time. Two additional questions: "Have you ever had a drinking problem?" and "When was your last drink?" along with a drink within 24 hours are suspicious for problem drinking.[20] The most widely used screening questions are the **CAGE** questions about **C**utting down, **A**nnoyance if criticized, **G**uilty feelings, and **E**ye-openers.

THE CAGE QUESTIONNAIRE

Have you ever felt the need to **Cut down** on drinking?
Have you ever felt **Annoyed** by criticism of your drinking?
Have you ever felt **Guilty** about drinking?
Have you ever taken a drink first thing in the morning (**Eye-opener**) to steady your nerves or get rid of a hangover?

Adapted from Mayfield D, McCleod G, Hall P. The CAGE questionnaire: validation of a new alcoholism screening instrument. Am J Psychiatry 131:1121–1123, 1974.

Two or more affirmative answers to the CAGE Questionnaire suggest alcohol misuse and have a sensitivity that ranges from 43% to 94% and specificity that ranges from 70% to 96%.[21,22] If you detect misuse, you need to ask about blackouts (loss of memory about events during drinking), seizures, accidents or injuries while drinking, job problems, conflict in personal relationships, or legal problems. Also ask specifically about drinking while driving or operating machinery.

Illicit Drugs. As with alcohol, your questions about drugs should generally become more focused if you are to get accurate answers that help you distinguish use from misuse. A good opening question is, "Have you ever used any drugs other than those required for medical reasons?"[23] From there, you can ask specifically about either patterns of use (last use, how often, substances used, amount) or inquire about modes of consumption. "Have you ever injected a drug?" "Have you ever smoked or inhaled a drug?" "Have you ever taken a pill for nonmedical reasons?" As fashions in drugs of abuse change it is important to stay up to date about the most current hazards and risks from overdose.

Another approach is to adapt the CAGE questions to screening for substance abuse by adding "or drugs" to each question. Once you identify substance abuse, continue with further questions like "Are you always able to control your use of drugs?" "Have you had any bad reactions?" "What happened . . . Any drug-related accidents, injuries, or arrests? Job or family problems?" . . . "Have you ever tried to quit? Tell me about it."

Family Violence. Because of the high prevalence of physical, sexual, and emotional abuse, many authorities recommend the routine screening of all female patients for domestic violence. Other patients at increased risk are children and the elderly.[24] As with other sensitive topics, start this part of the interview with general "normalizing" questions: "Because abuse is common in many women's lives, I've begun to ask about it routinely." "Are there times in your relationships that you feel unsafe or afraid?" "Many women tell me that someone at home is hurting them in some way. Is this true for you?" "Within the last year, have you been hit, kicked, punched, or otherwise hurt by someone you know? If so, by whom?" As with other segments of the history, use a pattern that goes from general to specific, less difficult to more difficult.

Physical abuse—often not mentioned by either victim or perpetrator—should be considered in the following settings:

CLUES TO POSSIBLE PHYSICAL ABUSE

- If injuries are unexplained, seem inconsistent with the patient's story, are concealed by the patient, or cause embarrassment
- If the patient has delayed getting treatment for trauma
- If there is a past history of repeated injuries or "accidents"
- If the patient or person close to the patient has a history of alcohol or drug abuse
- If the partner tries to dominate the interview, will not leave the room, or seems unusually anxious or solicitous

---

When you suspect abuse, it is important to spend part of the encounter alone with the patient. You can use the transition to the physical examination as an excuse to ask the other person to leave the room. If the patient is also resistant, you should not force the situation, potentially placing the victim in jeopardy. Be attuned to diagnoses that have a higher association with abuse, such as pregnancy and somatization disorder.

Child abuse is unfortunately also common. Asking parents about their approach to discipline is a routine part of well-child care (see Chapter 18: Assessing Children: Infancy Through Adolescence). You can also ask parents how they cope with a baby who will not stop crying or a child who misbehaves: "Most parents get very upset when their baby cries (or their child has been naughty). How do you feel when your baby cries?" "What do you do when your baby won't stop crying?" "Do you have any fears that you might hurt your child?" Find out how other caretakers or companions handle these situations as well.

Death and the Dying Patient. There is a growing and important emphasis in health care education on improving clinician training related to death and dying. Many clinicians avoid talking about death because of their own discomforts and anxieties. Work through your own feelings with the help of reading and discussion. Basic concepts of care are appropriate even for beginning students because you will come into contact with patients of all ages near the end of their lives. (For a discussion of end-of-life decision making, grief and bereavement, and advance directives, turn to Chapter 20, The Older Adult, p. 854.)

Kubler-Ross has described five stages in a person's response to loss or the anticipatory grief of impending death: denial and isolation, anger, bargaining, depression or sadness, and acceptance.[25] These stages may occur sequentially or overlap in any order or combination. At each stage, follow the same approach. Be sensitive to the patient's feelings about dying; watch for cues that the patient is open to talking about them. Make openings for patients to ask questions: "I wonder if you have any concerns about the procedure? . . . your illness? . . . what it will be like when you go home?" Explore these concerns and provide whatever information the patient requests. Avoid unwarranted reassurance. If you explore and accept patients' feelings, answer their questions, and demonstrate your commitment to staying with them throughout their illness, reassurance will grow where it really matters—within the patients themselves.

Dying patients rarely want to talk about their illnesses at each encounter, nor do they wish to confide in everyone they meet. Give them opportunities to talk, and listen receptively, but if they stay at a social level, respect their preferences. Remember that illness—even a terminal one—is only one small part of the total person. A smile, a touch, an inquiry about a family member, a comment on the day's events, or even some gentle humor affirms and sustains the unique individual you are caring for. Communicating effectively means getting to know the whole patient; that is part of the helping process.

Understanding the patient's wishes about treatment at the end of life is an important clinician responsibility. Failing to establish communication about end-of-life decisions is widely viewed as a flaw in clinical care. Even if discussions of death and dying are difficult for you, you must learn to ask specific questions. The condition of the patient and the health care setting often determine what needs to be discussed. For patients who are acutely ill and in the hospital, discussions about what the patient wants to have done in the event of a cardiac or respiratory arrest are usually mandatory. Asking about *Do Not Resuscitate (DNR) status* is often difficult when you have no previous relationship with the patient or lack knowledge of the patient's values and life experience. Find out about the patient's frame of reference because the media gives many patients an unrealistic view of the effectiveness of resuscitation. "What experiences have you had with the death of a close friend or relative?" "What do you know about cardiopulmonary resuscitation (CPR)?" Educate patients about the likely success of CPR, especially if they are chronically ill or advanced in age. Assure them that relieving pain and taking care of their other spiritual and physical needs will be a priority.

In general, it is important to encourage any adult, but especially the elderly or chronically ill, to establish a *health proxy,* who can act as the patient's health decision maker (see p. 52). This part of the interview can be a "values history" that identifies what is important to the patient and makes life worth living, and the point when living would no longer be worthwhile. Ask how patients spend their time every day, what brings them joy, and what they look forward to. Make sure to clarify the meaning of statements like, "You said that you don't want to be a burden to your family. What exactly do you mean by that?" Explore the patient's religious or spiritual frame of reference so that you and the patient can make the most appropriate decisions about health care.

SOCIETAL ASPECTS OF INTERVIEWING

Achieving Cultural Competence. Communicating effectively with patients from every background has always been an important professional skill. Nevertheless, disparities in health care resulting from factors such as class, education, ethnicity, and race have fueled renewed efforts to raise the standards of cultural competence among clinicians.[26]

Working well with diverse patients is a career-long process built on genuine interest in learning about others, appreciation of the value of diverse cultures, and the practice of reflecting on how your own perspectives are equally shaped by culture. The following examples illustrate how cultural differences and unconscious bias can unwittingly lead to poor communication and influence the quality of patient care.

CULTURAL COMPETENCE: SCENARIO 1

A 28-year-old taxi driver from Ghana who had recently moved to the United States complained to a friend about U.S. medical care. He had gone to the clinic because of fever and fatigue. He described being weighed, having his temperature taken, and having a cloth wrapped tightly, to the point of pain, around his arm. The clinician, a 36-year-old woman from Washington, D.C., had asked the patient many questions, examined him, and wanted to take blood, which the patient had refused. The patient's final comment was ". . . and she didn't even give me chloroquine!"—his primary reason for seeking care. The man from Ghana was expecting few questions, no examination, and treatment for malaria, which is what fever usually means in Ghana.

In this example, cross-cultural miscommunication is understandable and so less threatening to explore. Unconscious bias leading to miscommunication, however, occurs in many clinical interactions. Consider the scenario below that is closer to daily practice.

CULTURAL COMPETENCE: SCENARIO 2

A 16-year-old high school student came to the local teen health center because of painful menstrual cramps that were interfering with concentrating at school. She was dressed in a tight top and short skirt and had multiple piercings, including in her eyebrow. The 30-year-old male clinician asked the following questions: "Are you passing all of your classes? What kind of job do you want after high school? What kind of birth control do you want?" The teenager felt pressured into accepting birth control pills, even though she had clearly stated that she had never had intercourse and planned to postpone it until she got married. She was an honor student and planning to go to college, but the clinician did not elicit these goals. The clinician glossed over her cramps by saying, "Oh, you can just take some ibuprofen. Cramps usually get better as you get older." The patient will not take the birth control pills that were prescribed, nor will she seek health care soon again. She experienced the encounter as an interrogation, so failed to gain trust in her clinician. In addition, the questions made assumptions about her life and did not treat her health concern with respect. Even though the provider pursued the important psychosocial domains, she received ineffective health care because of conflicting cultural values and unreflected clinician bias.

In both of these cases, the failure stems from mistaken assumptions or biases. In the first case, the clinician did not consider the many variables affecting patient beliefs about health and expectations for care. In the second case, the clinician allowed stereotypes to dictate the agenda instead of listening to the patient and respecting her as an individual. Each of us has our own cultural background and our own biases. These do not simply fade away as we become clinicians.

As you provide care for an ever-expanding and diverse group of patients, you must recognize how culture shapes not just the patient's beliefs, but your own. *Culture* is the system of shared ideas, rules, and meanings that influences how we view the world, experience it emotionally, and behave in relation to other people. It can be understood as the "lens" through which we perceive and make sense out of the world we inhabit. The meaning of culture is much broader than the term "ethnicity." Cultural influences are not limited to minority groups; they are relevant to everyone. They reflect factors like geography, age, religion, gender, sexual orientation, ethnicity, race, and socioeconomic status.

Although learning about specific cultural groups is important, avoid allowing this knowledge to turn into stereotyping rather than understanding. For example, you may have learned that Hispanic patients convey their pain in a more dramatic fashion. However, it is still important for you to evaluate each patient with pain as an individual, not decreasing the amount of analgesic you would typically use, but being aware of your reactions to the patient's style. Work on an appropriate and informed clinical approach to all patients by becoming aware of your own values and biases, developing communication skills that transcend cultural differences, and building therapeutic partnerships based on respect for each patient's life experience. This type of framework, described in the section below, will allow you to approach each patient as unique and distinct.

THE THREE DIMENSIONS OF CULTURAL COMPETENCE

- *Self-awareness.* Learn about your own biases . . . we all have them.
- *Respectful communication.* Work to eliminate assumptions about what is "normal." Learn directly from your patients—they are the experts on their culture and illness.
- *Collaborative partnerships.* Build your patient relationships on respect and mutually acceptable plans.

Self-Awareness. Start by exploring your own cultural identity. How do you describe yourself in terms of ethnicity, class, region or country of origin, religion, and political affiliation? Don't forget the characteristics that we often take for granted—gender, life roles, sexual orientation, physical ability, and race—especially if we are in majority groups. What aspects of your family of origin do you identify with, and how are you different from your family of origin? How do these identities influence your beliefs and behaviors?

A more challenging task in learning about ourselves is to bring our own values and biases to a conscious level. *Values* are the standards we use to measure our own and others' beliefs and behaviors. These may appear to be absolutes. *Biases* are the attitudes or feelings that we attach to perceived differences. Being attuned to difference is normal; in fact, in the distant past, detecting differences may have preserved life. Intuitively knowing members of one's own group is a survival skill that we may have outgrown as a society but that is still actively at work.

Feeling guilty about our biases makes it hard to recognize and acknowledge them. Start with less threatening constructs, like the way an individual relates to time, a culturally determined phenomenon. Are you always on time—a positive value in the dominant Western culture? Or do you tend to run a little late? How do you feel about people whose habits are opposite to yours? Next time you attend a meeting or class, notice who is early, on time, or late. Is it predictable? Think about the role of physical appearance. Do you consider yourself thin, mid-size, or heavy? How do you feel about your weight? What does prevailing U.S. culture teach us to value in physique? How do you feel about people who have different weights?

Respectful Communication.   Given the complexity of culture, no one can possibly know the health beliefs and practices of every culture and subculture. Let your patients be the experts on their own unique cultural perspectives. Even if patients have trouble describing their values or beliefs in the abstract, they should be able to respond to specific questions. Find out about the patient's cultural background. Use some of the same questions discussed earlier in the section, Creating a Shared Understanding of the Problem (see p. 33). Maintain an open, respectful, and inquiring attitude. "What did you hope to get from this visit?" If you have established rapport and trust, patients will be willing to teach you. Be aware of questions that contain assumptions. And always be ready to acknowledge your areas of ignorance or bias. "I know very little about Ghana. What would have happened at a clinic there if you had these concerns?" Or, with the second patient and with much more difficulty, "I mistakenly made assumptions about you that are not right. I apologize. Would you be willing to tell me more about yourself and your future goals?"

Learning about specific cultures is valuable because it broadens what you, as a clinician, identify as areas you need to explore. Do some reading about the life experiences of individuals in ethnic or racial groups that live in your area. Go to movies that are filmed in different countries or explicitly present the perspective of different cultures. Learn about the concerns of different consumer groups with visible health agendas. Get to know healers of different disciplines and learn about their practices. Most importantly, be open to learning from your patients. Do not assume that what you have learned about a cultural group applies to the individual before you.

Collaborative Partnerships.   Through continual work on self-awareness and seeing through the "lens" of others, the clinician lays the foundation for the collaborative relationship that best supports the patient's health. Communication based on trust, respect, and a willingness to reexamine assumptions allows patients to express aspects of their concerns that may run counter to the dominant culture. These concerns may be associated with strong feelings such as anger or shame. You, the clinician, must be willing to listen to and validate these feelings, and not let your own feelings prevent you from exploring painful areas. You must also be willing to reexamine your beliefs about what is the "right approach" to clinical care in a given situation. Make every effort to be flexible and creative in your plans and respectful of patients' knowledge about their own best interests. By consciously distinguishing what is truly important to the patient's health from what is just the standard advice, you and your patients can construct the unique approach to their health care that is in concert with their beliefs and effective clinical care. Remember that if the patient stops listening, fails to follow your advice, or does not return, your health care has not been successful.

Sexuality in the Clinician–Patient Relationship. Clinicians of both genders occasionally find themselves physically attracted to their patients. Similarly, patients may make sexual overtures or exhibit flirtatious behavior toward clinicians. The emotional and physical intimacy of the clinician–patient relationship may lend itself to these sexual feelings.

If you become aware of such feelings in yourself, accept them as a normal human response, and bring them to conscious level so they will not affect your behavior. Denying these feelings makes it more likely for you to act inappropriately. *Any* sexual contact or romantic relationship with patients is *unethical;* keep your relationship with the patient within professional bounds, and seek help if you need it.

Sometimes clinicians meet patients who are frankly seductive or make sexual advances. You may be tempted to ignore this behavior because you are not sure that it really happened, or you are just hoping it will go away. Calmly but firmly, make it clear that your relationship is professional, not personal. If unwelcome overtures continue, leave the room and find a chaperone to continue the interview. You should also reflect on your image. Has your clothing or demeanor been unconsciously seductive? Have you been overly warm with the patient? Although it is your responsibility to avoid contributing to these problems, usually you are not at fault. Often these problems reflect the patient's discomfort with feeling less powerful.

ETHICS AND PROFESSIONALISM

You may wonder why an introductory chapter on interviewing contains a section on clinical ethics. The potential power of clinician–patient communication calls for guidance beyond our innate sense of morality. *Ethics* are a set of principles crafted through reflection and discussion to define right and wrong. *Medical ethics,* which guide our professional behavior, are neither static nor simple, but several principles have guided clinicians throughout the ages. Although in most situations your gut sense of right and wrong will be all that you need, even as students, you will face decisions that call for the application of ethical principles.

Some of the traditional and still fundamental maxims embedded in the healing professions are listed below.

BUILDING BLOCKS OF PROFESSIONAL ETHICS IN PATIENT CARE

- **Nonmaleficence or primum non nocere** is commonly stated as, "First, do no harm." In the context of an interview, giving information that is incorrect or not really related to the patient's problem can do harm. Avoiding relevant topics or creating barriers to open communication can also do harm.

(continued)

> **BUILDING BLOCKS OF PROFESSIONAL ETHICS IN PATIENT CARE** (Continued)
>
> - **Beneficence** is the dictum that the clinician needs to "do good" for the patient. As clinicians, your actions need to be motivated by what is in the patient's best interest.
> - **Autonomy** reminds us that patients have the right to determine what is in their own best interest. This principle has become increasingly important over time and is consistent with collaborative rather than paternalistic clinician–patient relationships.
> - **Confidentiality** can be one of the most challenging principles. As a clinician, you are obligated not to repeat what you learn from or know about a patient. This privacy is fundamental to our professional relationships with patients. In the daily flurry of activity in a hospital, it is all too easy to let something slip. You must be on your guard.

As students, you are exposed to some of the ethical challenges that you will confront later as practicing clinicians. However, there are dilemmas unique to students that you will face from the time that you begin taking care of patients. The following vignettes capture some of the most common experiences. They raise a variety of ethical and practical issues that are overlapping.

> **ETHICS AND PROFESSIONALISM: SCENARIO 1**
>
> You are a third-year medical student on your first clinical rotation in the hospital. It is late in the evening when you are finally assigned to the patient you are to "work up" and present the next day at preceptor rounds. You go to the patient's room and find the patient exhausted from the day's events and clearly ready to settle down for the night. You know that your intern and attending physician have already done their evaluations. Do you proceed with a history and physical that is likely to take 1 to 2 hours? Is this process only for your education? Do you ask permission before you start? What do you include?

Here you are confronted with the tension between *the need to learn by doing* and *doing no harm to patients*. There is a utilitarian ethical principle that reminds us that if clinicians-in-training do not learn, there will be no future caregivers. Yet the dictums to do no harm and prioritize what is in the patient's best interests are clearly in conflict with that future need. As a student, this dilemma will arise often.

Obtaining *informed consent* is the means to address this ethical dilemma. Making sure the patient realizes that you are in training and new at patient evaluation is always important. It is impressive how often patients willingly let students be involved in their care. It is an opportunity for patients to give back to their caregivers. Even when clinical activities appear to be purely for educational purposes, there may be a benefit to the patient. Multiple caregivers provide multiple perspectives, and the experience of being heard can be therapeutic.

ETHICS AND PROFESSIONALISM: SCENARIO 2

It is after 10 PM, and you and your resident are on the way to complete the required advance directives form with a frail, elderly patient who was admitted earlier that day with bilateral pneumonia. The form, which includes a discussion of Do Not Resuscitate orders, must be completed before the team can sign out and leave for the day. Just then, your resident is paged to an emergency and asks you to go ahead and meet with the patient to complete the form; the resident will cosign it later. You had a lecture on advance directives and end-of-life discussions in your first year of school but have never seen a clinician discuss this with a patient. You have not yet met the patient, nor have you had a chance to really look at the form. What should you do? Do you inform the resident that you have never done this before nor even seen it done? Do you need to inform the patient that this is totally new for you? Who should decide whether you are competent to do this independently?

In this situation, you are being asked to take responsibility for clinical care that exceeds your level of comfort and maybe your competence. This can happen in a number of situations, such as being asked to evaluate a clinical situation without proper back-up or to draw blood or start an IV before you have done one under supervision. For the patient above, you may have many of the following thoughts: "the patient needs to have this completed before going to sleep and so will benefit"; "the risk to the patient from discussing advance directives is minimal"; "you are pretty good with elderly patients and think that you might be able to do this"; "what if the patient actually arrests that night and you are responsible for what happens"; and finally, "if you bother the resident now he or she will be angry and that may affect your evaluation." There is educational value to the learner in being pushed to the limits of his or her knowledge to solve problems and to gain confidence in functioning independently. But what is the right thing to do in this situation?

The principles listed above only partially help you sort this out because only part of your quandary relates to your relationship with the patient. Much of the tension in this scenario has to do with the dynamics of a health care team and your role on that team. You are there to help with the work of the team, but you are primarily there to learn. Current formulations of medical ethics address those issues and others. One such formulation is the Tavistock Principles.[27] These principles construct a framework for analyzing health care situations that extends beyond our direct care of individual patients to complicated choices about the interactions of health care teams and the distribution of resources for the well-being of society. A broadly representative group that initially met in Tavistock Square in London in 1998 has continued to elaborate an evolving document of ethical principles for guiding health care behavior for both individuals and institutions across the health care spectrum. A current iteration of the Tavistock Principles follows.

THE TAVISTOCK PRINCIPLES

Rights: People have a right to health and health care.
Balance: Care of the individual patient is central, but the health of populations is also our concern.
Comprehensiveness: In addition to treating illness, we have an obligation to ease suffering, minimize disability, prevent disease, and promote health.
Cooperation: Health care succeeds only if we cooperate with those we serve, each other, and those in other sectors.
Improvement: Improving health care is a serious and continuing responsibility.
Safety: Do no harm.
Openness: Being open, honest, and trustworthy is vital in health care.

In the second scenario, think about the Tavistock Principles of *openness and cooperation,* in addition to the balance between *do no harm* and *beneficence.* You need to work with your team in a way that is honest and reliable to do the best for the patient. You can also see that there are no clear or easy answers in such situations. What responses are available to you to address these and other quandaries?

You need to reflect on your beliefs and assess your level of comfort with a given situation. Sometimes there may be alternative solutions. For example, in Scenario 1, the patient may really be willing to have the history and physical examination done at that late hour, or perhaps you can renegotiate the time for the next morning. In Scenario 2, you might find another person who is more qualified to complete the form or to supervise when you do it. Alternatively, you may choose to go ahead and complete the form, alerting the patient to your inexperience and obtaining the patient's consent. You will need to choose which situations warrant voicing your concerns, even at the risk of a bad evaluation.

Seek coaching on how to express your reservations in a way that ensures that they will be heard. As a clinical student, you will need settings for discussing these immediately relevant ethical dilemmas with other students and with more senior trainees and faculty. Small groups that are structured to address these kinds of issues are particularly useful in providing validation and support. Take advantage of such opportunities whenever possible.

ETHICS AND PROFESSIONALISM: SCENARIO 3

You are the student on the clinical team that has been taking care of Ms. Robbins, a 64-year-old woman admitted for an evaluation of weight loss and weakness. During the hospitalization, she had a biopsy of a mass in her chest in addition to many other tests. You have gotten to know her well, spending a lot of time with her to answer questions, explain procedures, and learn about her and her family. You have discussed her fears about what

(continued)

"they" will find and know that she likes to know everything possible about her health and medical care. You have even heard her express frustrations with her attending physician at not always being given the "straight story." It is late Friday afternoon, but you promised Ms. Robbins that you would come by one more time before the weekend and let her know if the results of the biopsy were back yet. Just before you go to her room, the resident tells you that the pathology is back from her biopsy and shows metastatic cancer, but the attending physician does not want the team to say anything until he comes in on Monday.

What are you going to do? You feel that it is wrong to avoid the situation by not going to her room. You also believe that the patient's preference and anxiety are best served by finding out then and not waiting for 3 days. You do not want to go against the attending physician's clear instructions, however, both because you respect the fact that it is his patient and because that feels dishonest.

In this situation, telling the patient about her biopsy results is dictated by several ethical principles: the patient's best interests, autonomy, and your integrity. The other part of the ethical dilemma concerns communicating your plan to the attending. Sometimes the most challenging part of such dilemmas tests your will to follow through with the right course of action. Although it may appear to be a lose-lose situation, a respectful and honest discussion with the attending, respectfully articulating what is in the patient's best interest, will usually be heard. Enlist the support of your resident or other helpful attendings if that is possible. Learning how to navigate difficult discussions will be a useful professional skill.

Bibliography

CITATIONS

1. Cohen-Cole SA: The Medical Interview: The Three-Function Approach. St. Louis, Mosby–Year Book, 1991.
2. Bird J, Cohen-Cole SA: The three-function model of the medical interview. Adv Psychosom Med 20:65–88, 1990.
3. Lazare A, Putnam SM, Lipkin M Jr: Three functions of the medical interview. In Lipkin M Jr, Putnam SM, Lazare A, et al (eds): The Medical Interview: Clinical Care, Education, and Research. New York, Springer-Verlag, 1995.
4. Novack DH: Therapeutic aspects of the clinical encounter. In Lipkin M Jr, Putnam SM, Lazare A, et al (eds). The Medical Interview: Clinical Care, Education, and Research, p. 32. New York, Springer-Verlag, 1995.
5. Suchman AL, Matthews DA. What makes the patient-doctor relationship therapeutic? Exploring the connectional dimension of medical care. Ann Intern Med 108(1):125–130, 1988.
6. Hastings C. The lived experiences of the illness: making contact with the patient. In Benne P, Wrubel J (eds): The Primacy of Caring: Stress and Coping in Health and Illness. Menlo Park, CA, Addison-Wesley, 1989.
7. Conant EB. Addressing patients by their first names. N Engl J Med 308(4):226, 1998.
8. Heller ME. Addressing patients by their first names. N Engl J Med 308(18):1107, 1987.
9. Delbanco TL. Enriching the doctor-patient relationship by inviting the patient's perspective. Ann Intern Med 116(5):414–418, 1993.
10. Beckman HB, Frankel RM. The effect of physician behavior on the collection of data. Ann Intern Med 101(5):692–696, 1984.
11. Kleinman A, Eisenberg L, Good B. Culture, illness, and care: clinical lessons from anthropological and cross-cultural research. Ann Intern Med 88(2):251–258, 1978.
12. Smith RC. Patient-Centered Interviewing: An Evidence-Based Method. Philadelphia, Lippincott Williams & Wilkins, 2002.
13. Smith RC, Lyles JS, Mettler J, et al. The effectiveness of an intensive teaching experience for residents in interviewing: a randomized controlled study. Ann Intern Med 128(2):118–126, 1998.

14. Engel GL. The need for a new medical model: a challenge for biomedicine. Science 196(4286):126–129, 1977.

15. Engel GL, Morgan WL Jr. Interviewing the Patient. Philadelphia, WB Saunders, 1973.

16. Bayer–Fetzer Conference on Physician–Patient Communication in Medical Education: Essential elements of communication in medical encounters: the Kalamazoo Consensus Statement. Acad Med 76(4):390–393, 2001.

17. Stewart M. Questions about patient-centered care: answers from quantitative research. In Stewart M, et al (eds): Patient Centered Medicine: Transforming the Clinical Method, pp. 263–268. Abington, UK: Radcliffe Medical Press, 2003.

18. U.S. Preventive Services Task Force. Screening for Depression: Recommendations and Rationale. Rockville, MD, Agency for Healthcare Research and Quality, May 2002.

19. Regier DA, Farmer ME, Rae DS, et al. Comorbidity of mental disorders with alcohol and other drug abuse. Results from the Epidemiologic Catchment Area (ECA) Study. JAMA 264(19):2511–2518, 1990.

20. Cyr MG, Wartman SA. The effectiveness of routine screening questions in the detection of alcoholism. JAMA 259(1):51–54, 1988.

21. U.S. Preventive Services Task Force: Screening and Behavioral Counseling Interventions in Primary Care to Reduce Alcohol Misuse: Recommendation Statement. Rockville, MD, Agency for Healthcare Research and Quality, April 2004. Available at: http://www.ahrq.gov/clinic/3rduspstf/alcohol/alcomisrs.htm.

22. Ewing JA. Detecting alcoholism: the CAGE questionnaire. JAMA 252(14):1905–1907, 1984.

23. Cocco KM, Carey KB. Psychometric properties of the Drug Abuse Screening Test in psychiatric outpatients. Psychol Assess 10(4):408–414, 1998.

24. U.S. Preventive Services Task Force: Screening for Family and Intimate Partner Violence: Recommendation Statement. Rockville, MD, Agency for Healthcare Research and Quality, March 2004.

25. Kubler-Ross E. On Death and Dying. New York, Macmillan, 1997.

26. Smedley BA, Stith AY, Nelson AR (eds): Committee on Understanding and Eliminating Racial and Ethnic Disparities in Health Care. Unequal Treatment: Confronting Racial and Ethnic Disparities in Health Care. Washington, DC: Institute of Medicine, 2003.

27. Berwick D, Davidoff F, Hiatt H, et al. Refining and implementing the Tavistock principles for everybody in health care. BMJ 323(7313):616–619, 2001.

ADDITIONAL REFERENCES

Building a Therapeutic Relationship: The Techniques of Skilled Interviewing

Billings JA, Stoeckle JD. The Clinical Encounter: A Guide to the Medical Interview and Case Presentation. Chicago, Year Book Medical Publishers, 1989.

Branch WT, Malik TK. Using "windows of opportunities" in brief interviews to understand patients' concerns. JAMA 269(13):1667–1668, 1993.

Fadiman A. The Spirit Catches You and You Fall Down. New York: Farrar, Straus and Giroux, 1997.

Frankel RM, Stein TS. The Four Habits of Highly Effective Clinicians: A Practical Guide. Oakland, CA, Kaiser Permanente Northern California Region Physician Education and Development, 1996.

Inui TS. Establishing the doctor–patient relationship: science, art, or competence? Schweiz Med Wochenschr 128(7):225–230, 1998.

Quill TE, Brody H. Physician recommendations and patient autonomy: finding a balance between physician power and patient choice. Ann Intern Med 125(9):763–769, 1996.

Silverman J, Kurtz S, Draper J. Skills for communicating with patients. Abingdon, UK: Radcliffe Medical Press Ltd, 1998.

Smith RC. The Patient's Story, Integrated Patient-Doctor Interviewing. Boston: Little, Brown, 1996.

Adapting Interviewing Techniques to Specific Situations

Barnett S. Cross-cultural communication with patients who use American Sign Language. Fam Med 34(5):376–382, 2002.

Committee on Disabilities of the Group for the Advancement of Psychiatry: Issues to consider in deaf and hard-of-hearing patients. Am Fam Phys 56(8):2057–2066, 1997.

Goldoft M. A piece of mind: another language. JAMA 268(24):3482, 1992.

Grantmakers in Health: In the right words: addressing language and culture in providing health care. Issues in Brief 18:1–54, 2003.

Mayeaux EJ Jr, Murphy PW, Arnold C, et al. Improving patient education for patients with low literacy skills. Am Fam Phys 53(1):205–211, 1996.

McDaniel SH, Campbell TL, Hepworth J, et al. Family-Oriented Primary Care, 2nd ed. New York: Springer, 2005.

National Work Group on Literacy and Health. Communicating with patients who have limited literacy skills. Report of the National Work Group on Literacy and Health. J Fam Pract 46(2):168–176, 1998.

Putsch RW. Cross-cultural communication: the special case of interpreters in health care. JAMA 254(23):3344–3348, 1985.

Rivadeneyra R, Elderkin-Thompson V, Silver RC, et al. Patient centeredness in medical encounters requiring an interpreter. Am J Med 108(6):470–474, 2000.

Sensitive Topics That Call for Specific Approaches

Council on Scientific Affairs, AMA: Health care needs of gay men and lesbians in the U.S. JAMA 275(17):1354–1357, 1996.

End of Life/Palliative Education Resource Center. Available at: http://www.eperc.mcw.edu/index.htm. Accessed February 10, 2005.

Fiellin DA, Reid MC, O'Connor PG. Screening for alcohol problems in primary care: a systematic review. Arch Intern Med 160(13):1977–1989, 2000.

Harrison AE. Primary care of lesbian and gay patients: educating ourselves and our students. Fam Med 28(1):10–23, 1996.

BIBLIOGRAPHY

Robinson GE, Stewart DE. A curriculum on physician-patient sexual misconduct and teacher-learner mistreatment. Part 1: Content. Can Med Assoc J 154(1):643–649, 1996.

Societal Aspects of Interviewing

Carrillo JE, Green AR, Betancourt JR. Cross-cultural primary care: a patient-based approach. Ann Intern Med 130:829–834, 1999.

Christakis DA, Feudtner C. Ethics in a short white coat: The ethical dilemmas that medical students confront. Acad Med 68(4):249–254, 1993.

Council on Ethical and Judicial Affairs, American Medical Association: Sexual misconduct in the practice of medicine. JAMA 266(19):2741–2745, 1991.

Doyal L. Closing the gap between professional teaching and practice. BMJ 322(7288):685–686, 2001.

Gabbard GO, Nadelson C. Professional boundaries in the physician-patient relationship. JAMA 273(18):1445–1449, 1995.

Lo B. Resolving Ethical Dilemmas: A Guide for Clinicians. Philadelphia, Lippincott Williams & Wilkins, 2000.

Tervalon M, Murray-Garcia J. Cultural humility versus cultural competence: a critical distinction in defining physician training outcomes in multicultural education. J Health Care Poor Underserved 9(2):117–125, 1998.

Waitzkin H. Doctor-patient communication: clinical implications of social scientific research. JAMA 252(17):2441–2446, 1984.

Clinical Reasoning, Assessment, and Plan

Now that you have gained your patient's trust, gathered a detailed history, and completed the requisite portions of the physical examination, you have reached the critical step of formulating your *Assessment(s)* and *Plan*. You must now analyze your findings and identify the patient's problems. You must also share your impressions with the patient, eliciting any concerns and making sure that he or she understands and agrees to the steps ahead. Finally, you must document your findings in the patient's record in a succinct and legible format. A clear and well-organized record is essential for communicating the patient's story and your clinical reasoning and plan to other members of the health care team.

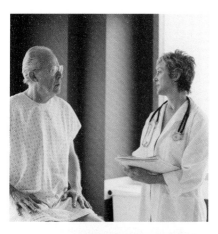

This chapter follows a step-wise approach designed to help you acquire the important skills of clinical reasoning, assessment, and recording your Assessment and Plan. Review the learning objectives below, which mirror the organization of this chapter, and test your understanding by returning to the history and physical examination of Mrs. N found in Chapter 1, pp. 16–20.

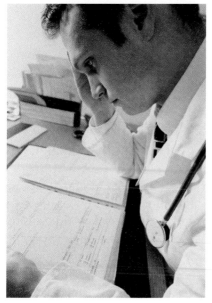

DEVELOPING AN ASSESSMENT AND PLAN:
OBJECTIVES FOR LEARNERS

- Understand the process of clinical reasoning and its component steps.
- Analyze this process using the written *Assessment* and *Plan* for Mrs. N (pp. 71–72).
- Address the challenges of clinical data by:
  - Clustering data into single versus multiple problems
  - Sifting through an extensive array of data
  - Assessing the quality of patient information, including how to ensure quality and principles for selecting and analyzing tests
- Integrate clinical reasoning with assessment of clinical data.
- Organize a clear and accurate patient record.

The comprehensive information you have collected, both *subjective* (the history, or what the patient or family has told you) and *objective* (the physical examination and laboratory tests), make up the core elements of your patient observations. This information is primarily factual and descriptive. As you move to *Assessment,* you go beyond description and observation to analysis and interpretation. You select and cluster relevant pieces of information, analyze their possible meanings, and try to explain them logically using principles of biopsychosocial and biomedical science. The *Assessment* and *Plan* include the patient's responses to the problems identified and to your diagnostic and therapeutic plans. A successful *Plan* requires good interpersonal skills and sensitivity to the patient's goals, economic means, competing responsibilities, and family structure and dynamics. Your patient record facilitates clinical thinking, promotes communication and coordination among the many professionals caring for your patient, and documents the patient's problems and management for medicolegal purposes.

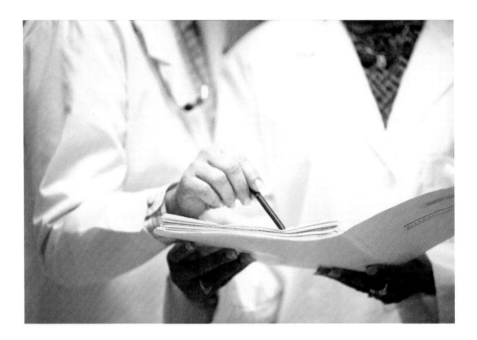

■ ASSESSMENT AND PLAN:
■ THE PROCESS OF CLINICAL REASONING

Because assessment takes place in the clinician's mind, the process of clinical reasoning often seems inaccessible and even mysterious to the beginning student. Experienced clinicians often think quickly, with little overt or conscious effort. They differ widely in personal style, communication skills, clinical training, experience, and interests. Some clinicians may find it difficult to explain the logic behind their clinical thinking. As an active learner, it is expected that you will ask teachers and clinicians to elaborate on the fine points of their clinical reasoning and decision making.[1,2]

As you gain experience, your thinking process will begin at the outset of the patient encounter, not at the end. Listed below are a set of principles that underlie the process of clinical reasoning and certain explicit steps to help guide your thinking as you analyze the information you have compiled. After reading through this section, review the case of Mrs. N, introduced in Chapter 1, and use this as a sample database to practice the process of clinical reasoning and assessment. As with all patients, focus on finding answers to the questions "What is wrong with this patient?" "What are the problems and diagnoses?" To reach these answers, try following the steps discussed below. Then turn to the *Assessment and Plan* for Mrs. N on pp. 71–72 and compare them with your own insights and clinical thinking.

Identifying Problems and Making Diagnoses: Steps in Clinical Reasoning

- Identify abnormal findings.
- Localize findings anatomically.
- Interpret findings in terms of probable process.
- Make hypotheses about the nature of the patient's problem.
- Test the hypotheses and establish a working diagnosis.
- Develop a plan agreeable to the patient.

■ **Identify abnormal findings.** Make a list of the patient's *symptoms,* the *signs* you observed during the physical examination, and any laboratory reports available to you.

■ **Localize these findings anatomically.** This step may be easy. The symptom of scratchy throat and the sign of an erythematous inflamed pharynx, for example, clearly localize the problem to the pharynx. For Mrs. N, the complaint of headache leads you quickly to the structures of the skull and brain. Other symptoms, however, may present greater difficulty. Chest pain, for example, can originate in the coronary arteries, the stomach and esophagus, or the muscles and bones of the chest. If the pain is exertional and relieved by rest, either the heart or the musculoskeletal components of the chest wall may be involved. If the patient notes pain only when carrying groceries with the left arm, the musculoskeletal system becomes the likely culprit.[3,4]

When localizing findings, be as specific as your data allow, but bear in mind that you may have to settle for a body region, such as the chest, or a body system, such as the musculoskeletal system. On the other hand, you may be able to define the exact structure involved, such as the left pectoral muscle. Some symptoms and signs cannot be localized, such as fatigue or fever, but are useful in the next set of steps.

■ **Interpret the findings in terms of the probable process.** Patient problems often stem from a *pathologic process* involving diseases of a body structure. There are a number of such processes, variably classified, including congenital, inflammatory or infectious, immunologic, neoplastic, metabolic, nutritional, degenerative, vascular, traumatic, and toxic. Possible pathologic causes of headache, for example, include concussion from trauma, subarachnoid hemorrhage, or even compression from a brain tumor. Fever and stiff neck, or nuchal rigidity, are two of the classic signs of headache from meningitis. Even without other signs, such as rash or papilledema, they strongly suggest an infectious process.

Other problems are *pathophysiologic,* reflecting derangements of biologic functions, such as congestive heart failure or migraine headache. Still other problems are *psychopathologic,* such as disorders of mood like depression or headache as an expression of a somatization disorder.

■ **Make hypotheses about the nature of the patient's problem.** Here you will draw on all the knowledge and experience you can muster, and it is here that reading will be most helpful for learning about patterns of abnormalities and diseases, and clustering your patient's findings accordingly.

By consulting the clinical literature, you will embark on the lifelong goal of **evidence-based decision-making.**[5,6]

Until you gain broader knowledge and experience, you may not be able to develop highly specific hypotheses, but proceed as far as you can with the data and knowledge you have. The following steps should help:

STEPS IN CLINICAL DECISION-MAKING

1. *Select the most specific and critical findings to support your hypothesis.* If the patient reports "the worst headache of her life," nausea, and vomiting, for example, and you find a change in mental status, papilledema, and meningismus, build your hypothesis around elevated intracranial pressure rather than gastrointestinal disorders. Although other symptoms are useful diagnostically, they are much less specific.
2. Using your inferences about the structures and processes involved, *match your findings against all the conditions you know that can produce them.* For example, you can match your patient's papilledema with a list of conditions affecting intracranial pressure. Or you can compare the symptoms and signs associated with the patient's headache with the various infectious, vascular, metabolic, or neoplastic conditions that might produce this kind of clinical picture.
3. *Eliminate the diagnostic possibilities that fail to explain the findings.* You might consider cluster headache as a cause of Mrs. N's headaches, but eliminate this hypothesis because it fails to explain the patient's throbbing bifrontal localization with intermittent nausea and vomiting. Also, the pain pattern is atypical for cluster headache—it is not unilateral, boring, or occurring repetitively at the same time over a period of days, nor is it associated with lacrimation or rhinorrhea.
4. *Weigh the competing possibilities and select the most likely diagnosis* from among the conditions that might be responsible for the patient's findings. You are looking for a close match between the patient's clinical presentation and a typical case of a given condition. Other clues help in this selection, too. The *statistical probability* of a given disease in a patient of this age, sex, ethnic group, habits, lifestyle, and locality should greatly influence your selection. You should consider the possi-

(continued)

STEPS IN CLINICAL DECISION-MAKING (Continued)

bilities of osteoarthritis and metastatic prostate cancer in a 70-year-old man with back pain, for example, but not in a 25-year-old woman with the same complaint. The *timing of the patient's illness* also makes a difference. Headache in the setting of fever, rash, and stiff neck that develops suddenly over 24 hours suggests quite a different problem than recurrent headache over a period of years associated with stress, visual scotoma, and nausea and vomiting relieved by rest.

5. Finally, as you develop possible explanations for the patient's problem, *give special attention to potentially life-threatening and treatable conditions* such as meningococcal meningitis, bacterial endocarditis, pulmonary embolus, or subdural hematoma. Here you make every effort to minimize the risk for missing conditions that may occur less frequently or be less probable but that, if present, would be particularly ominous. *One rule of thumb is always to include "the worst case scenario" in your list of differential diagnoses* and make sure you have ruled out that possibility based on your findings and patient assessment.

■ **Test your hypotheses.** Now that you have made a hypothesis about the patient's problem, you will usually want to *test your hypothesis*. You are likely to need further history, additional maneuvers on physical examination, or laboratory studies or x-rays to confirm or rule out your tentative diagnosis or to clarify which of two or three possible diagnoses are most likely. When the diagnosis seems clear-cut—a simple upper respiratory infection or a case of hives, for example—these steps may not be necessary.

■ **Establish a working diagnosis.** You are now ready to establish a working definition of the problem. Make this at the highest level of explicitness and certainty that the data allow. You may be limited to a symptom, such as "tension headache, cause unknown." At other times, you can define a problem explicitly in terms of its structure, process, and cause. Examples include "bacterial meningitis, pneumococcal," "subarachnoid hemorrhage, left temporoparietal lobe," or "hypertensive cardiovascular disease with left ventricular dilatation and congestive heart failure."

Although diagnoses are based primarily on identifying abnormal structures, altered processes, and specific causes, you will frequently see patients whose complaints do not fall neatly into these categories. Some symptoms defy analysis, and you may never be able to move beyond simple descriptive categories such as "fatigue" or "anorexia." Other problems relate to the patient's life, rather than to the body. Events such as losing a job or loved one may increase the risk for subsequent illness. Identifying these events and helping the patient develop coping strategies are just as important as managing a headache or a duodenal ulcer.

Another increasingly prominent item on problem lists is *Health Maintenance*. Routinely listing this category helps you track several important health concerns more effectively: immunizations, screening measures (e.g., mammograms, prostate examinations), instructions regarding nutrition and breast or testicular self-examinations, recommendations about exercise or use of seat belts, and responses to important life events.

■ **Develop a plan agreeable to the patient.** You should identify and record a *Plan* for each patient problem. Your *Plan* will flow logically from the problems or diagnoses you have identified and specify which steps are needed next. These steps range from tests to confirm or further evaluate a diagnosis; to consultations for subspecialty evaluation; to additions, deletions, or changes in medication; to arranging a family meeting. You will find that you will follow many of the same diagnoses over time; however, your *Plan* is often more fluid, encompassing changes and modifications that emerge from each patient visit. The *Plan* should make reference to diagnosis, therapy, and patient education.

Before finalizing your *Plan,* it is important to share your assessment and clinical thinking with the patient and seek out his or her opinions, concerns, and willingness to proceed with any further testing or evaluation. Remember that patients may need to hear the same information multiple times and ways before they comprehend it. You will enhance your relationship with the patient if the patient is an active participant in the plan of care.

THE CASE OF MRS. N: ASSESSMENT AND PLAN

As you study the *Assessment* and *Plan* for Mrs. N, think carefully about the clarity and organization of the clinical record. When creating a record, you do more than simply list the patient's story and your physical findings. You must review and organize your data, evaluate the importance and relevance of each item, and construct a clear, concise, yet comprehensive report. At first, it will be challenging to clearly and logically organize your patient assessment. Let the patient's story and symptoms serve as guides, examine the appropriate areas of the body, and apply the steps of clinical reasoning to deepen your knowledge, judgment, and clinical acumen.

Using Mrs. N's record, make a checklist of the features of a good medical record. Later, compare your list with the checklist on pp. 81–83. The following questions may help:

■ Are the data easy to follow, orderly, and presented in a readable format?

■ Is there sufficient detail, both positive and negative, to formulate an Assessment and Plan?

■ Is there excess repetition of information or redundancy?

■ Is the tone professional, avoiding disapproving or moralizing comments?

ASSESSMENT AND PLAN FOR MRS. N

1. **Migraine headaches.** A 54-year-old woman with migraine headaches since childhood, with a throbbing vascular pattern and frequent nausea and vomiting. Headaches are associated with stress and relieved by sleep and cold compresses. There is no papilledema, and there are no motor or sensory deficits on the neurologic examination. The differential diagnosis includes tension headache, also associated with stress, but there is no relief with massage, and the pain is more throbbing than aching. There are no fever, stiff neck, or focal findings to suggest meningitis, and the lifelong recurrent pattern makes subarachnoid hemorrhage unlikely (usually described as "the worst headache of my life").

   Plan:

   - Discuss features of migraine vs. tension headaches.
   - Discuss biofeedback and stress management.
   - Advise patient to avoid caffeine, including coffee, colas, and other carbonated beverages.
   - Start NSAIDs for headache, as needed.
   - If needed next visit, begin prophylactic medication because patient is having more than three migraines per month.

2. **Elevated blood pressure.** Systolic hypertension with wide cuff is present. May be related to obesity, also to anxiety from first visit. No evidence of end-organ damage to retina or heart.

   Plan:

   - Discuss standards for assessing blood pressure.
   - Recheck blood pressure in 1 month, using wide cuff.
   - Review urinalysis.
   - Introduce weight reduction and/or exercise programs (see #4).
   - Reduce salt intake.

3. **Cystocele with occasional stress incontinence.** Cystocele on pelvic examination, probably related to bladder relaxation. Patient is perimenopausal. Incontinence reported with coughing, suggesting alteration in bladder neck anatomy. No dysuria, fever, flank pain. Not taking any contributing medications. Usually involves small amounts of urine, no dribbling, so doubt urge or overflow incontinence.

   Plan:

   - Explain cause of stress incontinence.
   - Review urinalysis.
   - Recommend Kegel's exercises.
   - Consider topical estrogen cream to vagina next visit if no improvement.

4. **Overweight.** Patient 5'2", weighs 143 lbs. BMI is ~26.

   Plan:

   - Explore diet history, ask patient to keep food intake diary.
   - Explore motivation to lose weight, set target for weight loss by next visit.
   - Schedule visit with dietitian.
   - Discuss exercise program, specifically, walking 30 minutes most days a week.

(continued)

ASSESSMENT AND PLAN FOR MRS. N (Continued)

5. **Family stress.** Son-in-law with alcohol problem; daughter and grandchildren seeking refuge in patient's apartment, leading to tensions in these relationships. Patient also has financial constraints. Stress currently situational. No evidence of major depression at present.

   Plan:
   - Explore patient's views on strategies to cope with sources of stress.
   - Explore sources of support, including Al-Anon for daughter and financial counseling for patient.
   - Continue to monitor for depression.

6. **Occasional musculoskeletal low back pain.** Usually with prolonged standing. No history of trauma or motor vehicle accident. Pain does not radiate; no tenderness or motor-sensory deficits on examination. Doubt disc or nerve root compression, trochanteric bursitis, sacroiliitis.

   Plan:
   - Review benefits of weight loss and exercises to strengthen low back muscles.

7. **Tobacco abuse.** 1 pack per day for 36 years.

   Plan:
   - Check peak flow or FEV_1/FVC on office spirometry.
   - Give strong warning to stop smoking.
   - Offer referral to tobacco cessation program.
   - Offer patch, current treatment to enhance abstinence.

8. **Varicose veins, lower extremities.** No complaints currently.
9. **History of right pyelonephritis, 1982.**
10. **Ampicillin allergy.** Developed rash but no other allergic reaction.
11. **Health maintenance.** Last Pap smear 1998; has never had a mammogram.

    Plan:
    - Teach patient breast self-examination; schedule mammogram.
    - Schedule Pap smear next visit.
    - Provide three stool guaiac cards; next visit discuss screening colonoscopy.
    - Suggest dental care for mild gingivitis.
    - Advise patient to move medications and caustic cleaning agents to locked cabinet, if possible, above shoulder height.

APPROACHING THE CHALLENGES OF CLINICAL DATA

As you can see from the case of Mrs. N, organizing the patient's clinical data poses several challenges. The beginning student must decide whether to cluster the patient's symptoms and signs into one problem or into several problems. The amount of data may appear unmanageable. The quality of the data may be prone to error. Guidelines to help you address these challenges are provided in the following paragraphs.

Clustering Data into Single versus Multiple Problems. One of the greatest difficulties facing students is how to cluster the clinical data. Do selected data fit into one problem or several problems? The patient's *age* may help—young people are more likely to have a single disease, whereas older people tend to have multiple diseases. The *timing* of symptoms is often useful. For example, an episode of pharyngitis 6 weeks ago is probably unrelated to fever, chills, pleuritic chest pain, and cough that prompt an office visit today. To use timing effectively, you need to know the natural history of various diseases and conditions. A yellow penile discharge followed 3 weeks later by a painless penile ulcer suggests two problems: gonorrhea and primary syphilis. In contrast, a penile ulcer followed in 6 weeks by a maculopapular skin rash and generalized lymphadenopathy suggest two stages of the same problem: primary and secondary syphilis.

Involvement of *different body systems* may help you to cluster the clinical data. If symptoms and signs occur in a single system, one disease may explain them. Problems in different, apparently unrelated systems often require more than one explanation. Again, knowledge of disease patterns is necessary. You might decide, for example, to group a patient's high blood pressure and sustained apical impulse together with flame-shaped retinal hemorrhages, place them in the cardiovascular system, and label the constellation "hypertensive cardiovascular disease with hypertensive retinopathy." You would develop another explanation for the patient's mild fever, left lower quadrant tenderness, and diarrhea.

Some diseases involve more than one body system. As you gain knowledge and experience, you will become increasingly adept at recognizing *multisystem conditions* and building plausible explanations that link together their seemingly unrelated manifestations. To explain cough, hemoptysis, and weight loss in a 60-year-old plumber who has smoked cigarettes for 40 years, you probably even now would rank lung cancer high in your differential diagnosis. You might support your diagnosis with your observation of the patient's cyanotic fingernails. With experience and continued reading, you will recognize that his other symptoms and signs can be linked to the same diagnosis. Dysphagia would reflect extension of the cancer to the esophagus, pupillary asymmetry would suggest pressure on the cervical sympathetic chain, and jaundice could result from metastases to the liver.

In another case of multisystem disease, a young man who presents with odynophagia, fever, weight loss, purplish skin lesions, leukoplakia, generalized lymphadenopathy, and chronic diarrhea is likely to have AIDS. Related risk factors should be explored promptly.

Sifting Through an Extensive Array of Data. It is common to confront a relatively long list of symptoms and signs, and an equally long list of potential explanations. One approach is to *tease out separate clusters of observations and analyze one cluster at a time,* as just described. You can also *ask a series of key questions* that may steer your thinking in one direction and allow you to temporarily ignore the others. For example, you may ask what produces and relieves the patient's chest pain. If the answer is exercise and rest, you can focus on the cardiovascular and musculoskeletal systems and set the gastrointestinal system aside. If the pain is substernal, burning, and occurs only after meals, you can logically focus on the gastrointestinal tract. A series of discriminating questions helps you form a decision tree or algorithm that is helpful in collecting and analyzing clinical data and reaching logical conclusions and explanations.

Assessing the Quality of the Data. Almost all clinical information is subject to error. Patients forget to mention symptoms, confuse the events of their illness, avoid recounting facts that are embarrassing, and often slant their stories to what the clinician wants to hear. Clinicians misinterpret patient statements, overlook information, fail to ask "the one key question," jump prematurely to conclusions and diagnoses, or forget an important part of the examination, such as the testicular examination in a young man with asymptomatic testicular carcinoma. You can avoid some of these errors by acquiring the habits of skilled clinicians, summarized below.

TIPS FOR ENSURING THE QUALITY OF PATIENT DATA

- Ask open-ended questions and listen carefully and patiently to the patient's story.
- Craft a thorough and systematic sequence to history taking and physical examination.
- Keep an open mind toward both the patient and the data.
- Always include "the worst-case scenario" in your list of possible explanations of the patient's problem, and make sure it can be safely eliminated.
- Analyze any mistakes in data collection or interpretation.
- Confer with colleagues and review the pertinent medical literature to clarify uncertainties.
- Apply principles of data analysis to patient information and testing.

Symptoms, physical findings, tests, and x-rays should help you reduce uncertainty about whether a patient does or does not have a given condition. Clinical data, including laboratory work, however, are inherently imperfect. You can improve your assessment of clinical data and laboratory tests by applying several key principles for selecting and using clinical data and tests. Learn to apply the principles of *reliability, validity, sensitivity, specificity,* and *predictive value* to your clinical findings and the tests you order. These test characteristics will help you decide how confident you can be of your findings and test results as you assess the presence or absence of a disease or problem.

Displaying Clinical Data. To use these principles, it is important to display the data in the 2 × 2 format diagrammed on the following page. Always using this format will ensure the accuracy of your calculations of sensitivity, specificity, and predictive value. Note that the presence or absence of disease implies use of a *gold standard* to establish whether the disease is truly present or absent. This is usually the best test available, such as a coronary angiogram for assessing coronary artery disease or a tissue biopsy for malignancy.

PRINCIPLES OF TEST SELECTION AND USE

Reliability. Indicates how well repeated measurements of the same relatively stable phenomenon will give the same result, also known as precision. Reliability may be measured for one observer or for more than one observer.

Example: If on several occasions one clinician consistently percusses the same span of a patient's liver dullness, *intraobserver reliability* is good. If, on the other hand, several observers find quite different spans of liver dullness on the same patient, *interobserver reliability* is poor.

Validity. Indicates how closely a given observation agrees with "the true state of affairs," or the best possible measure of reality.

Example: Blood pressure measurements by mercury-based sphygmomanometers are less valid than intra-arterial pressure tracings.

Sensitivity. Identifies the proportion of people who test positive in a group of people known to have the disease or condition, or the proportion of people who are *true positives* compared with the total number of people who actually have the disease. When the observation or test is negative in persons who have the disease, the result is termed *false negative*. *Good observations or tests have a sensitivity of more than 90%, and help rule out disease because there are few false negatives. Such observations or tests are especially useful for screening.*

Example: The sensitivity of Homan's sign in the diagnosis of deep venous thrombosis (DVT) of the calf is 50%. In other words, compared with a group of patients with deep vein thrombosis confirmed by phlebogram, a much better test, only 50% will have a positive Homan's sign, so this sign, if absent, is not helpful because 50% of patients may have a DVT.

Specificity. Identifies the proportion of people who test negative in a group of people known to be *without* a given disease or condition, or the proportion of people who are "true negatives" compared with the total number of people without the disease. When the observation or test is positive in persons without the disease, the result is termed *false positive*. Good observations or tests have a specificity of more than 90% and help "rule in" disease because the test is rarely positive when disease is absent, and there are few false positives.

Example: The specificity of serum amylase in patients with possible acute pancreatitis is 70%. In other words, of 100 patients without pancreatitis, 70% will have a normal serum amylase; in 30%, the serum amylase will be falsely elevated.

Predictive Value. Indicates how well a given symptom, sign, or test result—either positive or negative—predicts the presence or absence of disease.

(continued)

PRINCIPLES OF TEST SELECTION AND USE (Continued)

Positive predictive value is the probability of disease in a patient with a positive (abnormal) test, or the proportion of "true positives" out of the total population tested.

Example: In a group of women with palpable breast nodules in a cancer screening program, the proportion with confirmed breast cancer would constitute the *positive predictive value* of palpable breast nodules for diagnosing breast cancer.

Negative predictive value is the probability of not having the condition or disease when the test is negative, or normal, or the proportion of "true negatives" out of the total population tested.

Example: In a group of women without palpable breast nodules in a cancer screening program, the proportion without confirmed breast cancer constitutes the *negative predictive value* of absence of breast nodules.

Note that the numbers related to presence or absence of disease, as determined by the gold standard, are always displayed **down the table** in the left and right columns (*present = a + c; absent = b + d*). Numbers related to the observation or test are always displayed **across the table** in the upper and lower rows (*test positive = a + b; test negative = c + d*).

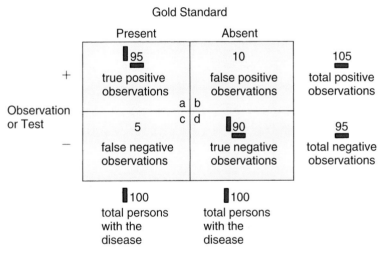

Now you are ready to make your calculations:

$$\text{Sensitivity} = \frac{a}{a+c} = \frac{\text{true positive observations (95)}}{\text{total persons with disease } (95+5)} \times 100 = 95\%$$

$$\text{Specificity} = \frac{d}{b+d} = \frac{\text{true negative observations (90)}}{\text{total persons with disease } (90+10)} \times 100 = 90\%$$

$$\text{Positive predictive value} = \frac{a}{a+b} = \frac{\text{true positive observations (95)}}{\text{total positive observations } (95+10)} \times 100 = 90.5\%$$

$$\text{Negative predictive value} = \frac{d}{c+d} = \frac{\text{true negative observations (90)}}{\text{total negative observations } (90+5)} \times 100 = 94.7\%$$

Now return to the table. *The **vertical red bars** designate sensitivity (a/a + c) and specificity (d/b + d), and the **horizontal red bars** designate positive predictive value (a/a + b) and negative predictive value (d/c + d).* The data displayed indicate that the hypothetical test has excellent test characteristics. The sensitivity and specificity of the test are both more than 90%, as are the positive and negative predictive values. Such a test would be clinically useful for assessing a disease or condition in your patient.

Note that the predictive value of a test or observation depends heavily on the *prevalence* of the condition within the population studied. Prevalence is the proportion of people in a defined population at any given point in time who have the condition in question. When the prevalence of a condition is *low*, the positive predictive value of the test will fall. When the prevalence is *high*, the sensitivity, specificity, and positive predictive value are high, and the negative predictive value approaches zero. To work further on these relationships, turn to the tables below on Prevalence and Predictive Value, and practice making the calculations described.

PREVALENCE AND PREDICTIVE VALUE

Two examples further illustrate these principles and show *how predictive values vary with prevalence.* Consider first (*Example 1*) an imaginary population *A* with 1,000 people. The prevalence of disease *X* in this population is high—40%. You can quickly calculate that 400 of these people have *X*. You then set out to detect these cases with an observation or test that is 90% sensitive and 80% specific. Of the 400 people with *X*, the observation reveals .90 × 400, or 360 (the true positives). It misses the other 40 (400 − 360, the false negatives). Out of the 600 people without *X*, the observation or test proves negative in .80 × 600, or 480. These people are truly free of *X*, as the observation suggests (the true negatives). But the observation misleads you in the remaining 120 (600 − 480). These people are falsely labeled as having *X* when they are really free of it (the false positives). These figures are summarized below:

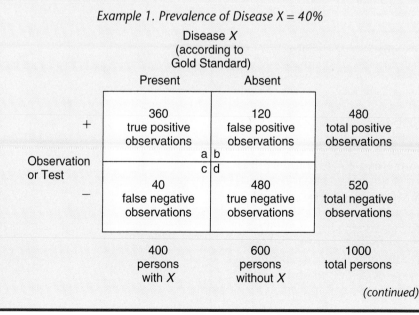

Example 1. Prevalence of Disease X = 40%

	Disease *X* (according to Gold Standard)		
	Present	Absent	
Observation or Test (+)	360 true positive observations	120 false positive observations	480 total positive observations
	a	b	
	c	d	
Observation or Test (−)	40 false negative observations	480 true negative observations	520 total negative observations
	400 persons with *X*	600 persons without *X*	1000 total persons

(continued)

PREVALENCE AND PREDICTIVE VALUE (Continued)

As a clinician who does not have perfect knowledge of who really does or does not have disease *X*, you are faced with a total of 480 people with positive observations. You must try to distinguish between the true and the false positives and will undoubtedly use additional kinds of data to help you in this task. Given only the sensitivity and specificity of your observation, however, you can determine the probability that a positive observation is a true positive, and you may wish to explain it to the concerned patient. This probability is calculated as follows:

$$\textit{Positive predictive value} = \frac{a}{a+b} = \frac{\text{true positives (360)}}{\text{total positives (360 + 120)}} \times 100 = 75\%$$

Thus, 3 out of 4 of the people with positive observations really have the disease, and 1 out of 4 does not.

By a similar calculation, you can determine the probability that a negative observation is a true negative. The results here are reasonably reassuring to the involved patient:

$$\textit{Negative predictive value} = \frac{d}{c+d} = \frac{\text{true negatives (480)}}{\text{total negatives (40 + 480)}} \times 100 = 92\%$$

As *prevalence* of the disease in a population diminishes, however, the predictive value of a positive observation diminishes remarkably, while the predictive value of a negative observation rises further. In *Example 2*, in a second population, *B*, of 1,000 people, only 1% have disease *X*. Now there are only 10 cases of *X* and 990 people without *X*. If this population is screened with the same observation, which has a 90% sensitivity and an 80% specificity, here are the results:

Example 2. Prevalence of Disease X = 1%

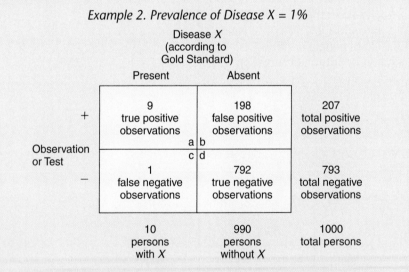

You are now confronted with possibly upsetting 207 people (all those with positive observations) to detect 9 out of the 10 real cases. The predictive value of a positive observation is only 4%. Improving the specificity of your observation without diminishing its sensitivity would be very helpful, if it were possible. For example, if you could increase the specificity of the observation from 80% to 98% (given the same prevalence of 1% and sensitivity of 90%), the positive predictive value of the observation would improve from 4% to 31%—scarcely ideal but certainly better. Good observations or tests have a sensitivity and specificity of 90%.

Because prevalence strongly affects the predictive value of an observation, prevalence too influences the assessment process. Because coronary artery disease is much more common in middle-aged men than in young women, you should pursue angina as a cause of chest pain more actively in the former group. The effect of prevalence on predictive value explains why your odds of making a correct assessment are better when you hypothesize a common condition rather than a rare one. The combination of fever, headache, myalgias, and cough probably has the same sensitivity and specificity for influenza throughout the year, but your chance of making this diagnosis correctly by using this cluster of symptoms is much greater during a winter flu epidemic than it is during a quiet August.

Prevalence varies importantly with clinical setting as well as with season. Chronic bronchitis is probably the most common cause of hemoptysis among patients seen in a general medical clinic. In the oncology clinic of a tertiary medical center, however, lung cancer might head the list, while in a group of postoperative patients on a general surgical service, irritation from an endotracheal tube or pulmonary infarction might be most likely. In certain parts of Asia, in contrast, one should think first of a worm called a lung fluke. When you hear hoofbeats in the distance, according to the familiar saying, bet on horses, not on zebras, unless, of course, you're visiting the zoo.

■ BUILDING YOUR CASE: INTEGRATING CLINICAL REASONING AND ASSESSMENT OF CLINICAL DATA

The concepts of sensitivity and specificity help in both the collection and analysis of data. They even underlie some of the basic strategies of interviewing. Questions with high sensitivity, if answered in the affirmative, may be particularly useful for screening and for gathering evidence to support a hypothesis. For example, "Have you had any discomfort or pain in your chest?" is a highly sensitive question for diagnosing angina pectoris. For patients with this condition, there would be few false-negative responses. Thus, it is a good first screening question. However, because there are many other causes of chest discomfort, it is not all that specific. Pain that is retrosternal, pressing, and less than 10 minutes in duration—each a reasonably sensitive attribute of angina—would add importantly to your growing evidence for the diagnosis. To confirm your hypothesis, a more specific question, if answered in the affirmative, is needed, such as "Is the pain precipitated by exertion?" or "Is the pain relieved by rest?"

Data for testing hypotheses also come from the physical examination. Heart murmurs are good examples of findings with varying sensitivity and specificity. The vast majority of patients with significant valvular *aortic stenosis* have systolic ejection murmurs audible in the aortic area. Presence of a systolic murmur has a high sensitivity for aortic stenosis. This finding is present in most cases. The false-negative rate is low. On the other hand, many other conditions produce systolic murmurs, such as increased blood flow across a normal valve, or the sclerotic changes associated with aging, termed aortic sclerosis, so the finding of a systolic murmur is not very specific. Using such a murmur as your only criterion for diagnosing aortic stenosis would lead to many false positives.

In contrast, a high-pitched, soft blowing decrescendo diastolic murmur best heard along the left sternal border is quite specific for *aortic regurgitation*. Such a murmur is almost never heard in normal people, and it is present in very few other conditions, so there are few false positives.

Combining data from the history and physical examination allows you to test your hypotheses, screen for selected conditions, build your case, and clinch a diagnosis even before obtaining further diagnostic tests. Consider the following list of evidence: cough, fever, a shaking chill, left-sided pleuritic chest pain, dullness throughout the left lower posterior lung field with crackles, bronchial breathing, and egophony. Cough and fever are good screening items for pneumonia, the next items support the hypothesis, and bronchial breathing with egophony in this distribution is very specific for lobar pneumonia. A chest x-ray would confirm the diagnosis.

Absence of selected symptoms and signs is also diagnostically useful, especially when they are usually present in a given condition (i.e., their sensitivity is high). For example, if a patient with cough and left-sided pleuritic chest pain does not have fever, bacterial pneumonia becomes much less likely (except possibly in infancy and old age). Likewise, in a patient with severe dyspnea, the absence of orthopnea makes left ventricular failure less probable as an explanation for shortness of breath.

Skilled clinicians use this kind of logic even if they are unaware of its statistical underpinnings. They start to generate tentative hypotheses as soon as the patient describes the *Chief Complaint,* then build evidence for one or more of these hypotheses and discard others as they continue with the history and examination. In developing a *Present Illness,* they borrow items from other parts of the history, such as the *Past Medical History,* the *Family History,* and the *Review of Systems.* In a 55-year-old man with chest pain, the skilled clinician does not stop with the attributes of pain, but moves on to probe risk factors from coronary artery disease such as family history, hypertension, diabetes, lipid abnormalities, and smoking. In both the history and physical examination, the clinician searches explicitly for other possible manifestations of cardiovascular disease such as congestive heart failure or the claudication or diminished lower extremity pulses of atherosclerotic peripheral vascular disease. By generating hypotheses early and testing them sequentially, experienced clinicians improve their efficiency and enhance the relevance and value of the data they collect. They dig and collect less ore but find more gold.

This sequence of collecting data and testing hypotheses is diagrammed below.

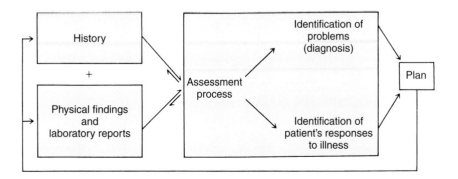

After the plan has been implemented, the process recycles. The clinician gathers more data, assesses the patient's progress, modifies the problem list if indicated, and adjusts the plan accordingly. As you gain experience, the interplay of assessment and data collection will become increasingly familiar. You will come to value the challenges and rewards of clinical reasoning and assessment that make patient care so meaningful.

ORGANIZING THE PATIENT RECORD

A clear, well-organized clinical record is one of the most important adjuncts to your patient care. Your skill in recording your patient's history and physical examination should evolve in parallel with your growing skills in clinical reasoning and your ability to formulate the patient's *Assessment* and *Plan*. Your goal should be a clear, concise, but comprehensive report that documents the key findings of your patient assessment and communicates the patient's problems in a succinct and *legible* format to other providers and members of the health care team. Note that a good record provides the supporting data for the problems or diagnoses identified.

Regardless of your experience, certain principles will help you to organize a good record. Think especially about the *order and readability* of the record and the *amount of detail* needed. How much detail to include often poses a vexing problem. As a student, you may wish (or you may be required) to be quite detailed. This helps to build your descriptive skills, vocabulary, and speed—admittedly a painful and tedious process. Pressures of time, however, will ultimately force some compromises.

Run through the following checklist to make sure your record is clear, informative, and easy to follow.

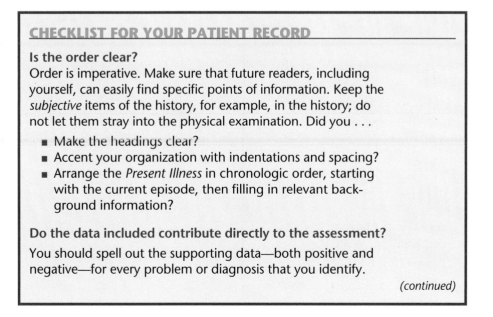

CHECKLIST FOR YOUR PATIENT RECORD

Is the order clear?
Order is imperative. Make sure that future readers, including yourself, can easily find specific points of information. Keep the *subjective* items of the history, for example, in the history; do not let them stray into the physical examination. Did you . . .

- Make the headings clear?
- Accent your organization with indentations and spacing?
- Arrange the *Present Illness* in chronologic order, starting with the current episode, then filling in relevant background information?

Do the data included contribute directly to the assessment?
You should spell out the supporting data—both positive and negative—for every problem or diagnosis that you identify.

(continued)

CHECKLIST FOR YOUR PATIENT RECORD (Continued)

Are pertinent negatives specifically described?

Often portions of the history or examination suggest that an abnormality might exist or develop in that area.

For the patient with notable bruises, record the "pertinent negatives," such as the absence of injury or violence, familial bleeding disorders, or medications or nutritional deficits that might lead to bruising.

For the patient who is depressed but not suicidal, record both facts. In the patient with a transient mood swing, on the other hand, a comment on suicide is unnecessary.

Are there overgeneralizations or omissions of important data?

Remember that data not recorded are data lost. No matter how vividly you can recall selected details today, you will probably not remember them in a few months. The phrase "neurologic exam negative," even in your own handwriting, may leave you wondering in a few months' time, "Did I really do the sensory exam?"

Is there too much detail?

Avoid burying important information in a mass of excessive detail, to be discovered by only the most persistent reader. *Omit most of your negative findings* unless they relate directly to the patient's complaints or to specific exclusions in your diagnostic assessment. *Do not list abnormalities that you did not observe. Instead, concentrate on a few major ones, such as* "no heart murmurs," and try to describe structures in a concise, positive way. You can omit certain body structures even though you examined them, such as normal eyebrows and eyelashes.

"Cervix pink and smooth" indicates you saw no redness, ulcers, nodules, masses, cysts or other suspicious lesions, but this description is shorter and readable.

Are phrases and short words used appropriately? Is there unnecessary repetition of data?

Omit unnecessary words, such as those in parentheses in the examples. This saves valuable time and space.

"Cervix is pink (in color)." "Lungs are resonant (to percussion)." "Liver is tender (to palpation)." "Both (right and left) ears with cerumen." "II/IV systolic ejection murmur (audible)." "Thorax symmetric (bilaterally)."

Omit repetitive introductory phrases such as "The patient reports no . . . " because readers assume the patient is the source of the history unless otherwise specified.
Use short words instead of longer, fancier ones when they mean the same thing, such as "felt" for "palpated" or "heard" for "auscultated."

(continued)

CHECKLIST FOR YOUR PATIENT RECORD (Continued)

Describe what you observed, not what you did. "Optic discs seen" is less informative than "disc margins sharp," even if it marks your first glimpse as an examiner!

Is the written style succinct? Is there excessive use of abbreviations?

Records are scientific and legal documents, so they should be clear and understandable.
Using words and brief phrases instead of whole sentences is common, but abbreviations and symbols should be used only if they are readily understood.
Likewise, an overly elegant style is less appealing than a concise summary.
Be sure your record is legible, otherwise, all that you have recorded is worthless to your readers.

Are diagrams and precise measurements included where appropriate?

Diagrams add greatly to the clarity of the record.

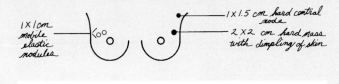

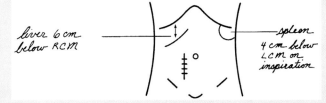

To ensure accurate evaluations and future comparisons, make measurements in centimeters, not in fruits, nuts, or vegetables.

"1 × 1 cm lymph node" versus a "pea-sized lymph node . . ."
Or "2 × 2 cm mass on the left lobe of the prostate" versus a "walnut-sized prostate mass."

Is the tone of the write-up neutral and professional?

It is important to be objective. Hostile, moralizing, or disapproving comments have no place in the patient's record.
Never use inflammatory or demeaning words, penmanship, or punctuation.

Comments such as "Patient DRUNK and LATE TO CLINIC AGAIN!!" are unprofessional and set a bad example for other providers reading the chart. They also might prove difficult to defend in a legal setting.

Your institution or agency may have printed forms for recording patient information, but you should always be able to create your own record. The record of Mrs. N may be longer than what you might see in patient charts, yet it still does not reflect every question and technique that you have learned to use. The amount of detail varies, depending on the patient's symptoms and signs and the complexity of the clinician's diagnoses and plans for management.

Generating the Problem List.   Once you have completed your assessment and written record, you will find it helpful to generate a *Problem List* that summarizes the patient's problems for the front of the office or hospital chart. *List the most active and serious problems first, and record their date of onset.* Some clinicians make separate lists for active or inactive problems; others make one list in order of priority. You will find that on follow-up visits the *Problem List* helps you remember to check the status of problems the patient may not mention. The *Problem List* also allows other members of the health care team to review the patient's health status at a glance.

A sample *Problem List* for Mrs. N is provided below. You may wish to give each problem a number and use the number when referring to specific problems in subsequent notes.

SAMPLE PROBLEM LIST

Date Entered	Problem No.	Problem
1/30/06	1	Migraine headaches
	2	Elevated blood pressure
	3	Cystocele with occasional stress incontinence
	4	Overweight
	5	Family stress
	6	Low back pain
	7	Tobacco abuse
	8	Varicose veins
	9	History of right pyelonephritis
	10	Allergy to ampicillin
	11	Health maintenance

Clinicians organize problem lists differently, even for the same patient. Your problem list for Mrs. N may look somewhat different from the one above. Note that problems can be symptoms, signs, or conditions. Good lists vary in emphasis, length, and detail, depending on the clinician's philosophy, specialty, and role as a provider. The list illustrated here includes problems that need attention now, such as the headaches, as well as problems that need future observation or attention, such as the blood pressure and cystocele. Listing the allergy to ampicillin warns you not to prescribe medications in the penicillin family.

Some of the items noted in the history and physical examination, such as the canker sores and hard stools, do not appear in this problem list because they are relatively common phenomena that do not currently demand attention. Such judgments may prove to be wrong; however, problem lists that are cluttered with relatively insignificant items diminish in value. Some clinicians would find this list too long; others would be more explicit about such problems as "family stress" or "varicose veins."

Writing the Progress Note. A month later, Mrs. N returns for a follow-up visit. The style of the progress note is also quite variable, but it should follow the same standards as the initial assessment. It should be clear, sufficiently detailed, and easy to follow. It should reflect your clinical thinking and delineate your assessment and plan. The following note follows the SOAP note format (**S**ubjective, **O**bjective, **A**ssessment, and **P**lan), but you will see many other styles and interest in making more "patient-centered" medical records.[7] Often clinicians record the history and physical examination, then give each patient problem *Assessment* and *Plan*.

SAMPLE SOAP NOTE

1. Migraine headaches.
   S: Has had only two headaches, both mild and without associated symptoms. These are less troubling. Cannot detect any precipitating factors.
   O: No tenderness over the temporal muscles. No papilledema.
   A: Headaches improved, now without migraine features.
   P: Call if symptoms recur.

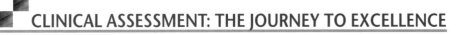

CLINICAL ASSESSMENT: THE JOURNEY TO EXCELLENCE

The process of learning about a patient continues far beyond the first few encounters. Your understanding of patient care will grow in depth and complexity throughout your clinical career. Your prowess in history taking, physical examination, clinical reasoning, evidence-based decision-making, and documenting the patient record is launched. Now you must embark on repetitive practice, with supervision, and on the lifelong pursuit of polishing your newly acquired skills.

Bibliography

CITATIONS

1. Peterson MC, Holbrook JH, Von Hales DE, et al. Contributions of the history, physical examination, and laboratory investigation in making medical diagnoses. West J Med 156:163–165, 1992.
2. Hampton JR, Harrison MJ, Mitchell JRA, et al. Relative contributions of history-taking, physical examination, and laboratory investigation to diagnosis and management of medical outpatients. BMJ 2:486–489, 1975.
3. McGee S. Evidence-Based Physical Diagnosis. Philadelphia: WB Saunders, 2001.
4. Schneiderman H. Bedside Diagnosis. An Annotated Bibliography of Literature on Physical Examination and Interviewing, 3rd ed. Philadelphia: American College of Physicians, 1997.
5. Evidence-Based Medicine Working Group. Evidence-based medicine: a new approach to teaching the practice of medicine. JAMA 268(17)2420–2425, 1992. [Launched the Rational Clinical Examination Series.]
6. Guyatt G, Rennie D. Users' Guides to the Medical Literature: A Manual for Evidence-Based Clinical Practice. Chicago: American Medical Association, 2001.
7. Donnelly WJ. Viewpoint: Patient-centered medical care requires a patient-centered medical record. Acad Med 80(1):33–38, 2005.

ADDITIONAL REFERENCES

Alfaro-LeFevre R. Critical Thinking and Clinical Judgment: A Practical Approach, 3rd ed. St. Louis, WB Saunders, 2004.

Carpenito LJ. Nursing Diagnosis: Application to Clinical Practice, 11th ed. Philadelphia, Lippincott Williams & Wilkins, 2005.

Cherry B, Jacob SR. Contemporary Nursing: Issues, Trends, and Management, 3rd ed. St. Louis, Elsevier Mosby, 2005.

Fletcher RH, Fletcher, SW. Clinical Epidemiology: The Essentials, 4th ed. Philadelphia, Lippincott Williams & Wilkins, 2005.

Innui TS. Establishing the doctor–patient relationship: science, art, or competence? Schweiz Med Wochenschr 128:225, 1998.

Laditka JN, Laditka SB, Mastanduno MP. Hospital utilization for ambulatory care sensitive conditions: health outcome disparities associated with race and ethnicity. Soc Sci Med 57(8):1429–1441, 2003.

Nettina SM. The Lippincott Manual of Nursing Practice, 7th ed. Philadelphia, Lippincott Williams & Wilkins, 2001.

Panzer RJ, Bordley DR, Cappuccio J, et al (eds). Diagnostic Strategies in Common Medical Problems, 3rd ed. Philadelphia: American College of Physicians, 2006.

Sackett DL. Evidence-based Medicine: How to Practice and Teach EBM, 2nd ed. New York, Churchill Livingstone, 2000.

Regional Examinations

4

Beginning the Physical Examination: General Survey and Vital Signs

Once you understand the patient's concerns and have elicited a careful history, you are ready to begin the physical examination. At first you may feel unsure of how the patient will relate to you. With practice, your skills in physical examination will grow, and you will gain confidence. Through study and repetition, the examination will flow more smoothly, and you will soon shift your attention from technique and how to handle instruments to what you hear, see, and feel. Touching the patient's body will seem more natural, and you will learn to minimize any discomfort to the patient. You will become more responsive to the patient's reactions and provide reassurance when needed. Before long, as you gain proficiency, what once took between 1 and 2 hours will take considerably less time.

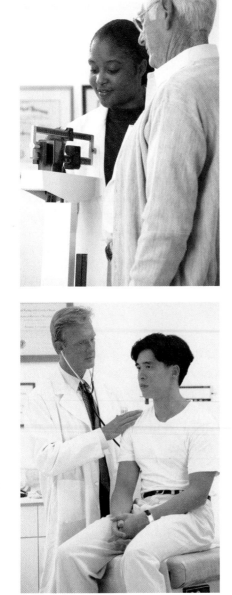

This chapter addresses skills and techniques needed for initial assessment as you begin the physical examination. Under Anatomy and Physiology, you will find information on how to measure height, weight, and Body Mass Index (BMI) and guidelines for nutritional assessment. There is clinical information on the relevant health history and on health promotion and counseling. The section on Techniques of Examination describes the initial steps of the physical examination: preparing for the examination, conducting the general survey, and taking the vital signs. Then follows an example of the written record relevant to the general survey and vital signs.

ANATOMY AND PHYSIOLOGY

As you begin the physical examination, you will survey the patient's general appearance and measure the patient's height and weight. These data provide information about the patient's nutritional status and amount of body fat. Body fat consists primarily of adipose in the form of triglyceride and is stored in subcutaneous, intra-abdominal, and intramuscular fat deposits. These stores are inaccessible and difficult to measure, so it will be important to compare your measurements of height and weight with standardized ranges of normal.

In the past, tables of desirable weight-for-height have been based on life insurance data, which often did not adjust for the effects of smoking and selected weight-inducing medical conditions such as diabetes and which tended to overstate desirable weight. Current practice, however, is to use the *Body Mass Index*, which incorporates estimated but more accurate measures of body fat than weight alone. BMI standards are derived from two surveys: the National Health Examination Survey, consisting of three survey cycles between 1960 and 1970, and the National Health and Nutrition Examination Survey, with three cycles from the 1970s to the 1990s.

More than half of U.S. adults are overweight (BMI >25), and nearly one fourth are obese (BMI >30), so assessing and educating patients about their BMI are vital for promoting health. These conditions are proven risk factors for diabetes, heart disease, stroke, hypertension, osteoarthritis, sleep apnea syndrome, and some forms of cancer. Remember that these BMI criteria are not rigid cutpoints but guidelines for increasing risks for health and well-being. Note that people older than age 65 have a disproportionate risk for undernutrition when compared with younger adults.

Height and weight in childhood and adolescence reflect the many behavioral, cognitive, and physiologic changes of growth and development. Developmental milestones, markers for growth spurts, and sexual maturity ratings can be found in Chapter 18, Assessing Children: Infancy Through Adolescence. With aging, some of these changes reverse, as described in Chapter 20, The Older Adult. Height may decrease, posture may become more stooping from kyphosis of the thoracic spine, and extension of the knees and hips may diminish. The abdominal muscles may relax, changing the abdominal contour, and fat may accumulate at the hips and lower abdomen. Be alert to these changes as you assess older patients.

Calculating the BMI.   There are several ways to calculate the BMI, as shown in the accompanying table. Choose the method most suited to your practice. The National Institutes of Health and the National Heart, Lung, and Blood Institute caution that people who are very muscular may have a high BMI but still be healthy.[1] Likewise, the BMI for people with low muscle mass and reduced nutrition may appear inappropriately "normal."

If the BMI is 35 or higher, measure the patient's *waist circumference*. With the patient standing, measure the waist just above the hip bones. The patient may have excess body fat if the waist measures:

- ≥35 inches for women

- ≥40 inches for men

■ Methods to Calculate Body Mass Index (BMI)

Unit of Measure	Method of Calculation
Weight *in pounds,* height *in inches*	(1) Body Mass Index Chart (see table below)
	(2) $\dfrac{\left(\dfrac{\text{Weight (lbs)} \times 700^*}{\text{Height (inches)}}\right)}{\text{Height (inches)}}$
Weight *in kilograms,* height *in meters squared*	(3) $\dfrac{\text{Weight (kg)}}{\text{Height }\left(\text{m}^2\right)}$
Either	(4) "BMI Calculator" at website www.nhlbisupport.com/bmi/bmicalc.htm

*Several organizations use 704.5, but the variation in BMI is negligible. Conversion formulas: 2.2 lbs = 1 kg; 1.0 inch = 2.54 cm; 100 cm = 1 meter.

Source: National Institutes of Health and National Heart, Lung, and Blood Institute: Body Mass Index Calculator. Available at: http://www.nhlbisupport.com/bmi/bmicalc.htm. Accessed December 12, 2004.

■ Body Mass Index Table

	Normal						Overweight					Obese									
BMI	19	20	21	22	23	24	25	26	27	28	29	30	31	32	33	34	35	36	37	38	39
Height (inches)										Body Weight (pounds)											
58	91	96	100	105	110	115	119	124	129	134	138	143	148	153	158	162	167	172	177	181	186
59	94	99	104	109	114	119	124	128	133	138	143	148	153	158	163	168	173	178	183	188	193
60	97	102	107	112	118	123	128	133	138	143	148	153	158	163	168	174	179	184	189	194	199
61	100	106	111	116	122	127	132	137	143	148	153	158	164	169	174	180	185	190	195	201	206
62	104	109	115	120	126	131	136	142	147	153	158	164	169	175	180	186	191	196	202	207	213
63	107	113	118	124	130	135	141	146	152	158	163	169	175	180	186	191	197	203	208	214	220
64	110	116	122	128	134	140	145	151	157	163	169	174	180	186	192	197	204	209	215	221	227
65	114	120	126	132	138	144	150	156	162	168	174	180	186	192	198	204	210	216	222	228	234
66	118	124	130	136	142	148	155	161	167	173	179	186	192	198	204	210	216	223	229	235	241
67	121	127	134	140	146	153	159	166	172	178	185	191	198	204	211	217	223	230	236	242	249
68	125	131	138	144	151	158	164	171	177	184	190	197	203	210	216	223	230	236	243	249	256
69	128	135	142	149	155	162	169	176	182	189	196	203	209	216	223	230	236	243	250	257	263
70	132	139	146	153	160	167	174	181	188	195	202	209	216	222	229	236	243	250	257	264	271
71	136	143	150	157	165	172	179	186	193	200	208	215	222	229	236	243	250	257	265	272	279
72	140	147	154	162	169	177	184	191	199	206	213	221	228	235	242	250	258	265	272	279	287
73	144	151	159	166	174	182	189	197	204	212	219	227	235	242	250	257	265	272	280	288	295
74	148	155	163	171	179	186	194	202	210	218	225	233	241	249	256	264	272	280	287	295	303
75	152	160	168	176	184	192	200	208	216	224	232	240	248	256	264	272	279	287	295	303	311
76	156	164	172	180	189	197	205	213	221	230	238	246	254	263	271	279	287	295	304	312	320

Source: Adapted from National Institutes of Health and National Heart, Lung, and Blood Institute: Clinical Guidelines on the Identification, Evaluation and Treatment of Overweight and Obesity in Adults: The Evidence Report. June 1998. Available at: www.nhlbi.nih.gov/guidelines/obesity/ob_gdlns.pdf. Accessed December 12, 2004.

Interpreting and Acting on the BMI.   Classify the BMI according to the national guidelines in the table below. If the BMI is *above 25,* assess the patient for *additional risk factors* for heart disease and other obesity-related diseases: hypertension, high LDL cholesterol, low HDL cholesterol, high triglycerides, high blood glucose, family history of premature heart disease, physical inactivity, and cigarette smoking. Patients with a BMI over 25 and two or more risk factors should pursue weight loss, especially if the waist circumference is elevated.

■ Classification of Overweight and Obesity by BMI		
	Obesity Class	BMI (kg/m²)
Underweight		<18.5
Normal		18.5–24.9
Overweight		25.0–29.9
Obesity	I	30.0–34.9
	II	35.0–39.9
Extreme obesity	III	≥40

Source: National Institutes of Health and National Heart, Lung, and Blood Institute: Clinical Guidelines on the Identification, Evaluation, and Treatment of Overweight and Obesity in Adults: The Evidence Report. NIH Publication 98-4083. June 1998.

Assessing Dietary Intake.   Advising patients about diet and weight loss is important, especially in light of the many, often contradictory dieting options in the popular press. Review three excellent guidelines for counseling your patients:

See Table 4-1, Healthy Eating: Food Groups and Servings per Day, p. 115. For screening tools, see Table 4-2, Rapid Screen for Dietary Intake, p. 115, and Table 4-4, Nutrition Screening Checklist, p. 117.

■ National Institutes of Health and National Heart, Lung, and Blood Institute: Clinical Guidelines on the Identification, Evaluation, and Treatment of Overweight and Obesity in Adults: The Evidence Report. September 1998. Available at: www.nhlbi.nih.gov/guidelines/obesity/ob_gdlns.pdf.[1]

■ U.S. Preventive Services Task Force: Screening for Obesity in Adults: Recommendations and Rationale. November 2003. Available at: www.ahrq.gov/clinic/3rduspstf/obesity/obesrr.htm.[2]

■ Department of Health and Human Services and the U.S. Department of Agriculture: Nutrition and Your Health. January 2005. Available at: www.health.gov/dietaryguidelines/dga2005/report/.[3]

Diet recommendations hinge on assessment of the patient's motivation and readiness to lose weight and individual risk factors. The *Clinical Guidelines on the Identification, Evaluation, and Treatment of Overweight and Obesity in Adults*[1] recommend the following general guidelines:

■ A 10% weight reduction over 6 months, or a decrease of 300 to 500 kcal/day, for people with BMIs between 27 and 35

- A weight loss goal of ½ to 1 pound per week because more rapid weight loss does not lead to better results at 1 year.[1]

These guidelines recommend low-calorie diets of 800 to 1500 kcal per day. Interventions that combine nutrition education, diet, and moderate exercise with behavioral strategies are most likely to succeed (see pp. 95–97). The *Clinical Guidelines* cite evidence supporting the role of moderate physical activity in weight loss and weight loss maintenance programs: it enhances and may assist with maintenance of weight; it increases cardiorespiratory fitness; and it may decrease abdominal fat.

If the BMI falls *below 18.5,* be concerned about possible anorexia nervosa, bulimia, or other medical conditions. These conditions are summarized in Table 4-3, Eating Disorders and Excessively Low BMI, p. 116. (See also pp. 95–97 for health promotion and counseling for overweight or underweight patients.)

THE HEALTH HISTORY

Common or Concerning Symptoms

- Changes in weight
- Fatigue and weakness
- Fever, chills, night sweats

Changes in Weight.   Changes in weight result from changes in body tissues or body fluid. Good opening questions include "How often do you check your weight?" "How is it compared to a year ago?" For changes, ask, "Why do you think it has changed?" "What would you like to weigh?" If weight gain or loss appears to be a problem, ask about the amount of change, its timing, the setting in which it occurred, and any associated symptoms.

Weight gain occurs when caloric intake exceeds caloric expenditure over time and typically appears as increased body fat. Weight gain may also reflect abnormal accumulation of body fluids. When the retention of fluid is relatively mild, it may not be visible, but several pounds of fluid usually appear as *edema.*

In the overweight patient, for example, when did the weight gain begin? Was the patient heavy as an infant or a child? Using milestones appropriate to the patient's age, inquire about weight at the following times: birth, kindergarten, high school or college graduation, discharge from military service, marriage, after each pregnancy, menopause, and retirement. What were the patient's life circumstances during the periods of weight gain? Has the patient tried to lose weight? How? With what results?

Rapid changes in weight (over a few days) suggest changes in body fluids, not tissues.

Weight loss is an important symptom with many causes. Mechanisms include one or more of the following: decreased intake of food for reasons such as anorexia, dysphagia, vomiting, and insufficient supplies of food; defective absorption of nutrients through the gastrointestinal tract; increased metabolic requirements; and loss of nutrients through the urine, feces, or injured skin. A person may also lose weight when a fluid-retaining state improves or responds to treatment.

Try to determine whether the drop in weight is proportional to any change in food intake, or whether it has remained normal or even increased.

Symptoms associated with weight loss often suggest a cause, as does a good psychosocial history. Who cooks and shops for the patient? Where does the patient eat? With whom? Are there any problems with obtaining, storing, preparing, or chewing food? Does the patient avoid or restrict certain foods for medical, religious, or other reasons?

Throughout the history, be alert for signs of malnutrition. Symptoms may be subtle and nonspecific, such as weakness, easy fatigability, cold intolerance, flaky dermatitis, and ankle swelling. Securing a good history of eating patterns and quantities is mandatory. It is important to ask general questions about intake at different times throughout the day, such as "Tell me what you typically eat for lunch." "What do you eat for a snack?" "When?"

Fatigue and Weakness. Like weight loss, *fatigue* is a nonspecific symptom with many causes. It refers to a sense of weariness or loss of energy that patients describe in various ways. "I don't feel like getting up in the morning" . . . "I don't have any energy" . . . "I just feel blah". . . "I'm all done in" . . . "I can hardly get through the day" . . . "By the time I get to the office I feel as if I've done a day's work." Because fatigue is a normal response to hard work, sustained stress, or grief, try to elicit the life circumstances in which it occurs. Fatigue unrelated to such situations requires further investigation.

Use open-ended questions to explore the attributes of the patient's fatigue, and encourage the patient to fully describe what he or she is experiencing. Important clues about etiology often emerge from a good psychosocial history, exploration of sleep patterns, and a thorough review of systems.

Causes of weight loss include gastrointestinal diseases; endocrine disorders (diabetes mellitus, hyperthyroidism, adrenal insufficiency); chronic infections; malignancy; chronic cardiac, pulmonary, or renal failure; depression; and anorexia nervosa or bulimia (see Table 4-3, Eating Disorders and Excessively Low BMI, p. 116).

Weight loss with relatively high food intake suggests diabetes mellitus, hyperthyroidism, or malabsorption. Consider also binge eating (bulimia) with clandestine vomiting.

Poverty, old age, social isolation, physical disability, emotional or mental impairment, lack of teeth, ill-fitting dentures, alcoholism, and drug abuse increase the likelihood of malnutrition.

See Table 4-4, Nutrition Screening Checklist, p. 117.

Fatigue is a common symptom of depression and anxiety states, but also consider infections (such as hepatitis, infectious mononucleosis, and tuberculosis); endocrine disorders (hypothyroidism, adrenal insufficiency, diabetes mellitus, panhypopituitarism); heart failure; chronic disease of the lungs, kidneys, or liver; electrolyte imbalance; moderate to severe anemia; malignancies; nutritional deficits; and medications.

Weakness is different from fatigue. It denotes a demonstrable loss of muscle power and will be discussed later with other neurologic symptoms (see pp. 608–609).

Weakness, especially if localized in a neuroanatomic pattern, suggests possible neuropathy or myopathy.

Fever, Chills and Night Sweats. *Fever* refers to an abnormal elevation in body temperature (see p. 112 for definitions of normal). Ask about fever if patients have an acute or chronic illness. Find out whether the patient has used a thermometer to measure the temperature. Bear in mind that errors in technique can lead to unreliable information. Has the patient felt feverish or unusually hot, noted excessive sweating, or felt chilly and cold? Try to distinguish between subjective *chilliness,* and a *shaking chill* with shivering throughout the body and chattering of teeth.

Recurrent shaking chills suggest more extreme swings in temperature and systemic bacteremia.

Feeling cold, goosebumps, and shivering accompany a rising temperature, while feeling hot and sweating accompany a falling temperature. Normally the body temperature rises during the day and falls during the night. When fever exaggerates this swing, *night sweats* occur. Malaise, headache, and pain in the muscles and joints often accompany fever.

Feelings of heat and sweating also accompany menopause. Night sweats occur in tuberculosis and malignancy.

Fever has many causes. Focus your questions on the timing of the illness and its associated symptoms. Become familiar with patterns of infectious diseases that may affect your patient. Inquire about travel, contact with sick people, or other unusual exposures. Be sure to inquire about medications because they may cause fever. In contrast, recent ingestion of aspirin, acetaminophen, corticosteroids, and nonsteroidal anti-inflammatory drugs may mask fever and affect the temperature recorded at the time of the physical examination.

HEALTH PROMOTION AND COUNSELING

Important Topics for Health Promotion and Counseling

- Optimal weight and nutrition
- Exercise
- Blood pressure and diet

Optimal Weight and Nutrition. Less than half of U.S. adults maintain a healthy weight (BMI ≥19 but ≤25). Obesity has increased in every segment of the population, regardless of age, gender, ethnicity, or socioeconomic group. More than half of people with non-insulin-dependent diabetes and roughly 20% of those with hypertension or elevated cholesterol are overweight or obese. Increasing obesity in children has been linked to rising rates of childhood diabetes. Once you detect excess weight or unhealthy nutritional patterns, take advantage of the excellent materials available to promote weight loss and good nutrition. Even reducing weight by

5% to 10% can improve blood pressure, lipid levels, and glucose tolerance and reduce the risk for developing diabetes or hypertension.

Once you have assessed food intake, nutritional status, and motivation to adopt healthy eating behaviors or lose weight, give patients the "nine major messages" of the 2005 Dietary Guidelines Advisory Committee to the Secretaries of HHS and USDA, as summarized and adapted below[3]:

See Table 4-1, Healthy Eating: Food Groups and Servings per Day, p. 115.

- Consume a variety of foods within and among the basic food groups while staying within energy needs.

- Control calorie intake and portion size to manage body weight.

- Maintain moderate physical activity for at least 30 minutes each day, for example, walking 3 to 4 miles per hour.

- Increase daily intake of fruits and vegetables, whole grains, and nonfat or low-fat milk and milk products.

- Choose fats wisely, keeping intake of saturated fat, *trans* fat found in partially hydrogenated vegetable oils, and cholesterol low.

- Choose carbohydrates—sugars, starches, and fibers—wisely for good health.

- Choose and prepare foods with little salt.

- If you drink alcoholic beverages, do so in moderation.

- Keep food safe to eat.

Be prepared to help adolescent females and women of childbearing age increase intake of iron and folic acid. Assist adults older than age 50 to identify foods rich in vitamin B12 and calcium. Advise older adults and those with dark skin or low exposure to sunlight to increase intake of vitamin D.

See Table 4-5, Nutrition Counseling: Sources of Nutrients, p. 117.

Exercise. Fitness is a key component of both weight control and weight loss. Currently, 30 minutes of moderate activity, defined as walking 2 miles in 30 minutes on most days of the week or its equivalent, is recommended. Patients can increase exercise by such simple measures as parking further away from their place of work or using stairs instead of elevators. A safe goal for weight loss is ½ to 2 pounds per week.

Blood Pressure and Diet. With respect to blood pressure, there is reliable evidence that regular and frequent exercise, decreased sodium intake and increased potassium intake, and maintenance of a healthy weight will reduce the risk for developing hypertension as well as lower blood pressure in adults who are already hypertensive. Explain to patients that most of the sodium in our diet comes from salt (sodium chloride). The recommended daily allowance (RDA) of sodium is <2400 mg, or 1 teaspoon, per day. Patients need to read food labels closely, especially the Nutrition Facts panel. Low-sodium foods are those with sodium listed at less than 5% of the RDA of <2400 mg. For nutritional interventions to reduce the risk for cardiac disease, turn to p. 118.

See Table 4-6, Patients With Hypertension: Recommended Changes in Diet, p. 118.

TECHNIQUES OF EXAMINATION

BEGINNING THE EXAMINATION: SETTING THE STAGE

Preparing for the Physical Examination

- Reflect on your approach to the patient.
- Adjust the lighting and the environment.
- Determine the scope of the examination.
- Choose the sequence of the examination.
- Observe the correct examining position and handedness.
- Make the patient comfortable.

Before you begin the physical examination, take time to prepare for the tasks ahead. Think through your approach to the patient, your professional demeanor, and how to make the patient feel comfortable and relaxed. Review the measures that promote the patient's physical comfort and make any adjustments needed in the lighting and the surrounding environment. *Make sure that you wash your hands in the presence of the patient before beginning the examination. This is a subtle yet much appreciated gesture of concern for the patient's welfare.*

Reflect on Your Approach to the Patient.   When first examining patients, feelings of insecurity are inevitable, but these will soon diminish with experience. Be straightforward. Identify yourself as a student. Try to appear calm, organized, and competent, even when you feel differently. If you forget to do part of the examination, this is not uncommon, especially at first! Simply examine that area out of sequence, but smoothly. It is not unusual to go back to the bedside and ask to check one or two items that you might have overlooked.

As a beginner, you will need to spend more time than experienced clinicians on selected portions of the examination, such as the ophthalmoscopic examination or cardiac auscultation. To avoid alarming the patient, warn the patient ahead of time by saying, for example, "I would like to spend extra time listening to your heart and the heart sounds, but this doesn't mean I hear anything wrong."

Most patients view the physical examination with at least some anxiety. They feel vulnerable, physically exposed, apprehensive about possible pain, and uneasy about what the clinician may find. At the same time, they appreciate the clinician's concern about their problems and respond to your attentiveness. With these considerations in mind, the skillful clinician is thorough without wasting time, systematic without being rigid, gentle yet not afraid to cause discomfort should this be required. In applying the techniques of inspection, palpation, auscultation, and percussion, the skillful clinician examines each region of the body, and at the same time senses the whole patient, notes the wince or worried glance, and shares information that calms, explains, and reassures.

Over time, you will begin sharing your findings with the patient. As a beginner, avoid interpreting your findings. You are not the patient's primary caretaker, and your views may be conflicting or wrong. As you grow in experience and responsibility, sharing findings will become more appropriate. If the patient has specific concerns, you may even provide reassurance as you finish examining the relevant area. Be selective, however—if you find an unexpected abnormality, you may wish you had kept a judicious silence. At times, you may discover abnormalities such as an ominous mass or a deep oozing ulcer. Always avoid showing distaste, alarm, or other negative reactions.

Adjust the Lighting and the Environment. Surprisingly, several environmental factors affect the calibre and reliability of your physical findings. To achieve superior techniques of examination, it is important to "set the stage" so that both you and the patient are comfortable. As the examiner, you will find that awkward positions impair the quality of your observations. Take the time to adjust the bed to a convenient height (but be sure to lower it when finished!), and ask the patient to move toward you if this makes it easier to examine a region of the body more carefully.

Good lighting and a quiet environment make important contributions to what you see and hear but may be hard to arrange. Do the best you can. If a television interferes with listening to heart sounds, politely ask the nearby patient to lower the volume. Most people cooperate readily. Be courteous and remember to thank the patient as you leave.

Tangential lighting is optimal for inspecting structures such as the jugular venous pulse, the thyroid gland, and the apical impulse of the heart. It casts light across body surfaces that throws contours, elevations, and depressions, whether moving or stationary, into sharper relief.

When light is perpendicular to the surface or diffuse, shadows are reduced and subtle undulations across the surface are lost. Experiment with focused,

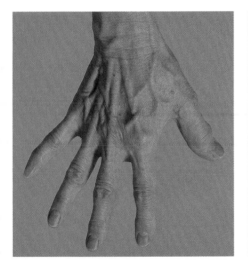

TANGENTIAL LIGHTING

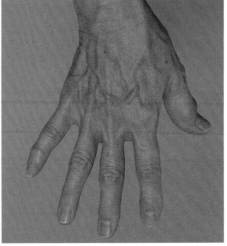

PERPENDICULAR LIGHTING

tangential lighting across the tendons on the back of your hand; try to see the pulsations of the radial artery at your wrist.

Determine the Scope of the Examination: Comprehensive or Focused? With each patient visit, you will ponder "How complete should I make the physical examination?" There is no simple answer to this common question. Chapter 1 provides initial guidelines for selecting a comprehensive examination or a focused examination (see p. 4). Review the table below to clarify your thinking as you enter the realm of patient assessment.

■ *The Physical Examination: Comprehensive or Focused?*
General Guidelines

The Comprehensive Examination	The Focused Examination
■ Is appropriate for new patients in the office or hospital ■ Provides fundamental and personalized knowledge about the patient ■ Strengthens the clinician-patient relationship ■ Helps identify or rule out physical causes related to patient concerns ■ Provides baselines for future assessments ■ Creates platform for health promotion through education and counseling ■ Develops proficiency in the essential skills of physical examination	■ Is appropriate for established patients, especially during routine or urgent care visits ■ Addresses focused concerns or symptoms ■ Assesses symptoms restricted to a specific body system ■ Applies examination methods relevant to assessing the concern or problem as precisely and carefully as possible

---

As you can see, the *comprehensive examination* does more than assess body systems. It is a source of fundamental and personalized knowledge about the patient that strengthens the clinician-patient relationship. Most people seeking your care have specific worries or symptoms. The comprehensive examination provides a more complete basis for assessing patient concerns and answering patient questions.

For the focused examination, you will select the methods relevant to thorough assessment of the targeted problem. The patient's symptoms, age, and health history help determine the scope of your examination, as does your knowledge of disease patterns. Of all the patients with sore throat, for example, you will need to decide who may have infectious mononucleosis and warrants careful palpation of the liver and spleen and who, in contrast, has a common cold and does not need this examination. The clinical thinking that underlies and guides such decisions is discussed in Chapter 3.

What about the *routine clinical check-up,* or *periodic physical examination?* The usefulness of the comprehensive physical examination for the purposes of screening and prevention of illness, in contrast to evaluation of symptoms, has been scrutinized in several studies.[4–6] Findings have validated the importance of physical examination techniques: blood pressure measurement, assessment of central venous pressure from the jugular venous pulse, listening to the heart for evidence of valvular disease, the clinical breast examination, detection of hepatic and splenic enlargement, and the pelvic examination with Papanicolaou smears. Recommendations for examination and screening have been further expanded by various consensus panels and expert advisory groups. Bear in mind, however, that when used for screening (rather than assessment of complaints), not all components of the examination have been validated as ways to reduce future morbidity and mortality.

Choose the Sequence of the Examination. It is important to recognize that *the key to a thorough and accurate physical examination is developing a systematic sequence of examination.* Organize your comprehensive or focused examination around three general goals:

- Maximize the patient's comfort.

- Avoid unnecessary changes in position.

- Enhance clinical efficiency.

In general, move from "head to toe." Avoid examining the patient's feet, for example, before checking the face or mouth. You will quickly see that some segments of the examination are best obtained while the patient is sitting, such as examination of the head and neck and of the thorax and lungs, whereas others are best obtained with the patient supine, such as the cardiovascular and abdominal examinations.

Often you will need to examine a patient *at bed rest,* as often occurs in the hospital, where patients frequently cannot sit up in bed or stand. This often dictates changes in your sequence of examination. You can examine the head, neck, and anterior chest with the patient lying supine. Then roll the patient onto each side to listen to the lungs, examine the back, and inspect the skin. Roll the patient back and finish the rest of the examination with the patient again supine.

With practice, you will develop your own sequence of examination, keeping the need for thoroughness and patient comfort in mind. At first, you may need notes to remind you what to look for as you examine each region of the body, but with a few months of practice, you will acquire a routine sequence of your own. This sequence will become habit and often prompt you to return to a segment of the examination you may have inadvertently skipped, helping you to become thorough.

Turn to Chapter 1, pp. 11–15, to review the examination sequence suggested there, and study the outline of this sequence summarized below. After you study and practice the techniques described in the regional examination chapters, reread these overviews to see how each segment of the examination fits into an integrated whole.

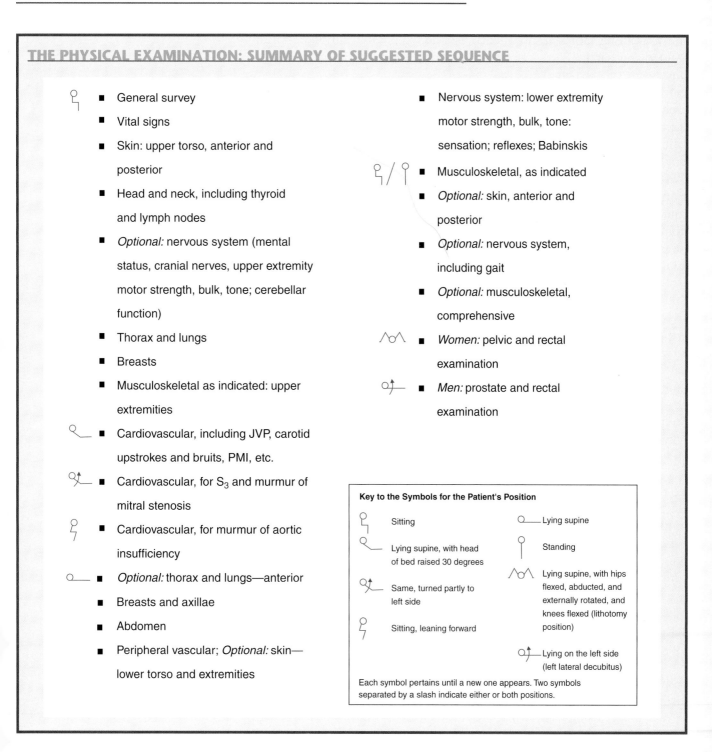

THE PHYSICAL EXAMINATION: SUMMARY OF SUGGESTED SEQUENCE

- General survey
- Vital signs
- Skin: upper torso, anterior and posterior
- Head and neck, including thyroid and lymph nodes
- *Optional:* nervous system (mental status, cranial nerves, upper extremity motor strength, bulk, tone; cerebellar function)
- Thorax and lungs
- Breasts
- Musculoskeletal as indicated: upper extremities
- Cardiovascular, including JVP, carotid upstrokes and bruits, PMI, etc.
- Cardiovascular, for S_3 and murmur of mitral stenosis
- Cardiovascular, for murmur of aortic insufficiency
- *Optional:* thorax and lungs—anterior
- Breasts and axillae
- Abdomen
- Peripheral vascular; *Optional:* skin— lower torso and extremities

- Nervous system: lower extremity motor strength, bulk, tone: sensation; reflexes; Babinskis
- Musculoskeletal, as indicated
- *Optional:* skin, anterior and posterior
- *Optional:* nervous system, including gait
- *Optional:* musculoskeletal, comprehensive
- *Women:* pelvic and rectal examination
- *Men:* prostate and rectal examination

Key to the Symbols for the Patient's Position

Sitting

Lying supine, with head of bed raised 30 degrees

Same, turned partly to left side

Sitting, leaning forward

Lying supine

Standing

Lying supine, with hips flexed, abducted, and externally rotated, and knees flexed (lithotomy position)

Lying on the left side (left lateral decubitus)

Each symbol pertains until a new one appears. Two symbols separated by a slash indicate either or both positions.

Observe the Correct Examining Position and Handedness. *This book recommends examining the patient from the patient's **right side,** moving to the opposite side or foot of the bed or examining table as necessary.* This is the standard position for the physical examination and has several advantages compared with the left side: it is more reliable to estimate jugular venous pressure from the right, the palpating hand rests more comfortably on the apical impulse, the right kidney is more frequently palpable than the left, and examining tables are frequently positioned to accommodate a right-handed approach.

Left-handed students are encouraged to adopt right-sided positioning, even though at first it may seem awkward. It still may be easier to use the left hand for percussing or for holding instruments such as the otoscope or reflex hammer.

Make the Patient Comfortable. Your access to the patient's body is a unique and time-honored privilege of your role as a clinician. Showing concern for privacy and patient modesty must be ingrained in your professional behavior. These attributes help the patient feel respected and at ease. Be sure to close nearby doors and draw the curtains in the hospital or examining room before the examination begins.

You will acquire the art of *draping the patient* with the gown or draw sheet as you learn each segment of the examination in the chapters ahead. *Your goal is to visualize one area of the body at a time.* This preserves the patient's modesty but also helps you to focus on the area being examined. With the patient sitting, for example, untie the gown in back to better listen to the lungs. For the breast examination, uncover the right breast but keep the left chest draped. Redrape the right chest, then uncover the left chest and proceed to examine the left breast and heart. For the abdominal examination, only the abdomen should be exposed. Adjust the gown to cover the chest and place the sheet or drape at the inguinal area.

To help the patient prepare for segments that might be awkward, it is considerate to briefly describe your plans before starting the examination. As you proceed with the examination, keep the patient informed, especially when you anticipate embarrassment or discomfort, as when checking for the femoral pulse. Also try to gauge how much the patient wants to know. Is the patient curious about the lung findings or your method for assessing the liver or spleen?

Make sure your instructions to the patient at each step in the examination are courteous and clear. For example, "I would like to examine your heart now, so please lie down."

As in the interview, be sensitive to the patient's feelings and physical comfort. Watching the patient's facial expressions and even asking "Is it okay?" as you move through the examination often reveals unexpressed worries or sources of pain. To ease discomfort, it may help to adjust the slant of the patient's bed or examining table. Rearranging the pillows or adding blankets for warmth shows your attentiveness to the patient's well-being.

When you have completed the examination, tell the patient your general impressions and what to expect next. For hospitalized patients, make sure the patient is comfortable and rearrange the immediate environment to his or her satisfaction. Be sure to lower the bed to avoid risk for falls and raise the bedrails if needed. As you leave, wash your hands, clean your equipment, and dispose of any waste materials.

THE GENERAL SURVEY

The *General Survey* of the patient's build, height, and weight begins with the opening moments of the patient encounter, but you will find that your observations of the patient's appearance crystallize as you start the physical examination. The best clinicians continually sharpen their powers of observation and description, like naturalists identifying birds from silhouettes backlit against the sky. It is important to heighten the acuity of your clinical perceptions of the patient's mood, build, and behavior. These details enrich and deepen your emerging clinical impression. A skilled observer can depict distinguishing features of the patient's general appearance so well in words that a colleague could spot the patient in a crowd of strangers.

Many factors contribute to the patient's body habitus—socioeconomic status, nutrition, genetic makeup, degree of fitness, mood state, early illnesses, gender, geographic location, and age cohort. Recall that the patient's nutritional status affects many of the characteristics you scrutinize during the *General Survey:* height and weight, blood pressure, posture, mood and alertness, facial coloration, dentition and condition of the tongue and gingiva, color of the nail beds, and muscle bulk, to name a few. Be sure to make the assessment of height, weight, BMI, and risk for obesity a routine part of your clinical practice.

You should now recapture the observations you have been making since the first moments of your interaction and sharpen them throughout your assessment. Does the patient hear you when greeted in the waiting room or examination room? Rise with ease? Walk easily or stiffly? If hospitalized when you first meet, what is the patient doing—sitting up and enjoying television? . . . or lying in bed? . . . What occupies the bedside table—a magazine? . . . a flock of "get well" cards? . . . a Bible or a rosary? . . . an emesis basin? . . . or nothing at all? Each of these observations should raise one or more tentative hypotheses about the patient for you to consider during future assessments.

Apparent State of Health.   Try to make a general judgment based on observations throughout the encounter. Support it with the significant details.

Acutely or chronically ill, frail, feeble

Level of Consciousness.   Is the patient awake, alert, and responsive to you and others in the environment? If not, promptly assess the level of consciousness (see p. 579).

Signs of Distress.   For example, does the patient show evidence of these problems?

■ Cardiac or respiratory distress

Clutching the chest, pallor, diaphoresis; labored breathing, wheezing, cough

■ Pain

Wincing, sweating, protectiveness of painful area

■ Anxiety or depression

Anxious face, fidgety movements, cold and moist palms; inexpressive or flat affect, poor eye contact, psychomotor slowing

Height and Build.   If possible, measure the patient's height in stocking feet. Is the patient unusually short or tall? Is the build slender and lanky, muscular, or stocky? Is the body symmetric? Note the general body proportions and look for any deformities.

Very short stature is seen in Turner's syndrome, childhood renal failure, and achondroplastic and hypopituitary dwarfism. Long limbs in proportion to the trunk are seen in hypogonadism and Marfan's syndrome. Height loss occurs with osteoporosis and vertebral compression fractures.

Weight.   Is the patient emaciated, slender, plump, obese, or somewhere in between? If the patient is obese, is the fat distributed evenly or concentrated over the trunk, the upper torso, or around the hips?

Generalized fat in simple obesity; truncal fat with relatively thin limbs in Cushing's syndrome and metabolic, or insulin resistance, syndrome

Whenever possible, weigh the patient with shoes off. Weight provides one index of caloric intake, and changes over time yield other valuable diagnostic data. Remember that changes in weight can occur with changes in body fluid status, as well as in fat or muscle mass.

Causes of weight loss include malignancy, diabetes mellitus, hyperthyroidism, chronic infection, depression, diuresis, and successful dieting.

Use weight and height measurements to calculate the BMI (see pp. 90–92).

Skin Color and Obvious Lesions.   See Chapter 5, The Skin, Hair, and Nails, for details.

Pallor, cyanosis, jaundice, rashes, bruises

Dress, Grooming, and Personal Hygiene.   How is the patient dressed? Is clothing appropriate to the temperature and weather? Is it clean, properly buttoned, and zipped? How does it compare with clothing worn by people of comparable age and social group?

Excess clothing may reflect the cold intolerance of hypothyroidism, hide skin rash or needle marks, or signal personal lifestyle preferences.

Glance at the patient's shoes. Have holes been cut in them? Are the laces tied? Or is the patient wearing slippers?

Cut-out holes or slippers may indicate gout, bunions, or other painful foot conditions. Untied laces or slippers also suggest edema.

Is the patient wearing any unusual jewelry? Where? Is there any body piercing?

Copper bracelets are sometimes worn for arthritis. Piercing may appear on any part of the body.

Note the patient's hair, fingernails, and use of cosmetics. They may be clues to the patient's personality, mood, or lifestyle. Nail polish and hair coloring that have "grown out" may signify decreased interest in personal appearance.

"Grown-out" hair and nail polish can help you estimate the length of an illness if the patient cannot give a history. Fingernails chewed to the quick may reflect stress.

Do personal hygiene and grooming seem appropriate to the patient's age, lifestyle, occupation, and socioeconomic group? These are norms that vary widely, of course.	Unkempt appearance may be seen in depression and dementia, but this appearance must be compared with the patient's probable norm.

Facial Expression.   Observe the facial expression at rest, during conversation about specific topics, during the physical examination, and in interaction with others. Watch for eye contact. Is it natural? Sustained and unblinking? Averted quickly? Absent?

The stare of hyperthyroidism; the immobile face of parkinsonism; the flat or sad affect of depression. Decreased eye contact may be cultural, or may suggest anxiety, fear, or sadness.

Odors of the Body and Breath.   Odors can be important diagnostic clues, such as the fruity odor of diabetes or the scent of alcohol. (For the scent of alcohol, the CAGE questions, p. 50, will help you determine possible misuse.)

Breath odors of alcohol, acetone (diabetes), pulmonary infections, uremia, or liver failure

Never assume that alcohol on a patient's breath explains changes in mental status or neurologic findings.

People with alcoholism may have other serious and potentially correctable problems such as hypoglycemia, subdural hematoma, or post-ictal state

Posture, Gait, and Motor Activity.   What is the patient's preferred posture?

Preference for sitting up in left-sided heart failure, and for leaning forward with arms braced in chronic obstructive pulmonary disease

Is the patient restless or quiet? How often does the patient change position? How fast are the movements?

Fast, frequent movements of hyperthyroidism; slowed activity of hypothyroidism

Is there any apparent involuntary motor activity? Are some body parts immobile? Which ones?

Tremors or other involuntary movements; paralyses. See Table 17-3, Tremors and Involuntary Movements (pp. 653–654).

Does the patient walk smoothly, with comfort, self-confidence, and balance, or is there a limp or discomfort, fear of falling, loss of balance, or any movement disorder?

See Table 17-8, Abnormalities of Gait and Posture (pp. 663–664).

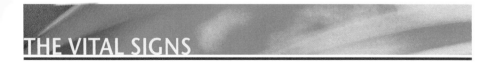

THE VITAL SIGNS

Now you are ready to measure the *Vital Signs*—the blood pressure, heart rate, respiratory rate, and temperature. You may find that the vital signs are already taken and recorded in the chart; if abnormal, you may wish to repeat them yourself. You can also make these important measurements later as you start the cardiovascular and thorax and lung examinations, but often they provide important initial information that influences the direction of your evaluation.

Check either the blood pressure or the pulse first. If the blood pressure is high, measure it again later in the examination. Count the radial pulse with your fingers, or the apical pulse with your stethoscope at the cardiac apex. Continue either of these techniques and count the respiratory rate without alerting the patient; because breathing patterns may change if the patient becomes aware that someone is watching. The temperature is taken with glass thermometers, tympanic thermometers, or digital electronic probes. Further details on techniques for ensuring accuracy of the vital signs are provided in the following pages.

See Table 4-7, Abnormalities of the Arterial Pulse and Pressure Waves (p. 119). See Table 4-8, Abnormalities in Rate and Rhythm of Breathing (p. 120).

BLOOD PRESSURE

Choice of Blood Pressure Cuff (Sphygmomanometer). As many as 50 million Americans have elevated blood pressure.[7] To measure blood pressure accurately, you must carefully choose a cuff of appropriate size. The blood pressure gauge may be either the aneroid or the mercury type. Because an aneroid instrument can become inaccurate with repeated use, it should be recalibrated regularly.

Cuffs that are too short or too narrow may give falsely high readings. Using a regular-size cuff on an obese arm may lead to a false diagnosis of hypertension.

The guidelines below will help you to select the best size blood pressure cuff and also to advise patients wishing to purchase home measurement devices. Urge patients to have such devices checked routinely for accuracy.

SELECTING THE CORRECT BLOOD PRESSURE CUFF

- Width of the inflatable bladder of the cuff should be about 40% of upper arm circumference (about 12–14 cm in the average adult).
- Length of the inflatable bladder should be about 80% of upper arm circumference (almost long enough to encircle the arm).

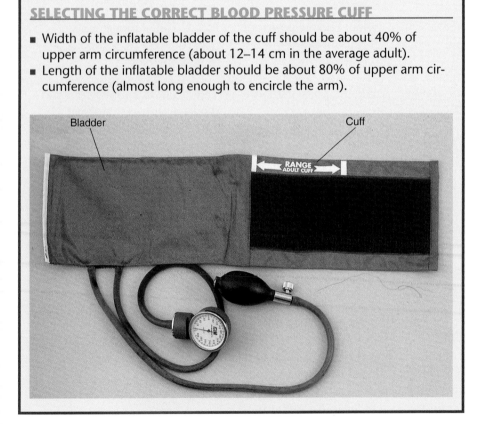

Technique for Measuring Blood Pressure. Before assessing the blood pressure, you should take several steps to make sure your measurement will be accurate. Once these steps are taken, you are ready to measure the blood pressure. Proper technique is important and reduces the inherent variability arising from the patient or examiner, the equipment, and the procedure itself.

GETTING READY TO MEASURE BLOOD PRESSURE

- Ideally, instruct the patient to avoid smoking or drinking caffeinated beverages for 30 minutes before the blood pressure is measured.
- Check to make sure the examining room is quiet and comfortably warm.
- Ask the patient to sit quietly for at least 5 minutes in a chair, rather than on the examining table, with feet on the floor. The arm should be supported at heart level.
- Make sure the arm selected is *free of clothing.* There should be no arteriovenous fistulas for dialysis, scarring from prior brachial artery cutdowns, or signs of lymphedema (seen after axillary node dissection or radiation therapy).
- Palpate the brachial artery to confirm that it has a viable pulse.
- Position the arm so that the brachial artery, at the antecubital crease, is *at heart level*—roughly level with the 4th interspace at its junction with the sternum.
- If the patient is seated, rest the arm on a table a little above the patient's waist; if standing, try to support the patient's arm at the midchest level.

If the brachial artery is much below heart level, blood pressure appears falsely high. The patient's own effort to support the arm may raise the blood pressure.

Now you are ready to measure the blood pressure.

- Center the inflatable bladder over the brachial artery. The lower border of the cuff should be about 2.5 cm above the antecubital crease. Secure the cuff snugly. Position the patient's arm so that it is slightly flexed at the elbow.

  A loose cuff or a bladder that balloons outside the cuff leads to falsely high readings.

- To determine how high to raise the cuff pressure, first estimate the systolic pressure by palpation. As you feel the radial artery with the fingers of one hand, rapidly inflate the cuff until the radial pulse disappears. Read this pressure on the manometer and add 30 mm Hg to it. Use of this sum as the target for subsequent inflations prevents discomfort from unnecessarily high cuff pressures. It also avoids the occasional error caused by an *auscultatory gap*—a silent interval that may be present between the systolic and the diastolic pressures.

  An unrecognized auscultatory gap may lead to serious underestimation of systolic pressure (e.g., 150/98 in the example on the next page) or overestimation of diastolic pressure.

- Deflate the cuff promptly and completely and wait 15 to 30 seconds.

- Now place the bell of a stethoscope lightly over the brachial artery, taking care to make an air seal with its full rim. Because the sounds to be heard, the *Korotkoff sounds,* are relatively low in pitch, they are heard better with the bell.

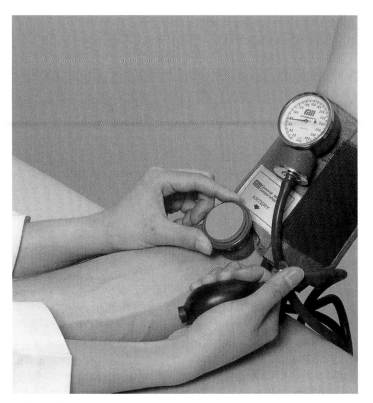

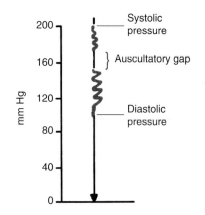

If you find an auscultatory gap, record your findings completely (e.g., 200/98 with an auscultatory gap from 170–150).

An auscultatory gap is associated with arterial stiffness and athero-sclerotic disease.[8]

■ Inflate the cuff rapidly again to the level just determined, and then deflate it slowly at a rate of about 2 to 3 mm Hg per second. Note the level at which you hear the sounds of at least two consecutive beats. This is the systolic pressure.

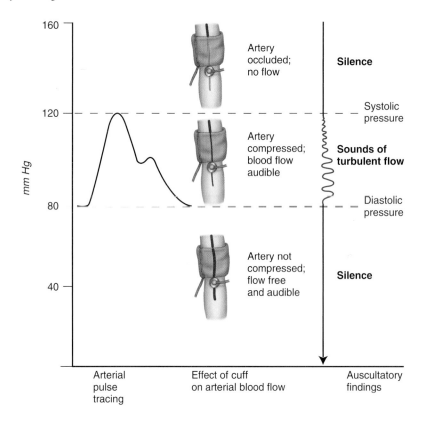

■ Continue to lower the pressure slowly until the sounds become muffled and then disappear. To confirm the disappearance of sounds, listen as the pressure falls another 10 to 20 mm Hg. Then deflate the cuff rapidly to zero. The disappearance point, which is usually only a few mm Hg below the muffling point, provides the best estimate of true diastolic pressure in adults.

In some people, the muffling point and the disappearance point are farther apart. Occasionally, as in aortic regurgitation, the sounds never disappear. If there is more than 10 mm Hg difference, record both figures (e.g., 154/80/68).

■ Read both the systolic and the diastolic levels to the nearest 2 mm Hg. Wait 2 or more minutes and repeat. Average your readings. If the first two readings differ by more than 5 mm Hg, take additional readings.

■ When using a mercury sphygmomanometer, keep the manometer vertical (unless you are using a tilted floor model) and make all readings at eye level with the meniscus. When using an aneroid instrument, hold the dial so that it faces you directly. Avoid slow or repetitive inflations of the cuff, because the resulting venous congestion can cause false readings.

By making the sounds less audible, venous congestion may produce artificially low systolic and high diastolic pressures.

■ Blood pressure should be taken in both arms at least once. Normally, there may be a difference in pressure of 5 mm Hg and sometimes up to 10 mm Hg. Subsequent readings should be made on the arm with the higher pressure.

Pressure difference of more than 10–15 mm Hg suggests arterial compression or obstruction on the side with the lower pressure.

Classification of Normal and Abnormal Blood Pressure. In its seventh report in 2003, the Joint National Committee on Prevention, Detection, Evaluation, and Treatment of High Blood Pressure recommended using the mean of two or more properly measured seated blood pressure readings, taken on two or more office visits, for diagnosis of hypertension.[7] Blood pressure measurement should be verified in the contralateral arm.

The Joint National Committee has identified four levels of systolic and diastolic hypertension. Note that either component may be high.

■ Blood Pressure Classification (Adults Older Than 18 Years)		
Category	Systolic (mm Hg)	Diastolic (mm Hg)
Normal	<120	<80
Prehypertension	120–139	80–89
Hypertension		
Stage 1	140–159	90–99
Stage 2	≥160	≥100

Assessment of hypertension also includes its effects on target organs—the eyes, the heart, the brain, and the kidneys. Look for evidence of hypertensive retinopathy, left ventricular hypertrophy, and neurologic deficits suggesting a stroke. Renal assessment requires urinalysis and blood tests.

When the systolic and diastolic levels fall in different categories, use the higher category. For example, 170/92 mm Hg is Stage 2 hypertension; 135/100 mm Hg is Stage 1 hypertension. In *isolated systolic hypertension*, systolic blood pressure is ≥140 mm Hg, and diastolic blood pressure is <90 mm Hg.[9]

Relatively low levels of blood pressure should always be interpreted in the light of past readings and the patient's present clinical state.

A pressure of 110/70 mm Hg would usually be normal, but could also indicate significant hypotension if past pressures have been high.

If indicated, assess *orthostatic*, or *postural*, *blood pressure* (see Chapter 20, the Older Adult, p. 861). Measure blood pressure and heart rate in two positions—supine after the patient is resting up to 10 minutes, then within 3 minutes after the patient stands up. Normally, as the patient rises from the horizontal to the standing position, systolic pressure drops slightly or remains unchanged, while diastolic pressure rises slightly. Orthostatic hypotension is a drop in systolic blood pressure of ≥20 mm Hg or in diastolic blood pressure of ≥ 10 mm Hg within 3 minutes of standing.[10,11]

A fall in systolic pressure of 20 mm Hg or more, especially when accompanied by symptoms, indicates orthostatic (postural) hypotension. Causes include drugs, loss of blood, prolonged bed rest, and diseases of the autonomic nervous system.

Special Situations

Weak or Inaudible Korotkoff Sounds.   Consider technical problems such as erroneous placement of your stethoscope, failure to make full skin contact with the bell, and venous engorgement of the patient's arm from repeated inflations of the cuff. Consider also the possibility of shock.

When you cannot hear Korotkoff sounds at all, you may be able to estimate the systolic pressure by palpation. Alternative methods such as Doppler techniques or direct arterial pressure tracings may be necessary.

To intensify Korotkoff sounds, one of the following methods may be helpful:

- Raise the patient's arm before and while you inflate the cuff. Then lower the arm and determine the blood pressure.

- Inflate the cuff. Ask the patient to make a fist several times, and then determine the blood pressure.

Arrhythmias.   Irregular rhythms produce variations in pressure and therefore unreliable measurements. Ignore the effects of an occasional premature contraction. With frequent premature contractions or atrial fibrillation, determine the average of several observations and note that your measurements are approximate.

The Anxious Patient and Isolated Office Hypertension (or "white coat hypertension").   Anxiety is a frequent cause of diastolic blood pressure readings in the office that are higher than those at home or during normal activities, occurring in 12% to 25% of patients.[12,13] This effect may last for several visits. Try to relax the patient and measure the blood pressure again later in the encounter.

Isolated home or ambulatory hypertension, unlike isolated office hypertension, is associated with increased risk for cardiovascular disease.[12–15]

The Obese or Very Thin Patient.   For the obese arm, it is important to use a wide cuff of 15 cm. If the arm circumference exceeds 41 cm, use a thigh cuff of 18 cm. For the very thin arm, a pediatric cuff may be indicated.

Use of a cuff that is too small can lead to overestimation of systolic blood pressure in obese patients.

The Hypertensive Patient With Unequal Blood Pressures in the Arms and Legs. To detect coarctation of the aorta, make two further blood pressure measurements at least once in every hypertensive patient:

- Compare blood pressures in the arms and legs.

- Compare the volume and timing of the radial and femoral pulses. Normally, volume is equal and the pulses occur simultaneously.

Coarctation of the aorta arises from narrowing of the thoracic aorta, usually proximal but sometimes distal to the left subclavian artery.

Coarctation of the aorta and *occlusive aortic disease* are distinguished by hypertension in the upper extremities and low blood pressure in the legs and by diminished or delayed femoral pulses.[16]

To determine blood pressure in the leg, use a wide, long thigh cuff that has a bladder size of 18×42 cm, and apply it to the midthigh. Center the bladder over the posterior surface, wrap it securely, and listen over the popliteal artery. If possible, the patient should be prone. Alternatively, ask the supine patient to flex one leg slightly, with the heel resting on the bed. When cuffs of the proper size are used for both the leg and the arm, blood pressures should be equal in the two areas. (The usual arm cuff, improperly used on the leg, gives a falsely high reading.)

HEART RATE AND RHYTHM

Examine the arterial pulses, the heart rate and rhythm, and the amplitude and contour of the pulse wave.

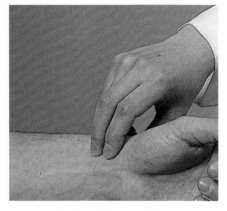

Heart Rate. The radial pulse is commonly used to assess the heart rate. With the pads of your index and middle fingers, compress the radial artery until a maximal pulsation is detected. If the rhythm is regular and the rate seems normal, count the rate for 15 seconds and multiply by 4. If the rate is unusually fast or slow, however, count it for 60 seconds.

When the rhythm is irregular, evaluate the heart rate by cardiac auscultation. Beats that occur earlier than others may not be detected peripherally, and the heart rate can thus be seriously underestimated.

Irregular rhythms include atrial fibrillation and atrial or ventricular premature contractions.

Rhythm. To begin your assessment of rhythm, feel the radial pulse. If there are any irregularities, check the rhythm again by listening with your stethoscope at the cardiac apex. Is the rhythm regular or irregular? If irregular, try to identify a pattern: (1) Do early beats appear in a basically regular rhythm? (2) Does the irregularity vary consistently with respiration? (3) Is the rhythm totally irregular?

See Table 8-1, Selected Heart Rates and Rhythms (p. 324) and Table 8-2, Selected Irregular Rhythms (p. 325).

Palpation of an irregularly irregular rhythm reliably indicates *atrial fibrillation.* For all other irregular patterns, an ECG is needed to identify the arrhythmia.

RESPIRATORY RATE AND RHYTHM

Observe the *rate, rhythm, depth,* and *effort of breathing.* Count the number of respirations in 1 minute either by visual inspection or by subtly listening over the patient's trachea with your stethoscope during your examination of the head and neck or chest. Normally, adults take 14 to 20 breaths per minute in a quiet, regular pattern. An occasional sigh is normal. Check to see if expiration is prolonged.

See Table 4-8, Abnormalities in Rate and Rhythm of Breathing (p. 120).

Prolonged expiration suggests narrowing in the bronchioles.

TEMPERATURE

Although you may choose to omit measuring the temperature in ambulatory patients, it should be checked whenever you suspect an abnormality. The average *oral temperature,* usually quoted at 37°C (98.6°F), fluctuates considerably. In the early morning hours, it may fall as low as 35.8°C (96.4°F), and in the late afternoon or evening, it may rise as high as 37.3°C (99.1°F). *Rectal temperatures* are *higher* than oral temperatures by an average of 0.4 to 0.5°C (0.7 to 0.9°F), but this difference is also quite variable. In contrast, *axillary temperatures* are *lower* than oral temperatures by approximately 1°, but take 5 to 10 minutes to register and are generally considered less accurate than other measurements.

Fever or pyrexia refers to an elevated body temperature. *Hyperpyrexia* refers to extreme elevation in temperature, above 41.1°C (106°F), while *hypothermia* refers to an abnormally low temperature, below 35°C (95°F) rectally.

Most patients prefer oral to rectal temperatures. However, taking oral temperatures is not recommended when patients are unconscious, restless, or unable to close their mouths. Temperature readings may be inaccurate and thermometers may be broken by unexpected movements of the patient's jaws.

Rapid respiratory rates tend to increase the discrepancy between oral and rectal temperatures. In this situation, rectal temperatures are more reliable.

For *oral temperatures,* you may choose either a glass or electronic thermometer. When using a glass thermometer, shake the thermometer down to 35°C (96°F) or below, insert it under the tongue, instruct the patient to close both lips, and wait 3 to 5 minutes. Then read the thermometer, reinsert it for a minute, and read it again. If the temperature is still rising, repeat this procedure until the reading remains stable. Note that hot or cold liquids, and even smoking, can alter the temperature reading. In these situations, it is best to delay measuring the temperature for 10 to 15 minutes.

Causes of *fever* include infection, trauma such as surgery or crush injuries, malignancy, blood disorders such as acute hemolytic anemia, drug reactions, and immune disorders such as collagen vascular disease.

If using an electronic thermometer, carefully place the disposable cover over the probe and insert the thermometer under the tongue. Ask the patient to close both lips, and then watch closely for the digital readout. An accurate temperature recording usually takes about 10 seconds.

The chief cause of *hypothermia* is exposure to cold. Other predisposing causes include reduced movement as in paralysis, interference

For a *rectal temperature*, ask the patient to lie on one side with the hip flexed. Select a rectal thermometer with a stubby tip, lubricate it, and insert it about 3 cm to 4 cm (1½ inches) into the anal canal, in a direction pointing to the umbilicus. Remove it after 3 minutes, then read. Alternatively, use an electronic thermometer after lubricating the probe cover. Wait about 10 seconds for the digital temperature recording to appear.

Taking the *tympanic membrane temperature* is an increasingly common practice and is quick, safe, and reliable if performed properly. Make sure the external auditory canal is free of cerumen. Position the probe in the canal so that the infrared beam is aimed at the tympanic membrane (otherwise the measurement will be invalid). Wait 2 to 3 seconds until the digital temperature reading appears. This method measures core body temperature, which is higher than the normal oral temperature by approximately 0.8°C (1.4°F).

with vasoconstriction as from sepsis or excess alcohol, starvation, hypothyroidism, and hypoglycemia. Elderly people are especially susceptible to hypothermia and also less likely to develop fever.

RECORDING YOUR FINDINGS

Your write-up of the physical examination begins with a general description of the patient's appearance, based on the General Survey. Note that initially you may use sentences to describe your findings; later you will use phrases. The style below contains phrases appropriate for most write-ups.

Recording the Physical Examination—The General Survey and Vital Signs

Choose vivid and graphic adjectives, as if you are painting a picture in words. Avoid cliches such as "well-developed" or "well-nourished" or "in no acute distress," because they could apply to any patient and do not convey the special features of the patient before you.

Record the vital signs taken at the time of your examination. They are preferable to those taken earlier in the day by other providers. (Common abbreviations for blood pressure, heart rate, and respiratory rate are self-explanatory.)

"Mrs. Scott is a young, healthy-appearing woman, well-groomed, fit, and in good spirits. Height is 5'4", weight 135 lbs, BMI 24, BP 120/80, HR 72 and regular, RR 16, temperature 37.5°C."

OR

"Mr. Jones is an elderly male who looks pale and chronically ill. He is alert, with good eye contact but unable to speak more than two or three words at a time due to shortness of breath. He has intercostal muscle retraction when breathing and sits upright in bed. He is thin, with diffuse muscle wasting. Height is 6'2", weight 175 lbs, BP 160/95, HR 108 and irregular, RR 32 and labored, temperature 101.2°F."

Suggests exacerbation of *chronic obstructive pulmonary disease*

Bibliography

CITATIONS

1. National Institutes of Health and National Heart, Lung, and Blood Institute. Clinical Guidelines on the Identification, Evaluation, and Treatment of Overweight and Obesity in Adults: The Evidence Report. NIH Publication 98-4083. June 1998. Available at: www.nhlbi.nih.gov/guidelines/obesity/ob_gdlns.pdf. Accessed December 12, 2004.

2. U.S. Preventive Services Task Force. Screening for Obesity in Adults: Recommendations and Rationale. Rockville, MD. Agency for Healthcare Research and Quality, November 2003. Available at: www.ahrq.gov/clinic/3rduspstf/obesity/obesrr.htm. Accessed December 12, 2004.

3. 2005 Dietary Guidelines Advisory Committee to the Secretaries of Health and Human Services and the U.S. Department of Agriculture. Nutrition and Your Health. January 2005. Available at: www.health/gov/dietaryguidelines/dga2005/report/. Accessed December 13, 2004.

4. U.S. Preventive Services Task Force. Clinician's Handbook of Preventive Services: Put Prevention Into Practice, 2nd ed. Washington, DC, Office of Public Health and Science, Office of Disease Prevention and Health Promotion, 1998.

5. Hensrud DD. Clinical preventive medicine in primary care: background and practice. Rational and current preventive practices. Mayo Clin Proc 75:165–172, 2000.

6. Culica D, Rohrer J, Ward M, et al. Medical check-ups: who does not get them? Am J Public Health 92(1):8890, 2002.

7. Chobanion AV, Bakris GL, Black HR, et al. The Seventh Report of the Joint National Committee on Prevention, Detection, Evaluation, and Treatment of High Blood Pressure—The JNC 7 Report. JAMA 289(19):2560–2572, 2003. Available at: www.nhlbi.nih.gov/guidelines/hypertension/jncintro.htm.

8. Cavallini MC, Roman MJ, Blank SG, et al. Association of the auscultatory gap with vascular disease in hypertensive patients. Ann Intern Med 124(10):877–883, 1996.

9. Chaudhry SI, Krumholz HM, Foody JM. Systolic hypertension in older persons. JAMA 292(9):1074–1080, 2004.

10. Carlson JE. Assessment of orthostatic blood pressure: measurement technique and clinical applications. South Med J 92(2):167–173, 1999.

11. Consensus Committee of the American Autonomic Society and the American Academy of Neurology. Consensus statement on the definition of orthostatic hypotension, pure autonomic failure, and multiple system atrophy. Neurology 46:1470, 1996.

12. Kaplan NM, Rose BD. Ambulatory blood pressure monitoring and white coat hypertension in adults. Available at: www.utdol.com. Accessed December 11, 2004.

13. Bobrie G, Genes N, Vaur L, et al. Is "isolated home" hypertension as opposed to "isolated office" hypertension a sign of greater cardiovascular risk? Arch Intern Med 161(18):2205–2211, 2001.

14. Clement DL, De Buyzere ML, De Bacquer DA, et al. Prognostic value of ambulatory blood-pressure recordings in patients with treated hypertension. N Engl J Med 348(24):2407–2415, 2003.

15. Rickerby J. The role of home blood pressure measurement in managing hypertension: an evidence-based review. J Hum Hypertens 16(7):469–472, 2002.

16. Brickner ME, Hillis LD, Lange RA. Congenital heart disease in adults. First of two parts. N Engl J Med 342(4):256–263, 2000.

ADDITIONAL REFERENCES

Weight and Nutrition

American Academy of Family Physicians. Nutrition Screening Initiative. Available at: http://www.aafp.org/preBuilt/NSI_DETERMINE.pdf. Accessed December 12, 2004.

Beevers G, Lip GY, O'Brien E. ABC of hypertension. Blood pressure measurement. Part I. Sphygmomanometry: factors common in all techniques. BMJ 322(7292):981–985, 2001.

Beevers G, Lip GY, O'Brien E. ABC of hypertension. Blood pressure measurement. Part II. Conventional sphygmomanometry: technique of auscultatory blood pressure measurement. BMJ 322(7293):1043–1047, 2001.

Ford ES, Wayne G, Dietz WH, Ford ES, Giles WH, Dietz WH. Prevalence of the metabolic syndrome among U.S. adults: findings from the Third National Health and Nutrition Examination Survey. JAMA 287(3):356–359, 2002.

Gail SM, Castracacane VD, Mantazoros. Energy homeostasis, obesity and eating disorders: recent advances in endocrinology. J. Nutr 134:295–298, 2004.

Mehler PS. Bulimia nervosa. N Engl J Med 349(9):875–880, 2003.

Sacks FM, Svetkey LP, Vollmer WM, et al. Effects on blood pressure of reduced dietary sodium and the dietary approaches to stop hypertension (DASH) diet. N Engl J Med 344(1):3–10, 2001.

Samaha FF, Iqbal N, Seshadri P, et al. A low-carbohydrate as compared with a low-fat diet in severe obesity. N Engl J Med 34(21):2074–2081, 2003.

McAlister FA, Straus SE. Evidence-based treatment of hypertension. Measurement of blood pressure: an evidence based review. BMJ 322:908–911, 2001.

Pearson TA, Blair SN, Daniels SR, et al. AHA guidelines for primary prevention of cardiovascular disease and stroke: 2002 update. Circulation 106:388–391, 2002.

Blood Pressure

Perry HM, Davis BR, Price TR, et al, for the Systolic Hypertension in the Elderly Program Cooperative Research Group. Effect of treating isolated systolic hypertension on the risk of developing various types and subtypes of stroke: the Systolic Hypertension in the Elderly Program (SHEP). JAMA 284(4):465–471, 2000.

Tholl U, Forstner K, Anlauf M. Measuring blood pressure: pitfalls and recommendations. Nephrol Dial Transplant 19:766, 2004.

U.S. Preventive Services Task Force. Screening for High Blood Pressure: Recommendations and Rationale. Rockville, MD, Agency for Healthcare Research and Quality, July 2003. Available at: http://www.ahrq.gov/clinic/3rduspstf/hibloodrr.htm. Accessed December 9, 2004.

Writing Group of the PREMIER Collaborative Research Group. Effects of comprehensive lifestyle modification on blood pressure control: main results of the PREMIER clinical trial. JAMA 289(16): 2083–2093, 2003.

TABLE 4-1 ■ Healthy Eating: Food Groups and Servings per Day

Food Group	Women, Some Older Adults, Children Ages 2–6 yrs (about 1,600 cal)*	Active Women, Most Men, Older Children, Teen Girls (about 2,200 cal)*	Active Men, Teen Boys (about 2,800 cal)*
Bread, rice, cereal, pasta (grains) group, especially whole grain	6	9	11
Vegetable group	3	4	5
Fruit group	2	3	4
Milk, yogurt, and cheese (dairy) group—preferably fat free or low fat	2–3**	2–3**	2–3**
Dry beans, eggs, nuts, fish, and meat and poultry group—preferably lean or low fat	2, for a total of 5 oz	2, for a total of 6 oz	3, for a total of 7 oz

Source: Adapted from U.S. Department of Agriculture, Center for Nutrition Policy and Promotion. The Food Guide Pyramid, Home and Garden Bulletin Number 252, 1996.

*These are the calorie levels if low-fat, lean foods are chosen from the 5 major food groups and foods from the fats, oil, and sweets group are used sparingly.

**Older children and teenagers (ages 9–18 yrs) and adults older than the age of 50 need 3 servings daily. During pregnancy and lactation, the recommended number of dairy group servings is the same as for nonpregnant women.

TABLE 4-2 ■ Rapid Screen for Dietary Intake

	Portions Consumed by Patient	Recommended
Grains, cereals, bread group	_____	6–11
Fruit group	_____	2–4
Vegetable group	_____	3–5
Meat/meat substitute group	_____	2–3
Dairy group	_____	2–3
Sugars, fats, snack foods	_____	—
Soft drinks	_____	—
Alcoholic beverages	_____	<2

Instructions. Ask the patient for a 24-hour dietary recall (perhaps two of these) before completing the form.

Source: Nestle M: Nutrition. In: Woolf SH, Jonas S, Lawrence RS, eds. Health Promotion and Disease Prevention in Clinical Practice. Baltimore, Williams & Wilkins, 1996.

TABLE 4-3 **Eating Disorders and Excessively Low BMI**

In the United States an estimated 5 to 10 million women and 1 million men suffer from eating disorders. These severe disturbances of eating behavior are often difficult to detect, especially in teens wearing baggy clothes or in individuals who binge then induce vomiting or evacuation. Be familiar with the two principal eating disorders, *anorexia nervosa* and *bulimia nervosa*. Both conditions are characterized by distorted perceptions of body image and weight. Early detection is important, because prognosis improves when treatment occurs in the early stages of these disorders.

Clinical Features

Anorexia Nervosa	Bulimia Nervosa
■ Refusal to maintain minimally normal body weight (or BMI above 17.5 kg/m²)	■ Repeated binge eating followed by self-induced vomiting, misuse of laxatives, diuretics or other medications, fasting; or excessive exercise
■ Afraid of appearing fat	■ Often with normal weight
■ Frequently starving but in denial; lacking insight	■ Overeating at least twice a week during 3-month period; large amounts of food consumed in short period (~2 hrs)
■ Often brought in by family members	
■ May present as failure to make expected weight gains in childhood or adolescence, amenorrhea in women, loss of libido or potency in men	■ Preoccupation with eating; craving and compulsion to eat; lack of control over eating; alternating with periods of starvation
■ Associated with depressive symptoms such as depressed mood, irritability, social withdrawal, insomnia, decreased libido	■ Dread of fatness but may be obese
■ Additional features supporting diagnosis: self-induced vomiting or purging, excessive exercise, use of appetite suppressants and/or diuretics	■ Subtypes of
	■ *Purging:* bulimic episodes accompanied by self-induced vomiting or use of laxatives, diuretics, or enemas
■ Biologic complications	
■ *Neuroendocrine changes:* amenorrhea, increased corticotropin-releasing factor, cortisol, growth hormone, serotonin; decreased diurnal cortisol fluctuation, luteinizing hormone, follicle-stimulating hormone, thyroid-stimulating hormone	■ *Nonpurging:* bulimic episodes accompanied by compensatory behavior such as fasting, exercise, but without purging
	■ Biologic complications
■ *Cardiovascular disorders:* bradycardia, hypotension, arrhythmias, cardiomyopathy	See changes listed for anorexia nervosa, especially weakness, fatigue, mild cognitive disorder; also erosion of dental enamel, parotitis, pancreatic inflammation with elevated amylase, mild neuropathies, seizures, hypokalemia, hypochloremic metabolic acidosis, hypomagnesemia
■ *Metabolic disorders:* hypokalemia, hypochloremic metabolic alkalosis, increased BUN, edema	
■ *Other:* dry skin, dental caries, delayed gastric emptying, constipation, anemia, osteoporosis	

Sources: World Health Organization: The ICD-10 Classification of Mental and Behavioral Disorders: Diagnostic Criteria for Research. Geneva, World Health Organization, 1993. American Psychiatric Association: DSM-IV-TR: Diagnostic and Statistical Manual of Mental Disorders, 4th ed. Washington, DC, American Psychiatric Association, 1994. Halmi KA: Eating Disorders: In: Kaplan HI, Sadock BJ, eds. Comprehensive Textbook of Psychiatry, 7th ed. Philadelphia, Lippincott Williams & Wilkins, 1663–1676, 2000. Mehler PS. Bulimia nervosa. N Engl J Med 349(9):875–880, 2003.

TABLE 4-4	Nutrition Screening Checklist

I have an illness or condition that made me change the kind and/or amount of food I eat.	Yes (2 pts)	_____
I eat fewer than 2 meals per day.	Yes (3 pts)	_____
I eat few fruits or vegetables, or milk products.	Yes (2 pts)	_____
I have 3 or more drinks of beer, liquor, or wine almost every day.	Yes (2 pts)	_____
I have tooth or mouth problems that make it hard for me to eat.	Yes (2 pts)	_____
I don't always have enough money to buy the food I need.	Yes (4 pts)	_____
I eat alone most of the time.	Yes (1 pt)	_____
I take 3 or more different prescribed or over-the-counter drugs each day.	Yes (1 pt)	_____
Without wanting to, I have lost or gained 10 pounds in the last 6 months.	Yes (2 pts)	_____
I am not always physically able to shop, cook, and/or feed myself.	Yes (2 pts)	_____
	TOTAL	_____

Instructions. Check "yes" for each condition that applies, then total the nutritional score. For total scores between 3–5 points (moderate risk) or ≥6 points (high risk), further evaluation is needed (especially for the elderly).

Source: American Academy of Family Physicians: The Nutrition Screening Initiative. Available at: www.aafp.org/PreBuilt/NSI_DETERMINE.pdf. Accessed December 12, 2004.

TABLE 4-5	Nutrition Counseling: Sources of Nutrients

Nutrient	Food Source
Calcium	Dairy foods such as yogurt, milk, and natural cheeses Breakfast cereal, fruit juice with calcium supplements Dark green leafy vegetables such as collards, turnip greens
Iron	Shellfish Lean meat, dark turkey meat Cereals with iron supplements Spinach, peas, lentils Enriched and whole-grain bread
Folate	Cooked dried beans and peas Oranges, orange juice Dark-green leafy vegetables
Vitamin D	Milk (fortified) Eggs, butter, margarine Cereals (fortified)

Source: Adapted from Dietary Guidelines Committee, 2000 Report. Nutrition and Your Health: Dietary Guidelines for Americans. Washington, DC, Agricultural Research Service, U.S. Department of Agriculture, 2000.

TABLE 4-6 — Patients With Hypertension: Recommended Changes in Diet

Dietary Change	Food Source
Increase foods high in potassium	Baked white or sweet potatoes, cooked greens such as spinach Bananas, plantains, many dried fruits, orange juice
Decrease foods high in sodium	Canned foods (soups, tuna fish) Pretzels, potato chips, pickles, olives Many processed foods (frozen dinners, ketchup, mustard) Batter-fried foods Table salt, including for cooking

Source: Adapted from Dietary Guidelines Committee, 2000 Report. Nutrition and Your Health: Dietary Guidelines for Americans. Washington, DC, Agricultural Research Service, U.S. Department of Agriculture, 2000.

Normal

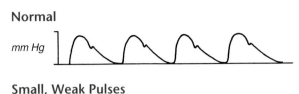

The pulse pressure is about 30–40 mm Hg. The pulse contour is smooth and rounded. (The notch on the descending slope of the pulse wave is not palpable.)

Small, Weak Pulses

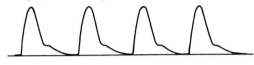

The pulse pressure is diminished, and the pulse feels weak and small. The upstroke may feel slowed, the peak prolonged. Causes include (1) decreased stroke volume, as in heart failure, hypovolemia, and severe aortic stenosis, and (2) increased peripheral resistance, as in exposure to cold and severe congestive heart failure.

Large, Bounding Pulses

The pulse pressure is increased, and the pulse feels strong and bounding. The rise and fall may feel rapid, the peak brief. Causes include (1) an increased stroke volume, a decreased peripheral resistance, or both, as in fever, anemia, hyperthyroidism, aortic regurgitation, arteriovenous fistulas, and patent ductus arteriosus; (2) an increased stroke volume due to slow heart rates, as in bradycardia and complete heart block; and (3) decreased compliance (increased stiffness) of the aortic walls, as in aging or atherosclerosis.

Bisferiens Pulse

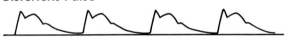

A bisferiens pulse is an increased arterial pulse with a double systolic peak. Causes include pure aortic regurgitation, combined aortic stenosis and regurgitation, and, though less commonly palpable, hypertrophic cardiomyopathy.

Pulsus Alternans

The pulse alternates in amplitude from beat to beat even though the rhythm is basically regular (and must be for you to make this judgment). When the difference between stronger and weaker beats is slight, it can be detected only by sphygmomanometry. Pulsus alternans indicates left ventricular failure and is usually accompanied by a left-sided S_3.

Bigeminal Pulse

Premature contractions

This is a disorder of rhythm that may masquerade as pulsus alternans. A bigeminal pulse is caused by a normal beat alternating with a premature contraction. The stroke volume of the premature beat is diminished in relation to that of the normal beats, and the pulse varies in amplitude accordingly.

Paradoxical Pulse

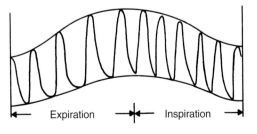

Expiration   Inspiration

A paradoxical pulse may be detected by a palpable decrease in the pulse's amplitude on quiet inspiration. If the sign is less pronounced, a blood pressure cuff is needed. Systolic pressure decreases by more than 10 mm Hg during inspiration. A paradoxical pulse is found in pericardial tamponade, constrictive pericarditis (though less commonly), and obstructive lung disease.

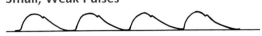

TABLE 4-8   Abnormalities in Rate and Rhythm of Breathing

When observing respiratory patterns, think in terms of *rate, depth,* and *regularity* of the patient's breathing. Describe what you see in these terms. Traditional terms, such as tachypnea, are given below so that you will understand them, but simple descriptions are recommended for use.

Normal

The respiratory rate is about 14–20 per min in normal adults and up to 44 per min in infants.

Slow Breathing (*Bradypnea*)

Slow breathing may be secondary to such causes as diabetic coma, drug-induced respiratory depression, and increased intracranial pressure.

Sighing Respiration

Breathing punctuated by frequent sighs should alert you to the possibility of hyperventilation syndrome—a common cause of dyspnea and dizziness. Occasional sighs are normal.

Rapid Shallow Breathing (*Tachypnea*)

Rapid shallow breathing has a number of causes, including restrictive lung disease, pleuritic chest pain, and an elevated diaphragm.

Cheyne-Stokes Breathing

Periods of deep breathing alternate with periods of apnea (no breathing). Children and aging people normally may show this pattern in sleep. Other causes include heart failure, uremia, drug-induced respiratory depression, and brain damage (typically on both sides of the cerebral hemispheres or diencephalon).

Obstructive Breathing

In obstructive lung disease, expiration is prolonged because narrowed airways increase the resistance to air flow. Causes include asthma, chronic bronchitis, and COPD.

Rapid Deep Breathing (*Hyperpnea, Hyperventilation*)

Rapid deep breathing has several causes, including exercise, anxiety, and metabolic acidosis. In the comatose patient, consider infarction, hypoxia, or hypoglycemia affecting the midbrain or pons. *Kussmaul breathing* is deep breathing due to metabolic acidosis. It may be fast, normal in rate, or slow.

Ataxic Breathing (*Biot's Breathing*)

Ataxic breathing is characterized by unpredictable irregularity. Breaths may be shallow or deep, and stop for short periods. Causes include respiratory depression and brain damage, typically at the medullary level.

CHAPTER 5

The Skin, Hair, and Nails

ANATOMY AND PHYSIOLOGY

The major function of the skin is to keep the body in homeostasis despite the daily assaults of the environment. The skin provides boundaries for body fluids while protecting underlying tissues from microorganisms, harmful substances, and radiation. It modulates body temperature and synthesizes vitamin D. **Hair, nails,** and **sebaceous** and **sweat glands** are considered appendages of the skin. The skin and its appendages undergo many changes during aging. Turn to Chapter 20, The Older Adult (pp. 841–842), to review normal and abnormal changes of the skin with aging.

Skin. The skin is the heaviest single organ of the body, accounting for approximately 16% of body weight and covering an area of roughly 1.2 to 2.3 meters squared. It contains three layers: the epidermis, the dermis, and the subcutaneous tissues.

The most superficial layer, the *epidermis,* is thin, devoid of blood vessels, and itself divided into two layers: an outer horny layer of dead keratinized cells and an inner cellular layer where both melanin and keratin are formed. Migration from the inner layer to the top layer of the epidermis takes approximately 1 month.

The epidermis depends on the underlying *dermis* for its nutrition. The dermis is well supplied with blood. It contains connective tissue, sebaceous glands, sweat glands, and hair follicles. It merges below with *subcutaneous tissue,* or *adipose,* also known as fat.

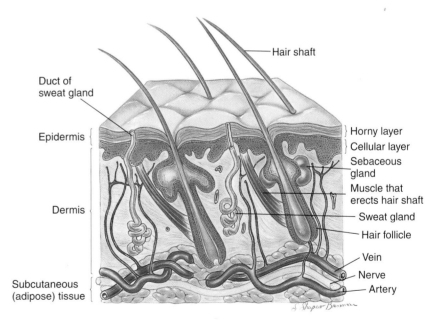

The color of normal skin depends primarily on four pigments: melanin, carotene, oxyhemoglobin, and deoxyhemoglobin. The amount of *melanin*, the brownish pigment of the skin, is genetically determined and is increased by sunlight. *Carotene* is a golden yellow pigment that exists in subcutaneous fat and in heavily keratinized areas such as the palms and soles.

Hemoglobin, which circulates in the red cells and carries most of the oxygen of the blood, exists in two forms. *Oxyhemoglobin*, a bright red pigment, predominates in the arteries and capillaries. An increase in blood flow through the arteries to the capillaries of the skin causes a reddening of the skin, whereas the opposite change usually produces pallor. The skin of light-colored people is normally redder on the palms, soles, face, neck, and upper chest.

As blood passes through the capillary bed, oxyhemoglobin loses its oxygen to the tissues and changes to *deoxyhemoglobin*—a darker and somewhat bluer pigment. An increased concentration of deoxyhemoglobin in cutaneous blood vessels gives the skin a bluish cast known as *cyanosis*.

Cyanosis is of two kinds, depending on the oxygen level in the arterial blood. If this level is low, cyanosis is *central*. If it is normal, cyanosis is *peripheral*. Peripheral cyanosis occurs when cutaneous blood flow decreases and slows, and tissues extract more oxygen than usual from the blood. Peripheral cyanosis may be a normal response to anxiety or a cold environment.

Skin color is affected not only by pigments but also by the scattering of light as it is reflected back through the turbid superficial layers of the skin or vessel walls. This scattering makes the color look more blue and less red. The bluish color of a subcutaneous vein is a result of this effect; it is much bluer than the venous blood obtained on venipuncture.

Hair. Adults have two types of hair: *vellus hair*, which is short, fine, inconspicuous, and relatively unpigmented; and *terminal hair*, which is coarser, thicker, more conspicuous, and usually pigmented. Scalp hair and eyebrows are examples of terminal hair.

Nails. Nails protect the distal ends of the fingers and toes. The firm, rectangular, and usually curving *nail plate* gets its pink color from the vascular *nail bed* to which the plate is firmly attached. Note the whitish moon, or *lunula*, and the free edge of the nail plate. Roughly one fourth of the nail plate (the *nail root*) is covered by the *proximal nail fold*. The *cuticle* extends from this fold and, functioning as a seal, protects the space between the fold and the plate from external moisture. *Lateral nail folds* cover the sides of the nail plate. Note that the angle between the proximal nail fold and the nail plate is normally less than 180°.

Fingernails grow approximately 0.1 mm daily; toenails grow more slowly.

Sebaceous Glands and Sweat Glands. *Sebaceous glands* produce a fatty substance that is secreted onto the skin surface through the hair follicles. These glands are present on all skin surfaces except the palms and soles.

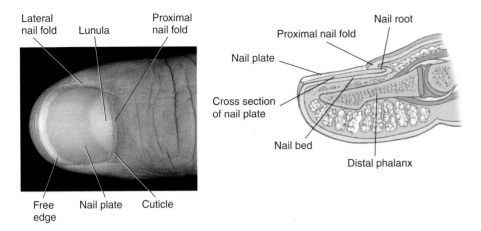

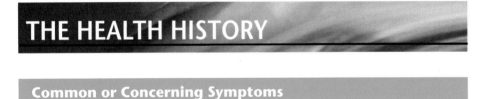

Sweat glands are of two types: eccrine and apocrine. The *eccrine glands* are widely distributed, open directly onto the skin surface, and by their sweat production help to control body temperature. In contrast, the *apocrine glands* are found chiefly in the axillary and genital regions, usually open into hair follicles, and are stimulated by emotional stress. Bacterial decomposition of apocrine sweat is responsible for adult body odor.

THE HEALTH HISTORY

Common or Concerning Symptoms

- Hair loss
- Rash
- Moles

Start your inquiry about the skin with a few open-ended questions: "Have you noticed any changes in your skin?". . . your hair? . . . your nails?. . . "Have you had any rashes? . . . sores? . . . lumps? . . . itching?"

Ask, "Have you noticed any moles you are concerned about? Do you have any moles that have changed in size, shape, color, or sensation? What about any new moles?" If patients have such moles, pursue any personal or family history of melanoma and results of any prior biopsies of the skin.

You may wish to defer further questions about the skin until the physical examination, when you inspect the skin and identify the lesions that the patient is concerned about.

Causes of generalized itching without obvious reason include dry skin, aging, pregnancy, uremia, jaundice, lymphomas and leukemia, drug reaction, and lice.

Approximately half of *melanomas* are initially detected by the patient.[1]

HEALTH PROMOTION AND COUNSELING

Important Topics for Health Promotion and Counseling

- Risk factors for melanoma
- Avoidance of excessive sun exposure

Clinicians play an important role in educating patients about early detection of suspicious moles, protective measures for skin care, and the hazards of excessive sun exposure. Skin cancers are the most common cancers in the United States and usually arise on sun-exposed areas, particularly the head, neck, and hands. Almost all skin cancers are of three types[2, 3]:

- *Basal cell carcinoma,* arising in the lowest, or basal, level of the epidermis, accounts for approximately 80% of skin cancers. These cancers are shiny and translucent, tend to grow slowly, and rarely metastasize.

- *Squamous cell carcinoma,* in the upper layer of the epidermis, accounts for approximately 16% of skin cancers. These cancers are often crusted and scaly with a red inflamed or ulcerated appearance; they can metastasize.

- *Melanoma,* arising from the pigment-producing melanocytes in the epidermis that give the skin its color, accounts for approximately 4% of skin cancers and is the most lethal type. Although rare, melanomas are the most rapidly increasing U.S. malignancy. Lifetime risk for invasive melanoma is now 1 in 65, and is 1 in 37 for noninvasive melanoma. Melanomas can spread rapidly to the lymph system and internal organs. Mortality rates are highest in white men, approximately 3.6% per year, possibly because of lower "skin awareness" and lower rates of self-examination.[4]

Educate your patients about *risk factors for melanoma:* 50 or more common moles; 1–4 or more atypical or unusual moles, especially if dysplastic[5, 6]; red or light hair; actinic lentigenes, or macular brown or tan spots usually on sun-exposed areas, such as freckles; heavy sun exposure; light eye or skin color, especially skin that freckles or burns easily; and family history of melanoma.[4] Early detection of melanoma when less than 3 mm improves prognosis.

The most commonly recommended screening measure for skin cancer is *total-body skin examination* by a clinician, although data on utility of this method for nondermatologists are limited. Although the U.S. Preventive Services Task Force has found insufficient evidence to recommend inspection for routine screening, the American Cancer Society recommends skin examination as part of a routine cancer-related check-up every 3 years for people aged 20–40, and yearly for those older than 40.[7, 8] Only a few studies have shown that *skin self-examination* enhances detection,[9–11] but this low-cost method of patient education can promote health awareness in at-risk patients. (See Techniques for Skin Self-Examination on pp. 128–129.)

There is also value in use of the ***ABCDE method*** for screening moles for melanoma by clinicians and patients. Sensitivity ranges from 50% to 97%, and specificity from 96% to 99%[1, 12] (see Table 5-8, Benign and Malignant Nevi, p. 143).

ABCDE: SCREENING MOLES FOR POSSIBLE MELANOMA

- **A** for *asymmetry*
- **B** for irregular *borders,* especially ragged, notched, or blurred
- **C** for variation or change in *color,* especially blue or black
- **D** for *diameter ≥ 6 mm* or *different from others,* especially if changing, itching, or bleeding
- **E** for *elevation* or *enlargement*

You may also wish to counsel patients about such preventive strategies as reducing sun exposure and using sunscreens (though these are not conclusively validated as effective[9]). Caution patients to minimize direct sun exposure, especially at midday when ultraviolet B rays (UV-B), the most common cause of skin cancer, are most intense. Sunscreens fall into two categories—thick, pastelike ointments that block all solar rays, and light-absorbing sunscreens rated by "sun protective factor" (SPF). The SPF is a ratio of the number of minutes for treated versus untreated skin to redden with exposure to UV-B. An SPF of at least 15 is recommended and protects against 93% of UV-B. (There is no scale for UV-A, which causes photoaging, or UV-C, the most carcinogenic ray but blocked in the atmosphere by ozone.) Water-resistant sunscreens that remain on the skin for prolonged periods are preferable. Be aware, however, that use of sunscreens may give patients a false sense of security and increase sun exposure.

TECHNIQUES OF EXAMINATION

Your examination of the skin, hair, and nails begins with the General Survey and continues throughout the physical examination. Take time, however, to ensure that the patient wears a gown and is draped accordingly to facilitate close inspection of the hair, anterior and posterior surfaces of the body, palms and soles, and webspaces between the fingers and toes.

Inspect the entire skin surface in good light, preferably natural light or artificial light that resembles it. Correlate your findings with observations of the mucous membranes, especially when assessing skin color, because diseases may appear in both areas. Techniques for examining these membranes are described in later chapters.

Artificial light often distorts colors and masks jaundice.

To sharpen your observations, you may wish to turn now to the tables at the end of the chapter to better identify skin colors and patterns and types of lesions that you may encounter during the examination.

 ## SKIN

Inspect and palpate the skin. Note these characteristics:

Color. Patients may notice a change in their skin color before the clinician does. Ask about it. Look for increased pigmentation (brownness), loss of pigmentation, redness, pallor, cyanosis, and yellowing of the skin.

See Table 5-1, Skin Colors (pp. 132–133).

The red color of oxyhemoglobin and the pallor in its absence are best assessed where the horny layer of the epidermis is thinnest and causes the least scatter: the fingernails, the lips, and the mucous membranes, particularly those of the mouth and the palpebral conjunctiva. In dark-skinned people, inspecting the palms and soles may also be useful.

Pallor from decreased redness in *anemia* and in decreased blood flow, as occurs in fainting or arterial insufficiency

Central cyanosis is best identified in the lips, oral mucosa, and tongue. The lips, however, may turn blue in the cold, and melanin in the lips may simulate cyanosis in darker-skinned people.

Causes of *central cyanosis* include advanced lung disease, congenital heart disease, and abnormal hemoglobins.

Cyanosis of the nails, hands, and feet may be central or peripheral in origin. Anxiety or a cold examining room may cause peripheral cyanosis.

Cyanosis in congestive heart failure is usually peripheral, reflecting decreased blood flow, but in pulmonary edema, it may also be central. Venous obstruction may cause peripheral cyanosis.

Look for the yellow color of jaundice in the sclera. Jaundice may also appear in the palpebral conjunctiva, lips, hard palate, undersurface of the tongue, tympanic membrane, and skin. To see jaundice more easily in the lips, blanch out the red color by pressure with a glass slide.

Jaundice suggests liver disease or excessive hemolysis of red blood cells.

For the yellow color that accompanies high levels of carotene, look at the palms, soles, and face.

Carotenemia

Moisture.   Examples are dryness, sweating, and oiliness.

Dryness in hypothyroidism; oiliness in acne

Temperature.   Use the backs of your fingers to make this assessment. In addition to identifying generalized warmth or coolness of the skin, note the temperature of any red areas.

Generalized warmth in fever, *hyperthyroidism;* coolness in *hypothyroidism.* Local warmth of inflammation or cellulitis

Texture.   Examples arc roughness and smoothness.

Roughness in hypothyroidism; velvety texture in hyperthyroidism

Mobility and Turgor.   Lift a fold of skin and note the ease with which it lifts up (mobility) and the speed with which it returns into place (turgor).

Decreased mobility in edema, *scleroderma;* decreased turgor in dehydration

Lesions.   Observe any lesions of the skin, noting their characteristics:

- Their *anatomic location and distribution* over the body. Are they generalized or localized? Do they, for example, involve the exposed surfaces, the intertriginous or skin fold areas, extensor or flexor areas, or acral (peripheral) areas? Do they involve areas exposed to specific allergens or irritants, such as wrist bands, rings, or industrial chemicals?

Many skin diseases have typical distributions. Acne affects the face, upper chest, and back; psoriasis, the knees and elbows (among other areas); and *Candida* infections, the intertriginous areas. See patterns in Table 5-2, Skin Lesions—Anatomic Location and Distribution (p. 134).

- Their *patterns and shapes.* For example, are they linear, clustered, annular (in a ring), arciform (in an arc), geographic, or serpiginous (serpent or worm-like)? Are they dermatomal, covering a skin band that corresponds to a sensory nerve root (see pp. 605–606)?

Vesicles in a unilateral dermatomal pattern are typical of herpes zoster.[13] See patterns in Table 5-3, Skin Lesions—Patterns and Shapes (p. 135).

- The *types of skin lesions* (e.g., macules, papules, vesicles, nevi). If possible, find representative and recent lesions that have not been traumatized by scratching or otherwise altered. Inspect them carefully and feel them.

See Table 5-4, Elevated Skin Lesions (pp. 136–139); Table 5-5, Depressed Skin Lesions (p. 140); Table 5-6, Vascular and Purpuric Lesions of the Skin (p. 141); Table 5-7, Skin Tumors (p. 142); and Table 5-8, Benign and Malignant Nevi (p. 143).

- Their *color.*

SKIN LESIONS IN CONTEXT

After familiarizing yourself with the basic types of lesions, review their appearances in Tables 5-9 and 5-10 and in a well-illustrated textbook of dermatology. Whenever you see a skin lesion, look it up in such a text. The type of lesions, their location, and their distribution, together with other infor-

See Table 5-9, Skin Lesions in Context (pp. 144–145), and Table 5-10, Diseases and Related Skin Conditions (pp. 146–147).

mation from the history and the examination, should equip you well for this search and, in time, for arriving at specific dermatologic diagnoses.

Evaluating the Bedbound Patient. People who are confined to bed, especially when they are emaciated, elderly, or neurologically impaired, are particularly susceptible to skin damage and ulceration. *Pressure sores* result when sustained compression obliterates arteriolar and capillary blood flow to the skin. Sores may also result from the shearing forces created by bodily movements. When a person slides down in bed from a partially sitting position, for example, or is dragged rather than lifted up from a supine position, the movements may distort the soft tissues of the buttocks and close off the arteries and arterioles within. Friction and moisture further increase the risk.

See Table 5-11, Pressure Ulcers (p. 148).

Assess every susceptible patient by carefully inspecting the skin that overlies the sacrum, buttocks, greater trochanters, knees, and heels. Roll the patient onto one side to see the sacrum and buttocks.

Local redness of the skin warns of impending necrosis, although some deep pressure sores develop without antecedent redness. Ulcers may be seen.

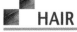

HAIR

Inspect and palpate the hair. Note its quantity, distribution, and texture.

Alopecia refers to hair loss—diffuse, patchy, or total. Sparse hair in hypothyroidism; fine silky hair in hyperthyroidism

See Table 5-12, Hair Loss (p. 149).

NAILS

Inspect and palpate the fingernails and toenails. Note their color and shape and any lesions. Longitudinal bands of pigment may be seen in the nails of normal people who have darker skin.

See Table 5-13, Findings In or Near the Nails (pp. 150–151).

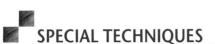

SPECIAL TECHNIQUES

Instructions for the Skin Self-Examination. The American Academy of Dermatology recommends regular self-examination of the skin using the techniques below. The patient will need a full-length mirror, a hand-held mirror, and a well-lit room that provides privacy. Teach the patient the **ABCDE** method for assessing moles (see p. 125), and show the patient the photos of benign and malignant nevi in Table 5-8 on p. 143.

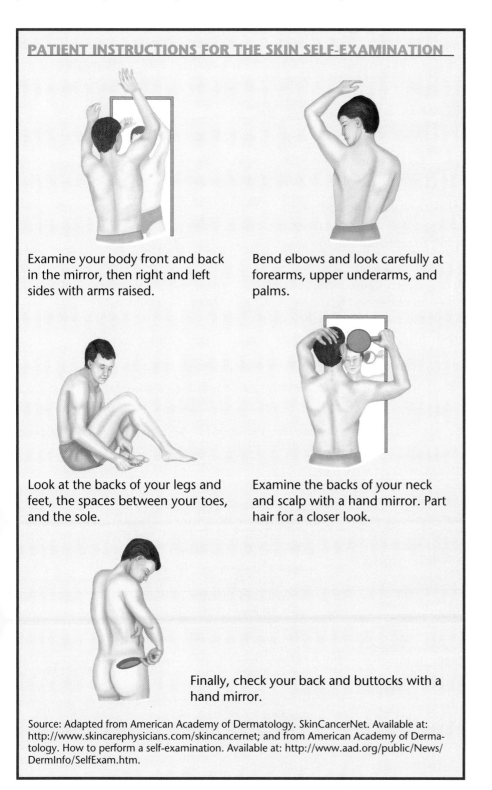

PATIENT INSTRUCTIONS FOR THE SKIN SELF-EXAMINATION

Examine your body front and back in the mirror, then right and left sides with arms raised.

Bend elbows and look carefully at forearms, upper underarms, and palms.

Look at the backs of your legs and feet, the spaces between your toes, and the sole.

Examine the backs of your neck and scalp with a hand mirror. Part hair for a closer look.

Finally, check your back and buttocks with a hand mirror.

Source: Adapted from American Academy of Dermatology. SkinCancerNet. Available at: http://www.skincarephysicians.com/skincancernet; and from American Academy of Dermatology. How to perform a self-examination. Available at: http://www.aad.org/public/News/DermInfo/SelfExam.htm.

RECORDING YOUR FINDINGS

Note that initially you may use sentences to describe your findings; later you will use phrases. The style below contains phrases appropriate for most write-ups.

Recording the Physical Examination—The Skin

"Color good. Skin warm and moist. Nails without clubbing or cyanosis. No suspicious nevi. No rash, petechiae, or ecchymoses."

OR

"Marked facial pallor, with circumoral cyanosis. Palms cold and moist. Cyanosis in nailbeds of fingers and toes. One raised blue-black nevus, 1×2 cm, with irregular border on right forearm. No rash."

Suggests central cyanosis and possible melanoma

OR

"Facial plethora. Skin icteric. Spider angioma over anterior torso. Palmar erythema. Single pearly papule with depressed center and telangiectasias, 1×1 cm, on posterior neck above collarline. No suspicious nevi. Nails with clubbing but no cyanosis."

Suggests possible liver disease and basal cell carcinoma

Bibliography

CITATIONS

1. Whited JD, Grichnik JM. Does this patient have a mole or a melanoma? The rational clinical examination. JAMA 279(9): 696–701, 1998.
2. American Academy of Dermatology. Public Resource Center: 2004 Melanoma fact sheet. Available at: http://www.aad.org/public/News/DermInfo/2004MelanomaFAQ.htm. Accessed January 29, 2005.
3. American Academy of Dermatology. What is skin cancer? Skincare.net. Available at: http://www.skincarephysicians.com/skincancernet/whatis.html. Accessed January 29, 2005.
4. Helfand M, Krages KP. Counseling to Prevent Skin Cancer: A Summary of the Evidence for the U.S. Preventive Services Task Force. Rockville, MD, Agency for Healthcare Research and Quality, 2003. Available at: http://www.ahrq.gov/clinic/3rduspstf/skcacoun/skcounsum.htm. Accessed January 29, 2005.
5. Naeyaert JM, Broches L. Dysplastic nevi. N Engl J Med 349(23):2233–2240, 2003.
6. Tucker MA, Halpern A, Holly EA, et al. Clinically recognized dysplastic nevi: A central risk factor for cutaneous melanoma. JAMA 277(18):1439–1444, 1997.
7. U.S. Preventive Services Task Force. Screening for Skin Cancer: Recommendations and Rationale. [Article originally published in Am J Prev Med 20(3S):44–46, 2001.] Rockville, MD, Agency for Healthcare Research and Quality. Available at: http://www.ahrq.gov/clinic/ajpmsuppl/skcarr.htm. Accessed January 29, 2005.
8. American Cancer Society. Skin cancer, 2005. Available at: http://www.cancer.org/downloads/PRO/SkinCancer.pdf. Accessed January 19, 2005.
9. U.S. Preventive Services Task Force: Counseling to Prevent Skin Cancer: Recommendations and Rationale. Rockville, MD, Agency for Healthcare Research and Quality, 2003. Available at: http://www.ahrq.gov/clinic/3rduspstf/skcacoun/skcarr.htm. Accessed January 28, 2005.
10. Berwick M, Begg CB, Fine JA, et al. Screening for cutaneous melanoma by skin self-examination. J Natl Cancer Inst 88: 17–23, 1996.
11. Robinson JK, Fisher SG, Turrisi RJ. Predictors of skin self-examination performance. Cancer 95(1):135–146, 2002.
12. U.S. Preventive Services Task Force: Screening for Skin Cancer: Summary of the Evidence. [Article originally published in Am J Prev 20(3S):47–58, 2001.] Rockville, MD, Agency for Healthcare Research and Quality, 2001. Available at: http://www.ahrq.gov/clinic/ajpmsuppl/helfand1.htm. Accessed January 29, 2005.
13. Gnann JG, Whitley RJ: Herpes zoster. N Engl J Med 3247(5):340–346, 2002.

BIBLIOGRAPHY

ADDITIONAL REFERENCES

Fitzpatrick TB, Freedberg IM. Fitzpatrick's Dermatology in General Medicine, 6th ed. New York, McGraw-Hill, 2003.

Fitzpatrick TB, Wolff K, Johnson RA, Suurmond D. Fitzpatrick's Color Atlas and Synopsis of Clinical Dermatology, 5th ed. New York, McGraw-Hill, 2005.

Grimes P. New insights and new therapies in vitiligo. JAMA 293(6):730–735, 2005.

Habif TP. Clinical Dermatology: A Color Guide to Diagnosis and Therapy, 4th ed. New York, Mosby, 2004.

Habif TP. Skin Disease: Diagnosis and Treatment, 2nd ed. Philadelphia, Elsevier Mosby, 2005.

Hall JC, Sauer GC. Sauer's Manual of Skin Diseases, 8th ed. Philadelphia, Lippincott Williams & Wilkins, 2000.

Hordinsky M, Sawaya M, Roberts JL. Hirsutism and hair loss in the elderly. Clin Geriatr Med 18(1):121–133, 2002.

Lyder CH. Pressure ulcer prevention and management. JAMA 289(2):223–226.

Myers KA, Farquhar DRE. Does this patient have clubbing? JAMA 2001(2863):341–347.

Scanlon E, Stubbs N. Pressure ulcer risk assessment in patients with darkly pigmented skin. Professional Nurse 19(6):339–341, 2004.

Schon MP, Henning-Boehncke W. Psoriasis. N Engl J Med 352(18): 1899–1912, 2005.

Singer AJ, Clark RAF. Cutaneous wound healing. N Engl J Med 341(10):738–746, 1999.

Singh N, Armstrong DG, Lipsky BA. Preventing foot ulcers in patients with diabetes. JAMA 293(2):217–228, 2005.

Swartz MN. Cellulitis. N Engl J Med 350(9):904–912, 2004.

Yancey KB, Egan GA. Pemphigoid: clinical, histologic, immunopathologic, and therapeutic considerations. JAMA 284(3): 350–356, 2000.

TABLE 5-1   **Skin Colors**

Changes in Pigmentation

A widespread increase in *melanin* may be caused by Addison's disease (hypofunction of the adrenal cortex) or some pituitary tumors. More common are local areas of increased or decreased pigment:

Café-Au-Lait Spot

A slightly but uniformly pigmented macule or patch with a somewhat irregular border, usually 0.5 to 1.5 cm in diameter and of no consequence. Six or more such spots, each with a diameter of >1.5 cm, however, suggest neurofibromatosis (p. 799). (The small, darker macules are unrelated.)

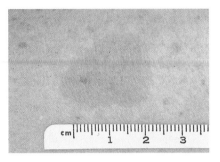

Tinea Versicolor

Common superficial fungus infection of the skin, causing hypopigmented, slightly scaly macules on the trunk, neck, and upper arms (short-sleeved shirt distribution). They are easier to see in darker skin and in some are more obvious after tanning. In lighter skin, macules may look reddish or tan instead of pale.

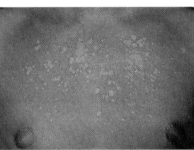

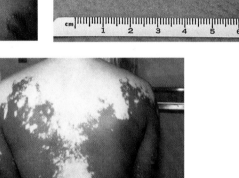

Vitiligo

In vitiligo, depigmented macules appear on the face, hands, feet, extensor surfaces, and other regions and may coalesce into extensive areas that lack melanin. The brown pigment is normal skin color; the pale areas are vitiligo. The condition may be hereditary. These changes may be distressing to the patient.

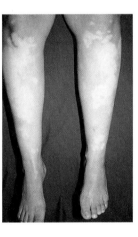

Cyanosis

Cyanosis is the somewhat bluish color that is visible in these toenails and toes. Compare this color with the normally pink fingernails and fingers of the same patient. Impaired venous return in the leg caused this example of peripheral cyanosis. Cyanosis, especially when slight, may be hard to distinguish from normal skin color.

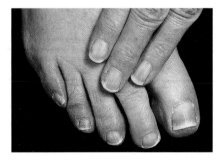

(table continues next page)

TABLE 5-1 **Skin Colors** *(Continued)*

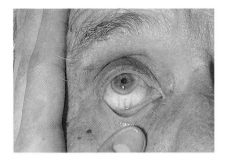

Jaundice

Jaundice makes the skin diffusely yellow. Note this patient's skin color, contrasted with the examiner's hand. The color of jaundice is seen most easily and reliably in the sclera, as shown here. It may also be visible in mucous membranes. Causes include liver disease and hemolysis of red blood cells.

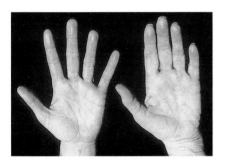

Carotenemia

The yellowish palm of carotenemia is compared with a normally pink palm, sometimes a subtle finding. Unlike jaundice, carotenemia does not affect the sclera, which remains white. The cause is a diet high in carrots and other yellow vegetables or fruits. Carotenemia is not harmful but indicates the need for assessing dietary intake.

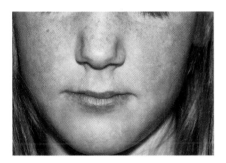

Erythema

Red hue, increased blood flow, seen here as the "slapped cheeks" of erythema infectiosum ("fifth disease").

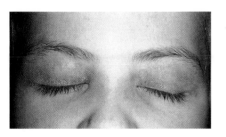

Heliotrope

Violaceous eruption over the eyelids in the collagen vascular disease dermatomyositis.

(Sources of photos: *Tinea Versicolor*—Ostler HB, Mailbach HI, Hoke AW, Schwab IR. Diseases of the Eye and Skin: A Color Atlas. Philadelphia, Lippincott Williams & Wilkins, 2004; *Vitiligo, Erythema*—Goodheart HP. Goodheart's Photoguide of Common Skin Disorders: Diagnosis and Management, 2nd ed. Philadelphia, Lippincott Williams & Wilkins, 2003; *Heliotrope*—Hall JC. Sauer's Manual of Skin Diseases, 8th ed. Philadelphia, Lippincott Williams & Wilkins, 2000)

TABLE 5-2	Skin Lesions—Anatomic Location and Distribution

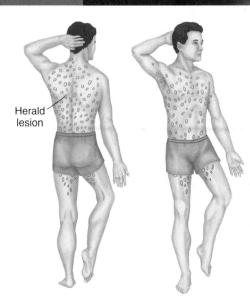

Pityriasis Rosea
Reddish oval ringworm-like lesions

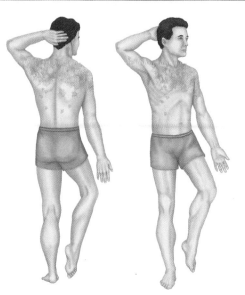

Tinea Versicolor
Tan, flat, scaly lesions

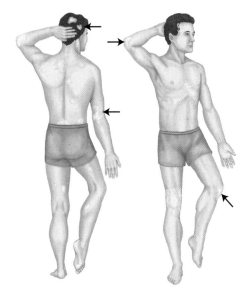

Psoriasis
Silvery scaly lesions, mainly on the extensor surfaces

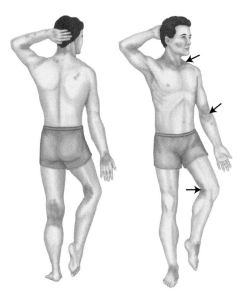

Atopic Eczema (adult form)
Appears mainly on flexor surfaces

(Source: Hall JC. *Sauer's Manual of Skin Diseases*, 8th ed. Philadelphia, Lippincott Williams & Wilkins, 2000)

TABLE 5-3   Skin Lesions—Patterns and Shapes

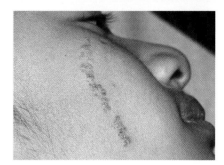

Linear
Example: Linear epidermal nevus

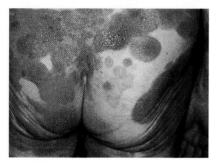

Geographic
Example: Mycosis fungoides

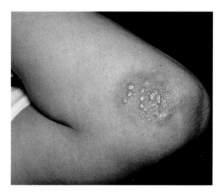

Clustered
Example: Grouped lesions of herpes simplex

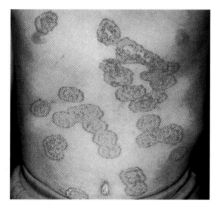

Serpiginous
Example: Tinea corporis

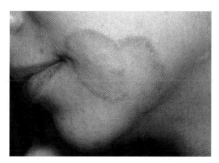

Annular, arciform
Example: Annular lesion of tinea faciale (ringworm)

(Sources of photos: *Linear Epidermal Nevus, Herpes Simplex, Tinea Faciale*—Goodheart HP. Goodheart's Photoguide of Common Skin Disorders: Diagnosis and Management, 2nd ed. Philadelphia, Lippincott Williams & Wilkins, 2003; *Mycosis Fungoides, Tinea Corporis*—Hall JC. Sauer's Manual of Skin Diseases, 8th ed. Philadelphia, Lippincott Williams & Wilkins, 2000)

TABLE 5-4   Elevated Skin Lesions

Primary Lesions

Flat, Nonpalpable Lesions With Changes in Skin Color
Macule—Small flat spot, up to 1.0 cm

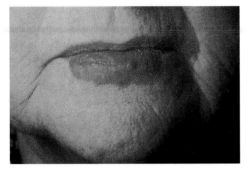

Hemangioma

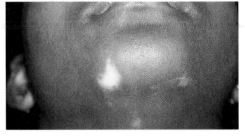

Vitiligo

Patch—Flat spot, 1.0 cm or larger

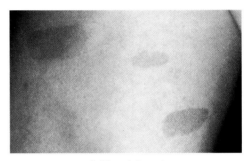

Café-au-lait spot

Palpable Elevations: Solid Masses
Plaque—Elevated superficial lesion 1.0 cm or larger, often formed by coalescence of papules

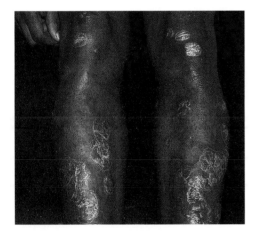

Psoriasis

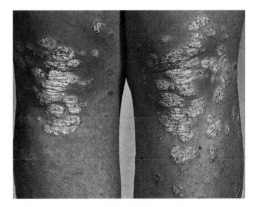

Psoriasis

(table continues next page)

TABLE 5-4   Elevated Skin Lesions *(Continued)*

Papule—Up to 1.0 cm

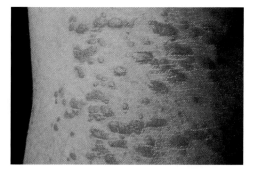

Psoriasis

Nodule—Marble-like lesion larger than 0.5 cm, often deeper and firmer than a papule

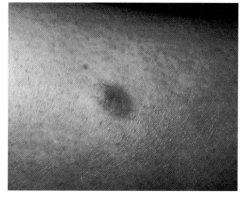

Dermatofibroma

Cyst—Nodule filled with expressible material, either liquid or semisolid

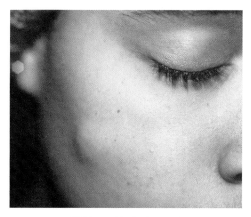

Epidermal inclusion cyst

Wheal—A somewhat irregular, relatively transient, superficial area of localized skin edema

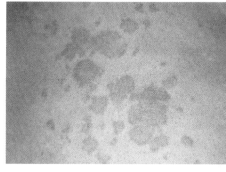

Urticaria

Palpable Elevations With Fluid-Filled Cavities
Vesicle—Up to 1.0 cm; filled with serous fluid

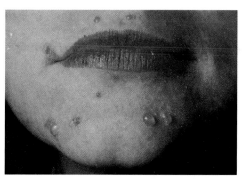

Herpes simplex

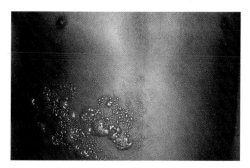

Herpes simplex

(table continues next page)

TABLE 5-4   **Elevated Skin Lesions** (*Continued*)

Bulla—1.0 cm or larger; filled with serous fluid

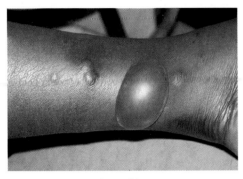

Insect bite

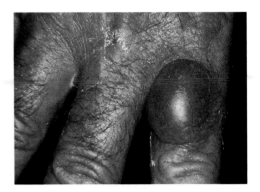

Insect bite

Pustule—Filled with pus

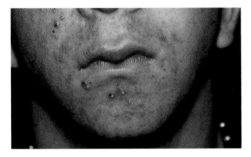

Acne

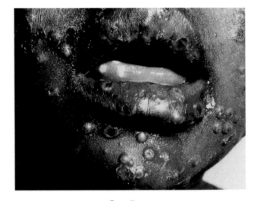

Small pox

Burrow (scabies)—A minute, slightly raised tunnel in the epidermis, commonly found on the finger webs and on the sides of the fingers. It looks like a short (5–15 mm), linear or curved gray line and may end in a tiny vesicle. Skin lesions include small papules, pustules, lichenified areas, and excoriations. With a magnifying lens, look for the *burrow* of the mite that causes scabies.

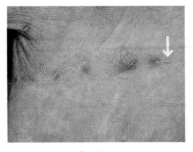

Scabies

(table continues next page)

TABLE 5-4   Elevated Skin Lesions *(Continued)*

Secondary Lesions (may arise from primary lesions)

Scale—A thin flake of dead exfoliated epidermis.

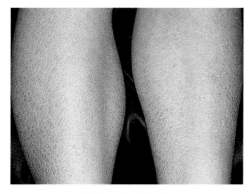

Ichthyosis vulgaris

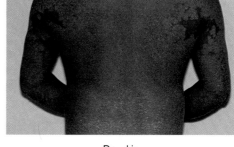

Dry skin

Crust—The dried residue of skin exudates such as serum, pus, or blood

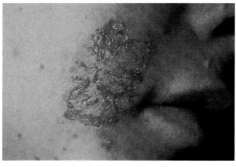

Impetigo

Lichenification—Visible and palpable thickening of the epidermis and roughening of the skin with increased visibility of the normal skin furrows (often from chronic rubbing)

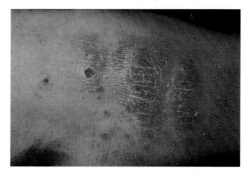

Neurodermatitis

Scars—Connective tissue that arises from injury or disease

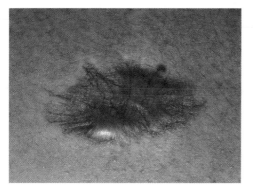

Hypertrophic scar from steroid injections

Keloids—Hypertrophic scarring that extends beyond the borders of the initiating injury

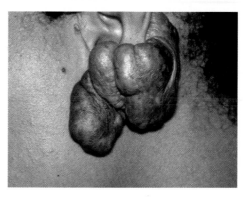

Keloid—ear lobe

Sources of photos: *Hemangioma, Café-au-Lait Spot, Elevated Nevus, Psoriasis (bottom), Dermatofibroma, Herpes Simplex, Insect Bite (bottom), Impetigo, Lichenification*—Hall JC. Sauer's Manual of Skin Diseases, 8th ed. Philadelphia, Lippincott Williams & Wilkins, 2000; *Vitiligo, Psoriasis (top), Epidermal Inclusion Cyst, Urticaria, Insect Bite (top), Acne, Ichthyosis, Psoriasis, Hypertrophic Scar, Keloids*—Goodheart HP. Goodheart's Photoguide of Common Skin Disorders: Diagnosis and Management, 2nd ed. Philadelphia, Lippincott Williams & Wilkins, 2003; *Small Pox*—Ostler HB, Mailbach HI, Hoke AW, Schwab IR. Diseases of the Eye and Skin: A Color Atlas. Philadelphia, Lippincott Williams & Wilkins, 2004)

TABLE 5-5	Depressed Skin Lesions*

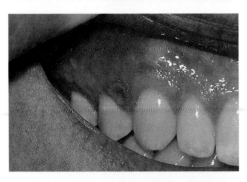

Erosion—Nonscarring loss of the superficial epidermis; surface is moist but does not bleed

   Example: Aphthous stomatitis, moist area after the rupture of a vesicle, as in chickenpox

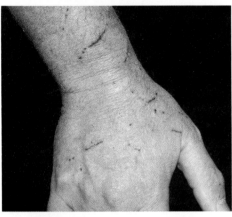

Excoriation—Linear or punctate erosions caused by scratching

   Example: Cat scratches

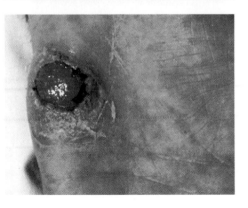

Fissure—A linear crack in the skin, often resulting from excessive dryness

   Example: Athlete's foot

Ulcer—A deeper loss of epidermis and dermis; may bleed and scar

   Examples: Stasis ulcer of venous insufficiency, syphilitic chancre

---

*These are secondary lesions (resulting from primary lesions).
(Sources of photos: *Erosion, Excoriation, Fissure*—Goodheart HP: Goodheart's Photoguide of Common Skin Disorders: Diagnosis and Management, 2nd ed. Philadelphia, Lippincott Williams & Wilkins, 2003; *Ulcer*—Hall JC: Sauer's Manual of Skin Diseases, 8th ed. Philadelphia, Lippincott Williams & Wilkins, 2000)

TABLE 5-6

Vascular and Purpuric Lesions of the Skin

Vascular Lesions

	Spider Angioma*	Spider Vein*	Cherry Angioma
Color and Size	Fiery red. From very small to 2 cm	Bluish. Size variable, from very small to several inches	Bright or ruby red; may become brownish with age. 1–3 mm
Shape	Central body, sometimes raised, surrounded by erythema and radiating legs	Variable. May resemble a spider or be linear, irregular, cascading	Round, flat or sometimes raised, may be surrounded by a pale halo
Pulsatility and Effect of Pressure	Often seen in center of the spider, when pressure with a glass slide is applied. Pressure on the body causes blanching of the spider.	Absent. Pressure over the center does not cause blanching, but diffuse pressure blanches the veins.	Absent. May show partial blanching, especially if pressure applied with edge of a pinpoint
Distribution	Face, neck, arms, and upper trunk; almost never below the waist	Most often on the legs, near veins; also on the anterior chest	Trunk; also extremities
Significance	Liver disease, pregnancy, vitamin B deficiency; also occurs normally in some people	Often accompanies increased pressure in the superficial veins, as in varicose veins	None; increase in size and numbers with aging

Purpuric Lesions

	Petechia/Purpura	Ecchymosis
Color and Size	Deep red or reddish purple, fading away over time. Petechia, 1–3 mm; purpura, larger	Purple or purplish blue, fading to green, yellow, and brown with time. Variable size, larger than petechiae, >3 mm
Shape	Rounded, sometimes irregular; flat	Rounded, oval, or irregular; may have a central subcutaneous flat nodule (a hematoma)
Pulsatility and Effect of Pressure	Absent. No effect from pressure	Absent. No effect from pressure
Distribution	Variable	Variable
Significance	Blood outside the vessels; may suggest a bleeding disorder or, if petechiae, emboli to skin; palpable purpura in *vasculitis*	Blood outside the vessels; often secondary to bruising or trauma; also seen in bleeding disorders

*These are telangiectasias, or dilated small vessels that look red or bluish.

(Sources of photos: *Spider Angioma*—Marks R: Skin Disease in Old Age. Philadelphia, JB Lippincott, 1987; *Petechia/Purpura*—Kelley WN: Textbook of Internal Medicine. Philadelphia, JB Lippincott, 1989)

TABLE 5-7 **Skin Tumors**

Actinic Keratosis

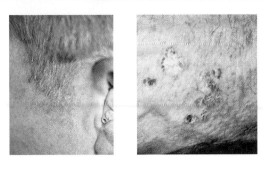

Superficial, flattened papules covered by a dry scale. Often multiple; can be round or irregular; pink, tan, or grayish. Appear on sun-exposed skin of older, fair-skinned persons. Though benign, 1 of every 1,000 per year develop into squamous cell carcinoma (suggested by rapid growth, induration, redness at the base, and ulceration). Keratoses on face and hand, typical locations, are shown.

Seborrheic Keratosis

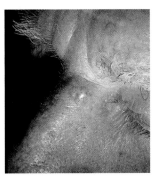

Common, benign, yellowish to brown raised lesions that feel slightly greasy and velvety or warty and have a "stuck on" appearance. Typically multiple and symmetrically distributed on the trunk of older people, but may also appear on the face and elsewhere. In black people, often younger women, may appear as small, deeply pigmented papules on the cheeks and temples (dermatosis papulosa nigra).

Basal Cell Carcinoma

A basal cell carcinoma, though malignant, grows slowly and seldom metastasizes. It is most common in fair-skinned adults over age 40, and usually appears on the face. An initial translucent nodule spreads, leaving a depressed center and a firm, elevated border. Telangiectatic vessels are often visible.

Squamous Cell Carcinoma

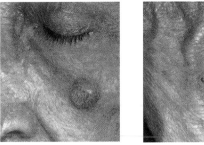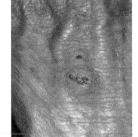

Usually appears on sun-exposed skin of fair-skinned adults older than 60. May develop in an actinic keratosis. Usually grows more quickly than a basal cell carcinoma, is firmer, and looks redder. The face and the back of the hand are often affected, as shown here.

(Sources of photos: *Basal Cell Carcinoma*—Rapini R. *Squamous Cell Carcinoma, Actinic Keratosis, Seborrheic Keratosis*—Sauer GC. Manual of Skin Diseases, 5th ed. Philadelphia, JB Lippincott, 1985)

TABLE 5-8   Benign and Malignant Nevi

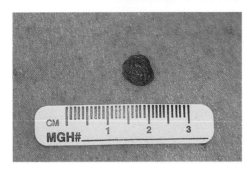

Benign Nevus

The *benign nevus*, or common mole, usually appears in the first few decades. Several nevi may arise at the same time, but their appearance usually remains unchanged. Note the following typical features and contrast them with those of atypical nevi and melanoma:

- Round or oval shape
- Sharply defined borders
- Uniform color, especially tan or brown
- Diameter <6 mm
- Flat or raised surface

Changes in these features raise the the spectre of *atypical (dysplastic) nevi*, or melanoma. Atypical nevi are varied in color but often dark and larger than 6 mm, with irregular borders that fade into the surrounding skin. Look for atypical nevi primarily on the trunk. They may number more than 50 to 100.

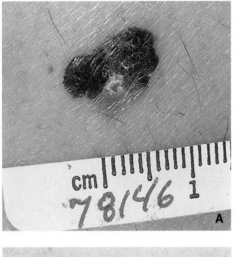

A

Malignant Melanoma

Learn the **ABCDEs** of melanoma from these reference standard photographs from the American Cancer Society:

- *Asymmetry* (Fig. A)
- Irregular *Borders*, especially notching (Fig. B)
- Variation in *Color*, especially mixtures of black, blue, and red (Figs. B, C)
- *Diameter* >6 mm (Fig. C)
- *Elevation*, though also may be flat (Fig. C)

Review *melanoma risk factors* such as intense year-round sun exposure, blistering sunburns in childhood, fair skin that freckles or burns easily (especially if blond or red hair), family history of melanoma, and nevi that are changing or atypical, especially if >50. Changing nevi may have new swelling or redness beyond the border, scaling, oozing, or bleeding, or sensations such as itching, burning, or pain.

On darker skin, look for melanomas under the nails, on the hands, or on the soles of the feet.

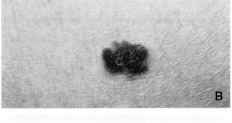

B

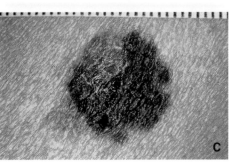

C

(Source: Courtesy of American Cancer Society; American Academy of Dermatology)

| TABLE 5-9 | Skin Lesions in Context |

This table shows a variety of primary and secondary skin lesions. Try to identify them, including those indicated by letters, before reading the accompanying text.

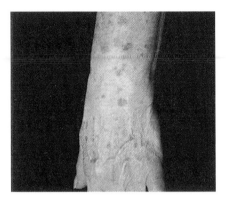

Macules on the dorsum of the hand, wrist, and forearm (*actinic lentigines*)

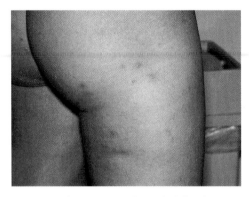

Papules and pustules (in hot tub folliculitis from *Pseudomonas*)

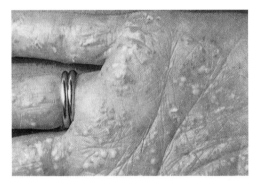

Pustules on the palm (in *pustular psoriasis*)

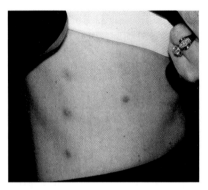

Vesicles (*chickenpox*)

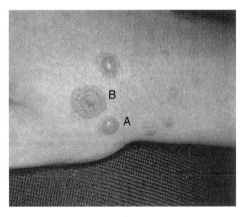

(A) Bulla, (B) target (or iris) lesion (in *erythema multiforme*)

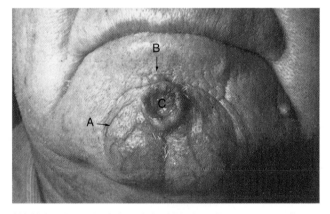

(A) Telangiectasia, (B) nodule, (C) ulcer (in *squamous cell carcinoma*)

(table continues next page)

TABLE 5-9   **Skin Lesions in Context** *(Continued)*

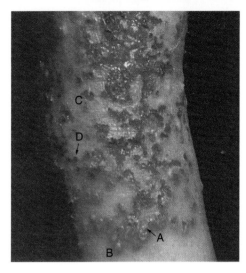

(A) Vesicle, (B) pustule, (C) erosions, (D) crust, on the back of a knee (in *infected atopic dermatitis*)

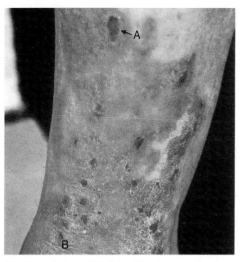

(A) Excoriation, (B) lichenification on the leg (in *atopic dermatitis*)

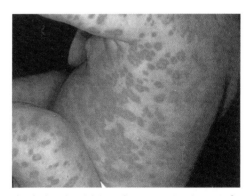

Wheals (*urticaria*) in a drug eruption in an infant

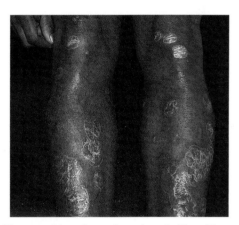

Plaques with scales on knee (*psoriasis*) and legs

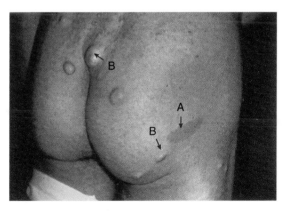

(A) Patch (café-au-lait spots), (B) nodules—a combination typical of neurofibromatosis.

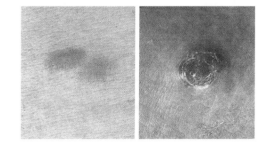

Kaposi's sarcoma in AIDS: This malignant tumor may appear in many forms: macules, papules, plaques, or nodules almost anywhere on the body. Lesions are often multiple and may involve internal structures. On left: ovoid, pinkish red plaques that typically lengthen along the skin line may become pigmented. On right: a purplish red nodule on the foot.

(Sources of photos: Sauer GC: Manual of Skin Diseases, 5th ed. Philadelphia, JB Lippincott, 1985; *Kaposi's Sarcoma in AIDS*—DeVita VT Jr, Hellman S, Rosenberg SA [eds]: AIDS: Etiology, Diagnosis, Treatment, and Prevention. Philadelphia, JB Lippincott, 1985; *Psoriasis, Papules, Vesicles (chickenpox)*—Goodheart HP. Goodheart's Photoguide of Common Skin Disorders: Diagnosis and Management, 2nd ed. Philadelphia, Lippincott Williams & Wilkins, 2003)

| TABLE 5-10 | Diseases and Related Skin Conditions |

Addison's disease	Hyperpigmentation of skin and mucous membranes
AIDS	Hairy leukoplakia, Kaposi's sarcoma, herpes simplex virus (HSV), human papillomavirus (HPV), cytomegalovirus (CMV), molluscum contagiosum, mycobacterial skin infections, candidiasis and other cutaneous fungal infections, oral and anal squamous cell carcinoma, acquired ichthyosis, bacterial abscesses, psoriasis (often severe), erythroderma, seborrheic dermatitis (often severe)
Chronic renal disease	Pallor, xerosis, pruritus, hyperpigmentation, uremic frost, metastatic calcification in the skin, calciphylaxis, "half and half" nails, hemodialysis-related skin disease
CREST syndrome	Calcinosis, Raynaud's phenomenon, sclerodactyly, telangiectasias
Crohn's disease	Erythema nodosum, pyoderma gangrenosum, enterocutaneous fistulas, aphthous ulcers
Cushing's disease	Striae, skin atrophy, purpura, ecchymoses, telangiectasias, acne, moon facies, buffalo hump, hypertrichosis
Dermatomyositis	Heliotrope rash, Gottron's papules, periungual telangiectasias, alopecia, poikiloderma in sun-exposed areas, Raynaud's phenomenon
Diabetes	Necrobiosis lipoidica diabeticorum, diabetic bullae, diabetic dermopathy, granuloma annulare, acanthosis nigricans, candidiasis, neuropathic ulcers, eruptive xanthomas, peripheral vascular disease
Disseminated intravascular coagulation	Skin necrosis, petechiae, ecchymoses, hemorrhagic bullae, purpura fulminans
Dyslipidemias	Xanthomas (tendon, eruptive, and tuberous), xanthelasma (may occur in healthy people)
Gonococcemia	Erythematous macules to hemorrhagic pustules; lesions in acral distribution that can involve palms and soles
Hemochromatosis	Skin bronzing and hyperpigmentation
Hypothyroidism	Dry, rough, and pale skin; coarse and brittle hair; myxedema; alopecia (lateral third of the eyebrows to diffuse); skin cool to touch; thin and brittle nails
Hyperthyroidism	Warm, moist, soft, and velvety skin; thin and fine hair; alopecia; vitiligo; pretibial myxedema (in Graves' disease); hyperpigmentation (local or generalized)
Infective endocarditis	Janeway lesions, Osler nodes, splinter hemorrhages, petechiae
Kawasaki disease	Mucosal erythema (lips, tongue, and pharynx), strawberry tongue, cherry red lips, polymorphous rash (primarily on trunk), erythema of palms and soles with later desquamation of fingertips
Liver disease	Jaundice, spider angiomas and other telangiectasias, palmar erythema, Terry's nails, pruritus, purpura, caput medusae
Leukemia/lymphoma	Pallor, exfoliative erythroderma, nodules, petechiae, ecchymoses, pruritus, vasculitis, pyoderma gangrenosum, bullous diseases
Meningococcemia	Pink macules and papules, petechiae, hemorrhagic petechiae, hemorrhagic bullae, purpura fulminans
Neurofibromatoses 1 (von Recklinghausen's syndrome)	Neurofibromas, café au lait, freckling in the axillary and inguinal areas, plexiform neurofibroma
Pancreatitis (hemorrhagic)	Grey Turner sign, Cullen's sign, panniculitis
Pancreatic carcinoma	Panniculitis, migratory thrombophlebitis
Peripheral vascular disease	Dry, scaly, shiny atrophic skin; dystrophic, brittle toenails; cool skin; hairless shins; ulcers; pallor; cyanosis; gangrene
Pregnancy (physiologic changes)	Melasma, increased pigmentation of areolae, linea nigra, palmar erythema, varicose veins, striae, spider angiomas, hirsutism, pyogenic granuloma
Reiter's syndrome	Psoriasis-like skin and mucous membrane lesions, keratoderma blennorrhagicum, balanitis circinata

(table continues next page)

TABLE 5-10   **Diseases and Related Skin Conditions** *(Continued)*

TABLE 5

Rheumatoid arthritis	Vasculitis, Raynaud's phenomenon, rheumatoid nodules, pyo... rheumatoid papules, erythematous to salmon-colored rashes
Rocky Mountain spotted fever	Erythematous rash that begins on wrists and ankles, then s... becomes more purpuric as it generalizes
Scleroderma	Thickened, taut, and shiny skin; ulcerations and pitted scars on finge... telangiectasias; Raynaud's phenomenon
Sickle cell	Jaundice, leg ulcers (malleolar regions), pallor
Syphilis	*1°:* Chancre (painless) *2°:* Rash ("the great imitator")—ham- to bronze-colored, generalized, maculopapular rash that involves the palms and soles, pustules, condylomata lata, alopecia ("moth-eaten"), white plaques on oral and genital mucosa *3°:* Gummas, granulomas
Systemic lupus erythematosus	Photosensitivity, malar (butterfly) rash, discoid rash, alopecia, vasculitis, oral ulcers, Raynaud's phenomenon
Thrombocytopenic purpura	Petechiae, ecchymoses
Tuberous sclerosis	Adenoma sebaceum (angiofibromas), ash-leaf spots, shagreen patch, perungual fibromas
Ulcerative colitis	Erythema nodosum, pyoderma gangrenosum
Viral exanthems	*Coxsackie A (hand, foot, and mouth):* Oral ulcers; macules, papules, and vesicles on hands, feet, and buttocks *Erythema infectiosum (fifth disease):* Erythema of cheeks ("slapped cheeks") followed by erythematous, pruritic, reticulated (net-like) rash that starts on trunk and proximal extremities (rash worsens with sun, fever, and temperature changes) *Roseola infantum (HSV 6):* Erythematous, maculopapular, discrete rash (often fever present) that begins on head and spreads to involve trunk and extremities, petechiae on soft palate *Rubella (German measles):* Erythematous, maculopapular, discrete rash (often fever present) that begins on head and spreads to involve trunk and extremities, petechiae on soft palate *Rubeola (measles):* Erythematous, maculopapular rash that begins on head and spreads to involve trunk and extremities (lesions become confluent on face and trunk, but are discrete on extremities), Koplik spots on buccal mucosa *Varicella (chickenpox):* Generalized, pruritic, vesicular (vesicles on an erythematous base, "dewdrop on a rose petal") rash begins on trunk and spreads peripherally, lesions appear in crops and are in different stages of healing *Herpes zoster (shingles):* Pruritic, vesicular rash (vesicles on an erythematous base) in a dermatomal distribution

[Press]ure ulcers, also termed *decubitus* ulcers, usually develop over body prominences subject to unrelieved pressure, resulting in [isch]emic damage to underlying tissue. Prevention is important: inspect the skin thoroughly for *early warning signs* of erythema that [bl]anches with pressure, especially in patients with risk factors.

Pressure ulcers form most commonly over the sacrum, ischial tuberosities, greater trochanters, and heels. A commonly applied staging system, based on depth of destroyed tissue, is illustrated below. Note that necrosis or eschar must be débrided before ulcers can be staged; and ulcers may not progress sequentially through the four stages.

Inspect ulcers for signs of infection (drainage, odor, cellulitis, or necrosis). Fever, chills, and pain suggest underlying osteomyelitis. Address the patient's overall health, including *comorbid conditions* such as vascular disease, diabetes, immune deficiencies, collagen vascular disease, malignancy, psychosis, or depression; nutritional status; pain and level of analgesia; risk for recurrence; psychosocial factors such as learning ability, social supports, and lifestyle; and evidence of polypharmacy, overmedication, or abuse of alcohol, tobacco, or illicit drugs.

Risk Factors for Pressure Ulcers

- Decreased mobility, especially if accompanied by increased pressure or movement causing friction or shear stress
- Decreased sensation, from brain or spinal cord lesions or peripheral nerve disease

- Decreased blood flow from hypotension or microvascular disease such as diabetes or atherosclerosis
- Fecal or urinary incontinence
- Presence of fracture
- Poor nutritional status or low albumin

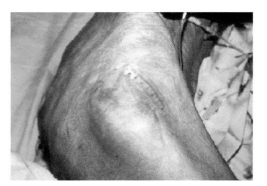

Stage I
Pressure-related alteration of intact skin, with changes in temperature (warmth or coolness), consistency (firm or boggy), sensation (pain or itching), or color (red, blue, or purple on darker skin; red on lighter skin)

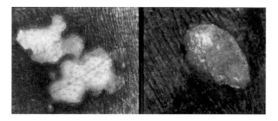

Stage II
Partial-thickness skin loss or ulceration involving the epidermis, dermis, or both

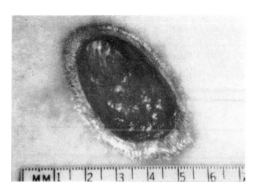

Stage III
Full-thickness skin loss, with damage to or necrosis of subcutaneous tissue that may extend to, but not through, underlying muscle

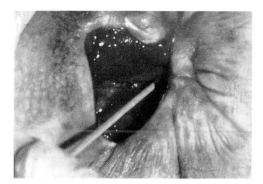

Stage IV
Full-thickness skin loss, with destruction, tissue necrosis, or damage to underlying muscle, bone, or supporting structures

(Source: National Pressure Ulcer Advisory Panel, Reston, VA)

TABLE 5-12 | **Hair Loss**

Alopecia Areata

Clearly demarcated round or oval patches of hair loss, usually affecting young adults and children. There is no visible scaling or inflammation.

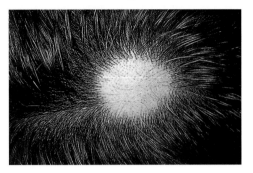
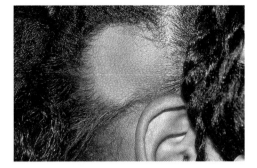

Trichotillomania

Hair loss from pulling, plucking, or twisting hair. Hair shafts are broken and of varying lengths. More common in children, often in settings of family or psychosocial stress.

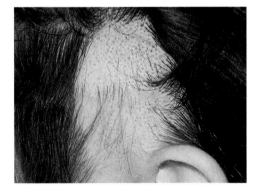
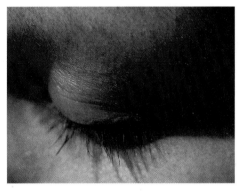

Tinea Capitis ("Ringworm")

Round scaling patches of alopecia. Hairs are broken off close to the surface of the scalp. Usually caused by fungal infection from *tinea tonsurans*. Mimics seborrheic dermatitis.

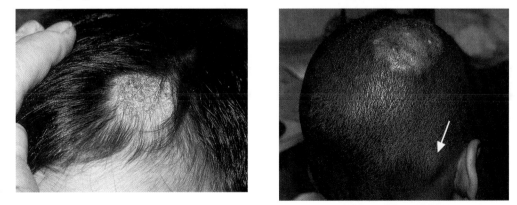

(Sources of photos: *Alopecia Areata (left)*, *Trichotillomania (top)*—Hall JC. Sauer's Manual of Skin Diseases, 8th ed. Philadelphia, Lippincott Williams & Wilkins, 2000; *Alopecia Areata (bottom)*, *Tinea Capitis*—Goodheart HP. Goodheart's Photoguide of Common Skin Disorders: Diagnosis and Management, 2nd ed. Philadelphia, Lippincott Williams & Wilkins, 2003; *Trichotillomania (bottom)*—Ostler HB, Mailbach HI, Hoke AW, Schwab IR. Diseases of the Eye and Skin: A Color Atlas. Philadelphia, Lippincott Williams & Wilkins, 2004)

TABLE 5-13   **Findings in or Near the Nails**

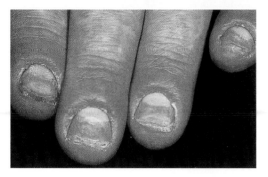

Paronychia

An inflammation of the proximal and lateral nail folds that may be acute or, as illustrated, chronic. The folds are red, swollen, and often tender. The cuticle may not be visible. People who frequently immerse their nails in water are especially susceptible. Multiple nails are often affected.

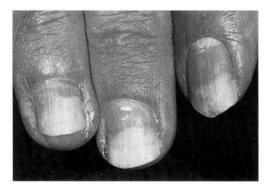

Onycholysis

A painless separation of the nail plate from the nail bed. It starts distally, enlarging the free edge of the nail to a varying degree. Several or all nails are usually affected. There are many causes.

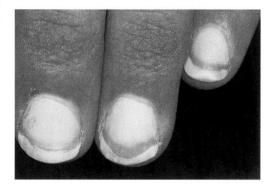

Terry's Nails

Nails are mostly whitish with a distal band of reddish brown. The lunulae of the nails may not be visible. Seen with aging and in people with chronic diseases such as cirrhosis of the liver, congestive heart failure, and non-insulin-dependent diabetes.

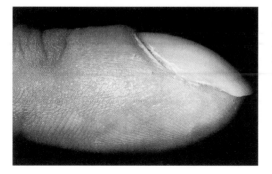

Clubbing of the Fingers

The distal phalanx of each finger is rounded and bulbous. The nail plate is more convex, and the angle between the plate and the proximal nail fold increases to 180° or more. The proximal nail fold, when palpated, feels spongy or floating. Causes are many, including chronic hypoxia from heart disease or lung cancer and hepatic cirrhosis.

(table continues next page)

TABLE 5-13 · **Findings in or Near the Nails** *(Continued)*

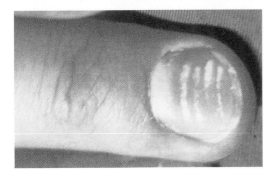

White Spots *(Leukonychia)*

Trauma to the nails is commonly followed by white spots that grow slowly out with the nail. Spots in the pattern illustrated are typical of overly vigorous and repeated manicuring. The curves in this example resemble the curve of the cuticle and proximal nail fold.

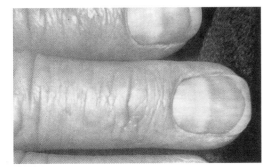

Transverse White Lines *(Mees' Lines)*

These are transverse lines, not spots, and their curves are similar to those of the lunula, not the cuticle. These uncommon lines may follow an acute or severe illness. They emerge from under the proximal nail folds and grow out with the nails.

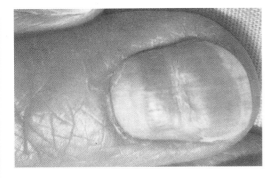

Beau's Lines

Beau's lines are transverse depressions in the nails associated with acute severe illness. The lines emerge from under the proximal nail folds weeks later and grow gradually out with the nails. As with Mees' lines, clinicians may be able to estimate the timing of a causal illness.

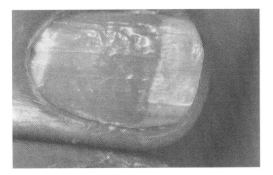

Psoriasis

Small pits in the nails may be early signs of psoriasis but are not specific for it. Additional findings, not shown here, include onycholysis and a circumscribed yellowish tan discoloration known as an "oil spot" lesion. Marked thickening of the nails may develop.

(Sources of photos: *Clubbing of the Fingers, Paronychia, Onycholysis, Terry's Nails*—Habif TP. Clinical Dermatology: A Color Guide to Diagnosis and Therapy, 2nd ed. St. Louis, CV Mosby, 1990; *White Spots, Transverse White Lines, Psoriasis, Beau's Lines*—Sams WM Jr, Lynch PJ. Principles and Practice of Dermatology. New York, Churchill Livingstone, 1990)

The Head and Neck

ANATOMY AND PHYSIOLOGY

THE HEAD

Regions of the head take their names from the underlying bones of the skull, for example, the frontal area. Knowing this anatomy helps to locate and describe physical findings.

Two paired salivary glands lie near the mandible: the *parotid gland,* superficial to and behind the mandible (both visible and palpable when enlarged), and the *submandibular gland,* located deep to the mandible. Feel for the latter as you bow and press your tongue against your lower incisors. Its lobular surface can often be felt against the tightened muscle. The openings of the parotid and submandibular ducts are visible within the oral cavity (see p. 167).

The *superficial temporal artery* passes upward just in front of the ear, where it is readily palpable. In many normal people, especially thin and elderly ones, the tortuous course of one of its branches can be traced across the forehead.

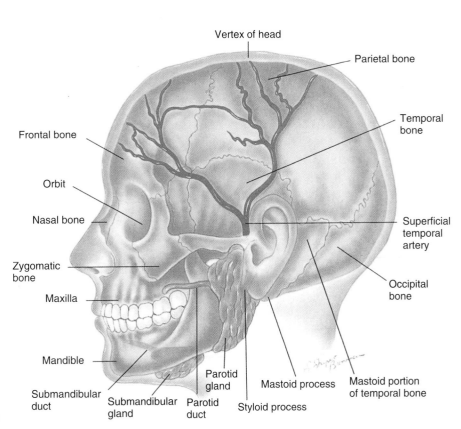

Vertex of head

Parietal bone

Temporal bone

Frontal bone

Orbit

Nasal bone

Superficial temporal artery

Zygomatic bone

Occipital bone

Maxilla

Mandible

Submandibular duct

Parotid gland

Mastoid process

Mastoid portion of temporal bone

Submandibular gland

Parotid duct

Styloid process

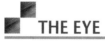

THE EYE

Anatomy. Begin by identifying the structures illustrated on this page. Note that the upper eyelid covers a portion of the iris but does not normally overlay the pupil. The opening between the eyelids is called the *palpebral fissure.* The white sclera may look somewhat buff colored at its periphery. Do not mistake this color for jaundice, which is a deeper yellow.

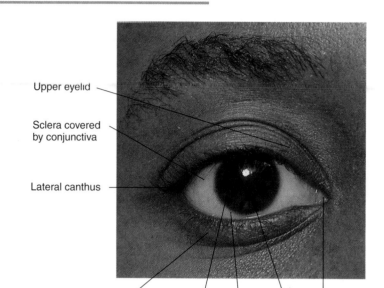

The *conjunctiva* is a clear mucous membrane with two easily visible components. The *bulbar conjunctiva* covers most of the anterior eyeball, adhering loosely to the underlying tissue. It meets the cornea at the *limbus.* The *palpebral conjunctiva* lines the eyelids. The two parts of the conjunctiva merge in a folded recess that permits movement of the eyeball.

Within the eyelids lie firm strips of connective tissue called *tarsal plates.* Each plate contains a parallel row of *meibomian glands,* which open on the lid margin. The *levator palpebrae* the muscle, which raises the upper eyelid, is innervated by the oculomotor nerve, Cranial Nerve III. Smooth muscle, innervated by the sympathetic nervous system, also contributes to lid elevation.

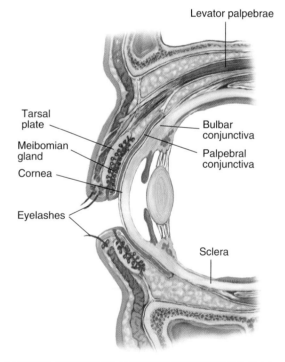

SAGITTAL SECTION OF ANTERIOR EYE WITH LIDS CLOSED

A film of tear fluid protects the conjunctiva and cornea from drying, inhibits microbial growth, and gives a smooth optical surface to the cornea. This fluid comes from the meibomian glands, conjunctival glands, and the lacrimal gland. The *lacrimal gland* lies mostly within the bony orbit, above and lateral to the eyeball. The tear fluid spreads across the eye and drains medially through two tiny holes called *lacrimal puncta*. The tears then pass into the *lacrimal sac* and on into the nose through the *nasolacrimal duct*. You can easily find a *punctum* atop the small elevation of the lower lid medially. The lacrimal sac rests in a small depression inside the bony orbit and is not visible.

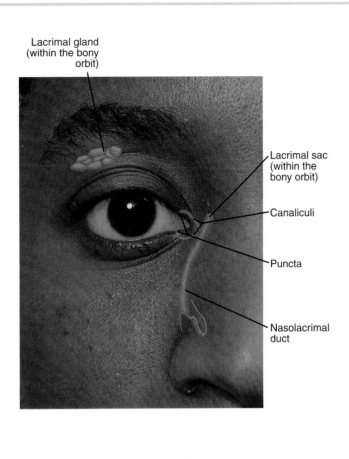

The eyeball is a spherical structure that focuses light on the neurosensory elements within the retina. The muscles of the iris control pupillary size. Muscles of the *ciliary body* control the thickness of the lens, allowing the eye to focus on near or distant objects.

A clear liquid called *aqueous humor* fills the anterior and posterior chambers of the eye. Aqueous humor is produced by the *ciliary body*, circulates from the posterior chamber through the pupil into the anterior chamber, and drains out through the *canal of Schlemm*. This circulatory system helps to control the pressure inside the eye.

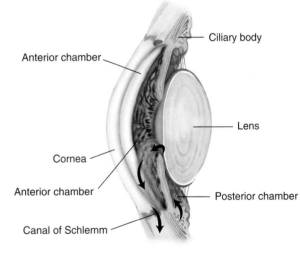

CIRCULATION OF AQUEOUS HUMOR

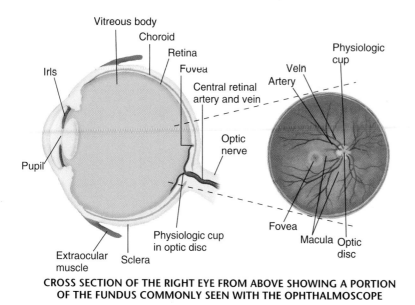

CROSS SECTION OF THE RIGHT EYE FROM ABOVE SHOWING A PORTION OF THE FUNDUS COMMONLY SEEN WITH THE OPHTHALMOSCOPE

The posterior part of the eye that is seen through an ophthalmoscope is often called the *fundus* of the eye. Structures here include the retina, choroid, fovea, macula, optic disc, and retinal vessels. The optic nerve with its retinal vessels enters the eyeball posteriorly. You can find it with an ophthalmoscope at the *optic disc*. Lateral and slightly inferior to the disc, there is a small depression in the retinal surface that marks the point of central vision. Around it is a darkened circular area called the *fovea*. The roughly circular *macula* (named for a microscopic yellow spot) surrounds the fovea but has no discernible margins. It does not quite reach the optic disc. You do not usually see the normal *vitreous body*, a transparent mass of gelatinous material that fills the eyeball behind the lens. It helps to maintain the shape of the eye.

Visual Fields.   A *visual field* is the entire area seen by an eye when it looks at a central point. Fields are conventionally diagrammed on circles from the patient's point of view. The center of the circle represents the focus of gaze. The circumference is 90° from the line of gaze. Each visual field, shown by the white areas below, is divided into quadrants. Note that the fields extend farthest on the temporal sides. Visual fields are normally limited by the brows above, the cheeks below, and the nose medially. A lack of retinal receptors at the optic disc produces an oval blind spot in the normal field of each eye, 15° temporal to the line of gaze.

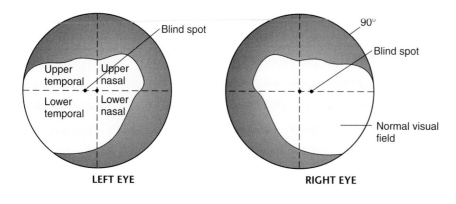

When a person is using both eyes, the two visual fields overlap in an area of binocular vision. Laterally, vision is monocular.

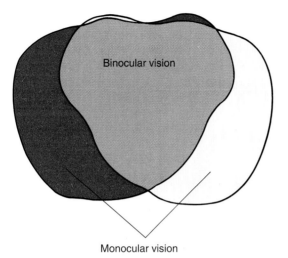

Binocular vision

Monocular vision

Visual Pathways. To see an image, light reflected from the image must pass through the pupil and be focused on sensory neurons in the retina. The image projected there is upside down and reversed right to left. An image from the upper nasal visual field thus strikes the lower temporal quadrant of the retina.

Nerve impulses, stimulated by light, are conducted through the retina, optic nerve, and optic tract on each side, then on through a curving tract called the *optic radiation*. This ends in the visual cortex, a part of the occipital lobe.

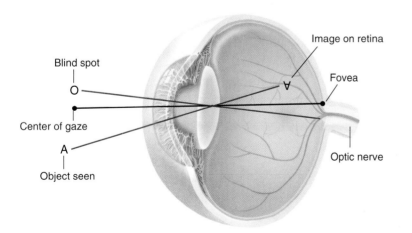

Blind spot

Image on retina

Fovea

O

Center of gaze

A

Object seen

Optic nerve

Pupillary Reactions. Pupillary size changes in response to light and to the effort of focusing on a near object.

The Light Reaction. A light beam shining onto one retina causes pupillary constriction in both that eye, termed the *direct reaction* to light, and in the opposite eye, the *consensual reaction*. The initial sensory pathways are similar to those described for vision: retina, optic nerve, and optic tract. The pathways diverge in the midbrain, however, and impulses are transmitted through the oculomotor nerve to the constrictor muscles of the iris of each eye.

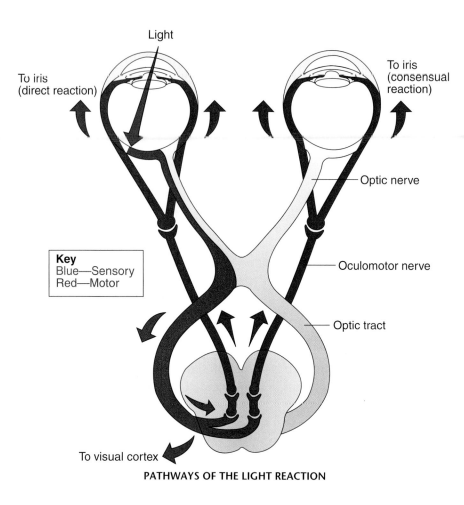

Key
Blue—Sensory
Red—Motor

PATHWAYS OF THE LIGHT REACTION

The Near Reaction. When a person shifts gaze from a far object to a near one, the pupils constrict. This response, like the light reaction, is mediated by the oculomotor nerve. Coincident with this pupillary reaction, but not part of it, are (1) *convergence* of the eyes, an extraocular movement; and (2) *accommodation*, an increased convexity of the lenses caused by contraction of the ciliary muscles. This change in shape of the lenses brings near objects into focus but is not visible to the examiner.

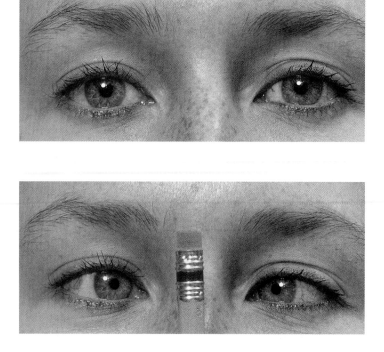

Autonomic Nerve Supply to the Eyes. Fibers travelling in the oculomotor nerve and producing pupillary constriction are part of the parasympathetic nervous system. The iris is also supplied by sympathetic fibers. When these are stimulated, the pupil dilates, and the upper eyelid rises a little, as if from fear. The sympathetic pathway starts in the hypothalamus and passes down through the brainstem and cervical cord into the neck. From there, it follows the carotid artery or its branches into the orbit. A lesion anywhere along this pathway may impair sympathetic effects on the pupil.

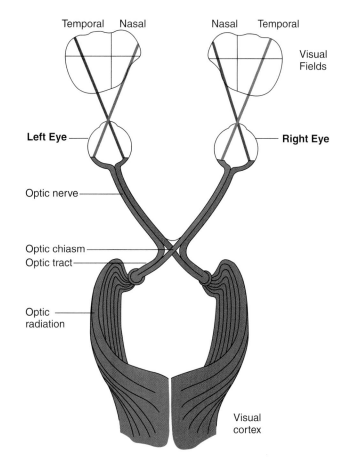

VISUAL PATHWAYS FROM THE RETINA TO THE VISUAL CORTEX

Extraocular Movements. The movement of each eye is controlled by the coordinated action of six muscles, the four rectus and two oblique muscles. You can test the function of each muscle and the nerve that supplies it by asking the patient to move the eye in the direction controlled by that muscle. There are six such *cardinal directions,* indicated by the lines on the figure below. When a person looks down and to the right, for example, the right inferior rectus (Cranial Nerve III) is principally responsible for moving the right eye, whereas the left superior oblique (Cranial Nerve IV) is principally responsible for moving the left. If one of these muscles is paralyzed, the eye will deviate from its normal position in that direction of gaze and the eyes will no longer appear conjugate, or parallel.

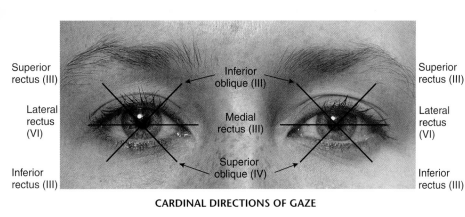

CARDINAL DIRECTIONS OF GAZE

THE EAR

Anatomy.　The ear has three compartments: the external ear, the middle ear, and the inner ear.

The *external ear* comprises the auricle and ear canal. The *auricle* consists chiefly of cartilage covered by skin and has a firm elastic consistency. Its prominent curved outer ridge is the *helix*. Parallel and anterior to the helix is another curved prominence, the *antihelix*. Inferiorly lies the fleshy projection of the earlobe, or *lobule*. The ear canal opens behind the *tragus*, a nodular eminence that points backward over the entrance to the canal.

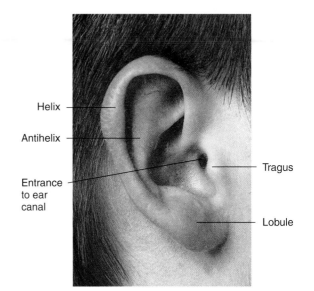

The *ear canal* curves inward approximately 24 mm. Cartilage surrounds its outer portion. The skin in this outer portion is hairy and contains glands that produce cerumen (wax). The inner portion of the canal is surrounded by bone and lined by thin, hairless skin. Pressure on this latter area causes pain—a point to remember when you examine the ear.

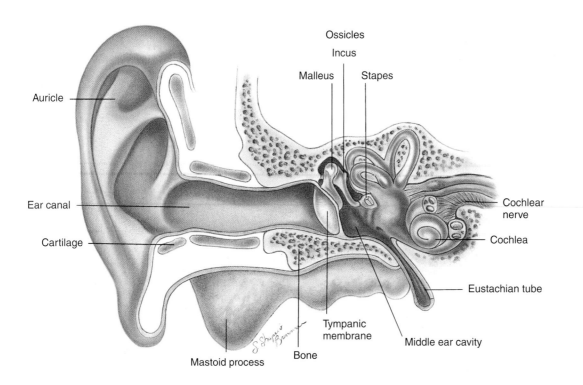

Behind and below the ear canal is the mastoid part of the temporal bone. The lowest portion of this bone, the *mastoid process,* is palpable behind the lobule.

At the end of the ear canal lies the *tympanic membrane,* or eardrum, marking the lateral limits of the middle ear. The *middle ear* is an air-filled cavity that transmits sound by way of three tiny bones, the *ossicles.* It is connected by the *eustachian tube* to the nasopharynx.

The eardrum is an oblique membrane held inward at its center by the *malleus,* one of its three ossicles. Find the *handle* and the *short process* of the malleus—the two chief landmarks. From the *umbo,* where the eardrum meets the tip of the malleus, a light reflection called the *cone of light* fans downward and anteriorly. Above the short process lies a small portion of the eardrum called the *pars flaccida.* The remainder of the drum is the *pars tensa.* Anterior and posterior malleolar folds, which extend obliquely upward from the short process, separate the pars flaccida from the pars tensa but are usually invisible unless the eardrum is retracted. A second ossicle, the *incus,* can sometimes be seen through the drum.

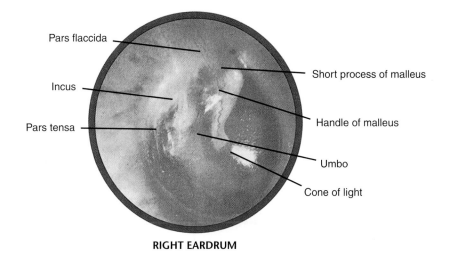

Pars flaccida

Incus

Pars tensa

Short process of malleus

Handle of malleus

Umbo

Cone of light

RIGHT EARDRUM

Much of the middle ear and all of the inner ear are inaccessible to direct examination. Some inferences concerning their condition can be made, however, by testing auditory function.

Pathways of Hearing. Vibrations of sound pass through the air of the external ear and are transmitted through the eardrum and ossicles of the middle ear to the *cochlea,* a part of the inner ear. The cochlea senses and codes the vibrations, and nerve impulses are sent to the brain through the cochlear nerve. The first part of this pathway—from the external ear through the middle ear—is known as the *conductive* phase, and a disorder here causes conductive hearing loss. The second part of the pathway, involving the cochlea and the cochlear nerve, is called the *sensorineural* phase; a disorder here causes sensorineural hearing loss.

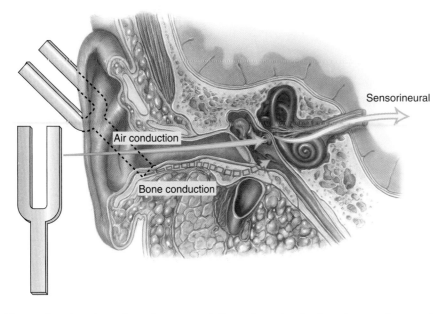

Air conduction describes the normal first phase in the hearing pathway. An alternate pathway, known as *bone conduction*, bypasses the external and the middle ear and is used for testing purposes. A vibrating tuning fork, placed on the head, sets the bone of the skull into vibration and stimulates the cochlea directly. In a normal person, air conduction is more sensitive.

Equilibrium. The labyrinth within the inner ear senses the position and movements of the head and helps to maintain balance.

◼ THE NOSE AND PARANASAL SINUSES

Review the terms used to describe the external anatomy of the nose.

Approximately the upper third of the nose is supported by bone, the lower two thirds by cartilage. Air enters the nasal cavity by way of the *anterior naris* on either side, then passes into a widened area known as the *vestibule* and on through the narrow nasal passage to the nasopharynx. The medial wall of each nasal cavity is formed by the *nasal septum,* which, like the external nose, is supported by both bone and cartilage. It is covered by a mucous membrane well supplied with blood. The vestibule, unlike the rest of the nasal cavity, is lined with hair-bearing skin, not mucosa.

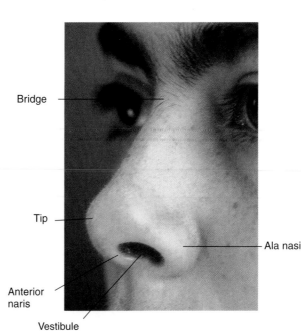

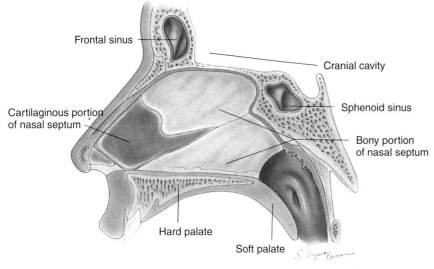

Frontal sinus

Cranial cavity

Cartilaginous portion
of nasal septum

Sphenoid sinus

Bony portion
of nasal septum

Hard palate

Soft palate

MEDIAL WALL—LEFT NASAL CAVITY (MUCOSA REMOVED)

Laterally, the anatomy is more complex. Curving bony structures, the *turbinates,* covered by a highly vascular mucous membrane, protrude into the nasal cavity. Below each turbinate is a groove, or meatus, each named according to the turbinate above it. Into the inferior meatus drains the nasolacrimal duct; into the middle meatus drain most of the paranasal sinuses. Their openings are not usually visible.

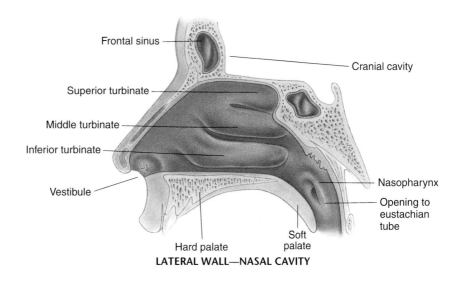

Frontal sinus

Cranial cavity

Superior turbinate

Middle turbinate

Inferior turbinate

Nasopharynx

Opening to
eustachian
tube

Vestibule

Hard palate

Soft
palate

LATERAL WALL—NASAL CAVITY

The additional surface area provided by the turbinates and the mucosa covering them aids the nasal cavities in their principal functions: cleansing, humidification, and temperature control of inspired air.

Inspection of the nasal cavity through the anterior naris is usually limited to the vestibule, the anterior portion of the septum, and the lower and middle turbinates. Examination with a nasopharyngeal mirror is required for detection of posterior abnormalities. This technique is beyond the scope of this book.

The *paranasal sinuses* are air-filled cavities within the bones of the skull. Like the nasal cavities into which they drain, they are lined with mucous membrane. Their locations are diagrammed below. Only the frontal and maxillary sinuses are readily accessible to clinical examination.

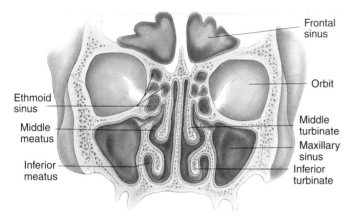

CROSS SECTION OF NASAL CAVITY—ANTERIOR VIEW

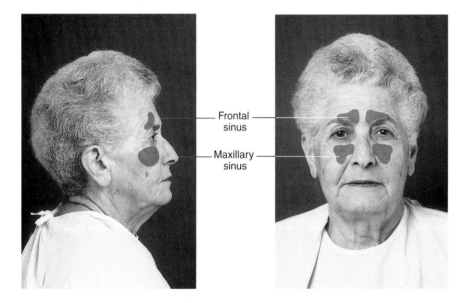

THE MOUTH AND PHARYNX

The *lips* are muscular folds that surround the entrance to the mouth. When opened, the gums (gingiva) and teeth are visible. Note the scalloped shape of the *gingival margins* and the pointed *interdental papillae*.

The *gingiva* is firmly attached to the teeth and to the maxilla or mandible in which they are seated. In lighter-skinned people, the gingiva is pale or coral pink and lightly stippled. In darker-skinned people, it may be diffusely or partly brown, as shown below. A midline mucosal fold, called a *labial frenulum*, connects each lip with the gingiva. A shallow *gingival sulcus* between the gum's thin margin and each tooth is not readily visible (but is probed and measured by dentists). Adjacent to the gingiva is the *alveolar mucosa*, which merges with the *labial mucosa* of the lip.

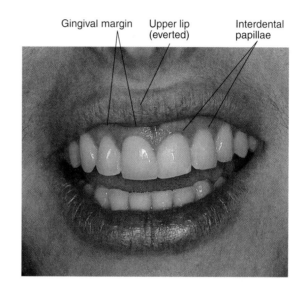

Gingival margin   Upper lip (everted)   Interdental papillae

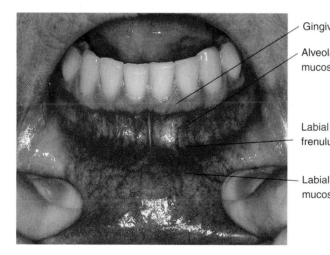

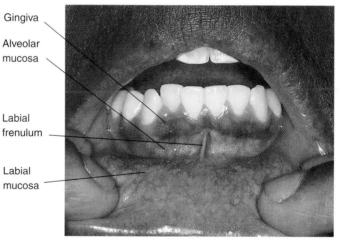

Gingiva

Alveolar mucosa

Labial frenulum

Labial mucosa

Each tooth, composed chiefly of dentin, lies rooted in a bony socket with only its enamel-covered crown exposed. Small blood vessels and nerves enter the tooth through its apex and pass into the pulp canal and pulp chamber.

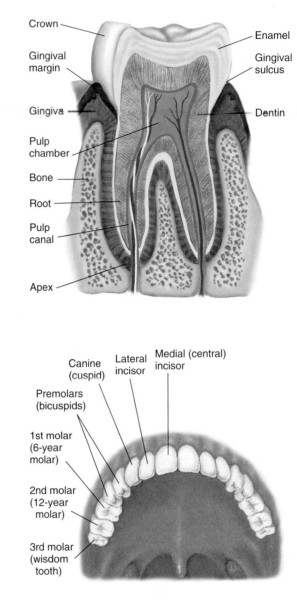

Note the terms designating the 32 adult teeth, 16 in each jaw.

The dorsum of the *tongue* is covered with papillae, giving it a rough surface. Some of these papillae look like red dots, which contrast with the thin white coat that often covers the tongue. The undersurface of the tongue has no papillae. Note the midline *lingual frenulum* that connects the tongue to the floor of the mouth. At the base of the tongue the *ducts of the submandibular gland* (Wharton's ducts) pass forward and medially. They open on papillae that lie on each side of the lingual frenulum.

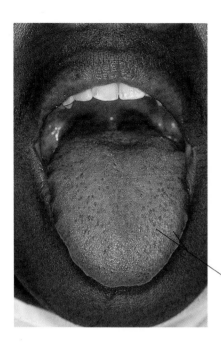

Papillae

Lingual frenulum

Vein

Duct of submandibular gland

Above and behind the tongue rises an arch formed by the *anterior* and *posterior pillars*, the *soft palate*, and the *uvula*. A meshwork of small blood vessels may web the soft palate. The *pharynx* is visible in the recess behind the soft palate and tongue.

In the adjacent photograph, note the right tonsil protruding from the hollowed *tonsillar fossa*, or cavity, between the anterior and posterior pillars. In adults, tonsils are often small or absent, as in the empty left tonsillar fossa here.

The *buccal mucosa* lines the cheeks. Each *parotid duct*, sometimes termed *Stenson's duct*, opens onto the buccal mucosa near the upper second molar. Its location is frequently marked by its own small papilla.

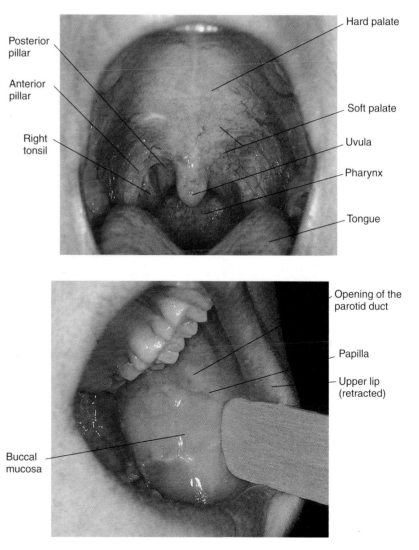

Posterior pillar

Anterior pillar

Right tonsil

Hard palate

Soft palate

Uvula

Pharynx

Tongue

Opening of the parotid duct

Papilla

Upper lip (retracted)

Buccal mucosa

THE NECK

For descriptive purposes, divide each side of the neck into two triangles bounded by the sternomastoid muscle. Visualize the borders of the two triangles as follows:

- For the *anterior triangle:* the mandible above, the sternomastoid laterally, and the midline of the neck medially

- For the *posterior triangle:* the sternomastoid muscle, the trapezius, and the clavicle. Note that a portion of the omohyoid muscle crosses the lower portion of this triangle and can be mistaken for a lymph node or mass.

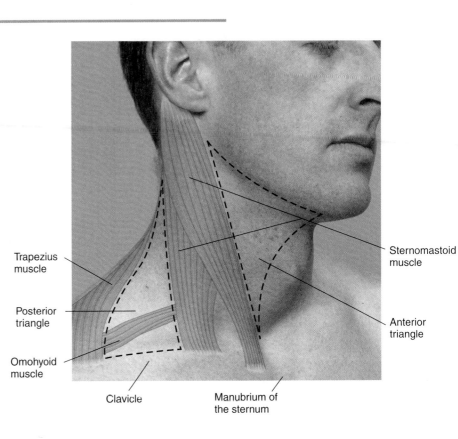

Trapezius muscle

Posterior triangle

Omohyoid muscle

Clavicle

Manubrium of the sternum

Sternomastoid muscle

Anterior triangle

Great Vessels. Deep to the sternomastoids run the great vessels of the neck: the *carotid artery* and the *internal jugular vein.* The *external jugular vein* passes diagonally over the surface of the sternomastoid and may be helpful when trying to identify the jugular venous pressure (see p. 290).

(see p. 290)

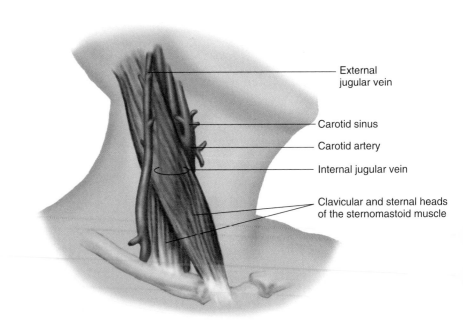

External jugular vein

Carotid sinus

Carotid artery

Internal jugular vein

Clavicular and sternal heads of the sternomastoid muscle

Midline Structures and Thyroid Gland. Now identify the following midline structures: (1) the mobile *hyoid bone* just below the mandible, (2) the *thyroid cartilage,* readily identified by the notch on its superior edge, (3) the *cricoid cartilage,* (4) the *tracheal rings,* and (5) the *thyroid gland.*

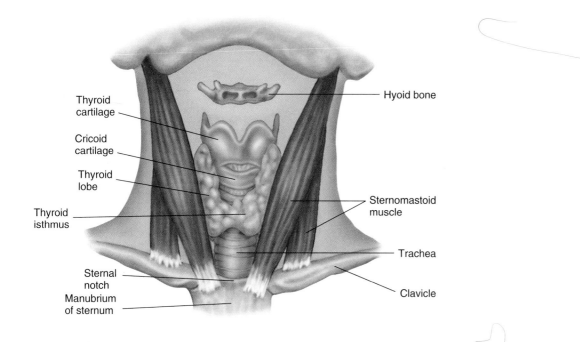

The isthmus of the thyroid gland lies across the trachea below the cricoid. The lateral lobes of this gland curve posteriorly around the sides of the trachea and the esophagus. Except in the midline, the thyroid gland is covered by thin straplike muscles, among which only the sternomastoids are visible. Women have larger and more easily palpable glands than men.

Lymph Nodes. The *lymph nodes* of the head and neck have been classified in a variety of ways. One classification is shown here, together with the directions of lymphatic drainage. The deep cervical chain is largely obscured by the overlying sternomastoid muscle, but at its two extremes, the tonsillar node and supraclavicular nodes may be palpable. The submandibular nodes lie superficial to the submandibular gland, from which they should be differentiated. Nodes are normally round or ovoid, smooth, and smaller than this gland. The gland is larger and has a lobulated, slightly irregular surface (see p. 153).

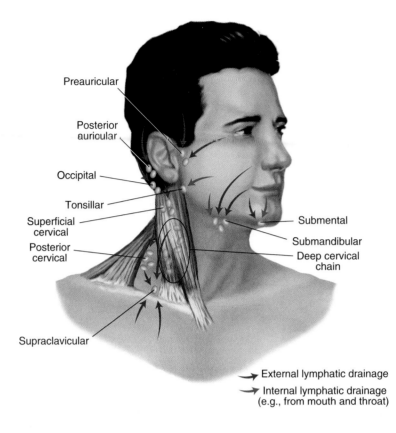

Preauricular

Posterior auricular

Occipital

Tonsillar

Superficial cervical

Posterior cervical

Supraclavicular

Submental

Submandibular

Deep cervical chain

External lymphatic drainage

Internal lymphatic drainage (e.g., from mouth and throat)

Note that the tonsillar, submandibular, and submental nodes drain portions of the mouth and throat as well as the face.

Knowledge of the lymphatic system is important to a sound clinical habit: whenever a malignant or inflammatory lesion is observed, look for involvement of the regional lymph nodes that drain it; whenever a node is enlarged or tender, look for a source such as infection in the area that it drains.

THE HEALTH HISTORY

Common or Concerning Symptoms

- Headache
- Change in vision: hyperopia, presbyopia, myopia, scotomas
- Double vision, or diplopia
- Hearing loss, earache; tinnitus
- Vertigo
- Nosebleed, or epistaxis
- Sore throat; hoarseness
- Swollen glands
- Goiter

THE HEAD

Headache is an extremely common symptom that always requires careful evaluation, because a small fraction of headaches arise from life-threatening conditions. It is important to elicit a full description of the headache and all seven attributes of the patient's pain (see p. 32). Is the headache one-sided or bilateral? Steady or throbbing? Continuous or comes and goes? After your usual open-ended approach, ask the patient to *point to the area of pain or discomfort.*

See Table 6-1, Headaches, pp. 206–209. *Tension* and *migraine headaches* are the most common kinds of recurring headaches.

Tension headaches often arise in the temporal areas; cluster headaches may be retro-orbital.

The most important attributes of headache are its *chronologic pattern* and *severity*. Is the problem new and acute? Chronic and recurring, with little change in pattern? Chronic and recurring, but with recent change in pattern or progressively severe? Does the pain recur at the same time every day?

Changing or progressively severe headaches increase the likelihood of *tumor, abscess,* or other *mass lesion.* Extremely severe headaches suggest *subarachnoid hemorrhage* or *meningitis.*

Ask about associated symptoms. Inquire specifically about associated nausea and vomiting and neurologic symptoms such as change in vision or motor-sensory deficits.

Visual aura or scintillating scotomas with *migraine.*[1] Nausea and vomiting common with migraine but also occur with brain tumors and subarachnoid hemorrhage.

Ask whether coughing, sneezing, or changing the position of the head have any effect (better, worse, or no effect) on the headache.

Such maneuvers may increase pain from brain tumor and acute sinusitis.

Ask about family history.

Family history may be positive in patients with migraine.

THE EYES

Start your inquiry about eye and vision problems with open-ended questions such as "How is your vision?" and "Have you had any trouble with your eyes?" If the patient reports a change in vision, pursue the related details:

Refractive errors most commonly explain gradual blurring. High blood glucose levels may cause blurring.[2]

■ Is the onset sudden or gradual?

Sudden visual loss suggests *retinal detachment, vitreous hemorrhage,* or *occlusion of the central retinal artery.*

■ Is the problem worse during close work or at distances?

Difficulty with close work suggests *hyperopia* (farsightedness) or *presbyopia* (aging vision); with distances, *myopia* (near-sightedness).

- Is there blurring of the entire field of vision or only parts of it? If the visual field defect is partial, is it central, peripheral, or only on one side?

Slow central loss in nuclear cataract (p. 216), *macular degeneration*[3] (p. 188); peripheral loss in advanced *open-angle glaucoma* (p. 181); one-sided loss in *hemianopsia* and *quadrantic defects* (p. 212).

- Are there specks in the vision or areas where the patient cannot see (*scotomas*)? If so, do they move around in the visual field with shifts in gaze or are they fixed?

Moving specks or strands suggest vitreous floaters; fixed defects (scotomas) suggest lesions in the retina or visual pathways.

- Has the patient seen lights flashing across the field of vision? Vitreous floaters may accompany this symptom.

Flashing lights or new vitreous floaters suggest detachment of vitreous from retina. Prompt eye consultation is indicated.

- Does the patient wear glasses?

Ask about *pain* in or around the eyes, *redness*, and *excessive tearing or watering* (see page 215).

Check for presence of *diplopia*, or double vision. If present, find out whether the images are side by side (horizontal diplopia) or on top of each other (vertical diplopia). Does diplopia persist with one eye closed? Which eye is affected?

Diplopia in adults may arise from a lesion in the brainstem or cerebellum, or from weakness or paralysis of one or more extraocular muscles, as in horizontal diplopia from palsy of CN III or VI, or vertical diplopia from palsy of CN III or IV. Diplopia in one eye, with the other closed, suggests a problem in the cornea or lens.

One kind of horizontal diplopia is physiologic. Hold one finger upright about 6 inches in front of your face, a second at arm's length. When you focus on either finger, the image of the other is double. A patient who notices this phenomenon can be reassured.

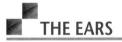

THE EARS

Opening questions are "How is your hearing?" and "Have you had any trouble with your ears?" If the patient has noticed a *hearing loss*, does it involve one or both ears? Did it start suddenly or gradually? What are the associated symptoms, if any? (See page 229.)

Try to distinguish between two basic types of hearing impairment: *conductive loss*, which results from problems in the external or middle ear, and *sensorineural loss*, from problems in the inner ear, the cochlear nerve, or its central connections in the brain. Two questions may be helpful . . . Does the patient have special difficulty understanding people as they talk? . . . What difference does a noisy environment make?

People with sensorineural loss have particular trouble understanding speech, often complaining that others mumble; noisy environments make hearing worse. In conductive loss, noisy environments may help.

Symptoms associated with hearing loss, such as earache or vertigo, help you to assess likely causes. In addition, inquire specifically about medications that might affect hearing and ask about sustained exposure to loud noise.

Medications that affect hearing include aminoglycosides, aspirin, NSAIDs, quinine, furosemide, and others.

Complaints of *earache,* or *pain in the ear,* are especially common. Ask about associated fever, sore throat, cough, and concurrent upper respiratory infection.

Pain suggests a problem in the external ear, such as *otitis externa,* or, if associated with symptoms of respiratory infection, in the inner ear, as in *otitis media.* It may also be referred from other structures in the mouth, throat, or neck.

Ask about *discharge from the ear,* especially if associated with earache or trauma.

Unusually soft wax, debris from inflammation or rash in the ear canal, or discharge through a perforated eardrum secondary to *acute* or *chronic otitis media*

Tinnitus is a perceived sound that has no external stimulus—commonly a musical ringing or a rushing or roaring noise. It can involve one or both ears. Tinnitus may accompany hearing loss and often remains unexplained. Occasionally, popping sounds originate in the temporomandibular joint, or vascular noises from the neck may be audible.

Tinnitus is a common symptom, increasing in frequency with age. When associated with hearing loss and vertigo, it suggests *Ménière's disease.*

Vertigo refers to the perception that the patient or the environment is rotating or spinning. These sensations point primarily to a problem in the labyrinths of the inner ear, peripheral lesions of CN VIII, or lesions in its central pathways or nuclei in the brain.

See Table 6-2, Vertigo, p. 210.

Vertigo is a challenging symptom for you as clinician, because patients differ widely in what they mean by the word "dizzy." "Are there times when you feel dizzy?" is an appropriate first question, but patients often find it difficult to be more specific. Ask "Do you feel unsteady, as if you are going to fall or black out? . . . Or do you feel the room is spinning (true vertigo)?" Get the story without biasing it. You may need to offer the patient several choices of wording. Ask if the patient feels pulled to the ground or off to one side. And if the dizziness is related to a change in body position. Pursue any associated feelings of clamminess or flushing, nausea, or vomiting. Check if any medications may be contributing.

Feeling unsteady, lightheaded, or "dizzy in the legs" sometimes suggests a cardiovascular etiology. A feeling of being pulled suggests true vertigo from an inner ear problem or a central or peripheral lesion of CN VIII.

THE NOSE AND SINUSES

Rhinorrhea refers to drainage from the nose and is often associated with *nasal congestion,* a sense of stuffiness or obstruction. These symptoms are frequently accompanied by *sneezing,* watery eyes, and throat discomfort, and also by *itching* in the eyes, nose, and throat.

Causes include viral infections, *allergic rhinitis* ("hay fever"), and *vasomotor rhinitis.* Itching favors an allergic cause.

Assess the chronology of the illness. Does it last for a week or so, especially when common colds and related syndromes are prevalent, or does it occur seasonally when pollens are in the air? Is it associated with specific contacts or environments? What remedies has the patient used? For how long? And how well do they work?

Relation to seasons or environmental contacts suggests allergy.

Excessive use of decongestants can worsen the symptoms, causing rhinitis medicamentosa.

Inquire about drugs that might cause stuffiness.

Oral contraceptives, reserpine, guanethidine, and alcohol

Are there symptoms in addition to rhinorrhea or congestion, such as pain and tenderness in the face or over the sinuses, local headache, or fever?

These together suggest *sinusitis*.[5-7]

Is the patient's nasal congestion limited to one side? If so, you may be dealing with a different problem that requires careful physical examination.

Consider a deviated nasal septum, foreign body, or tumor.

Epistaxis means bleeding from the nose. The blood usually originates from the nose itself, but may come from a paranasal sinus or the nasopharynx. The history is usually quite graphic! However, in patients who are lying down, or whose bleeding originates in posterior structures, blood may pass into the throat instead of out the nostrils. You must identify the source of the bleeding carefully—is it from the nose, or has it been coughed up or vomited? Assess the site of bleeding, its severity, and associated symptoms. Is it a recurrent problem? Has there been easy bruising or bleeding elsewhere in the body?

Local causes of epistaxis include trauma (especially nose picking), inflammation, drying and crusting of the nasal mucosa, tumors, and foreign bodies.

Bleeding disorders may contribute to epistaxis.

THE MOUTH, THROAT, AND NECK

Sore throat is a frequent complaint, usually associated with acute upper respiratory symptoms.

Fever, pharyngeal exudates, and anterior lymphadenopathy, especially in the absence of cough, suggest streptococcal pharyngitis, or *strep throat* (p. 232)

A *sore tongue* may be caused by local lesions as well as by systemic illness.

Aphthous ulcers (p. 238); sore smooth tongue of nutritional deficiency (p. 237)

Bleeding from the gums is a common symptom, especially when brushing teeth. Ask about local lesions and any tendency to bleed or bruise elsewhere.

Bleeding gums are most often caused by *gingivitis* (p. 235).

Hoarseness refers to an altered quality of the voice, often described as husky, rough, or harsh. The pitch may be lower than before. Hoarseness usually arises from disease of the larynx, but may also develop as extralaryngeal lesions press on the laryngeal nerves. Check for overuse of the voice, allergy, smoking or other inhaled irritants, and any associated symptoms. Is the problem acute or chronic? If hoarseness lasts more than 2 weeks, visual examination of the larynx by indirect or direct laryngoscopy is advisable.

Overuse of the voice (as in cheering) and acute infections are the most likely causes.

Causes of chronic hoarseness include smoking, allergy, voice abuse, hypothyroidism, chronic infections such as tuberculosis, and tumors.

Ask "Have you noticed any swollen glands or lumps in your neck?", since patients are more familiar with the lay terms than with "*lymph nodes.*"

Assess thyroid function and ask about any evidence of an enlarged thyroid gland or *goiter*. To evaluate thyroid function, ask about *temperature intolerance* and *sweating*. Opening questions include "Do you prefer hot or cold weather?" "Do you dress more warmly or less warmly than other people?" "What about blankets . . . do you use more or fewer than others at home?" "Do you perspire more or less than others?" "Any new palpitations or change in weight?" Note that as people grow older, they sweat less, have less tolerance for cold, and tend to prefer warmer environments.

Enlarged tender lymph nodes commonly accompany pharyngitis.

With goiter, thyroid function may be increased, decreased, or normal.

Intolerance to cold, preference for warm clothing and many blankets, and decreased sweating suggest *hypothyroidism*; the opposite symptoms, palpitations and involuntary weight loss, suggest *hyperthyroidism* (p. 239).

HEALTH PROMOTION AND COUNSELING

Important Topics for Health Promotion and Counseling

- Changes in vision: cataracts, macular degeneration, glaucoma
- Hearing loss
- Oral health

Vision and hearing, critical senses for experiencing the world around us, are two areas of special importance for health promotion and counseling. Oral health, often overlooked, also merits clinical attention.

Disorders of vision shift with age. Healthy young adults generally have refractive errors. Up to 25% of adults older than 65 have refractive errors; however, cataracts, macular degeneration, and glaucoma become more prevalent.[8] These disorders reduce awareness of the social and physical environment and contribute to falls and injuries. To improve detection of visual defects, test visual acuity with a Snellen chart or handheld card (p. 753). Examine the lens and fundi for clouding of the lens (*cataracts*); mottling of the *macula*, variations in the retinal pigmentation, subretinal hemorrhage or exudate (*macular degeneration*); and change in size and color of the optic cup (*glaucoma*). After diagnosis, review effective treatments—corrective lenses, cataract surgery, photocoagulation for choroidal neovascularization in macular degeneration, and topical medications for glaucoma.

Surveillance for glaucoma is especially important.[9] Glaucoma is the leading cause of blindness in African Americans and the second leading cause of blindness overall. There is gradual loss of vision with damage to the optic nerve, loss of visual fields beginning usually at the periphery, and pallor and increasing size of the optic cup (enlarging to more than half the diameter of the optic disc). Elevated intraocular pressure (IOP) is seen in up to 80% of cases and is linked to damage of the optic nerve. Risk factors include age older than 65, African American origin, diabetes mellitus, myopia, family history of glaucoma, and ocular hypertension (IOP ≥ 21 mm Hg). Screening tests include tonometry to measure IOP, ophthalmoscopy or slit-lamp examination of the optic nerve head, and perimetry to map the visual fields. In the hands of general clinicians, however, all three tests lack accuracy, so attention to risk factors and referral to eye specialists remain important tools for clinical care.

Hearing loss can also trouble the later years.[10] More than a third of adults older than age 65 have detectable hearing deficits, contributing to emotional isolation and social withdrawal. These losses may go undetected—unlike vision prerequisites for driving and vision, there is no mandate for widespread testing, and many seniors avoid use of hearing aids. Questionnaires and hand-held audioscopes work well for periodic screening. Less sensitive are the clinical "whisper test," rubbing fingers, or use of the tuning fork. Groups at risk are those with a history of congenital or familial hearing loss, syphilis, rubella, meningitis, or exposure to hazardous noise levels at work or on the battlefield.

Clinicians should play an active role in promoting oral health: up to half of all children ages 5 to 17 have from one to eight cavities, and the average U.S. adult has 10 to 17 teeth that are decayed, missing, or filled.[11] In adults, the prevalence of gingivitis and periodontal disease is 50% and 80%, respectively. In the United States, more than half of all adults older than age 65 have no teeth at all! Effective screening begins with careful examination of the mouth. Inspect the oral cavity for decayed or loose teeth, inflammation of the gingiva, and signs of periodontal disease (bleeding, pus, recession of the gums, and bad breath). Inspect the mucous membranes, the palate, the oral floor, and the surfaces of the tongue for ulcers and leukoplakia, warning signs for oral cancer and HIV disease.

To improve oral health, counsel patients to adopt daily hygiene measures. Use of fluoride-containing toothpastes reduces tooth decay, and brushing and flossing retard periodontal disease by removing bacterial plaques. Urge patients to seek dental care at least annually to receive the benefits of more specialized preventive care such as scaling, planing of roots, and topical fluorides.

Diet, tobacco and alcohol use, changes in salivary flow from medication, and proper use of dentures should also be addressed.[12] As with children, adults should avoid excessive intake of foods high in refined sugars, such as sucrose, which enhance attachment and colonization of cariogenic bacteria. Use of all tobacco products and excessive alcohol, the principal risk factors for oral cancers, should be avoided.

Saliva cleanses and lubricates the mouth. Many medications reduce salivary flow, increasing risk for tooth decay, mucositis, and gum disease from xerostomia, especially for the elderly. For those wearing dentures, be sure to counsel removal and cleaning each night to reduce bacterial plaque and risk of malodor. Regular massage of the gums relieves soreness and pressure from dentures on the underlying soft tissue.

TECHNIQUES OF EXAMINATION

◼ THE HEAD

Because abnormalities covered by the hair are easily missed, ask if the patient has noticed anything wrong with the scalp or hair. If you detect a hairpiece or wig, ask the patient to remove it.

Examine:

The Hair.   Note its quantity, distribution, texture, and pattern of loss, if any. You may see loose flakes of dandruff.

Fine hair in *hyperthyroidism*; coarse hair in *hypothyroidism*. Tiny white ovoid granules that adhere to hairs may be nits, or eggs of lice.

The Scalp.   Part the hair in several places and look for scaliness, lumps, nevi, or other lesions.

Redness and scaling in *seborrheic dermatitis, psoriasis; soft lumps of pilar cysts* (wens)

The Skull.   Observe the general size and contour of the skull. Note any deformities, depressions, lumps, or tenderness. Learn to recognize the irregularities in a normal skull, such as those near the suture lines between the parietal and occipital bones.

Enlarged skull in *hydrocephalus, Paget's disease* of bone. Tenderness after trauma

The Face.   Note the patient's facial expression and contours. Observe for asymmetry, involuntary movements, edema, and masses.

See Table 6-3, Selected Facies (p. 211).

The Skin.   Observe the skin, noting its color, pigmentation, texture, thickness, hair distribution, and any lesions.

Acne in many adolescents. *Hirsutism* (excessive facial hair) in some women with *polycystic ovary syndrome*

◼ THE EYES

Important Areas of Examination

- Visual acuity
- Visual fields
- Conjunctiva and sclera
- Cornea, lens, and pupils
- Extraocular movements

- Fundi, including:
  Optic disc and cup
  Retina
  Retinal vessels

Visual Acuity.   To test the acuity of central vision, use a Snellen eye chart, if possible, and light it well. Position the patient 20 feet from the chart.

Vision of 20/200 means that at 20 feet the patient can read print

Patients who use glasses other than for reading should put them on. Ask the patient to cover one eye with a card (to prevent peeking through the fingers) and to read the smallest line of print possible. Coaxing to attempt the next line may improve performance. A patient who cannot read the largest letter should be positioned closer to the chart; note the intervening distance. Determine the smallest line of print from which the patient can identify more than half the letters. Record the visual acuity designated at the side of this line, along with use of glasses, if any. Visual acuity is expressed as two numbers (e.g., 20/30): the first indicates the distance of patient from chart, and the second, the distance at which a normal eye can read the line of letters.

that a person with normal vision could read at 200 feet. The larger the second number, the worse the vision. "20/40 corrected" means the patient could read the 40 line with glasses (a correction).

Myopia is impaired far vision.

Testing near vision with a special hand-held card helps identify the need for reading glasses or bifocals in patients older than age 45. You can also use this card to test visual acuity at the bedside. Held 14 inches from the patient's eyes, the card simulates a Snellen chart. You may, however, let patients choose their own distance.

Presbyopia is the impaired near vision, found in middle-aged and older people. A presbyopic person often sees better when the card is farther away.

If you have no charts, screen visual acuity with any available print. If patients cannot read even the largest letters, test their ability to count your upraised fingers and distinguish light (such as your flashlight) from dark.

In the United States, a person is usually considered legally blind when vision in the better eye, corrected by glasses, is 20/200 or less. Legal blindness also results from a constricted field of vision: 20° or less in the better eye.

Visual Fields by Confrontation

Screening.   Screening starts in the temporal fields because most defects involve these areas. Imagine the patient's visual fields projected onto a

Field defects that are all or partly temporal include:

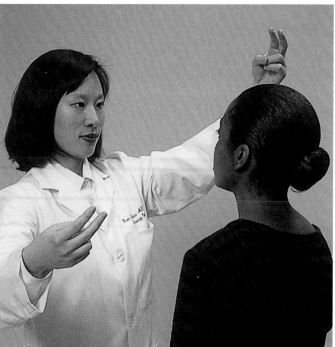

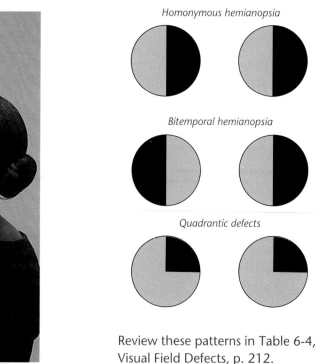

Homonymous hemianopsia

Bitemporal hemianopsia

Quadrantic defects

Review these patterns in Table 6-4, Visual Field Defects, p. 212.

glass bowl that encircles the front of the patient's head. Ask the patient to look with both eyes into your eyes. While you return the patient's gaze, place your hands about 2 feet apart, lateral to the patient's ears. Instruct the patient to point to your fingers as soon as they are seen. Then slowly move the wiggling fingers of both your hands along the imaginary bowl and toward the line of gaze until the patient identifies them. Repeat this pattern in the upper and lower temporal quadrants.

Usually a person sees both sets of fingers at the same time. If so, fields are usually normal.

Further Testing. If you find a defect, try to establish its boundaries. Test one eye at a time. If you suspect a temporal defect in the left visual field, for example, ask the patient to cover the right eye and, with the left one, to look into your eye directly opposite. Then slowly move your wiggling fingers from the defective area toward the better vision, noting where the patient first responds. Repeat this at several levels to define the border.

When the patient's left eye repeatedly does not see your fingers until they have crossed the line of gaze, a left temporal hemianopsia is present. It is diagrammed from the patient's viewpoint.

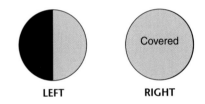

LEFT   RIGHT

A left homonymous hemianopsia may thus be established.

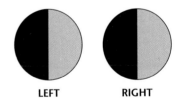

LEFT   RIGHT

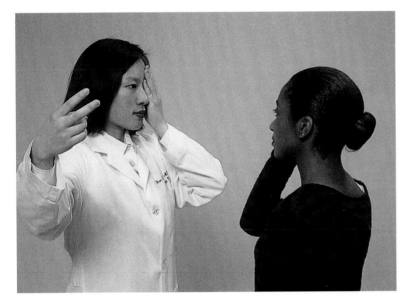

A temporal defect in the visual field of one eye suggests a nasal defect in the other eye. To test this hypothesis, examine the other eye in a similar way, again moving from the anticipated defect toward the better vision.

Small visual field defects and enlarged blind spots require a finer stimulus. Using a small red object such as a red-headed matchstick or the red eraser on a pencil, test one eye at a time. As the patient looks into your eye directly opposite, move the object about in the visual field. The normal blind spot can be found 15° temporal to the line of gaze—the small red object disappears. (Find your own blind spots for practice.)

An enlarged blind spot occurs in conditions affecting the optic nerve, e.g., *glaucoma, optic neuritis,* and *papilledema.*

Position and Alignment of the Eyes. Stand in front of the patient and survey the eyes for position and alignment with each other. If one or both eyes seem to protrude, assess them from above (see p. 200).

Inward or outward deviation of the eyes; abnormal protrusion in *Graves' disease* or ocular tumors

Eyebrows. Inspect the eyebrows, noting their quantity and distribution and any scaliness of the underlying skin.

Scaliness in *seborrheic dermatitis;* lateral sparseness in hypothyroidism

Eyelids. Note the position of the lids in relation to the eyeballs. Inspect for the following:

See Table 6-5, Variations and Abnormalities of the Eyelids (p. 213).

■ Width of the palpebral fissures

■ Edema of the lids

■ Color of the lids

Red inflamed lid margins in blepharitis, often with crusting

■ Lesions

■ Condition and direction of the eyelashes

■ Adequacy with which the eyelids close. Look for this especially when the eyes are unusually prominent, when there is facial paralysis, or when the patient is unconscious.

Failure of the eyelids to close exposes the corneas to serious damage.

Lacrimal Apparatus. Briefly inspect the regions of the lacrimal gland and lacrimal sac for swelling.

See Table 6-6, Lumps and Swellings in and Around the Eyes (p. 214).

Look for excessive tearing or dryness of the eyes. Assessment of dryness may require special testing by an ophthalmologist. To test for nasolacrimal duct obstruction, see p. 201.

Excessive tearing may be due to increased production or impaired drainage of tears. In the first group, causes include conjunctival inflammation and corneal irritation; in the second, ectropion (p. 213 and nasolacrimal duct obstruction.

Conjunctiva and Sclera. Ask the patient to look up as you depress both lower lids with your thumbs, exposing the sclera and conjunctiva. Inspect the sclera and palpebral conjunctiva for color, and note the vascular pattern against the white scleral background. Look for any nodules or swelling.

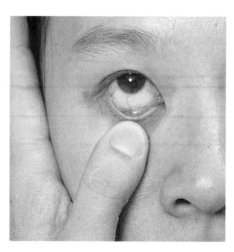
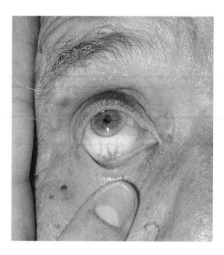

A yellow sclera indicates jaundice.

If you need a fuller view of the eye, rest your thumb and finger on the bones of the cheek and brow, respectively, and spread the lids.

Ask the patient to look to each side and down. This technique gives you a good view of the sclera and bulbar conjunctiva, but not of the palpebral conjunctiva of the upper lid. For this purpose, you need to evert the lid (see p. 201).

The local redness below is due to *nodular episcleritis:*

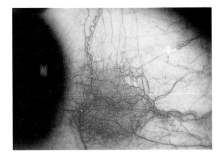

For comparisons, see Table 6-7, Red Eyes (p. 215).

Cornea and Lens. With oblique lighting, inspect the cornea of each eye for opacities and note any opacities in the lens that may be visible through the pupil.

See Table 6-8, Opacities of the Cornea and Lens (p. 216).

Iris. At the same time, inspect each iris. The markings should be clearly defined. With your light shining directly from the temporal side, look for a crescentic shadow on the medial side of the iris. Because the iris is normally fairly flat and forms a relatively open angle with the cornea, this lighting casts no shadow.

Occasionally the iris bows abnormally far forward, forming a very narrow angle with the cornea. The light then casts a crescentic shadow.

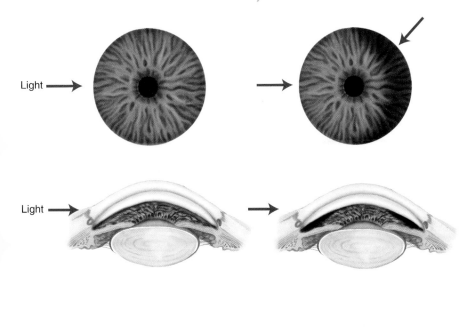

This narrow angle increases the risk for acute *narrow-angle glaucoma*—a sudden increase in intraocular pressure when drainage of the aqueous humor is blocked.

In *open-angle glaucoma*—the common form of glaucoma—the normal spatial relation between iris and cornea is preserved and the iris is fully lit.

Pupils. Inspect the *size, shape,* and *symmetry* of the pupils. If the pupils are large (>5 mm), small (<3 mm), or unequal, measure them. A card with black circles of varying sizes facilitates measurement.

Miosis refers to constriction of the pupils, *mydriasis* to dilation.

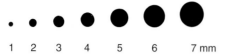

1 2 3 4 5 6 7 mm

Pupillary inequality of less than 0.5 mm (*anisocoria*) is visible in about 20% of normal people. If pupillary reactions are normal, anisocoria is considered benign.

Compare benign anisocoria with *Horner's syndrome, oculomotor nerve paralysis,* and *tonic pupil.* See Table 6-9, Pupillary Abnormalities (p. 217).

Test the *pupillary reaction to light.* Ask the patient to look into the distance, and shine a bright light obliquely into each pupil in turn. (Both the distant gaze and the oblique lighting help to prevent a near reaction.) Look for:

■ The *direct reaction* (pupillary constriction in the same eye)

■ The *consensual reaction* (pupillary constriction in the opposite eye)

Always darken the room and use a bright light before deciding that a light reaction is absent.

If the reaction to light is impaired or questionable, test the *near reaction* in normal room light. Testing one eye at a time makes it easier to concentrate on pupillary responses, without the distraction of extraocular movement. Hold your finger or pencil about 10 cm from the patient's eye. Ask the patient to look alternately at it and into the distance directly behind it. Watch for pupillary constriction with near effort.

Testing the near reaction is helpful in diagnosing *Argyll Robertson* and *tonic (Adie's) pupils* (see p. 217).

Extraocular Muscles. From about 2 feet directly in front of the patient, shine a light onto the patient's eyes and ask the patient to look at it. *Inspect the reflections in the corneas.* They should be visible slightly nasal to the center of the pupils.

Asymmetry of the corneal reflections indicates a deviation from normal ocular alignment. A temporal light reflection on one cornea, for example, indicates a nasal deviation of that eye. See Table 6-10, Dysconjugate Gaze (p. 218).

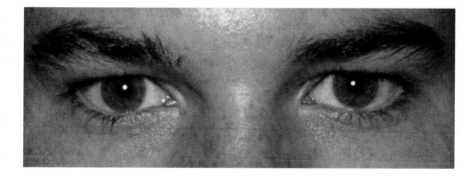

A *cover–uncover test* may reveal a slight or latent muscle imbalance not otherwise seen (see p. 218).

Now *assess the extraocular movements,* looking for:

■ The normal *conjugate movements* of the eyes in each direction, or any *deviation* from normal

See Table 6-10, Dysconjugate Gaze (p. 218).

■ *Nystagmus,* a fine rhythmic oscillation of the eyes. A few beats of nystagmus on extreme lateral gaze are normal. If you see it, bring your finger in to within the field of binocular vision and look again.

Sustained nystagmus within the binocular field of gaze is seen in a variety of neurologic conditions. See Table 17-4, Nystagmus (pp. 655–656).

■ *Lid lag* as the eyes move from up to down.

Lid lag of *hyperthyroidism*

To make these observations, *ask the patient to follow your finger or pencil* as you sweep through the six cardinal directions of gaze. Making a wide H in the air, lead the patient's gaze (1) to the patient's extreme right, (2) to the right and upward, and (3) down on the right; then (4) without pausing in the middle, to the extreme left, (5) to the left and upward, and (6) down on the left. Pause during upward and lateral gaze to detect nystagmus. Move your finger or pencil at a comfortable distance from the patient. Because middle-aged or older people may have difficulty focusing on near objects, make this distance greater for them than for young people. Some patients move their heads to follow your finger. If necessary, hold the head in the proper midline position.

In paralysis of the CN VI, illustrated below, the eyes are conjugate in right lateral gaze but not in left lateral gaze, *left infranuclear ophthalmoplegia*

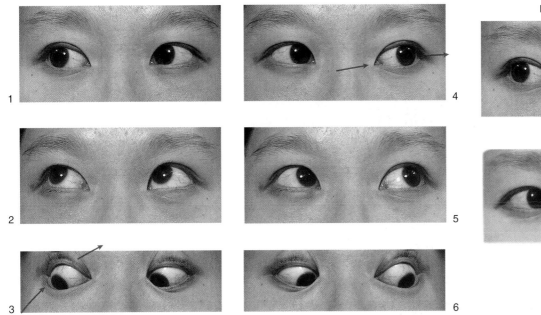

LOOKING RIGHT

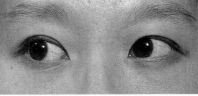

LOOKING LEFT

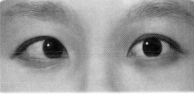

If you suspect a lid lag or hyperthyroidism, ask the patient to follow your finger again as you move it slowly from up to down in the midline. The lid should overlap the iris slightly throughout this movement.

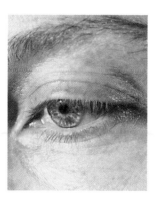

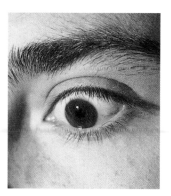

In the lid lag of hyperthyroidism, a rim of sclera is seen between the upper lid and iris; the lid seems to lag behind the eyeball.

Finally, test for *convergence*. Ask the patient to follow your finger or pencil as you move it in toward the bridge of the nose. The converging eyes normally follow the object to within 5 cm to 8 cm of the nose.

Poor convergence in *hyperthyroidism*

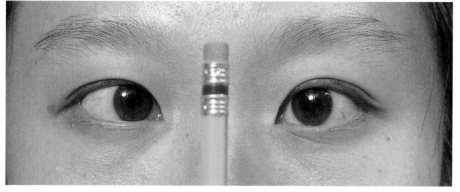

CONVERGENCE

Ophthalmoscopic Examination.
In general health care, you should usually examine your patients' eyes *without dilating their pupils.* Your view is therefore limited to the posterior structures of the retina. To see more peripheral structures, to evaluate the macula well, or to investigate unexplained visual loss, ophthalmologists dilate the pupils with mydriatic drops unless this is contraindicated.

At first, using the ophthalmoscope may seem awkward, and it may be difficult to visualize the fundus. With

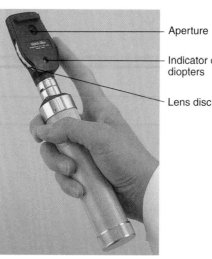

— Aperture

— Indicator of diopters

— Lens disc

Contraindications for mydriatic drops include (1) head injury and coma, in which continuing observations of pupillary reactions are essential, and (2) any suspicion of narrow-angle glaucoma.

patience and practice of proper technique, the fundus will come into view, and you will be able to assess important structures such as the optic disc and the retinal vessels. Remove your glasses unless you have marked nearsightedness or severe astigmatism. (However, if the patient's refractive errors make it difficult to focus on the fundi, it may be easier to keep your glasses on.)

Review the components of the ophthalmoscope pictured on the previous page. Then follow the steps for using the ophthalmoscope, and your examination skills will improve over time.

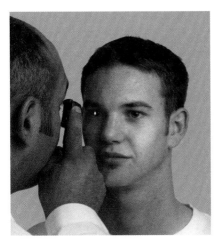

STEPS FOR USING THE OPHTHALMOSCOPE

- Darken the room. Switch on the ophthalmoscope light and turn the lens disc until you see the large round beam of white light.* Shine the light on the back of your hand to check the type of light, its desired brightness, and the electrical charge of the ophthalmoscope.
- Turn the lens disc to the 0 diopter (a diopter is a unit that measures the power of a lens to converge or diverge light). At this diopter, the lens neither converges nor diverges light. Keep your finger on the edge of the lens disc so you can turn the disc to focus the lens when you examine the fundus.
- Remember, hold the ophthalmoscope *in your right hand* to examine *the patient's right eye;* hold it *in your left hand* to examine *the patient's left eye.* This keeps you from bumping the patient's nose and gives you more mobility and closer range for visualizing the fundus. At first, you may have difficulty using the nondominant eye, but this will abate with practice.
- Hold the ophthalmoscope firmly braced against the medial aspect of your bony orbit, with the handle tilted laterally at about a 20° slant from the vertical. Check to make sure you can see clearly through the aperture. Instruct the patient to look slightly up and over your shoulder at a point directly ahead on the wall.
- Place yourself about 15 inches away from the patient and at an angle 15° lateral to the patient's line of vision. Shine the light beam on the pupil and look for the orange glow in the pupil—the *red reflex.* Note any opacities interrupting the red reflex.
- Now, place the thumb of your other hand across the patient's eyebrow (this technique helps keep you steady but is not essential). Keeping the light beam focused on the red reflex, move in with the ophthalmoscope on the 15° angle toward the pupil until you are very close to it, almost touching the patient's eyelashes.

    Try to keep both eyes open and relaxed, as if gazing into the distance, to help minimize any fluctuating blurriness as your eyes attempt to accommodate.

    You may need to lower the brightness of the light beam to make the examination more comfortable for the patient, avoid *hippus* (spasm of the pupil), and improve your observations.

Absence of a *red reflex* suggests an opacity of the lens (cataract) or possibly of the vitreous. Less commonly, a *detached retina* or, in children, a *retinoblastoma* may obscure this reflex. Do not be fooled by an artificial eye, which has no red reflex.

---

* Some clinicians like to use the large round beam for large pupils, the small round beam for small pupils. The other beams are rarely helpful. The slitlike beam is sometimes used to assess elevations or concavities in the retina, the green (or red-free) beam to detect small red lesions, and the grid to make measurements. Ignore the last three lights and practice with the large round white beam.

Now you are ready to inspect the *optic disc* and the *retina*. You should be seeing the optic disc—a yellowish orange to creamy pink oval or round structure that may fill your field of gaze or even exceed it. Of interest, the ophthalmoscope magnifies the normal retina about 15 times and the normal iris about 4 times. The optic disc actually measures about 1.5 mm. Follow the steps below for this important segment of the physical examination:

When the lens has been removed surgically, its magnifying effect is lost. Retinal structures then look much smaller than usual, and you can see a much larger expanse of fundus.

STEPS FOR EXAMINING THE OPTIC DISC AND THE RETINA

The Optic Disc

- First, *locate the optic disc.* Look for the round yellowish orange structure described above. If you do not see it at first, follow a blood vessel centrally until you do. You can tell which direction is central by noting the angles at which vessels branch—the vessel size becomes progressively larger at each junction as you approach the disc.

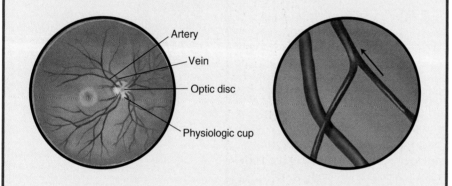

Artery

Vein

Optic disc

Physiologic cup

- Now, *bring the optic disc into sharp focus* by adjusting the lens of your ophthalmoscope. If both you and the patient have no refractive errors, the retina should be in focus at 0 diopters. If structures are blurred, rotate the lens disc until you find the sharpest focus.

  For example, if the patient is myopic (nearsighted), rotate the lens disc counterclockwise to the minus diopters; in a hyperopic (farsighted) patient, move the disc clockwise to the plus diopters. You can correct your own refractive error in the same way.

- *Inspect the optic disc.* Note the following features:

  – *The sharpness or clarity of the disc outline.* The nasal portion of the disc margin may be somewhat blurred, a normal finding.

  – *The color of the disc,* normally yellowish orange to creamy pink. White or pigmented crescents may ring the disc, a normal finding.

  – *The size of the central physiologic cup,* if present. It is usually yellowish white. The horizontal diameter is usually less than half the horizontal diameter of the disc.

  – *The comparative symmetry* of the eyes and findings in the fundi

(continued)

In a refractive error, light rays from a distance do not focus on the retina. In myopia, they focus anterior to it; in hyperopia, posterior to it. Retinal structures in a myopic eye look larger than normal.

See Table 6-11, Normal Variations of the Optic Disc (p. 219), and Table 6-12, Abnormalities of the Optic Disc (p. 220).

An enlarged cup suggests chronic open-angle glaucoma.

STEPS FOR EXAMINING THE OPTIC DISC AND THE RETINA (Continued)

Detecting Papilledema. *Papilledema* describes swelling of the optic disc and anterior bulging of the physiologic cup. Increased intracranial pressure is transmitted to the optic nerve, causing stasis of axoplasmic flow, intra-axonal edema, and swelling of the optic nerve head. Papilledema often signals serious disorders of the brain, such as meningitis, subarachnoid hemorrhage, trauma, and mass lesions, so searching for this important disorder is a priority during all your fundoscopic examinations.

If you detect papilledema, measure elevation of the optic disc by subtracting the difference in the diopters of the two lenses needed to focus clearly on the elevated disc and on the uninvolved retina. *Note that at the retina, 3 diopters = 1 mm.*

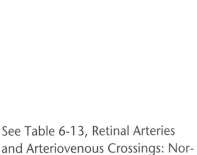

Clear focus here at −1 diopter   Clear focus here at + 3 diopters

+ 3 − (−1) = 4, therefore, a disc elevation of 4 diopters

PAPILLEDEMA

Photo from Tasman W, Jaeger E (eds.). The Wills Eye Hospital Atlas of Clinical Ophthalmology, 2nd ed. Philadelphia, Lippincott Williams & Wilkins, 2001.

Venous pulsations, seen in many but not all normal eyegrounds, may also be obliterated.

Loss of venous pulsations in pathologic conditions like head trauma, meningitis, or mass lesions may be an early sign of elevated intracranial pressure.

The Retina—Arteries, Veins, Fovea, and Macula

- *Inspect the retina,* including arteries and veins as they extend to the periphery, arteriovenous crossings, the fovea, and the macula. Distinguish arteries from veins based on the features listed below.

	Arteries	Veins
Color	Light red	Dark red
Size	Smaller (⅔ to ⅘ the diameter of veins)	Larger
Light Reflex (*reflection*)	Bright	Inconspicuous or absent

- *Follow the vessels peripherally in each of four directions,* noting their relative sizes and the character of the arteriovenous crossings.

  Identify any lesions of the surrounding *retina* and note their size, shape, color, and distribution. As you search the retina, *move your head and instrument as a unit,* using the patient's pupil as an imaginary fulcrum. At first, you may repeatedly lose your view of the retina because your light falls out of the pupil. You will improve with practice.

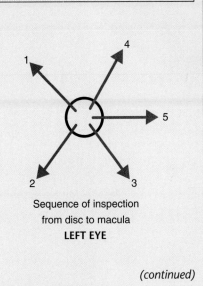

Sequence of inspection from disc to macula
LEFT EYE

See Table 6-13, Retinal Arteries and Arteriovenous Crossings: Normal and Hypertensive (p. 221); Table 6-14, Red Spots and Streaks in the Fundi (p. 222); Table 6-15, Ocular Fundi (pp. 223–224); Table 6-16, Light-Colored Spots in the Fundi (p. 225).

(continued)

STEPS FOR EXAMINING THE OPTIC DISC AND THE RETINA
(Continued)

Lesions of the retina can be measured in terms of "disc diameters" from the optic disc. For example, among the cotton-wool patches illustrated on the right, note the irregular patches between 11 and 12 o'clock, 1 to 2 disc diameters from the disc. Each measures about one-half by one-half disc diameters.

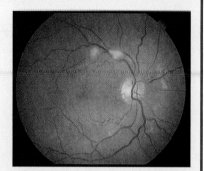

COTTON-WOOL PATCHES

■ Inspect the *fovea* and surrounding *macula*. Direct your light beam laterally or by asking the patient to look directly into the light. Except in older people, the tiny bright reflection at the center of the fovea helps to orient you. Shimmering light reflections in the macular area are common in young people.

Macular degeneration is an important cause of poor central vision in the elderly. Types include *dry atrophic* (more common but less severe) and *wet exudative,* or neovascular. Undigested cellular debris, called *drusen,* may be hard and sharply defined, as seen below, or soft and confluent with altered pigmentation (see p. 216).

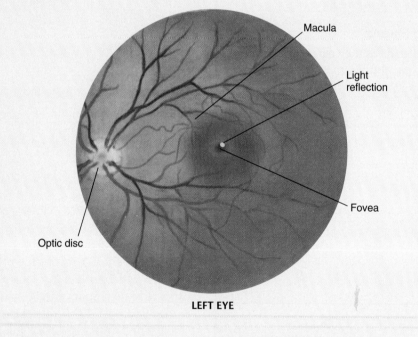

Macula

Light reflection

Fovea

Optic disc

LEFT EYE

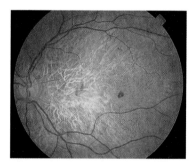

Photo from Tasman W, Jaeger E (eds). The Wills Eye Hospital Atlas of Clinical Ophthalmology, 2nd ed. Philadelphia, Lippincott Williams & Wilkins, 2001.

■ *Inspect the anterior structures.* Look for opacities in the *vitreous* or *lens* by rotating the lens disc progressively to diopters of around +10 or +12. This technique allows you to focus on the more anterior structures in the eye.

Vitreous floaters may be seen as dark specks or strands between the fundus and the lens. Cataracts are densities in the lens (see p. 216).

◼ THE EARS

The Auricle.   Inspect each auricle and surrounding tissues for deformities, lumps, or skin lesions.

If ear pain, discharge, or inflammation is present, move the auricle up and down, press the tragus, and press firmly just behind the ear.

Ear Canal and Drum.   To see the ear canal and drum, use an otoscope with the largest ear speculum that the canal will accommodate. Position the patient's head so that you can see comfortably through the instrument. To straighten the ear canal, grasp the auricle firmly but gently and pull it upward, backward, and slightly away from the head.

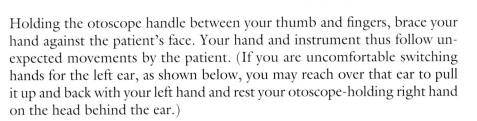

Holding the otoscope handle between your thumb and fingers, brace your hand against the patient's face. Your hand and instrument thus follow unexpected movements by the patient. (If you are uncomfortable switching hands for the left ear, as shown below, you may reach over that ear to pull it up and back with your left hand and rest your otoscope-holding right hand on the head behind the ear.)

Insert the speculum gently into the ear canal, directing it somewhat down and forward and through the hairs, if any.

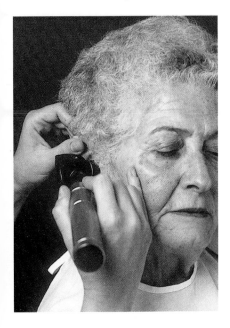
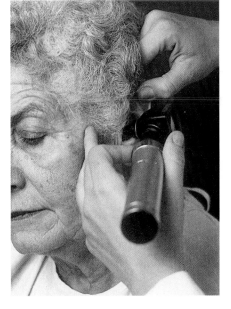

See Table 6-17, Lumps On or Near the Ear (p. 226).

Movement of the auricle and tragus (the "tug test") is painful in acute *otitis externa* (inflammation of the ear canal), but not in *otitis media* (inflammation of the middle ear). Tenderness behind the ear may be present in otitis media.

Nontender nodular swellings covered by normal skin deep in the ear canals suggest *exostoses*. These are nonmalignant overgrowths, which may obscure the drum.

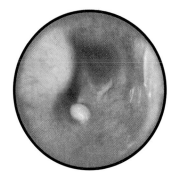

Inspect the ear canal, noting any discharge, foreign bodies, redness of the skin, or swelling. Cerumen, which varies in color and consistency from yellow and flaky to brown and sticky or even to dark and hard, may wholly or partly obscure your view.

In acute *otitis externa,* shown below, the canal is often swollen, narrowed, moist, pale, and tender. It may be reddened.

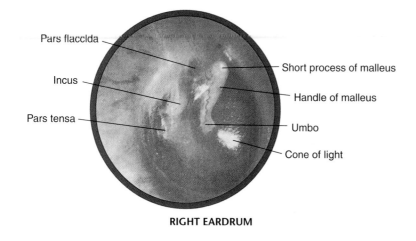

RIGHT EARDRUM

Labels: Pars flaccida, Incus, Pars tensa, Short process of malleus, Handle of malleus, Umbo, Cone of light

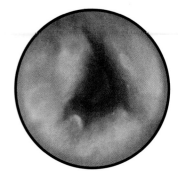

In *chronic otitis externa,* the skin of the canal is often thickened, red, and itchy.

Inspect the eardrum, noting its color and contour. The cone of light—usually easy to see—helps to orient you.

Red bulging drum of acute purulent otitis media, amber drum of a serous effusion

Identify the *handle of the malleus,* noting its position, and inspect the *short process of the malleus.*

An unusually prominent short process and a prominent handle that looks more horizontal suggest a retracted drum.

Gently move the speculum so that you can see as much of the drum as possible, including the *pars flaccida* superiorly and the margins of the *pars tensa.* Look for any perforations. The anterior and inferior margins of the drum may be obscured by the curving wall of the ear canal.

See Table 6-18, Abnormalities of the Eardrum (pp. 227–228).

Mobility of the eardrum can be evaluated with a pneumatic otoscope.

A serous effusion, a thickened drum, or purulent otitis media may decrease mobility.

Auditory Acuity. To estimate hearing, test one ear at a time. Ask the patient to occlude one ear with a finger, or better still, occlude it yourself. When auditory acuity on the two sides is different, move your finger rapidly, but gently, in the occluded canal. The noise so produced helps prevent the occluded ear from doing the work of the ear you wish to test. Then, standing 1 or 2 feet away, exhale fully (so as to minimize the intensity of your voice) and whisper softly toward the unoccluded ear. Choose numbers or other words with two equally accented syllables, such as "nine-four," or "baseball." If necessary, increase the intensity of your voice to a medium whisper, a loud whisper, and then a soft, medium, and loud voice. To make sure the patient does not read your lips, cover your mouth or obstruct the patient's vision.

Air and Bone Conduction. If hearing is diminished, *try to distinguish between conductive and sensorineural hearing loss.* You need a quiet room and a tuning fork, preferably of 512 Hz or possibly 1024 Hz. These frequencies fall within the range of human speech (300 Hz to 3000 Hz)—functionally the most important range. Forks with lower pitches may lead to overestimating bone conduction and can also be felt as vibration.

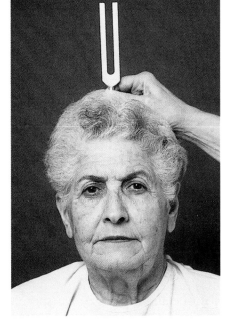

Set the fork into light vibration by briskly stroking it between the thumb and index finger ⇄ or by tapping it on your knuckles.

- *Test for lateralization* (Weber test). Place the base of the lightly vibrating tuning fork firmly on top of the patient's head or on the midforehead.

In unilateral *conductive hearing loss,* sound is heard in (lateralized to) the impaired ear. Visible explanations include acute otitis media, perforation of the eardrum, and obstruction of the ear canal, as by cerumen.

Ask where the patient hears it: on one or both sides. Normally the sound is heard in the midline or equally in both ears. If nothing is heard, try again, pressing the fork more firmly on the head.

In unilateral *sensorineural hearing loss,* sound is heard in the good ear.

- *Compare air conduction (AC) and bone conduction (BC)* (Rinne test). Place the base of a lightly vibrating tuning fork on the mastoid bone, behind the ear and level with the canal. When the patient can no longer hear the sound, quickly place the fork close to the ear canal and ascertain whether the sound can be heard again. Here the "U" of the fork should face forward, thus maximizing its sound for the patient. Normally the sound is heard longer through air than through bone (AC > BC).

In conductive hearing loss, sound is heard through bone as long as or longer than it is through air (BC = AC or BC > AC). In sensorineural hearing loss, sound is heard longer through air (AC > BC). See Table 6-19, Patterns of Hearing Loss (p. 229).

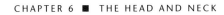

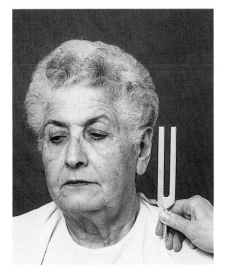

THE NOSE AND PARANASAL SINUSES

Inspect the anterior and inferior surfaces of the nose. Gentle pressure on the tip of the nose with your thumb usually widens the nostrils and, with the aid of a penlight or otoscope light, you can get a partial view of each nasal *vestibule*. If the tip is tender, be particularly gentle and manipulate the nose as little as possible.

Note any asymmetry or deformity of the nose.

Tenderness of the nasal tip or alae suggests local infection such as a furuncle.

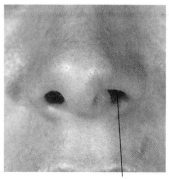

Vestibule

Test for nasal obstruction, if indicated, by pressing on each ala nasi in turn and asking the patient to breathe in.

Inspect the inside of the nose with an otoscope and the largest ear speculum available.‡ Tilt the patient's head back a bit and insert the speculum gently into the vestibule of each nostril, avoiding contact with the sensitive nasal septum. Hold the otoscope handle to one side to avoid the patient's chin and improve your mobility. By directing the speculum posteriorly, then upward in small steps, try to see the inferior and middle turbinates, the nasal septum, and the narrow nasal passage between them. Some asymmetry of the two sides is normal.

Deviation of the lower septum is common and may be easily visible, as illustrated above. Deviation seldom obstructs air flow.

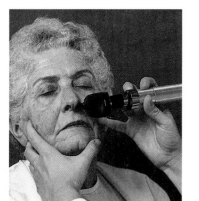
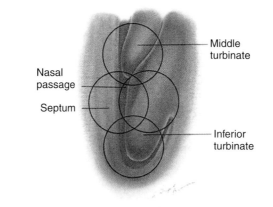

Nasal passage

Septum

Middle turbinate

Inferior turbinate

Observe the nasal mucosa, the nasal septum, and any abnormalities.

■ The *nasal mucosa* that covers the septum and turbinates. Note its color and any swelling, bleeding, or exudate. If exudate is present, note its character: clear, mucopurulent, or purulent. The nasal mucosa is normally somewhat redder than the oral mucosa.

In *viral rhinitis* the mucosa is reddened and swollen; in *allergic rhinitis* it may be pale, bluish, or red.

---

‡A nasal illuminator, equipped with a short wide nasal speculum but lacking an otoscope's magnification, may also be used, but structures look much smaller. Otolaryngologists use special equipment not widely available to others.

■ The *nasal septum*. Note any deviation, inflammation, or perforation of the septum. The lower anterior portion of the septum (where the patient's finger can reach) is a common source of *epistaxis* (nosebleed).

Fresh blood or crusting may be seen. Causes of septal perforation include trauma, surgery, and the intranasal use of cocaine or amphetamines.

■ Any *abnormalities* such as ulcers or polyps.

Make it a habit to place all nasal and ear specula outside your instrument case after use. Then discard them or clean and disinfect them appropriately. (Check the policies of your institution.)

Polyps are pale, semitranslucent masses that usually come from the middle meatus. Ulcers may result from nasal use of cocaine.

Palpate for sinus tenderness. Press up on the *frontal sinuses* from under the bony brows, avoiding pressure on the eyes. Then press up on the *maxillary sinuses.*

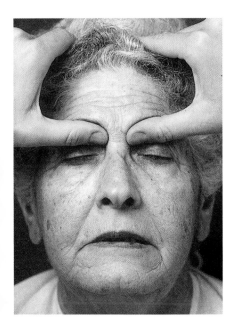
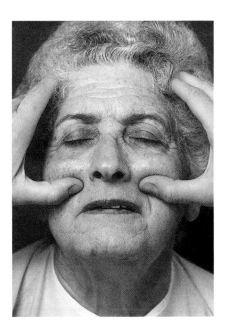

Local tenderness, together with symptoms such as pain, fever, and nasal discharge, suggest *acute sinusitis* involving the frontal or maxillary sinuses.[5-7] Transillumination may be diagnostically useful. For this technique, see p. 202.

THE MOUTH AND PHARYNX

If the patient wears dentures, offer a paper towel and ask the patient to remove them so that you can see the mucosa underneath. If you detect any suspicious ulcers or nodules, put on a glove and palpate any lesions, noting especially any thickening or infiltration of the tissues that might suggest malignancy.

Bright red edematous mucosa underneath a denture suggests denture sore mouth. There may be ulcers or papillary granulation tissue.

Inspect the following:

The Lips. Observe their color and moisture, and note any lumps, ulcers, cracking, or scaliness.

Cyanosis, pallor. See Table 6-20, Abnormalities of the Lips (pp. 230–231).

The Oral Mucosa. Look into the patient's mouth and, with a good light and the help of a tongue blade, inspect the oral mucosa for color, ulcers, white patches, and nodules. The wavy white line on this buccal mucosa developed where the upper and lower teeth meet. Irritation from sucking or chewing may cause or intensify it.

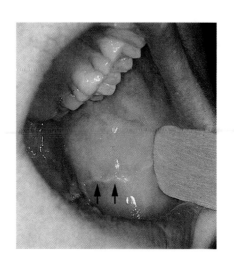

An *aphthous ulcer* on the labial mucosa is shown by the patient.

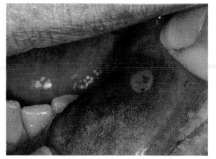

See Table 6-21, Findings in the Pharynx, Palate, and Oral Mucosa (pp. 232–234).

The Gums and Teeth. Note the color of the gums, normally pink. Patchy brownness may be present, especially but not exclusively in black people.

Redness of *gingivitis,* black line of *lead poisoning*

Inspect the gum margins and the interdental papillae for swelling or ulceration.

Swollen interdental papillae in *gingivitis.* See Table 6-22, Findings in the Gums and Teeth (pp. 235–236).

Inspect the teeth. Are any of them missing, discolored, misshapen, or abnormally positioned? You can check for looseness with your gloved thumb and index finger.

The Roof of the Mouth. Inspect the color and architecture of the hard palate.

Torus palatinus, a midline lump (see p. 233)

The Tongue and the Floor of the Mouth. Ask the patient to put out his or her tongue. Inspect it for symmetry—a test of the hypoglossal nerve (Cranial Nerve XII).

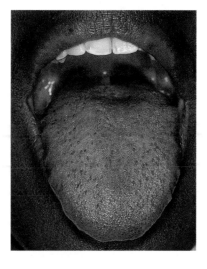

Asymmetric protrusion suggests a lesion of Cranial Nerve XII, as shown below.

Note the color and texture of the dorsum of the tongue.

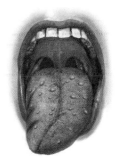

Inspect the sides and undersurface of the tongue and the floor of the mouth. These are the areas where cancer most often develops. Note any white or reddened areas, nodules, or ulcerations. Because cancer of the tongue is more

Cancer of the tongue is the second most common cancer of the mouth, second only to cancer of

common in men over age 50, especially in smokers and drinkers of alcohol, palpation is indicated. Explain what you plan to do and put on gloves. Ask the patient to protrude his tongue. With your right hand, grasp the tip of the tongue with a square of gauze and gently pull it to the patient's left. Inspect the side of the tongue, and then palpate it with your gloved left hand, feeling for any induration (hardness). Reverse the procedure for the other side.

the lip. Any persistent nodule or ulcer, red or white, must be suspect. Induration of the lesion further increases the possibility of malignancy. Cancer occurs most often on the side of the tongue, next most often at its base.

A carcinoma on the left side of a tongue:

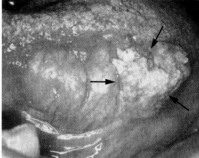

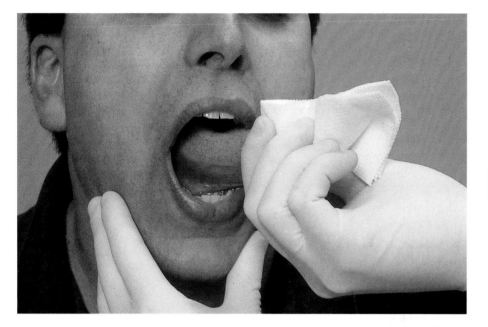

(Photo reprinted by permission of the New England Journal of Medicine, 328: 186, 1993—arrows added)

See Table 6-23, Findings In or Under the Tongue (pp. 237–238).

The Pharynx.   Now, with the patient's mouth open but the tongue not protruded, ask the patient to say "ah" or yawn. This action may let you see the pharynx well. If not, press a tongue blade firmly down upon the midpoint of the arched tongue—far enough back to get good visualization of the pharynx but not so far that you cause gagging. Simultaneously, ask for an "ah" or a yawn. Note the rise of the soft palate—a test of Cranial Nerve X (the vagal nerve).

In CN X paralysis, the soft palate fails to rise and the uvula deviates to the opposite side.

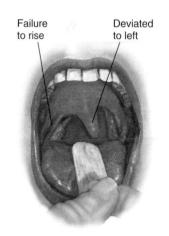

Failure to rise   Deviated to left

Inspect the soft palate, anterior and posterior pillars, uvula, tonsils, and pharynx. Note their color and symmetry and look for exudate, swelling, ulceration, or tonsillar enlargement. If possible, palpate any suspicious area for induration or tenderness. Tonsils have crypts, or deep infoldings of squamous epithelium. Whitish spots of normal exfoliating epithelium may sometimes be seen in these crypts.

Discard your tongue blade after use.

See Table 6-21, Findings in the Pharynx, Palate, and Oral Mucosa (pp. 232–234).

THE NECK

Inspect the neck, noting its symmetry and any masses or scars. Look for enlargement of the parotid or submandibular glands, and note any visible lymph nodes.

A scar of past thyroid surgery is often a clue to unsuspected thyroid disease.

The Lymph Nodes.   *Palpate the lymph nodes.* Using the pads of your index and middle fingers, move the skin over the underlying tissues in each area. The patient should be relaxed, with neck flexed slightly forward and, if needed, slightly toward the side being examined. You can usually examine both sides at once. For the submental node, however, it is helpful to feel with one hand while bracing the top of the head with the other.

Feel in sequence for the following nodes:

1. *Preauricular*—in front of the ear

2. *Posterior auricular*—superficial to the mastoid process

3. *Occipital*—at the base of the skull posteriorly

4. *Tonsillar*—at the angle of the mandible

A "tonsillar node" that pulsates is really the carotid artery. A small, hard, tender "tonsillar node" high and deep between the mandible and the sternomastoid is probably a styloid process.

5. *Submandibular*—midway between the angle and the tip of the mandible. These nodes are usually smaller and smoother than the lobulated submandibular gland against which they lie.

6. *Submental*—in the midline a few centimeters behind the tip of the mandible

7. *Superficial cervical*—superficial to the sternomastoid

8. *Posterior cervical*—along the anterior edge of the trapezius

9. *Deep cervical chain*—deep to the sternomastoid and often inaccessible to examination. Hook your thumb and fingers around either side of the sternomastoid muscle to find them.

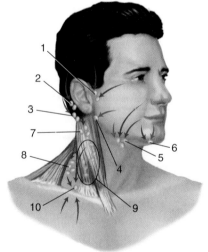

10. *Supraclavicular*—deep in the angle formed by the clavicle and the sternomastoid

→ External lymphatic drainage
→ Internal lymphatic drainage (e.g., from mouth and throat)

Enlargement of a supraclavicular node, especially on the left, suggests possible metastasis from a thoracic or an abdominal malignancy.

Note their size, shape, delimitation (discrete or matted together), mobility, consistency, and any tenderness. Small, mobile, discrete, nontender nodes, sometimes termed "shotty," are frequently found in normal persons.

Tender nodes suggest inflammation; hard or fixed nodes suggest malignancy.

- Using the pads of the 2nd and 3rd fingers, palpate the preauricular nodes with a gentle rotary motion. Then examine the posterior auricular and occipital lymph nodes.

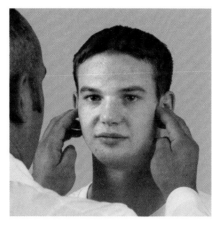

- Palpate the anterior cervical chain, located anterior and superficial to the sternomastoid. Then palpate the posterior cervical chain along the trapezius (anterior edge) and along the sternomastoid (posterior edge). Flex the patient's neck slightly forward toward the side being examined. Examine the supraclavicular nodes in the angle between the clavicle and the sternomastoid.

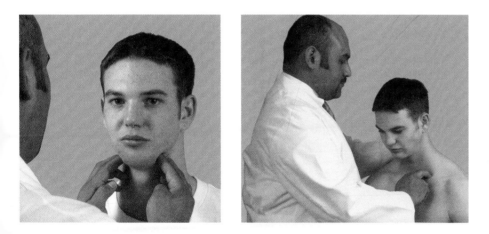

Enlarged or tender nodes, if unexplained, call for (1) reexamination of the regions they drain, and (2) careful assessment of lymph nodes elsewhere so that you can distinguish between regional and generalized lymphadenopathy.

Occasionally you may mistake a band of muscle or an artery for a lymph node. You should be able to roll a node in two directions: up and down, and side to side. Neither a muscle nor an artery will pass this test.

Diffuse lymphadenopathy raises the suspicion of HIV or AIDS.

The Trachea and the Thyroid Gland. To orient yourself to the neck, identify the thyroid and cricoid cartilages and the trachea below them.

■ *Inspect the trachea* for any deviation from its usual midline position. Then *feel for any deviation.* Place your finger along one side of the trachea and note the space between it and the sternomastoid. Compare it with the other side. The spaces should be symmetric.

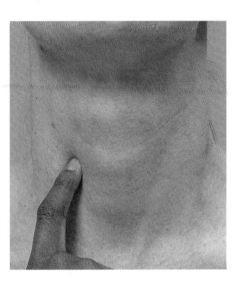

Masses in the neck may push the trachea to one side. Tracheal deviation may also signify important problems in the thorax, such as a mediastinal mass, atelectasis, or a large pneumothorax (see pp. 276–277).

■ *Inspect the neck for the thyroid gland.* Tip the patient's head back a bit. Using tangential lighting directed downward from the tip of the patient's chin, *inspect the region below the cricoid cartilage* for the gland. The lower, shadowed border of each thyroid gland shown here is outlined by arrows.

The lower border of this large thyroid gland is outlined by tangential lighting. *Goiter* is a general term for an enlarged thyroid gland.[13,14]

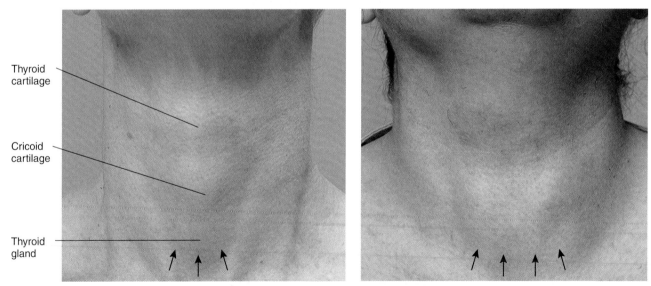

Thyroid cartilage

Cricoid cartilage

Thyroid gland

AT REST

Ask the patient to sip some water and to extend the neck again and swallow. Watch for upward movement of the thyroid gland, noting its contour and symmetry. The thyroid cartilage, the cricoid cartilage, and the thyroid gland all rise with swallowing and then fall to their resting positions.

With swallowing, the lower border of this large gland rises and looks less symmetric.

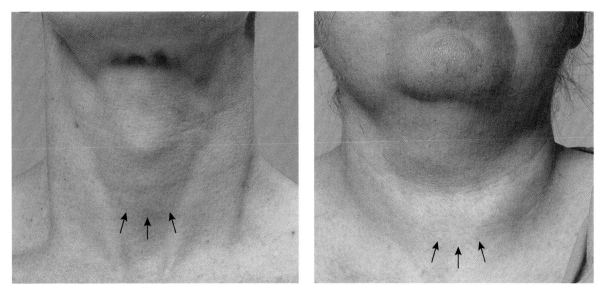

SWALLOWING

Until you become familiar with this examination, check your visual observations with your fingers from in front of the patient. This will orient you to the next step.

You are now ready to *palpate the thyroid gland*. This may seem difficult at first. Use the cues from visual inspection. Find your landmarks—the notched thyroid cartilage and the cricoid cartilage below it. Locate the *thyroid isthmus*, usually overlying the second, third, and fourth tracheal rings.

Adopt good technique, and follow the steps on the next page, which outline the posterior approach (technique for the anterior approach is similar). With experience you will become more adept. The thyroid gland is usually easier to feel in a long slender neck than in a short stocky one. In shorter necks, added extension of the neck may help. In some people, however, the thyroid gland is partially or wholly substernal and not amenable to physical examination.

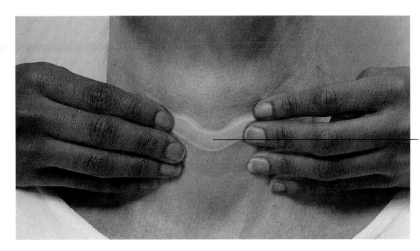

Cricoid cartilage

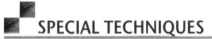

STEPS FOR PALPATING THE THYROID GLAND

- Ask the patient to flex the neck slightly forward to relax the sternomastoid muscles.
- Place the fingers of both hands on the patient's neck so that your index fingers are just below the cricoid cartilage.
- Ask the patient to sip and swallow water as before. Feel for the thyroid isthmus rising up under your finger pads. It is often but not always palpable.
- Displace the trachea to the right with the fingers of the left hand; with the right-hand fingers, palpate laterally for the right lobe of the thyroid in the space between the displaced trachea and the relaxed sternomastoid. Find the lateral margin. In similar fashion, examine the left lobe.

   The lobes are somewhat harder to feel than the isthmus, so practice is needed. The anterior surface of a lateral lobe is approximately the size of the distal phalanx of the thumb and feels somewhat rubbery.

- Note the *size, shape,* and *consistency* of the gland and identify any *nodules* or *tenderness.*

   If the thyroid gland is enlarged, listen over the lateral lobes with a stethoscope to detect a *bruit,* a sound similar to a cardiac murmur but of noncardiac origin.

Although physical characteristics of the thyroid gland, such as size, shape, and consistency, are diagnostically important, assessment of thyroid function depends upon symptoms, signs elsewhere in the body, and laboratory tests.[15,16] See Table 6-24, Thyroid Enlargement and Function (p. 239).

Soft in Graves' disease; firm in Hashimoto's thyroiditis, malignancy. Benign and malignant nodules,[17] tenderness in thyroiditis

A localized systolic or continuous bruit may be heard in hyperthyroidism.

The Carotid Arteries and Jugular Veins. Defer a detailed examination of these vessels until the patient lies down for the cardiovascular examination. Jugular venous distention, however, may be visible in the sitting position and should not be overlooked. You should also be alert to unusually prominent arterial pulsations. See Chapter 8 for further discussion.

Note: Many clinicians would complete examination of the cranial nerves (see pp. 611–616) at this point.

SPECIAL TECHNIQUES

For Assessing Protruding Eyes (Proptosis or Exophthalmos). For eyes that seem unusually prominent, stand behind the seated patient and inspect from above. Draw the upper lids gently upward, then compare the protrusion of the eyes and the relationship of the corneas to the lower lids. For objective measurement, use an exophthalmometer. This instrument measures the distance between the lateral angle of the orbit and an imaginary line across the most anterior point of the cornea. The upper limits of normal are 20 mm in whites and 22 mm in blacks.[18,19]

When protrusion exceeds normal, further evaluation by ultrasound or computerized tomography scan often follows.[20]

Exophthalmos is an abnormal protrusion of the eye.

For Nasolacrimal Duct Obstruction. This test helps identify the cause of excessive tearing. Ask the patient to look up. Press on the lower lid close to the medial canthus, just inside the rim of the bony orbit—this compresses the lacrimal sac. Look for fluid regurgitated out of the puncta into the eye. Avoid this test if the area is inflamed and tender.

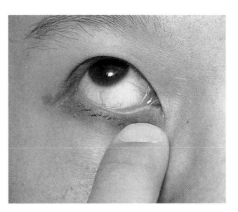

Discharge of mucopurulent fluid from the puncta suggests an obstructed nasolacrimal duct.

For Inspection of the Upper Palpebral Conjunctiva. Adequate examination of the eye in search of a foreign body requires eversion of the upper eyelid. Follow these steps:

- Instruct the patient to look down. Get the patient to relax the eyes— by reassurance and by gentle, assured, and deliberate movements. Raise the upper eyelid slightly so that the eyelashes protrude, and then grasp the upper eyelashes and pull them gently down and forward.

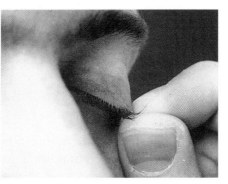

- Place a small stick such as an applicator or a tongue blade at least 1 cm above the lid margin (and therefore at the upper border of the tarsal plate). Push down on the stick as you raise the edge of the lid, thus everting the eyelid or turning it "inside out." Do not press on the eyeball itself.

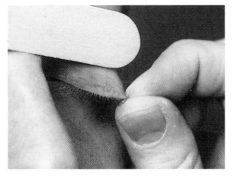

- Secure the upper lashes against the eyebrow with your thumb and inspect the palpebral conjunctiva. After your inspection, grasp the upper eyelashes and pull them gently forward. Ask the patient to look up. The eyelid will return to its normal position.

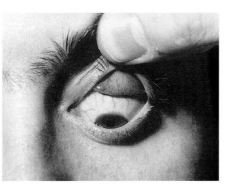

This view allows you to see the upper palpebral conjunctiva and look for a foreign body that might be lodged there.

Swinging Flashlight Test.   The swinging flashlight test is a clinical test for functional impairment in the optic nerves. In dim light, note the size of the pupils. After asking the patient to gaze into the distance, swing the beam of a penlight first into one pupil, then into the other. Normally, each illuminated eye looks or promptly becomes constricted. The opposite eye also constricts consensually.

When the optic nerve is damaged, as in the left eye below, the sensory or afferent stimulus sent to the brainstem is reduced. The pupil dilates instead of constricting when the light moves from the good right eye into the left eye. This response is an *afferent pupillary defect,* sometimes termed a *Marcus Gunn pupil.* The opposite eye responds consensually.

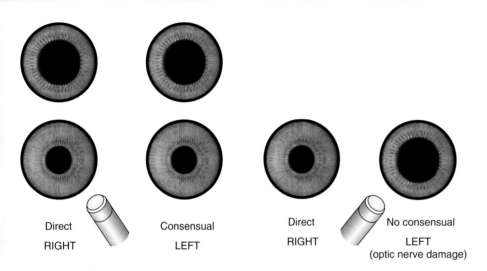

Direct	Consensual	Direct	No consensual
RIGHT	LEFT	RIGHT	LEFT
			(optic nerve damage)

Transillumination of the Sinuses.   When sinus tenderness or other symptoms suggest sinusitis, this test can at times be helpful but is not highly sensitive or specific for diagnosis. The room should be thoroughly darkened. Using a strong, narrow light source, place the light snugly deep under each brow, close to the nose. Shield the light with your hand. Look for a dim red glow as light is transmitted through the air-filled frontal sinus to the forehead.

Absence of glow on one or both sides suggests a thickened mucosa or secretions in the frontal sinus, but it may also result from developmental absence of one or both sinuses.

Ask the patient to tilt his or her head back with mouth opened wide. (An upper denture should first be removed.) Shine the light downward from just below the inner aspect of each eye. Look through the open mouth at the hard palate. A reddish glow indicates a normal air-filled maxillary sinus.

Absence of glow suggests thickened mucosa or secretions in the maxillary sinus. See p. 756 for an alternative method of transilluminating the maxillary sinuses.

RECORDING YOUR FINDINGS

Note that initially you may use sentences to describe your findings; later you will use phrases. The style below contains phrases appropriate for most write-ups.

Recording the Physical Examination— The Head, Eyes, Ears, Nose, and Throat (HEENT)

HEENT: Head—The skull is normocephalic/atraumatic (NC/AT). Hair with average texture. *Eyes*—Visual acuity 20/20 bilaterally. Sclera white, conjunctiva pink. Pupils are 4 mm constricting to 2 mm, equally round and reactive to light and accommodations. Disc margins sharp; no hemorrhages or exudates, no arteriolar narrowing. *Ears*—Acuity good to whispered voice. Tympanic membranes (TMs) with good cone of light. Weber midline. AC > BC. *Nose*—Nasal mucosa pink, septum midline; no sinus tenderness. *Throat (or Mouth)*—Oral mucosa pink, dentition good, pharynx without exudates.

Neck—Trachea midline. Neck supple; thyroid isthmus palpable, lobes not felt.

Lymph Nodes—No cervical, axillary, epitrochlear, inguinal adenopathy.

OR

Head—The skull is normocephalic/atraumatic. Frontal balding. *Eyes*—Visual acuity 20/100 bilaterally. Sclera white; conjunctiva injected. Pupils constrict 3 mm to 2 mm, equally round and reactive to light and accommodation. Disc margins sharp; no hemorrhages or exudates. Arteriolar-to-venous ratio (AV ratio) 2:4; no A-V nicking. *Ears*—Acuity diminished to whispered voice; intact to spoken voice. TMs clear. *Nose*—Mucosa swollen with erythema and clear drainage. Septum midline. Tender over maxillary sinuses. *Throat*—Oral mucosa pink, dental caries in lower molars, pharynx erythematous, no exudates.

Neck—Trachea midline. Neck supple; thyroid isthmus midline, lobes palpable but not enlarged.

Lymph Nodes—Submandibular and anterior cervical lymph nodes tender, 1 × 1 cm, rubbery and mobile; no posterior cervical, epitrochlear, axillary, or inguinal lymphadenopathy.

Suggests myopia and mild arteriolar narrowing. Also upper respiratory infection.

Bibliography

CITATIONS

1. Goadsby PJ, Lipton RB, Ferrari MD. Migraine: current understanding and treatment. N Engl J Med 346(4):257–270, 2002.
2. Shingleton BJ, O'Donoghue MW. Blurred vision. N Engl J Med 343(8):556–562, 2000.
3. Fine SL, Berger JW, Macguire MG, et al. Age-related macular degeneration. N Engl J Med 342(7):483–492, 2000.
4. Coleman AC. Glaucoma. Lancet 20:1803–1810, 1999.
5. Piccirillo JF. Acute bacterial sinusitis. N Engl J Med 351(9):902–910, 2004.
6. Spector SL, Bernstein IL, Li JT, et al. Parameters for the diagnosis and management of sinusitis. J Allergy Clin Immunol 102(6, part 2):S107–S144, 1998.
7. Williams JW, Simel DL, Roberts L, et al. Clinical evaluation for sinusitis: making the diagnosis by history and physical examination. Ann Intern Med 117:705–710, 1992.
8. U.S. Preventive Services Task Force. Screening for visual impairment. In Guide to Clinical Preventive Services, 2nd ed, pp. 373–382. Baltimore, Williams & Wilkins, 1996.
9. U.S. Preventive Services Task Force. Screening for glaucoma. In Guide to Clinical Preventive Services, 2nd ed., pp. 383–391. Baltimore, Williams & Wilkins, 1996.
10. U.S. Preventive Services Task Force. Screening for hearing impairment. In Guide to Clinical Preventive Services, 2nd ed., pp. 393–405. Baltimore, Williams & Wilkins, 1996.
11. U.S. Preventive Services Task Force. Counseling to prevent dental and periodontal disease. In Guide to Clinical Preventive Services, 2nd ed., pp. 711–721. Baltimore, Williams & Wilkins, 1996.
12. Greene JC, Greene AR. Oral health. In Woolf SH, Jonas S, Lawrence RS (eds). Health Promotion and Disease Prevention in Clinical Practice, pp. 315–334. Baltimore, Williams & Wilkins, 1996.
13. McGuirt WF. The neck mass. Med Clin N Am 83:219–234, 1989.
14. Siminoski K. Does this patient have a goiter? JAMA 273(10):813–817, 1995.
15. U.S. Preventive Services Task Force. Screening for thyroid disease: recommendation statement. Ann Intern Med 140(2):125–127, 2004.
16. Surks MI, Ortiz E, Daniels GH, et al. Subclinical thyroid disease: scientific review and guidelines for diagnosis and management. JAMA 291(2):228–238, 2004.
17. Hegedus L. The thyroid nodule. N Engl J Med 351(17):1764–1771, 2004.
18. Gladstone GJ. Ophthalmologic aspects of thyroid-related orbitopathy. Endocrinol Metab Clin North Am 27:91–100, 1998.
19. Bartley GB, et al. Clinical features of Graves' ophthalmopathy in an incidence cohort. Am J Ophthalmol 121:284–290, 1996.
20. Hallin ES, Feldon SE. Graves' ophthalmopathy. II. Correlation of clinical signs with measures derived from computed tomography. Br J Ophthalmol 72:678–682, 1988.
21. Headache Classification Subcommittee of the International Headache Society. The international headache classification. Cephalalgia 24(Suppl 1):1–160, 2004.
22. Rollnik JD, Karst M, Fink M, et al. Botulinum toxin type A and EMG: a key to the understanding of chronic tension-type headaches? Headache 41(10):985–989, 2001.
23. Smetana GW, Shmerling RH. Does this patient have temporal arteritis? JAMA 287(1):92–101, 2002.
24. Haas DC. Chronic post-traumatic headaches classified and compared with natural headaches. Cephalalgia 16(7):486–493, 1996.
25. Kroenke K, Lucas CA, Rosengerg ML, et al. Causes of persistent dizziness: a prospective study of 100 patients in ambulatory care. Ann Intern Med 117(11):898–904, 1992.
26. Kroenke K, Hoffman RM, Einstadter D. How common are various causes of dizziness? A critical review. South Med J 93(2):160–167, quiz 168, 2000.
27. Tusa RJ. Vertigo. Neurol Clin 19(1):23–55, 2001.
28. Branch W. Approach to the patient with dizziness. Available at: www.utdol.com. Accessed February 26, 2005.
29. Lockwood AH, Salvi RJ, Burkard RF. Tinnitus. N Engl J Med 347(12):904–910, 2002.
30. Matthies C, Samii M. Management of 1000 vestibular schwannomas (acoustic neuromas): clinical presentation. Neurosurgery 1:1–10, 1997.
31. Leibowitz HM. The red eye. N Engl J Med 342(5):345–351, 2000.
32. Wong TY, Mitchell P. Hypertensive retinopathy. N Engl J Med 351(22):2310–2317, 2004.

ADDITIONAL REFERENCES

Bahra A, May A. Cluster headache: a prospective clinical study with diagnostic implications. Neurology 58(3):354–361, 2002.

The Eye

Albert DM, Jakobiec FA. Principles and Practice of Ophthalmology, 2nd ed. Philadelphia, WB Saunders, 2000.

Congdon N, O'Colmain, Klaver CC, et al. Causes and prevalence of visual impairment among adults in the United States. Arch Ophthalmol 122(4):477–485, 2004.

Fong DS, Aiello LP, Ferris FL, et al. Diabetic retinopathy. Diabetes Care 27(10):2540–2553, 2004.

Gold DH, Weingeist TA. Color Atlas of the Eye in Systemic Disease. Philadelphia, Lippincott Williams & Wilkins, 2001.

McCluskey PJ, Towler HM, Lightman S. Management of chronic uveitis. BMJ 320(7234):555–558, 2000.

Ostler HB, Maibach HI, Hoke AW, Schwab IR. Diseases of the Eye and Skin. A Color Atlas. Philadelphia, Lippincott Williams & Wilkins, 2004.

Sheilds SR. Managing eye disease in primary care. Part 1. How to screen for occult disease. Postgrad Med 108(5):69–72, 75–78, 2000.

Spoor TC (ed). Atlas of Neuro-ophthalmology. New York, Taylor & Francis, 2004.

Tasman W, Jaeger EA. The Wills Eye Hospital Atlas of Clinical Ophthalmology, 2nd ed. Philadelphia, Lippincott Williams & Wilkins, 2001.

Yanoff M, Duker JS. Ophthalmology, 2nd ed. St. Louis, Mosby, 2004.

BIBLIOGRAPHY

The Ears, Nose, and Throat

Bevan Y, Shapiro N, MacLean CH, et al. Screening and management of adult hearing loss in primary care: scientific review. JAMA 289(15):1976–1985, 2003.

Bull TR. Color Atlas of ENT Diagnosis, 4th ed. New York, Thieme, 2003.

Doty RL (ed). Handbook of Olfaction and Gustation, 2nd ed. (Neurological Disease and Therapy, Vol 57). New York, Marcel Dekker, 2003.

Ebell MH, Smith MA, Barry HC, et al. Does this patient have strep throat? JAMA 284(22):2912–2918, 2000.

Hendley JO. Otitis media. N Engl J Med 347(15):1169–1174, 2002.

Kennedy DW. A 48-year-old man with recurrent sinusitis. JAMA 283(16):2143–2150, 2000.

O'Donoghue GM, Narula AA, Bates GJ. Clinical ENT: An Illustrated Textbook, 2nd ed. San Diego, Singular Pub Group, 2000.

Young T, Skatrud J, Peppard PE. Risk factors for obstructive sleep apnea in adults. JAMA 291(16):2013–2016, 2004.

The Mouth

Eisen D, Lynch DP. The Mouth: Diagnosis and Treatment. St. Louis, Mosby, 1998.

Field EA, Longman L, Tyldesley WR, et al. Tyldesley's Oral Medicine, 5th ed. New York, Oxford University Press, 2003.

Langlais RP, Miller CS. Color Atlas of Common Oral Diseases, 3rd ed. Philadelphia, Lippincott Williams & Wilkins, 2003.

Neville BW, Damm DD, White DK. Color Atlas of Clinical Oral Pathology, 2nd ed. Baltimore, Williams & Wilkins, 1999.

Newman MF, Carranza FA, Takei H. Carranza's Clinical Periodontology, 9th ed. Philadelphia, WB Saunders, 2002.

Regezi JA, Sciubba JJ, Jordan RCK. Oral Pathology: Clinical Pathologic Correlations, 4th ed. St. Louis, WB Saunders, 2003.

The Neck

Bliss SJ, Flanders SA, Saint S. A pain in the neck. N Engl J Med 350(10):1037–1042, 2004.

Henry PH, Long DL. Enlargement of the lymph nodes and spleen. In Kasper DL, Fauci AS, Longo DL, et al (eds). Harrison's Principles of Internal Medicine, 16th ed. New York, McGraw-Hill, 2005.

Prisco MK. Evaluating neck masses. Nurse Pract 25(4):30–32, 35–36, 38, 2000.

Schwetschenau E, Kelley DJ. The adult neck mass. Am Fam Physician 67(6):1190, 1192, 1195, 2003.

TABLE 6-1   **Headaches**[21]

Type	Process	Location	Quality and Severity
Primary Headaches			
Tension	Unclear—muscle contraction or vasoconstriction unlikely[22]	Usually bilateral; may be generalized or localized to the back of the head and upper neck or to the frontotemporal area	Pressing or tightening pain; mild to moderate intensity
Migraines ■ With aura ■ Without aura ■ Variants	Primary neuronal dysfunction, possibly of brainstem origin, causing imbalance of excitatory and inhibitory neurotransmitters and affecting craniovascular modulation[1]	Unilateral in ~70%; bifrontal or global in ~30%	Throbbing or aching, variable in severity
Cluster	Unclear—possibly extracranial vasodilation from neural dysfunction with trigeminovascular pain	Unilateral, usually behind or around the eye	Deep, continuous, severe
Secondary Headaches			
Analgesic Rebound	Withdrawal of medication	Previous headache pattern	Variable
Headaches From Eye Disorders			
Errors of Refraction (farsightedness and astigmatism, but not nearsightedness)	Probably the sustained contraction of the extraocular muscles, and possibly of the frontal, temporal, and occipital muscles	Around and over the eyes, may radiate to the occipital area	Steady, aching, dull
Acute Glaucoma	Sudden increase in intraocular pressure (see p. 181)	In and around one eye	Steady, aching, often severe
Headache From Sinusitis	Mucosal inflammation of the paranasal sinuses	Usually above the eye (frontal sinus) or over the maxillary sinus	Aching or throbbing, variable in severity; consider possible migraine
Meningitis	Infection of the meninges surrounding the brain	Generalized	Steady or throbbing, very severe

Timing			Associated Factors	Factors That Aggravate or Provoke	Factors That Relieve
Onset	*Duration*	*Course*			
Gradual	Minutes to days	Often recurrent or persistent over long periods; annual prevalence ~40%	Sometimes photophobia, phonophobia; nausea absent	Sustained muscle tension, as in driving or typing	Possible massage, relaxation
Fairly rapid, reaching a peak in 1–2 hours	4–72 hours	Peak incidence early to mid-adolescence; prevalence is ~6% in men and ~15% in women. Recurrent— usually monthly but weekly in ~10%	Nausea, vomiting, photophobia, phonophobia, visual auras (flickering zig-zagging lines), motor auras affecting hand or arm, sensory auras (numbness, tingling usually precede headache)	May be provoked by alcohol, certain foods, or tension. More common premenstrually. Aggravated by noise and bright light.	Quiet, dark room; sleep; sometimes transient relief from pressure on the involved artery, if early in the course
Abrupt, peaks within minutes	Up to 3 hours	Episodic, clustered in time with several each day for 4–8 weeks and then relief for 6–12 months; prevalence <1%, more common in men	Lacrimation, rhinorrhea, miosis, ptosis, eyelid edema, conjunctival infection	During attack, sensitivity to alcohol may increase	
Variable	Depends on prior headache pattern	Depends on frequency of "mini-withdrawals"	Depends on prior headache pattern	Fever, carbon monoxide, hypoxia, withdrawal of caffeine, other headache triggers	Depends on cause
Gradual	Variable	Variable	Eye fatigue, "sandy" sensations in the eyes, redness of the conjunctiva	Prolonged use of the eyes, particularly for close work	Rest of the eyes
Often rapid	Variable, may depend on treatment	Variable, may depend on treatment	Diminished vision, sometimes nausea and vomiting	Sometimes provoked by drops that dilate the pupils	
Variable	Often several hours at a time, recurring over days or longer	Often recurrent in a repetitive daily pattern	Local tenderness, nasal congestion, discharge, and fever	May be aggravated by coughing, sneezing, or jarring the head	Nasal decongestants, antibiotics
Fairly rapid	Variable, usually days	A persistent headache in an acute illness	Fever, stiff neck		

(table continues next page)

TABLE 6-1   **Headaches**[21] *(Continued)*

Type	Process	Location	Quality and Severity
Giant Cell (Temporal) Arteritis[23]	Vasculitis from cell-mediated immune response to elastic lamina of artery	Localized near the involved artery, most often the temporal, also the occipital; age related	Throbbing, generalized, persistent; often severe
Posttraumatic Headache	Mechanism unclear; episodes similar to tension-type and migraine without aura headaches[24]	May be localized to the injured area, but not necessarily	Generalized, dull, aching, constant
Subarachnoid Hemorrhage	Bleeding, most often from a ruptured intracranial aneurysm	Generalized	Very severe, "the worst of my life"
Brain Tumor	Displacement of or traction on pain-sensitive arteries and veins or pressure on nerves	Varies with the location of the tumor	Aching, steady, variable in intensity
Cranial Neuralgias *Trigeminal Neuralgia (CNV)*	Compression of CN V, often by aberrant loop or artery of vein	Cheek, jaws, lips, or gums; trigeminal nerve divisions 2 and 3 > 1	Shocklike, stabbing, burning; severe

Note: Blanks appear in these tables when the categories are not applicable or not usually helpful in assessing the problem.

Timing			Associated Factors	Factors That Aggravate or Provoke	Factors That Relieve
Onset	*Duration*	*Course*			
Gradual or rapid	Variable	Recurrent or persistent over weeks to months	Tenderness of the adjacent scalp; fever (in ~50%), fatigue, weight loss; new headache (~60%), jaw claudication (~50%), visual loss or blindness (~15%–20%), polymyalgia rheumatica (~50%)	Movement of neck and shoulders	
Within hours to 1–2 days of the injury	Weeks, months, or even years	Tends to diminish over time	Poor concentration, problems with memory, vertigo, irritability, restlessness, fatigue	Mental and physical exertion, straining, stooping, emotional excitement, alcohol	Rest
Usually abrupt, severe; prodromal symptoms may occur	Variable, usually days	A persistent headache in an acute illness	Nausea, vomiting, possibly loss of consciousness, neck pain		
Variable	Often brief	Often intermittent but progressive	May be aggravated by coughing, sneezing, or sudden movements of the head		
Abrupt, paroxysmal	Each jab lasts seconds but recurs at intervals of seconds or minutes	May last for months, then disappear for months, but often recurs. It is uncommon at night.	Exhaustion from recurrent pain	Touching certain areas of the lower face or mouth; chewing, talking, brushing teeth	

TABLE 6-2   Dizziness and Vertigo

"Dizziness" is a nonspecific term used by patients encompassing several disorders that clinicians must carefully sort out. A detailed history usually identifies the primary etiology.[25–30] It is important to learn the specific meanings of the following terms or conditions:

- *Vertigo*—a spinning sensation accompanied by nystagmus and ataxia; usually from *peripheral vestibular dysfunction* (~40% of "dizzy" patients) but may be from a *central brainstem lesion* (~10%; causes include atherosclerosis, multiple sclerosis, vertebrobasilar migraine, or TIA)
- *Presyncope*—a near faint from "feeling faint or lightheaded"; causes include orthostatic hypotension, especially from medication, arrhythmias, and vasovagal attacks (~5%)
- *Dysequilibrium*—unsteadiness or imbalance when walking, especially in older patients (see p. 858); causes include fear of walking, visual loss, weakness from musculoskeletal problems, and peripheral neuropathy (up to 15%)
- *Psychiatric*—causes include anxiety, panic disorder, hyperventilation, depression, somatization disorder, alcohol, and substance abuse (~10%)
- *Multifactorial or unknown*—(up to 20%)

Peripheral and Central Vertigo

	Onset	Duration and Course	Hearing	Tinnitus	Additional Features
Peripheral Vertigo					
Benign Positional Vertigo	Sudden, on rolling onto affected side or tilting head up	Onset a few seconds to <1 minute. Lasts a few weeks, may recur	Not affected	Absent	Sometimes nausea, vomiting. Nystagmus
Vestibular Neuronitis (acute labyrinthitis)	Sudden	Onset hours to up to 2 weeks. May recur over 12–18 months	Not affected	Absent	Nausea, vomiting, nystagmus
Ménière's Disease	Sudden	Onset several hours to ≥1 day. Recurrent	Sensorineural hearing loss—recurs, eventually progresses	Present, fluctuating	Pressure or fullness in affected ear; nausea, vomiting, nystagmus
Drug Toxicity	Insidious or acute—linked to loop diuretics, aminoglycosides, salicylates, alcohol	May or may not be reversible. Partial adaptation occurs	May be impaired	May be present	Nausea, vomiting
Acoustic Neuroma	Insidious from CN VIII compression, vestibular branch	Variable	Impaired, one side	Present	May involve CN V and VII
Central Vertigo	Often sudden (see causes above)	Variable but rarely continuous	Not affected	Absent	Usually with other brainstem deficits—dysarthria, ataxia, crossed motor and sensory deficits

TABLE 6-3　　**Selected Facies**

Facial Swelling

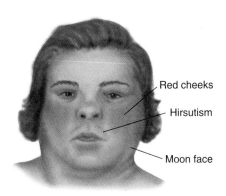

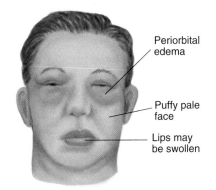

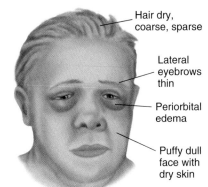

Cushing's Syndrome

The increased adrenal hormone production of Cushing's syndrome produces a round or "moon" face with red cheeks. Excessive hair growth may be present in the mustache and sideburn areas and on the chin.

Nephrotic Syndrome

The face is edematous and often pale. Swelling usually appears first around the eyes and in the morning. The eyes may become slitlike when edema is severe.

Myxedema

The patient with severe hypothyroidism (*myxedema*) has a dull, puffy facies. The edema, often particularly pronounced around the eyes, does not pit with pressure. The hair and eyebrows are dry, coarse, and thinned. The skin is dry.

Other Facies

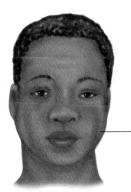

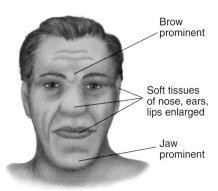

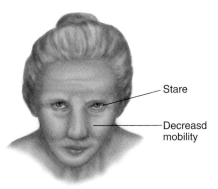

Parotid Gland Enlargement

Chronic bilateral asymptomatic parotid gland enlargement may be associated with obesity, diabetes, cirrhosis, and other conditions. Note the swellings anterior to the ear lobes and above the angles of the jaw. Gradual unilateral enlargement suggests neoplasm. Acute enlargement is seen in mumps.

Acromegaly

The increased growth hormone of acromegaly produces enlargement of both bone and soft tissues. The head is elongated, with bony prominence of the forehead, nose, and lower jaw. Soft tissues of the nose, lips, and ears also enlarge. The facial features appear generally coarsened.

Parkinson's Disease

Decreased facial mobility blunts expression. A masklike face may result, with decreased blinking and a characteristic stare. Since the neck and upper trunk tend to flex forward, the patient seems to peer upward toward the observer. Facial skin becomes oily, and drooling may occur.

TABLE 6-4 **Visual Field Defects**

Visual Field Defects

1 Horizontal Defect Occlusion of a branch of the central retinal artery may cause a horizontal (altitudinal) defect. Shown is the lower field defect associated with occlusion of the superior branch of this artery.

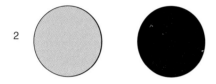

2 Blind Right Eye (right optic nerve) A lesion of the optic nerve, and of course of the eye itself, produces unilateral blindness.

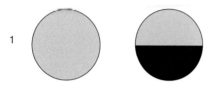

3 Bitemporal Hemianopsia (optic chiasm) A lesion at the optic chiasm may involve only fibers crossing over to the opposite side. Since these fibers originate in the nasal half of each retina, visual loss involves the temporal half of each field.

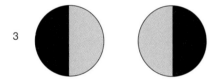

4 Left Homonymous Hemianopsia (right optic tract) A lesion of the optic tract interrupts fibers originating on the same side of both eyes. Visual loss in the eyes is therefore similar (homonymous) and involves half of each field (hemianopsia).

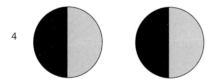

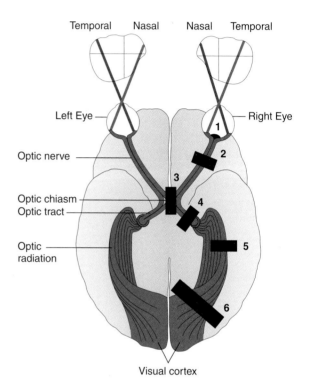

5 Homonymous Left Superior Quadrantic Defect (right optic radiation, partial) A partial lesion of the optic radiation in the temporal lobe may involve only a portion of the nerve fibers, producing, for example, a homonymous quadrantic defect.

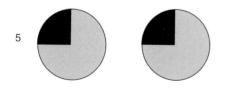

6 Left Homonymous Hemianopsia (right optic radiation) A complete interruption of fibers in the optic radiation produces a visual defect similar to that produced by a lesion of the optic tract.

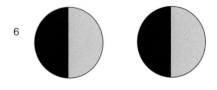

TABLE 6-5   Variations and Abnormalities of the Eyelids

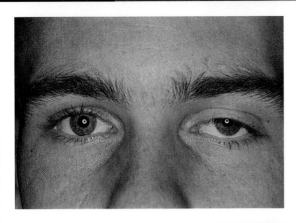

Ptosis

Ptosis is a drooping of the upper lid. Causes include myasthenia gravis, damage to the oculomotor nerve, and damage to the sympathetic nerve supply (*Horner's syndrome*). A weakened muscle, relaxed tissues, and the weight of herniated fat may cause senile ptosis. Ptosis may also be congenital.

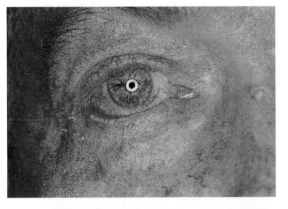

Entropion

Entropion, more common in the elderly, is an inward turning of the lid margin. The lower lashes, which are often invisible when turned inward, irritate the conjunctiva and lower cornea. Asking the patient to squeeze the lids together and then open them may reveal an entropion that is not obvious.

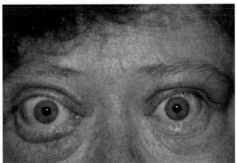

Ectropion

In ectropion the margin of the lower lid is turned outward, exposing the palpebral conjunctiva. When the punctum of the lower lid turns outward, the eye no longer drains satisfactorily, and tearing occurs. Ectropion is more common in the elderly.

Lid Retraction and Exophthalmos

A wide-eyed stare suggests retracted eyelids. Note the rim of sclera between the upper lid and the iris. Retracted lids and a lid lag (p. 183) are often due to hyperthyroidism.

In exophthalmos the eyeball protrudes forward. When bilateral, it suggests the infiltrative ophthalmopathy of Graves' hyperthyroidism. Edema of the eyelids and conjunctival injection may be associated. Unilateral exophthalmos seen in Graves' disease or a tumor or inflammation in the orbit.

(Source of photos: *Ptosis, Ectropion, Entropion*—Tasman W, Jaeger E (eds). The Wills Eye Hospital Atlas of Clinical Ophthalmology, 2nd ed. Philadelphia, Lippincott Williams & Wilkins, 2001.)

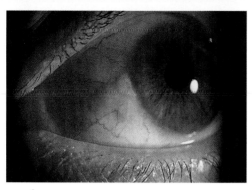

Pinguecula

A harmless yellowish triangular nodule in the bulbar conjunctiva on either side of the iris. Appears frequently with aging, first on the nasal and then on the temporal side.

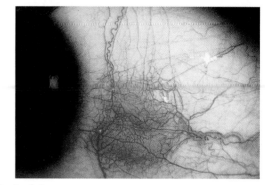

Episcleritis

A localized ocular redness from inflammation of the episcleral vessels. Vessels appear salmon pink and are movable over the scleral surface. May be nodular, as shown, or may show only redness and dilated vessels.

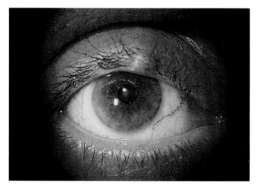

Sty

A painful, tender red infection in a gland at the margin of the eyelid.

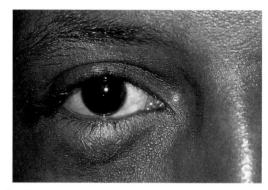

Chalazion

A subacute nontender and usually painless nodule involving a meibomian gland. May become acutely inflamed but, unlike a sty, usually points inside the lid rather than on the lid margin.

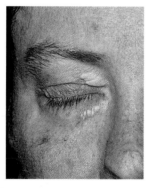

Xanthelasma

Slightly raised, yellowish, well-circumscribed plaques that appear along the nasal portions of one or both eyelids. May accompany lipid disorders.

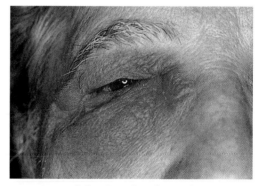

Inflammation of the Lacrimal Sac (Dacryocystitis)

A swelling between the lower eyelid and nose. An *acute* inflammation (illustrated) is painful, red, and tender. *Chronic* inflammation is associated with obstruction of the nasolacrimal duct. Tearing is prominent, and pressure on the sac produces regurgitation of material through the puncta of the eyelids.

(Source of photos: Tasman W, Jaeger E (eds). The Wills Eye Hospital Atlas of Clinical Ophthalmology, 2nd ed. Philadelphia, Lippincott Williams & Wilkins, 2001.)

TABLE 6-7   Red Eyes

Conjunctivitis

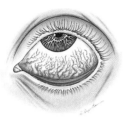

Subconjunctival Hemorrhage

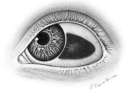

	Conjunctivitis	Subconjunctival Hemorrhage
Pattern of Redness	Conjunctival injection: diffuse dilatation of conjunctival vessels with redness that tends to be maximal peripherally	Leakage of blood outside of the vessels, producing a homogeneous, sharply demarcated, red area that fades over days to yellow and then disappears
Pain	Mild discomfort rather than pain	Absent
Vision	Not affected except for temporary mild blurring due to discharge	Not affected
Ocular Discharge	Watery, mucoid, or mucopurulent	Absent
Pupil	Not affected	Not affected
Cornea	Clear	Clear
Significance	Bacterial, viral, and other infections; allergy; irritation	Often none. May result from trauma, bleeding disorders, or a sudden increase in venous pressure, as from cough

Corneal Injury or Infection

Acute Iritis

Glaucoma

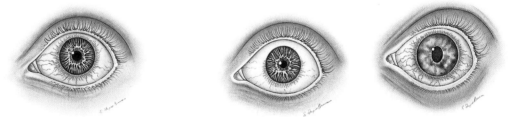

	Corneal Injury or Infection	Acute Iritis	Glaucoma
Pattern of Redness	Ciliary injection: dilation of deeper vessels that are visible as radiating vessels or a reddish violet flush around the limbus. Ciliary injection is an important sign of these three conditions but may not be apparent. The eye may be diffusely red instead. Other clues of these more serious disorders are pain, decreased vision, unequal pupils, and a less than perfectly clear cornea.		
Pain	Moderate to severe, superficial	Moderate, aching, deep	Severe, aching, deep
Vision	Usually decreased	Decreased	Decreased
Ocular Discharge	Watery or purulent	Absent	Absent
Pupil	Not affected unless iritis develops	May be small and, with time, irregular	Dilated, fixed
Cornea	Changes depending on cause	Clear or slightly clouded	Steamy, cloudy
Significance	Abrasions, and other injuries; viral and bacterial infections	Associated with many ocular and systemic disorders	Acute increase in intraocular pressure—an emergency

TABLE 6-8   Opacities of the Cornea and Lens

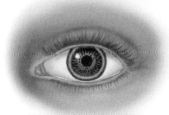

Corneal Arcus. A thin grayish white arc or circle not quite at the edge of the cornea. Accompanies normal aging but also seen in younger people, especially African Americans. In young people, suggests possible hyperlipoproteinemia. Usually benign.

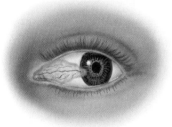

Corneal Scar. A superficial grayish white opacity in the cornea, secondary to an old injury or to inflammation. Size and shape are variable. Do not confuse with the opaque lens of a cataract, visible on a deeper plane and only through the pupil.

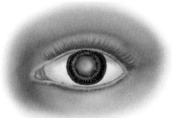

Pterygium. A triangular thickening of the bulbar conjunctiva that grows slowly across the outer surface of the cornea, usually from the nasal side. Reddening may occur. May interfere with vision as it encroaches on the pupil.

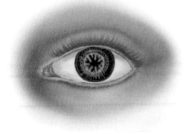

Cataracts. Opacities of the lenses visible through the pupil; most common in old age.

Nuclear cataract. A nuclear cataract looks gray when seen by a flashlight. If the pupil is widely dilated, the gray opacity is surrounded by a black rim. Through an ophthalmoscope, the cataract looks black against the red reflex.

Peripheral cataract. Produces spokelike shadows that point inward—gray against black as seen with a flashlight, or black against red with an ophthalmoscope. A dilated pupil, as shown here, facilitates this observation.

TABLE 6-9   **Pupillary Abnormalities**

Unequal Pupils (*Anisocoria*)—When anisocoria is greater in bright light than in dim light, the larger pupil cannot constrict properly. Causes include blunt trauma to the eye, open-angle glaucoma (p. 181), and impaired parasympathetic nerve supply to the iris, as in tonic pupil and oculomotor nerve paralysis. When anisocoria is greater in dim light, the smaller pupil cannot dilate properly, as in Horner's syndrome, caused by an interruption of the sympathetic nerve supply. See also Table 17-10, Pupils in Comatose Patients, p. 666.

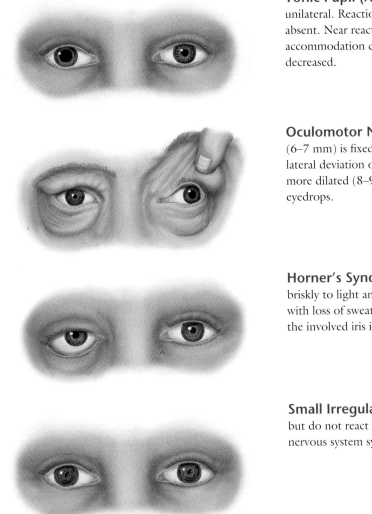

Tonic Pupil *(Adie's Pupil)*. Pupil is large, regular, and usually unilateral. Reaction to light is severely reduced and slowed, or even absent. Near reaction, although very slow, is present. Slow accommodation causes blurred vision. Deep tendon reflexes are often decreased.

Oculomotor Nerve (CN III) Paralysis. The dilated pupil (6–7 mm) is fixed to light and near effort. Ptosis of the upper eyelid and lateral deviation of the eye are often, but not always, present. An even more dilated (8–9 mm) and fixed pupil may result from atropine-like eyedrops.

Horner's Syndrome. The affected pupil, though small, reacts briskly to light and near effort. Ptosis of the eyelid is present, perhaps with loss of sweating on the forehead. In congenital Horner's syndrome, the involved iris is lighter in color than its fellow (*heterochromia*).

Small Irregular Pupils. Small, irregular pupils that accommodate but do not react to light indicate *Argyll Robertson pupils.* Seen in central nervous system syphilis.

Equal Pupils and One Blind Eye. Unilateral blindness does not cause anisocoria as long as the sympathetic and parasympathetic innervation to both irises is normal. A light directed into the seeing eye produces a direct reaction in that eye and a consensual reaction in the blind eye. A light directed into the blind eye, however, causes no response in either eye.

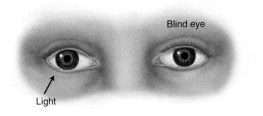

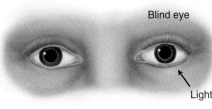

TABLE 6-10   **Dysconjugate Gaze**

There are a variety of gaze abnormality patterns that give clinicians clues about brainstem developmental disorders and cranial nerve abnormalities.

Developmental Disorders

Developmental dysconjugate gaze is caused by an imbalance in ocular muscle tone. This imbalance has many causes, may be hereditary, and usually appears in early childhood. These gaze deviations are classified according to direction:

Esotropia

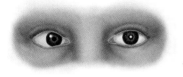

Exotropia

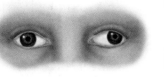

Cover–Uncover Test

A cover–uncover test may be helpful. Here is what you would see in the right monocular esotropia illustrated above.

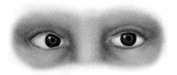

Corneal reflections are asymmetric.

COVER

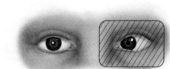

The right eye moves outward to fix on the light. (The left eye is not seen but moves inward to the same degree.)

UNCOVER

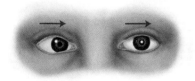

The left eye moves outward to fix on the light. The right eye deviates inward again.

Disorders of Cranial Nerves

New onset of dysconjugate gaze in adult life is usually the result of cranial nerve injuries, lesions, or abnormalities from such causes as trauma, multiple sclerosis, syphilis, and others.

A Left Cranial Nerve VI Paralysis

LOOKING TO THE RIGHT

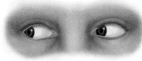

Eyes are conjugate.

LOOKING STRAIGHT AHEAD

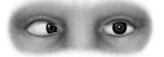

Esotropia appears.

LOOKING TO THE LEFT

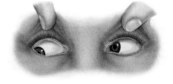

Esotropia is maximum.

A Left Cranial Nerve IV Paralysis

LOOKING DOWN AND TO THE RIGHT

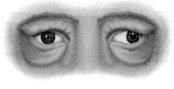

The left eye cannot look down when turned inward. Deviation is maximum in this direction.

A Left Cranial Nerve III Paralysis

LOOKING STRAIGHT AHEAD

The eye is pulled outward by action of the 6th nerve. Upward, downward, and inward movements are impaired or lost. Ptosis and pupillary dilation may be associated.

TABLE 6-11   **Normal Variations of the Optic Disc**

Physiologic Cupping

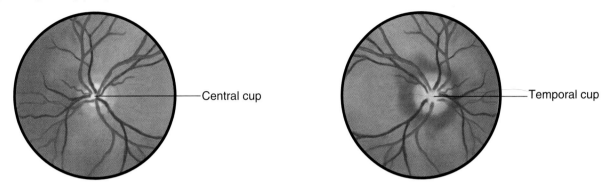

Central cup

Temporal cup

The physiologic cup is a small whitish depression in the optic disc from which the retinal vessels appear to emerge. Although sometimes absent, the cup is usually visible either centrally or toward the temporal side of the disc. Grayish spots are often seen at its base.

Rings and Crescents

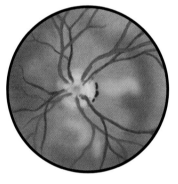

Medullated Nerve Fibers

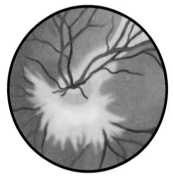

Rings and crescents are often seen around the optic disc. These are developmental variations in which you can glimpse either white sclera, black retinal pigment, or both, especially along the temporal border of the disc. Rings and crescents are not part of the disc itself and should not be included in your estimates of disc diameters.

Medullated nerve fibers are a much less common but dramatic finding. Appearing as irregular white patches with feathered margins, they obscure the disc edge and retinal vessels. They have no pathologic significance.

TABLE 6-12   **Abnormalities of the Optic Disc**

	Process	Appearance
Normal		
	Tiny disc vessels give normal color to the disc.	Color yellowish orange to creamy pink
		Disc vessels tiny
		Disc margins sharp (except perhaps nasally)
		The physiologic cup is located centrally or somewhat temporally. It may be conspicuous or absent. Its diameter from side to side is usually less than half that of the disc.
Papilledema		
	Venous stasis leads to engorgement and swelling.	Color pink, hyperemic
		Disc vessels more visible, more numerous, curve over the borders of the disc
		Disc swollen with margins blurred
		The physiologic cup is not visible.
Glaucomatous Cupping		
	Increased pressure within the eye leads to increased cupping (backward depression of the disc) and atrophy. The base of the enlarged cup is pale.	The physiologic cup is enlarged, occupying more than half of the disc's diameter, at times extending to the edge of the disc. Retinal vessels sink in and under it, and may be displaced nasally.
Optic Atrophy		
	Death of optic nerve fibers leads to loss of the tiny disc vessels.	Color white
		Disc vessels absent

(Source of photos: Tasman W, Jaeger E (eds). The Wills Eye Hospital Atlas of Clinical Ophthalmology, 2nd ed. Philadelphia, Lippincott Williams & Wilkins, 2001.)

Normal Retinal Artery and Arteriovenous (A-V) Crossing

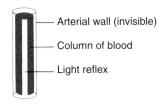

- Arterial wall (invisible)
- Column of blood
- Light reflex

The normal arterial wall is transparent. Only the column of blood within it can usually be seen. The normal light reflex is *narrow—about one fourth the diameter of the blood column.* Because the arterial wall is transparent, a vein crossing beneath the artery can be seen right up to the column of blood on either side.

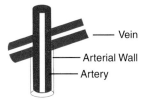

- Vein
- Arterial Wall
- Artery

Retinal Arteries in Hypertension

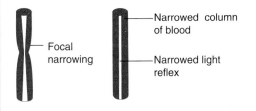

- Focal narrowing
- Narrowed column of blood
- Narrowed light reflex

In hypertension, the arteries may show areas of focal or generalized narrowing. The light reflex is also narrowed. The arterial wall thickens and becomes less transparent.

Copper Wiring

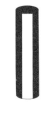

Sometimes the arteries, especially those close to the disc, become full and somewhat tortuous and develop an increased light reflex with a bright coppery luster.

Silver Wiring

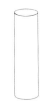

Occasionally a portion of a narrowed artery develops such an opaque wall that no blood is visible within it. It is then called a silver wire artery.

Arteriovenous Crossing

When the arterial walls lose their transparency, changes appear in the arteriovenous crossings. Decreased transparency of the retina probably also contributes to the first two changes shown below.

CONCEALMENT OR A-V NICKING

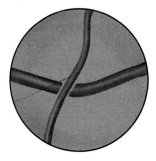

The vein appears to stop abruptly on either side of the artery.

TAPERING AND BANKING

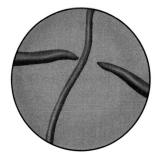

Tapering. The vein appears to taper down on either side of the artery.

BANKING

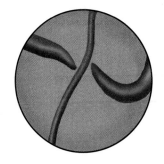

Banking. The vein is twisted on the distal side of the artery and forms a dark, wide knuckle.

TABLE 6-14   **Red Spots and Streaks in the Fundi**

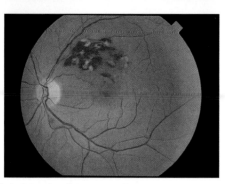

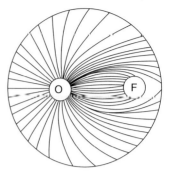

Superficial Retinal Hemorrhages—Small, linear, flame-shaped, red streaks in the fundi, shaped by the superficial bundles of nerve fibers that radiate from the optic disc in the pattern illustrated (O = optic disc; F = fovea). Sometimes the hemorrhages occur in clusters and look like a larger hemorrhage, but can be identified by the linear streaking at the edges. Superficial hemorrhages are seen in severe hypertension, papilledema, and occlusion of the retinal vein, among other conditions. An occasional superficial hemorrhage has a white center consisting of fibrin. White-centered retinal hemorrhages have many causes.

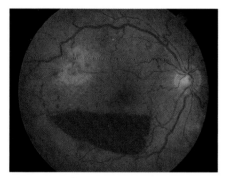

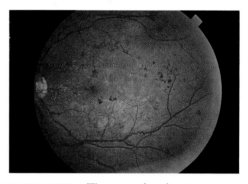

Preretinal Hemorrhage—Develops when blood escapes into the potential space between retina and vitreous. This hemorrhage is typically larger than retinal hemorrhages. Because it is anterior to the retina, it obscures any underlying retinal vessels. In an erect patient, red cells settle, creating a horizontal line of demarcation between plasma above and cells below. Causes include a sudden increase in intracranial pressure.

Microaneurysms—Tiny, round, red spots seen commonly but not exclusively in and around the macular area. They are minute dilatations of very small retinal vessels, but the vascular connections are too small to be seen ophthalmoscopically. They arise from diabetic retinopathy but have other causes.

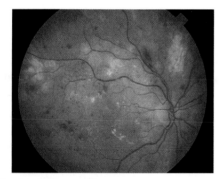

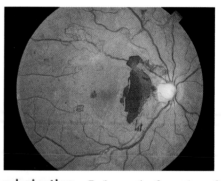

Neovascularization—Refers to the formation of new blood vessels. They are more numerous, more tortuous, and narrower than other blood vessels in the area and form disorderly looking red arcades. A common cause is the late, proliferative stage of diabetic retinopathy. The vessels may grow into the vitreous, where retinal detachment or hemorrhage may cause loss of vision.

Deep Retinal Hemorrhages—Small, rounded, slightly irregular red spots that are sometimes called dot or blot hemorrhages. They occur in a deeper layer of the retina than flame-shaped hemorrhages. Diabetes is a common cause.

TABLE 6-15   Ocular Fundi

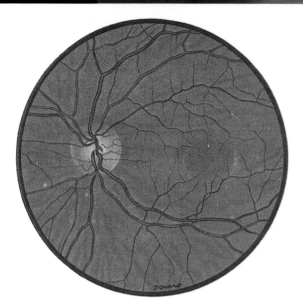

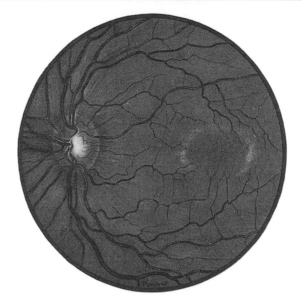

Normal Fundus of a Fair-Skinned Person

Inspect the optic disc. Follow the major vessels in four directions, noting their relative sizes and any arteriovenous crossings—both normal here. Inspect the macular area. The slightly darker fovea is just discernible; no light reflex is visible in this subject. Look for any lesions in the retina. Note the striped, or tessellated, character of the fundus, especially in the lower field that comes from normal underlying choroidal vessels.

Normal Fundus of a Dark-Skinned Person

Again, inspect the disc, vessels, macula, and retina. The ring around the fovea is a normal light reflection. The color of the fundus has a grayish brown, almost purplish cast, which comes from pigment in the retina and the choroid, that characteristically obscures the choroidal vessels; no tessellation is visible. The fundus of a light-skinned person with brunette coloring is redder.

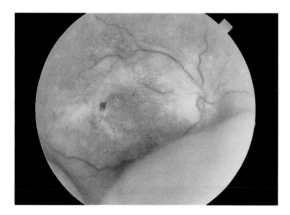

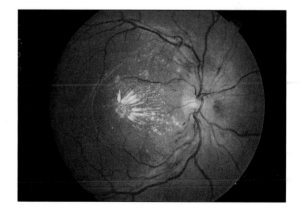

Hypertensive Retinopathy[32]

Inspect the fundus. The nasal border of the optic disc is blurred. The light reflexes from the arteries just above and below the disc are increased. Note venous tapering—at the A-V crossing, about 1 disc diameter above the disc.

Hypertensive Retinopathy With Macular Star

Punctate exudates are readily visible: some are scattered; others radiate from the fovea to form a macular star. Note the two small, soft exudates about 1 disc diameter from the disc. Find the flame-shaped hemorrhages sweeping toward 7 o'clock and 8 o'clock; a few more may be seen toward 10 o'clock. These fundi show changes typical of accelerated (malignant) hypertension and are often accompanied by a papilledema (p. 220).

(Source of photos: *Hypertensive Retinopathy, Hypertensive Retinopathy With Macular Star*—Tasman W, Jaeger E (eds). The Wills Eye Hospital Atlas of Clinical Ophthalmology, 2nd ed. Philadelphia, Lippincott Williams & Wilkins, 2001.)

(table continues next page)

TABLE 6-15   **Ocular Fundi** *(Continued)*

Diabetic Retinopathy

Study carefully the fundi in the series of photographs below. They represent a national standard used by ophthalmologists to assess diabetic retinopathy.

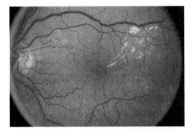

Nonproliferative Retinopathy, Moderately Severe

Note tiny red dots or microaneurysms. Note also the ring of hard exudates (white spots) located superotemporally. Retinal thickening or edema in the area of the hard exudates can impair visual acuity if it extends into the center of the macula (detection requires specialized stereoscopic examination).

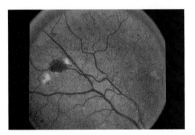

Nonproliferative Retinopathy, Severe

In the superior temporal quadrant, note the large retinal hemorrhage between two cotton-wool patches, beading of the retinal vein just above them, and tiny tortuous retinal vessels above the superior temporal artery.

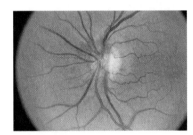

Proliferative Retinopathy, With Neovascularization

Note new preretinal vessels arising on the disc and extending across the disc margins. Visual acuity is still normal, but the risk for visual loss is high (photocoagulation reduces this risk by > 50%).

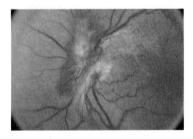

Proliferative Retinopathy, Advanced

This is the same eye, but 2 years later and without treatment. Neovascularization has increased, now with fibrous proliferations, distortion of the macula, and reduced visual acuity.

(Source of photos: *Nonproliferative Retinopathy, Moderately Severe; Proliferative Retinopathy, With Neovascularization; Nonproliferative Retinopathy, Severe; Proliferative Retinopathy, Advanced*—Early Treatment Diabetic Retinopathy Study Research Group. Courtesy of MF Davis, MD, University of Wisconsin, Madison.)

TABLE 6-16　　Light-Colored Spots in the Fundi

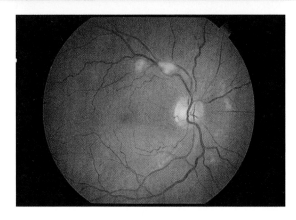

Cotton-Wool Patches (*Soft Exudates*)

Cotton-wool patches are white or grayish, ovoid lesions with irregular "soft" borders. They are moderate in size but usually smaller than the disc. They result from infarcted nerve fibers and are seen in hypertension and many other conditions.

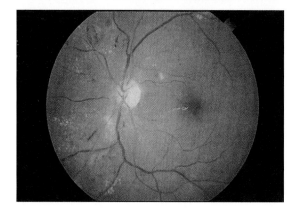

Hard Exudates

Hard exudates are creamy or yellowish, often bright lesions with well-defined "hard" borders. They are small and round (as shown in the lower group of exudates) but may coalesce into larger irregular spots (as shown in the upper group). They often occur in clusters or in circular, linear, or star-shaped patterns. Causes include diabetes and hypertension.

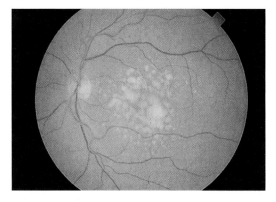

Drusen

Drusen are yellowish round spots that vary from tiny to small. The edges may be soft, as here, or hard (p. 188). They are haphazardly distributed but may concentrate at the posterior pole. Drusen appear with normal aging but may also accompany various conditions, including age-related macular degeneration.

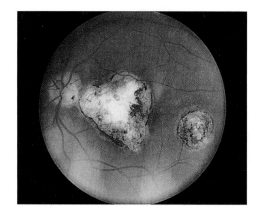

Healed Chorioretinitis

Here inflammation has destroyed the superficial tissues to reveal a well-defined, irregular patch of white sclera marked with dark pigment. Size varies from small to very large. *Toxoplasmosis* is illustrated. Multiple, small, somewhat similar-looking areas may be due to laser treatments. Here there is also a temporal scar near the macula.

(Source of photos: *Cotton-Wool Patches, Hard Exudates; Drusen, Healed Chorioretinitis*—Tasman W, Jaeger E (eds). The Wills Eye Hospital Atlas of Clinical Ophthalmology, 2nd ed. Philadelphia, Lippincott Williams & Wilkins, 2001.)

TABLE 6-17 **Lumps on or Near the Ear**

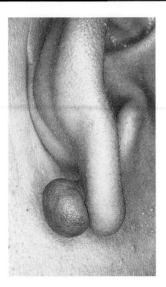

Keloid. A firm, nodular, hypertrophic mass of scar tissue extending beyond the area of injury. It may develop in any scarred area but is most common on the shoulders and upper chest. A keloid on a pierced earlobe may have troublesome cosmetic effects. Keloids are more common in darker-skinned people. Recurrence may follow treatment.

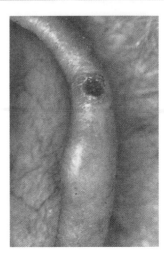

Chondrodermatitis Helicis. This chronic inflammatory lesion starts as a painful, tender papule on the helix or antihelix. Here the upper lesion is at a later stage of ulceration and crusting. Reddening may occur. Biopsy is needed to rule out carcinoma.

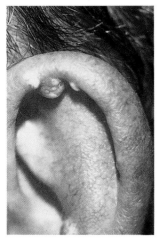

Tophi. A deposit of uric acid crystals characteristic of chronic tophaceous gout. It appears as hard nodules in the helix or antihelix and may discharge chalky white crystals through the skin. It also may appear near the joints: hands (p. 567), feet, and other areas. It usually develops after chronic sustained high blood levels of uric acid.

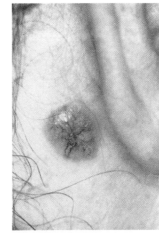

Basal Cell Carcinoma. This raised nodule shows the lustrous surface and telangiectatic vessels of basal cell carcinoma, a common slow-growing malignancy that rarely metastasizes. Growth and ulceration may occur. These are more frequent in fair-skinned people overexposed to sunlight.

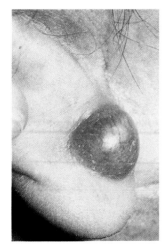

Cutaneous Cyst. Formerly called a *sebaceous cyst*, a dome-shaped lump in the dermis forms a benign closed firm sac attached to the epidermis. A dark dot (blackhead) may be visible on its surface. Histologically, it is usually either (1) an *epidermoid* cyst, common on the face and neck, or (2) a *pilar (trichilemmal)* cyst, common in the scalp. Both may become inflamed.

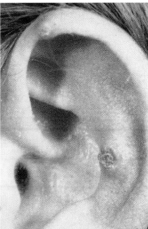

Rheumatoid Nodules. In chronic rheumatoid arthritis, look for small lumps on the helix or antihelix and additional nodules elsewhere on the hands, along the surface of the ulna distal to the elbow (p. 567), and on the knees and heels. Ulceration may result from repeated injuries. Such nodules may antedate the arthritis.

(Sources of photos: *Keloid*—Sams WM Jr, Lynch PJ (eds). Principles and Practice of Dermatology. Edinburgh, Churchill Livingstone, 1990; *Tophi*—du Vivier A. Atlas of Clinical Dermatology, 2nd ed. London, UK: Gower Medical Publishing, 1993; *Cutaneous Cyst, Chondrodermatitis Helicis*—Young EM, Newcomer VD, Kligman AM. Geriatric Dermatology: Color Atlas and Practitioner's Guide. Philadelphia, Lea & Febiger, 1993; *Basal Cell Carcinoma*—N Engl J Med, 326:169–170, 1992; *Rheumatoid Nodules*—Champion RH, Burton JL, Ebling FJG (eds). Rook/Wilkinson/Ebling Textbook of Dermatology, 5th ed. Oxford, UK: Blackwell Scientific, 1992.)

TABLE 6-18   Abnormalities of the Eardrum

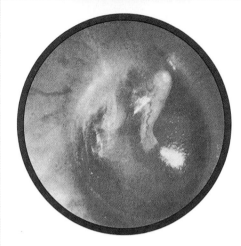

Normal Eardrum

This normal right eardrum (tympanic membrane) is pinkish gray. Note the malleus lying behind the upper part of the drum. Above the short process lies the *pars flaccida*. The remainder of the drum is the *pars tensa*. From the umbo, the bright cone of light fans anteriorly and downward. Posterior to the malleus, part of the incus is visible behind the drum. The small blood vessels along the handle of the malleus are normal.

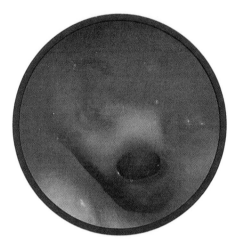

Perforation of the Drum

Perforations are holes in the eardrum that usually result from purulent infections of the middle ear. They are classified as *central* perforations, which do not extend to the margin of the drum, and *marginal* perforations, which do involve the margin.

The more common central perforation is illustrated here. A reddened ring of granulation tissue surrounds the perforation, indicating chronic infection. The eardrum itself is scarred, and no landmarks are visible. Discharge from the infected middle ear may drain out through such a perforation. A perforation often closes in the healing process, as in the next photo. The membrane covering the hole may be exceedingly thin and transparent.

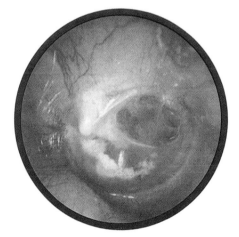

Tympanosclerosis

In the inferior portion of this left eardrum, there is a large, chalky white patch with irregular margins. It is typical of tympanosclerosis: a deposition of hyaline material within the layers of the tympanic membrane that sometimes follows a severe episode of otitis media. It does not usually impair hearing and is seldom clinically significant.

Other abnormalities in this eardrum include a *healed perforation* (the large oval area in the upper posterior drum) and signs of a *retracted drum*. A retracted drum is pulled medially, away from the examiner's eye, and the malleolar folds are tightened into sharp outlines. The short process often protrudes sharply, and the handle of the malleus, pulled inward at the umbo, looks foreshortened and more horizontal.

(Sources of photos: *Normal Eardrum*—Hawke M, Keene M, Alberti PW. Clinical Otoscopy: A Text and Colour Atlas. Edinburgh, Churchill Livingstone, 1984; *Perforation of the Drum, Tympanosclerosis*—Courtesy of Michael Hawke, MD, Toronto, Canada.)

(table continues next page)

TABLE 6-18   **Abnormalities of the Eardrum** *(Continued)*

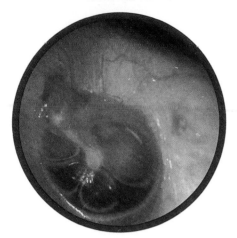

Serous Effusion

Serous effusions are usually caused by viral upper respiratory infections (*otitis media with serous effusion*) or by sudden changes in atmospheric pressure as from flying or diving (*otitic barotrauma*). The eustachian tube cannot equalize the air pressure in the middle ear with that of the outside air. Air is partly or completely absorbed from the middle ear into the bloodstream, and serous fluid accumulates there instead. Symptoms include fullness and popping sensations in the ear, mild conduction hearing loss, and perhaps some pain.

Amber fluid behind the eardrum is characteristic, as in this patient with otitic barotrauma. A fluid level, a line between air above and amber fluid below, can be seen on either side of the short process. Air bubbles (not always present) can be seen here within the amber fluid.

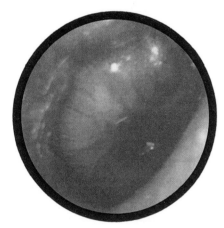

Acute Otitis Media With Purulent Effusion

Acute otitis media with purulent effusion is caused by bacterial infection. Symptoms include earache, fever, and hearing loss. The eardrum reddens, loses its landmarks, and bulges laterally, toward the examiner's eye.

Here the eardrum is bulging, and most landmarks are obscured. Redness is most obvious near the umbo, but dilated vessels can be seen in all segments of the drum. A diffuse redness of the entire drum often develops. Spontaneous rupture (perforation) of the drum may follow, with discharge of purulent material into the ear canal.

Hearing loss is of the conductive type. Acute purulent otitis media is much more common in children than in adults.

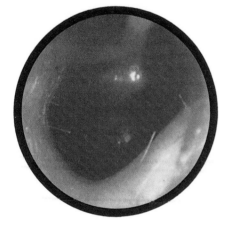

Bullous Myringitis

Bullous myringitis is a viral infection characterized by painful hemorrhagic vesicles that appear on the tympanic membrane, the ear canal, or both. Symptoms include earache, blood-tinged discharge from the ear, and hearing loss of the conductive type.

In this right ear, at least two large vesicles (bullae) are discernible on the drum. The drum is reddened, and its landmarks are obscured.

Several different viruses may cause this condition, including mycoplasma.

(Sources of photos: *Serous Effusion*—Hawke M, Keene M, Alberti PW. Clinical Otoscopy: A Text and Colour Atlas. Edinburgh, Churchill Livingstone, 1984; *Acute Otitis Media, Bullous Myringitis*—The Wellcome Trust, National Medical Slide Bank, London, UK.)

TABLE 6-19   **Patterns of Hearing Loss**

	Conductive Loss	Sensorineural Loss
	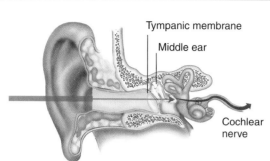	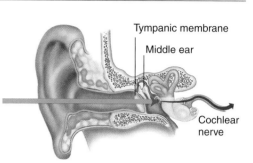
Pathophysiology	External or middle ear disorder impairs sound conduction to inner ear. Causes include foreign body, *otitis media*, perforated eardrum, and otosclerosis of ossicles.	Inner ear disorder involves cochlear nerve and neuronal impulse transmission to the brain. Causes include loud noise exposure, inner ear infections, trauma, tremors, congenital and familial disorders, and aging.
Usual Age of Onset	Childhood and young adulthood, up to age 40	Middle or later years
Ear Canal and Drum	Abnormality usually visible, except in otosclerosis	Problem not visible
Effects	■ Little effect on sound ■ Hearing seems to improve in noisy environment ■ Voice becomes soft because inner ear and cochlear nerve are intact	■ Higher registers are lost, so sound may be distorted. ■ Hearing worsens in noisy environment ■ Voice may be loud because hearing is difficult.
Weber Test *(in unilateral hearing loss)*	■ Tuning fork at vertex ■ Sound lateralizes to *impaired ear*—room noise not well heard, so detection of vibrations *improves.*	■ Tuning fork at vertex ■ Sound lateralizes to *good ear*—inner ear or cochlear nerve damage impairs transmission to affected ear
Rinne Test	■ Tuning fork at external auditory meatus then on mastoid bone ■ Bone conduction longer than or equal to air conduction (BC ≥ AC). While air conduction through the external or middle ear is impaired, vibrations through bone bypass the problem to reach the cochlea.	■ Tuning fork at external auditory meatus then on mastoid bone ■ Air conduction longer than bone conduction (AC > BC). The inner ear or cochlear nerve is less able to transmit impulses regardless of how the vibrations reach the cochlea. The normal pattern prevails.

TABLE 6-20   Abnormalities of the Lips

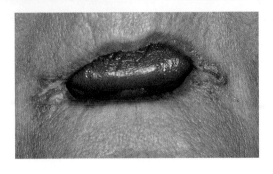

Angular Cheilitis

Angular cheilitis starts with softening of the skin at the angles of the mouth, followed by fissuring. It may be due to nutritional deficiency or, more commonly, to overclosure of the mouth, as in people with no teeth or with ill-fitting dentures. Saliva wets and macerates the infolded skin, often leading to secondary infection with *Candida,* as in this example.

Actinic Cheilitis

Actinic cheilitis results from excessive exposure to sunlight and affects primarily the lower lip. Fair-skinned men who work outdoors are most often affected. The lip loses its normal redness and may become scaly, somewhat thickened, and slightly everted. Because solar damage also predisposes to carcinoma of the lip, be alert to this possibility.

Herpes Simplex *(Cold Sore, Fever Blister)*

The herpes simplex virus (HSV) produces recurrent and painful vesicular eruptions of the lips and surrounding skin. A small cluster of vesicles first develops. As these break, yellow-brown crusts form, and healing ensues within 10 to 14 days. Both of these stages are visible here.

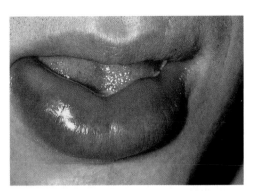

Angioedema

Angioedema is a diffuse, nonpitting, tense swelling of the dermis and subcutaneous tissue. It develops rapidly, and typically disappears over subsequent hours or days. Although usually allergic in nature and sometimes associated with hives, angioedema does not itch.

(Sources of photos: *Angular Cheilitis, Herpes Simplex, Angioedema*—Neville B, et al. Color Atlas of Clinical Oral Pathology. Philadelphia, Lea & Febiger, 1991; Used with permission; *Actinic Cheilitis*—Langlais RP, Miller CS. Color Atlas of Common Oral Diseases. Philadelphia, Lea & Febiger, 1992. Used with permission.)

(table continues next page)

TABLE 6-20   **Abnormalities of the Lips** *(Continued)*

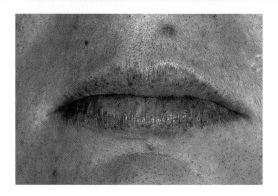

Hereditary Hemorrhagic Telangiectasia

Multiple small red spots on the lips strongly suggest hereditary hemorrhagic telangiectasia. Spots may also be visible on the face and hands and in the mouth. The spots are dilated capillaries and may bleed when traumatized. Affected people often have nosebleeds and gastrointestinal bleeding.

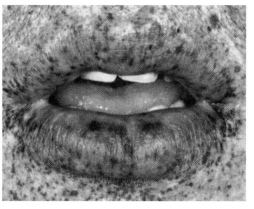

Peutz-Jeghers Syndrome

When pigmented spots on the lips are more prominent than freckling of the surrounding skin, suspect this syndrome. Pigment in the buccal mucosa helps to confirm the diagnosis. Pigmented spots may also be found on the face and hands. Multiple intestinal polyps are often associated.

Chancre of Syphilis

This lesion of primary syphilis may appear on the lip rather than on the genitalia. It is a firm, buttonlike lesion that ulcerates and may become crusted. A chancre may resemble a carcinoma or a crusted cold sore. Because it is infectious, use gloves to feel any suspicious lesion.

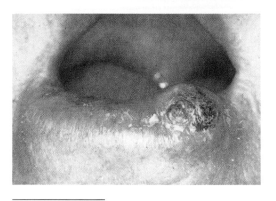

Carcinoma of the Lip

Like actinic cheilitis, carcinoma usually affects the lower lip. It may appear as a scaly plaque, as an ulcer with or without a crust, or as a nodular lesion, illustrated here. Fair skin and prolonged exposure to the sun are common risk factors.

(Sources of photos: *Hereditary Hemorrhagic Telangiectasia*—Langlais RP, Miller CS. Color Atlas of Common Oral Diseases. Philadelphia, Lea & Febiger, 1992; Used with permission; *Peutz-Jeghers Syndrome*—Robinson HBG, Miller AS. Colby, Kerr, and Robinson's Color Atlas of Oral Pathology. Philadelphia, JB Lippincott, 1990; *Chancre of Syphilis*—Wisdom A. A Colour Atlas of Sexually Transmitted Diseases, 2nd ed. London, Wolfe Medical Publications, 1989; *Carcinoma of the Lip*—Tyldesley WR. A Colour Atlas of Orofacial Diseases, 2nd ed. London, Wolfe Medical Publications, 1991.)

TABLE 6-21   **Findings in the Pharynx, Palate, and Oral Mucosa**

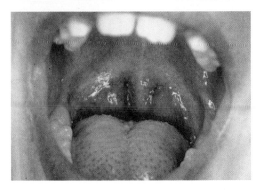

Large Normal Tonsils

Normal tonsils may be large without being infected, especially in children. They may protrude medially beyond the pillars and even to the midline. Here they touch the sides of the uvula and obscure the pharynx. Their color is within normal limits. The white marks are light reflections, not exudate.

Exudative Tonsillitis

This red throat has a white exudate on the tonsils. This, together with fever and enlarged cervical nodes, increases the probability of *group A streptococcal infection*, or infectious mononucleosis. Some anterior cervical lymph nodes are usually enlarged in the former, posterior nodes in the latter.

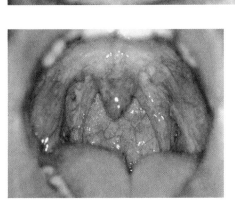

Pharyngitis

These two photos show reddened throats without exudate.

In **A**, redness and vascularity of the pillars and uvula are mild to moderate.

A

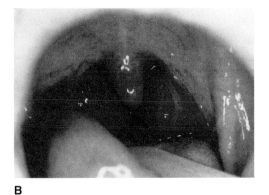

In **B**, redness is diffuse and intense. Each patient would probably complain of a sore throat, or at least a scratchy one. Possible causes include several kinds of viruses and bacteria. If the patient has no fever, exudate, or enlargement of cervical lymph node, the chances of infection by either of two common causes—*group A streptococci* and *Epstein Barr virus* (infectious mononucleosis)—are very small.

B

(Sources of photos: *Large Normal Tonsils, Exudative Tonsillitis, Pharyngitis [A and B]*—The Wellcome Trust, National Medical Slide Bank, London, UK.)

(table continues next page)

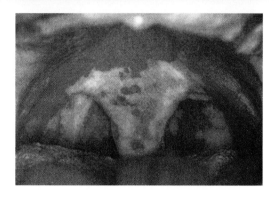

Diphtheria

Diphtheria (an acute infection caused by *Corynebacterium diphtheriae*) is now rare but still important. Prompt diagnosis may lead to life-saving treatment. The throat is dull red, and a gray exudate (pseudomembrane) is present on the uvula, pharynx, and tongue. The airway may become obstructed.

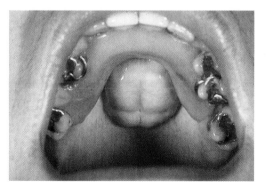

Thrush on the Palate (Candidiasis)

Thrush is a yeast infection due to *Candida*. Shown here on the palate, it may appear elsewhere in the mouth (see p. 237). Thick, white plaques are somewhat adherent to the underlying mucosa. Predisposing factors include (1) prolonged treatment with antibiotics or corticosteroids, and (2) AIDS.

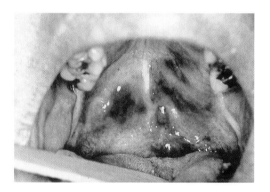

Kaposi's Sarcoma in AIDS

The deep purple color of these lesions, although not necessarily present, strongly suggests Kaposi's sarcoma. The lesions may be raised or flat. Among people with AIDS, the palate, as illustrated here, is a common site for this tumor.

Torus Palatinus

A torus palatinus is a midline bony growth in the hard palate that is fairly common in adults. Its size and lobulation vary. Although alarming at first glance, it is harmless. In this example, an upper denture has been fitted around the torus.

(Sources of photos: *Diphtheria*—Harnisch JP, et al. Diphtheria among alcoholic urban adults. Ann Intern Med 1989;111:77; *Thrush on the Palate*—The Wellcome Trust, National Medical Slide Bank, London, UK; *Kaposi's Sarcoma in AIDS*—Ioachim HL. Textbook and Atlas of Disease Associated With Acquired Immune Deficiency Syndrome. London, UK, Gower Medical Publishing, 1989.)

(table continues next page)

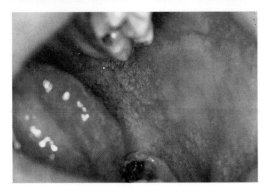

Fordyce Spots *(Fordyce Granules)*

Fordyce spots are normal sebaceous glands that appear as small yellowish spots in the buccal mucosa or on the lips. A worried person who has suddenly noticed them may be reassured. Here they are seen best anterior to the tongue and lower jaw. These spots are usually not so numerous.

Koplik's Spots

Koplik's spots are an early sign of measles (rubeola). Search for small white specks that resemble grains of salt on a red background. They usually appear on the buccal mucosa near the first and second molars. In this photo, look also in the upper third of the mucosa. The rash of measles appears within a day.

Petechiae

Petechiae are small red spots that result when blood escapes from capillaries into the tissues. Petechiae in the buccal mucosa, as shown, are often caused by accidentally biting the cheek. Oral petechiae may be due to infection or decreased platelets, as well as to trauma.

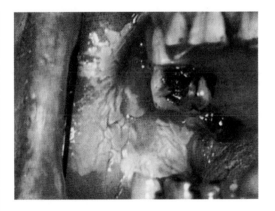

Leukoplakia

A thickened white patch (*leukoplakia*) may occur anywhere in the oral mucosa. The extensive example shown on this buccal mucosa resulted from frequent chewing of tobacco, a local irritant. This kind of irritation may lead to cancer.

(Sources of photos: *Fordyce Spots*—Neville B, et al. Color Atlas of Clinical Oral Pathology. Philadelphia, Lea & Febiger, 1991; Used with permission; *Koplik's Spots, Petechiae*—The Wellcome Trust, National Medical Slide Bank, London, UK; *Leukoplakia*—Robinson HBG, Miller AS. Colby, Kerr, and Robinson's Color Atlas of Oral Pathology. Philadelphia, JB Lippincott, 1990.)

TABLE 6-22 Findings in the Gums and Teeth

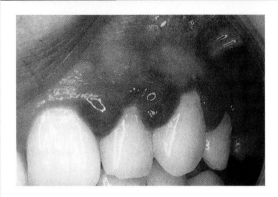

Marginal Gingivitis

Marginal gingivitis is common among teenagers and young adults. The gingival margins are reddened and swollen, and the interdental papillae are blunted, swollen, and red. Brushing the teeth often makes the gums bleed. *Plaque*—the soft white film of salivary salts, protein, and bacteria that covers the teeth and leads to gingivitis—is not readily visible.

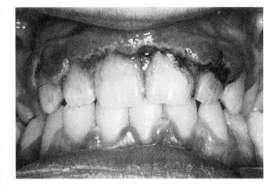

Acute Necrotizing Ulcerative Gingivitis

This uncommon form of gingivitis occurs suddenly in adolescents and young adults and is accompanied by fever, malaise, and enlarged lymph nodes. Ulcers develop in the interdental papillae. Then the destructive (necrotizing) process spreads along the gum margins, where a grayish pseudomembrane develops. The red, painful gums bleed easily; the breath is foul.

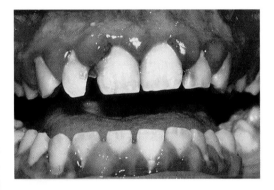

Gingival Hyperplasia

Gums enlarged by hyperplasia are swollen into heaped-up masses that may even cover the teeth. The redness of inflammation may coexist, as in this example. Causes include dilantin therapy (as in this case), puberty, pregnancy, and leukemia.

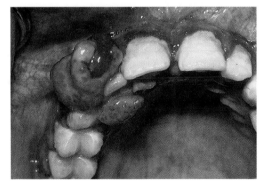

Pregnancy Tumor (Epulis, Pyogenic Granuloma)

Gingival enlargement may be localized, forming a tumorlike mass that usually originates in an interdental papilla. It is red and soft and usually bleeds easily. The estimated incidence of this lesion in pregnancy is about 1%. Note the accompanying gingivitis in this example.

(Sources of photos: *Marginal Gingivitis, Acute Necrotizing Ulcerative Gingivitis*—Tyldesley WR. A Colour Atlas of Orofacial Diseases, 2nd ed. London, Wolfe Medical Publications, 1991; *Gingival Hyperplasia*—Courtesy of Dr. James Cottone; *Pregnancy Tumor*—Langlais RP, Miller CS. Color Atlas of Common Oral Diseases. Philadelphia, Lea & Febiger, 1992. Used with permission.)

(table continues next page)

TABLE 6-22   **Findings in the Gums and Teeth** *(Continued)*

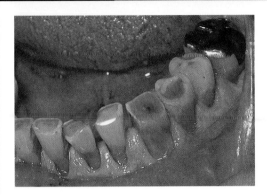

Attrition of Teeth; Recession of Gums

In many elderly people, the chewing surfaces of the teeth have been worn down by repetitive use so that the yellow-brown dentin becomes exposed—a process called *attrition*. Note also the *recession of the gums*, which has exposed the roots of the teeth, giving a "long in the tooth" appearance.

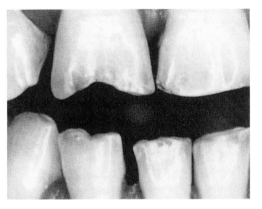

Erosion of Teeth

Teeth may be eroded by chemical action. Note here the erosion of the enamel from the lingual surfaces of the upper incisors, exposing the yellow-brown dentin. This results from recurrent regurgitation of stomach contents, as in bulimia.

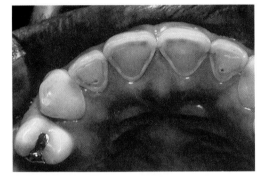

Abrasion of Teeth With Notching

The biting surface of the teeth may become abraded or notched by recurrent trauma, such as holding nails or opening bobby pins between the teeth. Unlike Hutchinson's teeth, the sides of these teeth show normal contours; size and spacing of the teeth are unaffected.

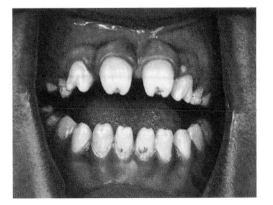

Hutchinson's Teeth

Hutchinson's teeth are smaller and more widely spaced than normal and are notched on their biting surfaces. The sides of the teeth taper toward the biting edges. The upper central incisors of the permanent (not the deciduous) teeth are most often affected. These teeth are a sign of congenital syphilis.

(Sources of photos: *Attrition of Teeth, Erosion of Teeth*—Langlais RP, Miller CS. Color Atlas of Common Oral Diseases. Philadelphia, Lea & Febiger, 1992. Used with permission; *Abrasion of Teeth, Hutchinson's Teeth*—Robinson HBG, Miller AS. Colby, Kerr, and Robinson's Color Atlas of Oral Pathology. Philadelphia, JB Lippincott, 1990.)

TABLE 6-23   Findings in or Under the Tongue

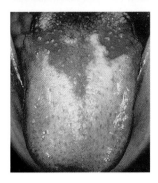

Geographic Tongue. In this benign condition, the dorsum shows scattered smooth red areas denuded of papillae. Together with the normal rough and coated areas, they give a maplike pattern that changes over time.

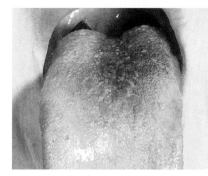

Hairy Tongue. Note the "hairy" yellowish to brown or black elongated papillae on the tongue's dorsum. This benign condition may follow antibiotic therapy; it also may occur spontaneously.

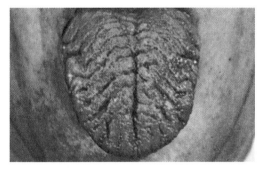

Fissured Tongue. Fissures appear with increasing age, sometimes termed *scrotal tongue*. Food debris may accumulate in the crevices and become irritating, but a fissured tongue is benign.

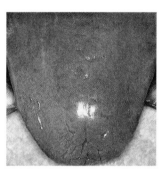

Smooth Tongue (Atrophic Glossitis). A smooth and often sore tongue that has lost its papillae suggests a deficiency in riboflavin, niacin, folic acid, vitamin B_{12}, pyridoxine, or iron, or treatment with chemotherapy.

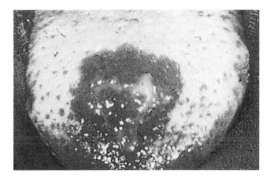

Candidiasis. Note the thick white coating from *Candida* infection. The raw red surface is where the coat was scraped off. Infection may also occur without the white coating. It is seen in immunosuppressed conditions.

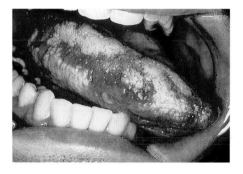

Hairy Leukoplakia. These whitish raised areas with a feathery or corrugated pattern most often affect the sides of the tongue. Unlike candidiasis, these areas cannot be scraped off. They are seen with HIV and AIDS.

(table continues next page)

TABLE 6-23   **Findings in or Under the Tongue** *(Continued)*

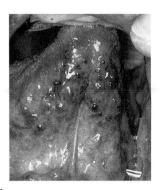

Varicose Veins. Small purplish or blue-black round swellings appear under the tongue with age. These dilatations of the lingual veins have no clinical significance.

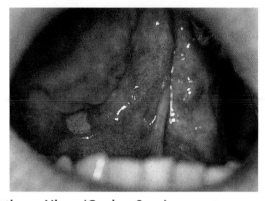

Aphthous Ulcer (Canker Sore). A painful, round or oval ulcer that is white or yellowish gray and surrounded by a halo of reddened mucosa. It may be single or multiple. It heals in 7–10 days, but may recur.

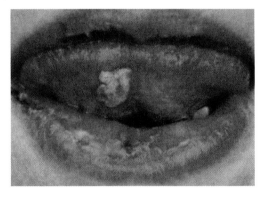

Mucous Patch of Syphilis. This painless lesion in the secondary stage of syphilis is highly infectious. It is slightly raised, oval, and covered by a grayish membrane. It may be multiple and occur elsewhere in the mouth.

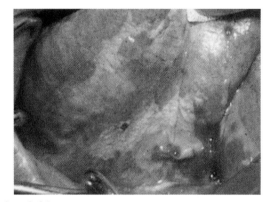

Leukoplakia. With this persisting painless white patch in the oral mucosa, the undersurface of the tongue appears painted white. Patches of any size raise the possibility of malignancy and require a biopsy.

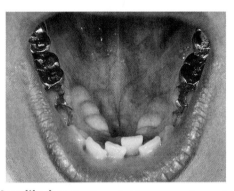

Tori Mandibulares. Rounded bony growths on the inner surfaces of the mandible are typically bilateral, asymptomatic, and harmless.

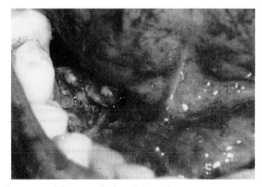

Carcinoma, Floor of the Mouth. This ulcerated lesion is in a common location for carcinoma. Medially, note the reddened area of mucosa, called *erythroplakia*, suggesting possible malignancy.

(Sources of photos: *Fissured Tongue, Candidiasis, Mucous Patch, Leukoplakia, Carcinoma*—Robinson HBG, Miller AS. Colby, Kerr, and Robinson's Color Atlas of Oral Pathology. Philadelphia, JB Lippincott, 1990; *Smooth Tongue*—Courtesy of Dr. R. A. Cawson, from Cawson RA. Oral Pathology, 1st ed. London, UK, Gower Medical Publishing, 1987; *Geographic Tongue*—The Wellcome Trust, National Medical Slide Bank, London, UK; *Hairy Leukoplakia*—Ioachim HL. Textbook and Atlas of Disease Associated With Acquired Immune Deficiency Syndrome. London, UK, Gower Medical Publishing, 1989; *Varicose Veins*—Neville B, et al. Color Atlas of Clinical Oral Pathology. Philadelphia, Lea & Febiger, 1991. Used with permission.)

TABLE 6-24   Thyroid Enlargement and Function

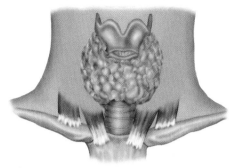

Diffuse Enlargement. Includes the isthmus and lateral lobes; there are no discretely palpable nodules. Causes include Graves' disease, Hashimoto's thyroiditis, and endemic goiter.

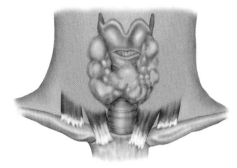

Single Nodule. May be a cyst, a benign tumor, or one nodule within a multinodular gland. It raises the question of malignancy. Risk factors are prior irradiation, hardness, rapid growth, fixation to surrounding tissues, enlarged cervical nodes, and occurrence in males.[17]

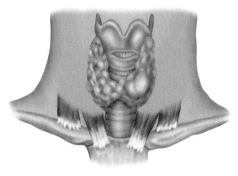

Multinodular Goiter. An enlarged thyroid gland with two or more nodules suggests a metabolic rather than a neoplastic process. Positive family history and continuing nodular enlargement are additional risk factors for malignancy.

	Hyperthyroidism	Hypothyroidism
Symptoms	Nervousness	Fatigue, lethargy
	Weight loss despite increased appetite	Modest weight gain with anorexia
	Excessive sweating and heat intolerance	Dry, coarse skin and cold intolerance
	Palpitations	Swelling of face, hands, and legs
	Frequent bowel movements	Constipation
	Muscular weakness of the proximal type and tremor	Weakness, muscle cramps, arthralgias, paresthesias, impaired memory and hearing
Signs	Warm, smooth, moist skin	Dry, coarse, cool skin, sometimes yellowish from carotene, with nonpitting edema and loss of hair
	With Graves' disease, eye signs such as stare, lid lag, and exophthalmos	Periorbital puffiness
	Increased systolic and decreased diastolic blood pressures	Decreased systolic and increased diastolic blood pressures
	Tachycardia or atrial fibrillation	Bradycardia and, in late stages, hypothermia
	Hyperdynamic cardiac pulsations with an accentuated S_1	Intensity of heart sounds sometimes decreased
	Tremor and proximal muscle weakness	Impaired memory, mixed hearing loss, somnolence, peripheral neuropathy, carpal tunnel syndrome

The Thorax and Lungs

CHAPTER

7

ANATOMY AND PHYSIOLOGY

Study the *anatomy of the chest wall,* identifying the structures illustrated. Note that an interspace between two ribs is numbered by the rib above it.

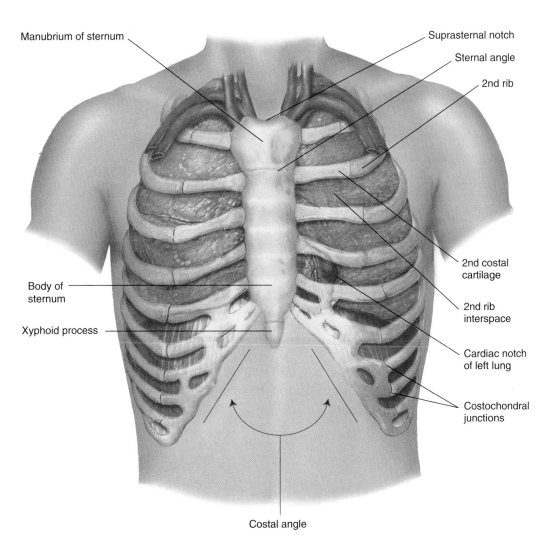

Manubrium of sternum

Suprasternal notch

Sternal angle

2nd rib

2nd costal cartilage

2nd rib interspace

Cardiac notch of left lung

Costochondral junctions

Body of sternum

Xyphoid process

Costal angle

Locating Findings on the Chest. Describe abnormalities of the chest in two dimensions: *along the vertical axis* and *around the circumference of the chest.*

To make *vertical* locations, you must be able to count the ribs and interspaces. The *sternal angle,* also termed the angle of Louis, is the best guide: place your finger in the hollow curve of the suprasternal notch, then move your finger down about 5 cm to the horizontal bony ridge joining the manubrium to the body of the sternum. Then move your finger laterally and find the adjacent 2nd rib and costal cartilage. From here, using two fingers, "walk down the interspaces," one space at a time, on an oblique line illustrated by the red numbers below. Do not try to count interspaces along the lower edge of the sternum; the ribs there are too close together. In a woman, to find the interspaces, either displace the breast laterally or palpate a little more medially than illustrated. Avoid pressing too hard on tender breast tissue.

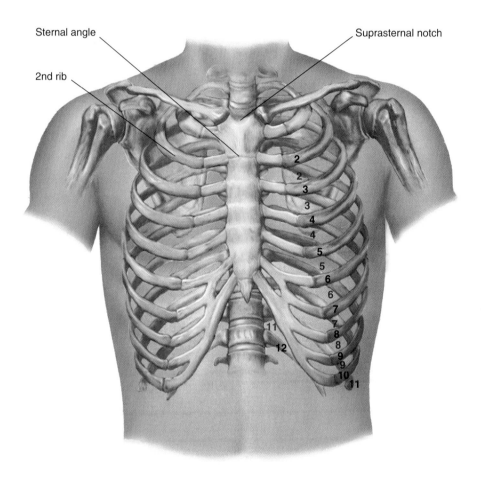

Note that the costal cartilages of the first seven ribs articulate with the sternum; the cartilages of the 8th, 9th, and 10th ribs articulate with the costal cartilages just above them. The 11th and 12th ribs, the "floating ribs," have no anterior attachments. The cartilaginous tip of the 11th rib can usually be felt laterally, and the 12th rib may be felt posteriorly. On palpation, costal cartilages and ribs feel identical.

Posteriorly, the 12th rib is another possible starting point for counting ribs and interspaces: it helps locate findings on the lower posterior chest and provides an option when the anterior approach is unsatisfactory. With the fingers of one hand, press in and up against the lower border of the 12th rib, then "walk up" the interspaces numbered in red below, or follow a more oblique line up and around to the front of the chest.

The inferior tip of the scapula is another useful bony marker—it usually lies at the level of the 7th rib or interspace.

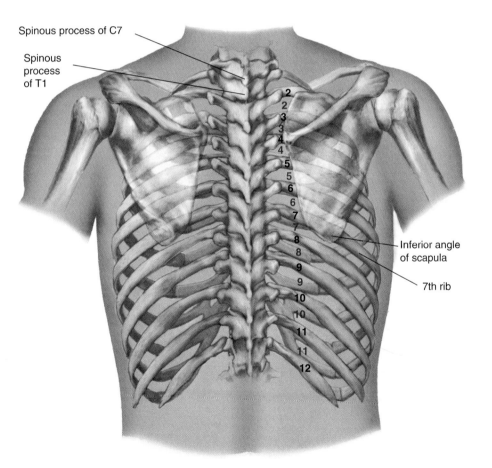

The spinous processes of the vertebrae are also useful anatomical landmarks. When the neck is flexed forward, the most protruding process is usually the vertebra of C7. If two processes are equally prominent, they are C7 and T1. You can often palpate and count the processes below them, especially when the spine is flexed.

To locate findings around the *circumference of the chest*, use a series of vertical lines, shown in the adjacent illustrations. The *midsternal* and *vertebral lines* are precise; the others are estimated. The *midclavicular line* drops vertically from the midpoint of the clavicle. To find it, you must identify both ends of the clavicle accurately (see p. 511).

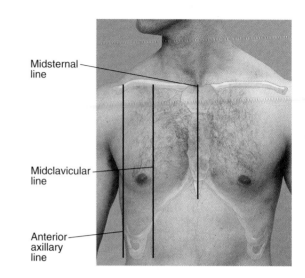

The *anterior* and *posterior axillary lines* drop vertically from the anterior and posterior axillary folds, the muscle masses that border the axilla. The *midaxillary line* drops from the apex of the axilla.

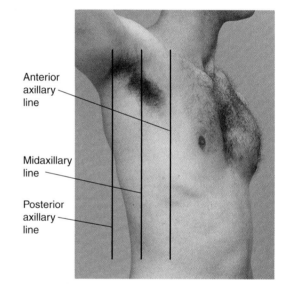

Posteriorly, the *vertebral line* overlies the spinous process of the vertebrae. The scapular line drops from the inferior angle of the scapula.

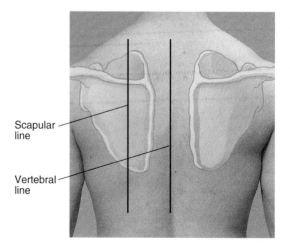

Lungs, Fissures, and Lobes.   Picture the lungs and their fissures and lobes on the chest wall. Anteriorly, the apex of each lung rises about 2 cm to 4 cm above the inner third of the clavicle. The lower border of the lung crosses the 6th rib at the midclavicular line and the 8th rib at the midaxillary line. Posteriorly, the lower border of the lung lies at about the level of the T10 spinous process. On inspiration, it descends farther.

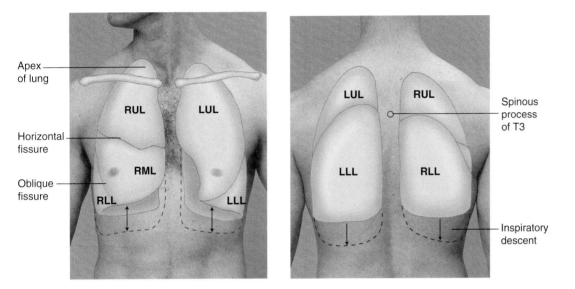

Each lung is divided roughly in half by an *oblique (major) fissure*. This fissure may be approximated by a string that runs from the T3 spinous process obliquely down and around the chest to the 6th rib at the midclavicular line. The right lung is further divided by the *horizontal (minor) fissure*. Anteriorly, this fissure runs close to the 4th rib and meets the oblique fissure in the midaxillary line near the 5th rib. The right lung is thus divided into *upper, middle,* and *lower lobes*. The left lung has only two lobes, upper and lower.

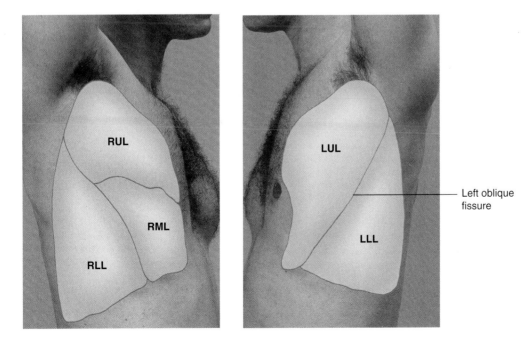

Locations on the Chest.   Learn the general anatomic terms used to locate chest findings, such as:

Supraclavicular—above the clavicles
Infraclavicular—below the clavicles
Interscapular—between the scapulae
Infrascapular—below the scapulae
Bases of the lungs—the lowermost portions
Upper, middle, and lower lung fields

You may then infer what parts of the lungs are affected by an abnormal process. Signs in the right upper lung field, for example, almost certainly originate in the right upper lobe. Signs in the right middle lung field laterally, however, could come from any of three different lobes.

The Trachea and Major Bronchi.   Breath sounds over the trachea and bronchi have a different quality than breath sounds over the lung parenchyma. Be sure you know the location of these structures. The trachea bifurcates into its mainstem bronchi at the levels of the sternal angle anteriorly and the T4 spinous process posteriorly.

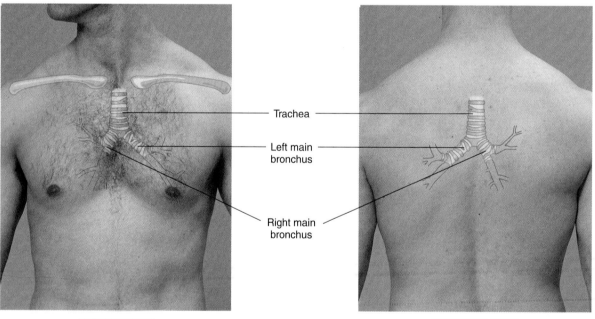

Trachea

Left main
bronchus

Right main
bronchus

ANTERIOR VIEW   **POSTERIOR VIEW**

The Pleurae.   The pleurae are serous membranes that cover the outer surface of each lung, the *visceral pleura,* and also line the inner rib cage and upper surface of the diaphragm, the *parietal pleura.* Their smooth opposing surfaces, lubricated by pleural fluid, allow the lungs to move easily within the rib cage during inspiration and expiration. The *pleural space* is the potential space between visceral and parietal pleurae.

Breathing.   Breathing is largely an automatic act, controlled in the brainstem and mediated by the muscles of respiration. The dome-shaped *diaphragm* is the primary muscle of inspiration. When it contracts, it descends in the chest and enlarges the thoracic cavity. At the same time, it compresses the abdominal contents, pushing the abdominal wall outward. Muscles in the rib cage and neck expand the thorax during inspiration, especially the *parasternals,* which run obliquely from sternum to ribs, and the *scalenes,* which run from the cervical vertebrae to the first two ribs.

During inspiration, as these muscles contract, the thorax expands. Intrathoracic pressure decreases, drawing air through the tracheobronchial tree into the *alveoli,* or distal air sacs, and expanding the lungs. Oxygen diffuses into the blood of adjacent pulmonary capillaries, and carbon dioxide diffuses from the blood into the alveoli.

After inspiratory effort stops, the expiratory phase begins. The chest wall and lungs recoil, the diaphragm relaxes and rises passively, air flows outward, and the chest and abdomen return to their resting positions.

Normal breathing is quiet and easy—barely audible near the open mouth as a faint whish. When a healthy person lies supine, the breathing movements of the thorax are relatively slight. In contrast, the abdominal movements are usually easy to see. In the sitting position, movements of the thorax become more prominent.

During exercise and in certain diseases, extra work is required to breathe, and accessory muscles join the inspiratory effort. The sternomastoids are the most important of these, and the scalenes may become visible. Abdominal muscles assist in expiration.

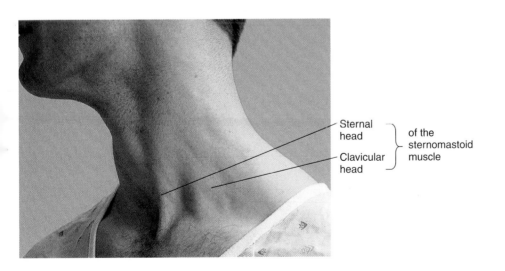

Sternal head
Clavicular head
of the sternomastoid muscle

THE HEALTH HISTORY

Common or Concerning Symptoms

- Chest pain
- Dyspnea
- Wheezing
- Cough
- Blood-streaked sputum (hemoptysis)

Complaints of *chest pain* or *chest discomfort* raise the specter of heart disease, but often arise from structures in the thorax and lung as well. To assess this symptom, you must pursue a dual investigation of both thoracic and cardiac causes. Sources of chest pain are listed below. For this important symptom, you must keep all of these in mind.

See Table 7-1. Chest Pain, pp. 268–269.

- The myocardium

Angina pectoris, myocardial infarction

- The pericardium

Pericarditis

- The aorta

Dissecting aortic aneurysm

- The trachea and large bronchi

Bronchitis

- The parietal pleura

Pericarditis, pneumonia

- The chest wall, including the musculoskeletal system and skin

Costochondritis, herpes zoster

- The esophagus

Reflux esophagitis, esophageal spasm

- Extrathoracic structures such as the neck, gallbladder, and stomach.

Cervical arthritis, biliary colic, gastritis

This section focuses on *pulmonary complaints*, including general questions about chest symptoms, dyspnea, wheezing, cough, and hemoptysis. For health history questions about exertional chest pain, palpitations, orthopnea, paroxysmal nocturnal dyspnea, and edema, see Chapter 8, The Cardiovascular System.

Your initial questions should be as broad as possible. "Do you have any discomfort or unpleasant feelings in your chest?" As you proceed to the full history, ask the patient to point to where the pain is in the chest. Watch for any

A clenched fist over the sternum suggests *angina pectoris;* a finger pointing to a tender area on the

gestures as the patient describes the pain. You should elicit all seven attributes of this symptom (see p. 32) to distinguish among the various causes of chest pain.

chest wall suggests musculo-skeletal pain; a hand moving from neck to epigastrum suggests heartburn.

Lung tissue itself has no pain fibers. Pain in lung conditions such as pneumonia or pulmonary infarction usually arises from inflammation of the adjacent parietal pleura. Muscle strain from prolonged recurrent coughing may also be responsible. The pericardium also has few pain fibers—the pain of pericarditis stems from inflammation of the adjacent parietal pleura. (Chest pain is commonly associated with anxiety, too, but the mechanism remains obscure.)

Anxiety is the most frequent cause of chest pain in children; costochondritis is also common.

Dyspnea is a nonpainful but uncomfortable awareness of breathing that is inappropriate to the level of exertion. This serious symptom warrants a full explanation and assessment because dyspnea commonly results from cardiac or pulmonary disease.

See Table 7-2, Dyspnea, pp. 270–271.

Ask "Have you had any difficulty breathing?" Find out when the symptom occurs, at rest or with exercise, and how much effort produces onset. Because of variations in age, body weight, and physical fitness, there is no absolute scale for quantifying dyspnea. Instead, make every effort *to determine its severity based on the patient's daily activities.* How many steps or flights of stairs can the patient climb before pausing for breath? What about work such as carrying bags of groceries, mopping the floor, or making the bed? Has dyspnea altered the patient's lifestyle and daily activities? How? Carefully elicit the timing and setting of dyspnea, any associated symptoms, and relieving or aggravating factors.

Most patients with dyspnea relate shortness of breath to their level of activity. Anxious patients present a different picture. They may describe difficulty taking a deep enough breath, or a smothering sensation with inability to get enough air, along with *paresthesias,* or sensations of tingling or "pins and needles" around the lips or in the extremities.

Anxious patients may have episodic dyspnea during both rest and exercise, and *hyperventilation,* or rapid, shallow breathing. At other times, they may have frequent sighs.

Wheezes are musical respiratory sounds that may be audible to the patient and to others.

Wheezing suggests partial airway obstruction from secretions, tissue inflammation, or a foreign body.

Cough is a common symptom that ranges in significance from trivial to ominous. Typically, cough is a reflex response to stimuli that irritate receptors in the larynx, trachea, or large bronchi. These stimuli include mucus, pus, and blood, as well as external agents such as dusts, foreign bodies, or even extremely hot or cold air. Other causes include inflammation of the respiratory mucosa and pressure or tension in the air passages from a tumor or enlarged peribronchial lymph nodes. Although cough typically signals a problem in the respiratory tract, it may also be cardiovascular in origin.

See Table 7-3, Cough and Hemoptysis, p. 272.

Cough can be a symptom of left-sided heart failure.

For complaints of cough, a thorough assessment is in order. Ask whether the cough is dry or produces *sputum*, or phlegm. Ask the patient to describe the volume of any sputum and its color, odor, and consistency.

Dry hacking cough in Mycoplasma pneumonia; productive cough in bronchitis, viral or bacterial pneumonia

Mucoid sputum is translucent, white, or gray; *purulent* sputum is yellowish or greenish.

Foul-smelling sputum in anaerobic lung abscess; tenacious sputum in cystic fibrosis

To help patients quantify volume, a multiple-choice question may be helpful . . . "How much do you think you cough up in 24 hours; a teaspoon, tablespoon, a quarter cup, half cup, cupful?" If possible, ask the patient to cough into a tissue; inspect the phlegm and note its characteristics. The symptoms associated with a cough often lead you to its cause.

Large volumes of purulent sputum in bronchiectasis or lung abscess

Diagnostically helpful symptoms include fever, chest pain, dyspnea, orthopnea, and wheezing.

Hemoptysis is the coughing up of blood from the lungs; it may vary from blood-streaked phlegm to frank blood. For patients reporting hemoptysis, assess the volume of blood produced as well as the other sputum attributes; ask about the related setting and activity and any associated symptoms.

See Table 7-3, Cough and Hemoptysis, p. 272. Hemoptysis is rare in infants, children, and adolescents; it is seen most often in cystic fibrosis.

Before using the term "hemoptysis," try to confirm the source of the bleeding by both history and physical examination. Blood or blood-streaked material may originate in the mouth, pharynx, or gastrointestinal tract and is easily mislabeled. When vomited, it probably originates in the gastrointestinal tract. Occasionally, however, blood from the nasopharynx or the gastrointestinal tract is aspirated and then coughed out.

Blood originating in the stomach is usually darker than blood from the respiratory tract and may be mixed with food particles.

HEALTH PROMOTION AND COUNSELING

Important Topics for Health Promotion and Counseling

- Tobacco cessation

Despite declines in smoking over the past several decades, 22.5% of all adults, or 46 million Americans, still smoke.[1] Eighty percent of smokers have their first cigarette before age 18, and smoking rates are highest among high school students and young adults ages 18 to 24. Smoking wreaks a heavy toll on health, accounting for approximately 440,000 deaths each year, or roughly 20% of annual U.S. mortality. These figures include an estimated

35,000 deaths from exposure to secondhand smoke. Risk for death from lung cancer is 22 times higher among male smokers and approximately 12 times higher among female smokers compared with those who have never smoked. Risk for death from chronic obstructive heart disease increases ten-fold for smokers. Smokers have a 2 to 4 times increased risk for heart disease, double the risk for stroke, and 10 times the risk for peripheral vascular disease. Nonsmokers exposed to smoke also have increased risk for lung cancer, ear and respiratory infection, asthma, low birth weight, and residential fires. Smoking exposes patients not only to carcinogens but also to nicotine, an addictive drug.

Smoking is the leading cause of preventable death in the United States. More than 70% of smokers express interest in quitting, although less than 10% are successful.[1] Clinicians should query smokers on every visit about quitting, especially teenagers and pregnant women, and should adopt the five "As":

- **A**sk about smoking at each visit.

- **A**dvise patients regularly to stop smoking using a clear personalized message.

- **A**ssess patient readiness to quit.

- **A**ssist patients to set stop dates and provide educational materials for self-help.

- **A**rrange for follow-up visits to monitor and support patient progress.

The disease risks of smoking drop significantly within 1 year of smoking cessation. Study the addictive features of nicotine: tolerance over time, physical dependence, and the features of withdrawal ranging from irritability, anger, and insomnia to anxiety and depressed mood. Learn to make effective interventions to promote sustained quit rates, including targeted messages, group counseling, and use of nicotine-replacement therapies.[2] Combining clinician and group counseling with nicotine replacement therapy is especially effective for highly addicted patients.

Relapses are common and should be expected. Nicotine withdrawal, weight gain, stress, social pressure, and use of alcohol are often cited as explanations. Help patients to learn from these experiences: work with the patient to pinpoint the precipitating circumstances and develop strategies for alternative responses and health-promoting behaviors.

TECHNIQUES OF EXAMINATION

It is helpful to examine the posterior thorax and lungs while the patient is sitting, and the anterior thorax and lungs with the patient supine. Proceed in an orderly fashion: inspect, palpate, percuss, and auscultate. Try to visualize the underlying lobes, and compare one side with the other, so that the patient serves as his or her own control. For men, arrange the patient's gown so that you can see the chest fully. For women, cover the anterior chest when you examine the back. For the anterior examination, drape the gown over each half of the chest as you examine the other half.

With the patient sitting, examine the posterior thorax and lungs. The patient's arms should be folded across the chest with hands resting, if possible, on the opposite shoulders. This position moves the scapulae partly out of the way and increases your access to the lung fields. Then ask the patient to lie down.

With the patient supine, examine the anterior thorax and lungs. The supine position makes it easier to examine women because the breasts can be gently displaced. Furthermore, wheezes, if present, are more likely to be heard. (Some authorities, however, prefer to examine both the back and the front of the chest with the patient sitting. This technique is also satisfactory).

For patients unable to sit up without aid, try to get help so that you can examine the posterior chest in the sitting position. If this is impossible, roll the patient to one side and then to the other. Percuss the upper lung, and auscultate both lungs in each position. Because ventilation is relatively greater in the dependent lung, your chances of hearing abnormal wheezes or crackles are greater on the dependent side (see p. 260).

■ INITIAL SURVEY OF RESPIRATION AND THE THORAX

Even though you may have already recorded the respiratory rate when you took the vital signs, it is wise to again *observe the rate, rhythm, depth, and effort of breathing.* A normal resting adult breathes quietly and regularly about 14 to 20 times a minute. An occasional sigh is to be expected. Note whether expiration lasts longer than usual.

See Table 4-8, Abnormalities in Rate and Rhythm of Breathing, p. 120.

Always inspect the patient for any signs of respiratory difficulty.

■ *Assess the patient's color* for cyanosis. Recall any relevant findings from earlier parts of your examination, such as the shape of the fingernails.

Cyanosis signals hypoxia. Clubbing of the nails (see p. 150) in lung abscesses or malignancy, congenital heart disease

■ *Listen to the patient's breathing.* Is there any *audible wheezing?* If so, where does it fall in the respiratory cycle?

Audible *stridor,* a high-pitched wheeze, is an ominous sign of airway obstruction in the larynx or trachea.

■ *Inspect the neck.* During inspiration, is there contraction of the sterno-mastoid or other accessory muscles, or supraclavicular retraction? Is the trachea midline?

Inspiratory contraction of the sternomastoids at rest signals severe difficulty breathing. Lateral displacement of the trachea in *pneumothorax, pleural effusion,* or *atelectasis*

Also *observe the shape of the chest.* The anteroposterior (AP) diameter may increase with aging.

The AP diameter also may increase in *chronic obstructive pulmonary disease* (COPD).

EXAMINATION OF THE POSTERIOR CHEST

INSPECTION

From a midline position behind the patient, note the *shape of the chest* and *the way in which it moves,* including:

■ Deformities or asymmetry

See Table 7-4, Deformities of the Thorax (p. 273).

■ Abnormal retraction of the interspaces during inspiration. Retraction is most apparent in the lower interspaces. Supraclavicular retraction is often present.

Retraction in severe asthma, COPD, or upper airway obstruction

■ Impaired respiratory movement on one or both sides or a unilateral lag (or delay) in movement.

Unilateral impairment or lagging of respiratory movement suggests disease of the underlying lung or pleura.

PALPATION

As you palpate the chest, focus on areas of tenderness and abnormalities in the overlying skin, respiratory expansion, and fremitus.

Intercostal tenderness over inflamed pleura

Identify tender areas. Carefully palpate any area where pain has been reported or where lesions or bruises are evident.

Bruises over a fractured rib

Assess any observed abnormalities such as masses or sinus tracts (blind, inflammatory, tubelike structures opening onto the skin).

Although rare, sinus tracts usually indicate infection of the underlying pleura and lung (as in tuberculosis, actinomycosis).

Test chest expansion. Place your thumbs at about the level of the 10th ribs, with your fingers loosely grasping and parallel to the lateral rib cage. As you position your hands, slide them medially just enough to raise a loose fold of skin on each side between your thumb and the spine.

Ask the patient to inhale deeply. Watch the distance between your thumbs as they move apart during inspiration, and feel for the range and symmetry of the rib cage as it expands and contracts.

Causes of unilateral decrease or delay in chest expansion include chronic fibrotic disease of the underlying lung or pleura, pleural effusion, lobar pneumonia, pleural pain with associated splinting, and unilateral bronchial obstruction.

Feel for tactile fremitus. Fremitus refers to the palpable vibrations transmitted through the bronchopulmonary tree to the chest wall when the patient speaks. To detect fremitus, use either the ball (the bony part of the palm at the base of the fingers) or the ulnar surface of your hand to optimize the vibratory sensitivity of the bones in your hand. Ask the patient to repeat the words "ninety-nine" or "one-one-one." If fremitus is faint, ask the patient to speak more loudly or in a deeper voice.

Use one hand until you have learned the feel of fremitus. Some clinicians find using one hand more accurate. The simultaneous use of both hands to compare sides, however, increases your speed and may facilitate detection of differences.

Fremitus is decreased or absent when the voice is soft or when the transmission of vibrations from the larynx to the surface of the chest is impeded. Causes include an obstructed bronchus; COPD; separation of the pleural surfaces by fluid (pleural effusion), fibrosis (pleural thickening), air (pneumothorax), or an infiltrating tumor; and a very thick chest wall.

Palpate and compare symmetric areas of the lungs in the pattern shown in the photograph. Identify and locate any areas of increased, decreased, or absent fremitus. Fremitus is typically more prominent in the interscapular area than in the lower lung fields and is often more prominent on the right side than on the left. It disappears below the diaphragm.

Tactile fremitus is a relatively rough assessment tool, but as a scouting technique, it directs your attention to possible abnormalities. Later in

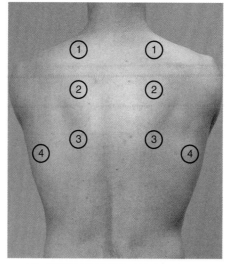

LOCATIONS FOR FEELING FREMITUS

the examination you will check any suggested findings by listening for breath sounds, voice sounds, and whispered voice sounds. All these attributes tend to increase or decrease together.

PERCUSSION

Percussion is one of the most important techniques of physical examination. Percussion of the chest sets the chest wall and underlying tissues into motion, producing audible sound and palpable vibrations. Percussion helps you establish whether the underlying tissues are air-filled, fluid-filled, or solid. It penetrates only about 5 cm to 7 cm into the chest, however, and will not help you to detect deep-seated lesions.

The technique of percussion can be practiced on any surface. As you practice, listen for changes in percussion notes over different types of materials or different parts of the body. The key points for good technique, described for a right-handed person, are as follows:

- Hyperextend the middle finger of your left hand, known as the pleximeter finger. Press its distal interphalangeal joint firmly on the surface to be percussed. Avoid surface contact by any other part of the hand, because this dampens out vibrations. Note that the thumb and 2nd, 4th, and 5th fingers are not touching the chest.

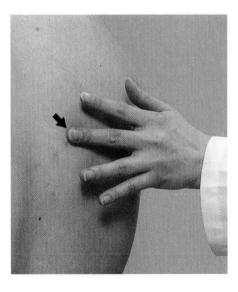

- Position your right forearm quite close to the surface, with the hand cocked upward. The middle finger should be partially flexed, relaxed, and poised to strike.

- With a *quick sharp but relaxed wrist motion,* strike the pleximeter finger with the right middle finger, or plexor finger. Aim at your distal interphalangeal joint. You are trying to transmit vibrations through the bones of this joint to the underlying chest wall.

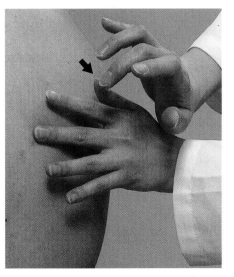

Strike using the *tip of the plexor finger,* not the finger pad. Your finger should be almost at right angles to the pleximeter. A short fingernail is recommended to avoid self-injury.

■ Withdraw your striking finger quickly to avoid damping the vibrations you have created.

In summary, the movement is at the wrist. It is directed, brisk yet relaxed, and a bit bouncy.

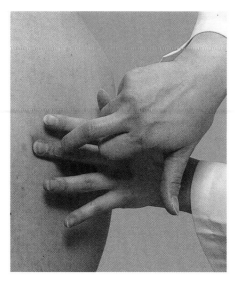

Percussion Notes.   With your plexor or tapping finger, use the lightest percussion that produces a clear note. A thick chest wall requires stronger percussion than a thin one. However, if a *louder* note is needed, apply more pressure with the *pleximeter* finger (this is more effective for increasing percussion note volume than tapping harder with the plexor finger).

When percussing the lower posterior chest, stand somewhat to the side rather than directly behind the patient. This allows you to place your pleximeter finger more firmly on the chest and your plexor is more effective, making a better percussion note.

When comparing two areas, use the same percussion technique in both areas. Percuss or strike twice in each location. It is easier to detect differences in percussion notes by comparing one area with another than by striking repetitively in one place.

Learn to identify five percussion notes. You can practice four of them on yourself. These notes differ in their basic qualities of sound: intensity, pitch, and duration. Train your ear to distinguish these differences by concentrating on one quality at a time as you percuss first in one location, then in another. Review the table below. Normal lungs are *resonant.*

■ *Percussion Notes and Their Characteristics*

	Relative Intensity	Relative Pitch	Relative Duration	Example of Location	Pathologic Examples
Flatness	Soft	High	Short	Thigh	Large pleural effusion
Dullness	Medium	Medium	Medium	Liver	Lobar pneumonia
Resonance	Loud	Low	Long	Normal lung	Simple chronic bronchitis
Hyperresonance	Very loud	Lower	Longer	None normally	Emphysema, pneumothorax
Tympany	Loud	High*	*	Gastric air bubble or puffed-out cheek	Large pneumothorax

* Distinguished mainly by its musical timbre.

While the patient keeps both arms crossed in front of the chest, percuss the thorax in symmetric locations from the apices to the lung bases.

Percuss one side of the chest and then the other at each level in a ladder-like pattern, as shown by the numbers below. Omit the areas over the scapulae—the thickness of muscle and bone alters the percussion notes over the lungs. Identify and locate the area and quality of any abnormal percussion note.

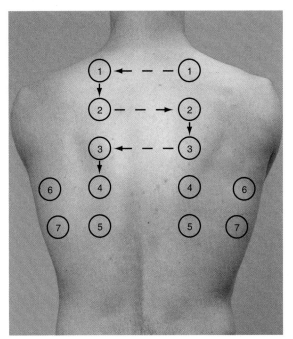

"LADDER" PATTERNS FOR PERCUSSION AND AUSCULTATION

Identify the descent of the diaphragms, or *diaphragmatic excursion.* First, *determine the level of diaphragmatic dullness* during quiet respiration. Holding the pleximeter finger *above and parallel* to the expected level of dullness, percuss downward in progressive steps until dullness clearly replaces resonance. Confirm this level of change by percussion near the middle of the hemothorax and also more laterally.

Dullness replaces resonance when fluid or solid tissue replaces air-containing lung or occupies the pleural space beneath your percussing fingers. Examples include: lobar pneumonia, in which the alveoli are filled with fluid and blood cells; and pleural accumulations of serous fluid (pleural effusion), blood (hemothorax), pus (empyema), fibrous tissue, or tumor.

Generalized hyperresonance may be heard over the hyperinflated lungs of emphysema or asthma, but it is not a reliable sign. *Unilateral hyperresonance* suggests a large pneumothorax or possibly a large air-filled bulla in the lung.

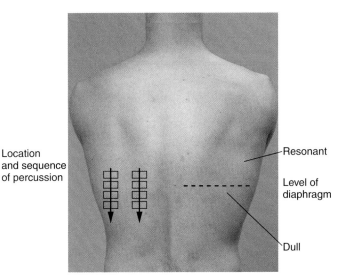

Location and sequence of percussion

Resonant

Level of diaphragm

Dull

An abnormally high level suggests pleural effusion, or a high diaphragm as in atelectasis or diaphragmatic paralysis.

Note that with this technique, you are identifying the boundary between the resonant lung tissue and the duller structures below the diaphragm. You are not percussing the diaphragm itself. You can infer the probable location of the diaphragm from the level of dullness.

Now, *estimate the extent of diaphragmatic excursion* by determining the distance between the level of dullness on full expiration and the level of dullness on full inspiration, normally about 5 or 6 cm. This estimate does not correlate well, however, with radiologic assessment of diaphragmatic movement.

AUSCULTATION

Auscultation of the lungs is the most important examining technique for assessing air flow through the tracheobronchial tree. Together with percussion, it also helps the clinician to assess the condition of the surrounding lungs and pleural space. Auscultation involves (1) listening to the sounds generated by breathing, (2) listening for any adventitious (added) sounds, and (3) if abnormalities are suspected, listening to the sounds of the patient's spoken or whispered voice as they are transmitted through the chest wall.

Sounds from bedclothes, paper gowns, and the chest itself can generate confusion in auscultation. Hair on the chest may cause crackling sounds. Either press harder or wet the hair. If the patient is cold or tense, you may hear muscle contraction sounds—muffled, low-pitched rumbling or roaring noises. A change in the patient's position may eliminate this noise. You can reproduce this sound on yourself by doing a Valsalva maneuver (straining down) as you listen to your own chest.

Breath Sounds (Lung Sounds).   You will learn to identify patterns of breath sounds by their intensity, their pitch, and the relative duration of their inspiratory and expiratory phases. Normal breath sounds are:

- *Vesicular,* or soft and low pitched. They are heard through inspiration, continue without pause through expiration, and then fade away about one third of the way through expiration.

- *Bronchovesicular,* with inspiratory and expiratory sounds about equal in length, at times separated by a silent interval. Detecting differences in pitch and intensity is often easier during expiration.

- *Bronchial,* or louder and higher in pitch, with a short silence between inspiratory and expiratory sounds. Expiratory sounds last longer than inspiratory sounds.

The characteristics of these three kinds of breath sounds are summarized in the table below. Also shown are the *tracheal* breath sounds—very loud, harsh sounds that are heard by listening over the trachea in the neck.

Listen to the breath sounds with the diaphragm of a stethoscope after instructing the patient to breathe deeply through an open mouth. Use the pattern suggested for percussion, moving from one side to the other and comparing symmetric areas of the lungs. If you hear or suspect abnormal sounds, auscultate adjacent areas so that you can fully describe the extent of any abnormality. Listen to at least one full breath in each location. Be alert for patient discomfort due to hyperventilation (e.g., lightheadedness, faintness), and allow the patient to rest as needed.

Note the *intensity* of the breath sounds. Breath sounds are usually louder in the lower posterior lung fields and may also vary from area to area. If the

Breath sounds may be decreased when air flow is decreased (as by

■ *Characteristics of Breath Sounds*

	Duration of Sounds	Intensity of Expiratory Sound	Pitch of Expiratory Sound	Locations Where Heard Normally
Vesicular*	Inspiratory sounds last longer than expiratory ones.	Soft	Relatively low	Over most of both lungs
Broncho-vesicular	Inspiratory and expiratory sounds are about equal.	Intermediate	Intermediate	Often in the 1st and 2nd interspaces anteriorly and between the scapulae
Bronchial	Expiratory sounds last longer than inspiratory ones.	Loud	Relatively high	Over the manubrium, if heard at all
Tracheal	Inspiratory and expiratory sounds are about equal.	Very loud	Relatively high	Over the trachea in the neck

* The thickness of the bars indicates intensity; the steeper their incline, the higher the pitch.

breath sounds seem faint, ask the patient to breathe more deeply. You may then hear them easily. When patients do not breathe deeply enough or have a thick chest wall, as in obesity, breath sounds may remain diminished.

If bronchovesicular or bronchial breath sounds are heard in locations distant from those listed, suspect that air-filled lung has been replaced by fluid-filled or solid lung tissue. See Table 7-5, Normal and Altered Breath and Voice Sounds (p. 274).

obstructive lung disease or muscular weakness) or when the transmission of sound is poor (as in pleural effusion, pneumothorax, or emphysema).

Is there a *silent gap* between the inspiratory and expiratory sounds?

A gap suggests bronchial breath sounds.

Listen for the *pitch, intensity, and duration of the expiratory and inspiratory sounds.* Are vesicular breath sounds distributed normally over the chest wall? Or are there bronchovesicular or bronchial breath sounds in unexpected places? If so, where are they?

Adventitious (Added) Sounds. Listen for any added, or adventitious, sounds that are superimposed on the usual breath sounds. Detection of adventitious sounds—*crackles* (sometimes called *rales*), *wheezes,* and *rhonchi*— is an important part of your examination, often leading to diagnosis of cardiac and pulmonary conditions. The most common kinds of these sounds are described on the next page:

For further discussion and other added sounds, see Table 7-6, Adventitious (Added) Lung Sounds: Causes and Qualities (p. 275).

■ Adventitious or Added Breath Sounds

Crackles (or Rales)	Wheezes and Rhonchi
■ **Discontinuous**	■ **Continuous**
■ Intermittent, nonmusical, and brief	■ >250 msec, musical, prolonged (but not necessarily persisting throughout the respiratory cycle)
■ Like dots in time	■ Like dashes in time
■ *Fine crackles:* soft, high-pitched, very brief (5–10 msec) · · · · ·	■ *Wheezes:* relatively high-pitched (≥400 Hz) with hissing or shrill quality
Coarse crackles: somewhat louder, lower in pitch, brief (20–30 msec) ● ● ● ● ●	■ *Rhonchi:* relatively low-pitched (≤200 Hz) with snoring quality

Crackles may be due to abnormalities of the lungs (pneumonia, fibrosis, early congestive heart failure) or of the airways (bronchitis, bronchiectasis).

Wheezes suggest narrowed airways, as in asthma, COPD, or bronchitis.

Rhonchi suggest secretions in large airways.

If you hear *crackles,* especially those that do not clear after cough, listen carefully for the following characteristics. These are clues to the underlying condition:

■ Loudness, pitch, and duration (summarized as fine or coarse crackles)

■ Number (few to many)

■ Timing in the respiratory cycle

■ Location on the chest wall

■ Persistence of their pattern from breath to breath

■ Any change after a cough or a change in the patient's position

Fine late inspiratory crackles that persist from breath to breath suggest abnormal lung tissue.

Clearing of crackles, wheezes, or rhonchi after cough or position change suggests inspissated secretions, as in bronchitis or atelectasis.

In some normal people, crackles may be heard at the lung bases anteriorly after maximal expiration. Crackles in dependent portions of the lungs may also occur after prolonged recumbency.

If you hear *wheezes* or *rhonchi,* note their timing and location. Do they change with deep breathing or coughing?

Transmitted Voice Sounds.   If you hear abnormally located bronchovesicular or bronchial breath sounds, assess transmitted voice sounds. With a stethoscope, listen in symmetric areas over the chest wall as you:

Increased transmission of voice sounds suggests that air-filled lung has become airless. See Table 7-5, Normal and Altered Breath and Voice Sounds (p. 274).

- Ask the patient to say "ninety-nine." Normally the sounds transmitted through the chest wall are muffled and indistinct.

Louder, clearer voice sounds are called *bronchophony.*

- Ask the patient to say "ee." You will normally hear a muffled long E sound.

When "ee" is heard as "ay," an *E-to-A change (egophony)* is present, as in lobar consolidation from pneumonia. The quality sounds nasal.

- Ask the patient to whisper "ninety-nine" or "one-two-three." The whispered voice is normally heard faintly and indistinctly, if at all.

Louder, clearer whispered sounds are called *whispered pectoriloquy.*

■ EXAMINATION OF THE ANTERIOR CHEST

When examined in the supine position, the patient should lie comfortably with arms somewhat abducted. A patient who is having difficulty breathing should be examined in the sitting position or with the head of the bed elevated to a comfortable level.

Persons with severe COPD may prefer to sit leaning forward, with lips pursed during exhalation and arms supported on their knees or a table.

INSPECTION

Observe *the shape of the patient's chest* and *the movement of the chest wall.* Note:

- Deformities or asymmetry

See Table 7-4, Deformities of the Thorax (p. 273).

- Abnormal retraction of the lower interspaces during inspiration

Severe asthma, COPD, or upper airway obstruction

- Local lag or impairment in respiratory movement

Underlying disease of lung or pleura

PALPATION

Palpation has four potential uses:

- *Identification of tender areas*

Tender pectoral muscles or costal cartilages tend to corroborate, but do not prove, that chest pain has a musculoskeletal origin.

- *Assessment of observed abnormalities*

- *Further assessment of chest expansion.* Place your thumbs along each costal margin, your hands along the lateral rib cage. As you position your hands, slide them medially a bit to raise loose skin folds between your thumbs. Ask the patient to inhale deeply. Observe how far your thumbs diverge as the thorax expands, and feel for the extent and symmetry of respiratory movement.

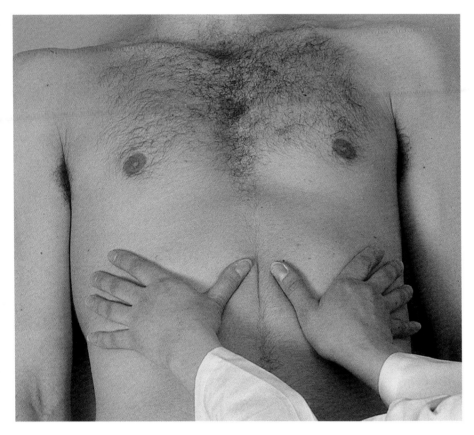

■ *Assessment of tactile fremitus.* Compare both sides of the chest, using the ball or ulnar surface of your hand. Fremitus is usually decreased or absent over the precordium. When examining a woman, gently displace the breasts as necessary.

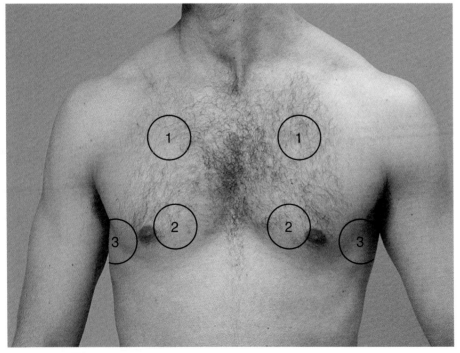

LOCATIONS FOR FEELING FREMITUS

PERCUSSION

Percuss the anterior and lateral chest, again comparing both sides. The heart normally produces an area of dullness to the left of the sternum from the 3rd to the 5th interspaces. Percuss the left lung lateral to it.

Dullness replaces resonance when fluid or solid tissue replaces air-containing lung or occupies the pleural space. Because pleural fluid usually sinks to the lowest part of the pleural space (posteriorly in a supine patient), only a very large effusion can be detected anteriorly.

The hyperresonance of COPD may totally replace cardiac dullness.

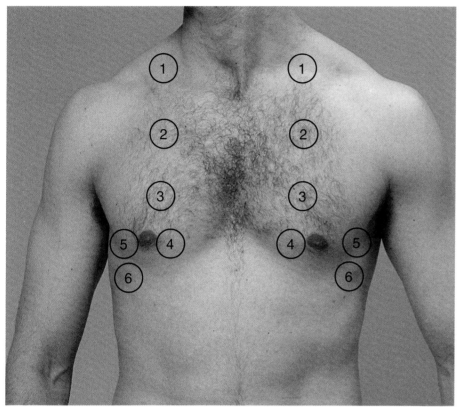

LOCATIONS FOR PERCUSSION AND AUSCULTATION

In a woman, to enhance percussion, gently displace the breast with your left hand while percussing with the right.

The dullness of right middle lobe pneumonia typically occurs behind the right breast. Unless you displace the breast, you may miss the abnormal percussion note.

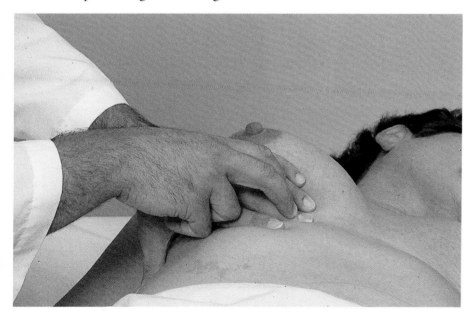

Alternatively, you may ask the patient to move her breast for you.

Identify and locate any area with an abnormal percussion note.

With your pleximeter finger above and parallel to the expected upper border of liver dullness, percuss in progressive steps downward in the right midclavicular line. Identify the upper border of liver dullness. Later, during the abdominal examination, you will use this method to estimate the size of the liver. As you percuss down the chest on the left, the resonance of normal lung usually changes to the tympany of the gastric air bubble.

A lung affected by COPD often displaces the upper border of the liver downward. It also lowers the level of diaphragmatic dullness posteriorly.

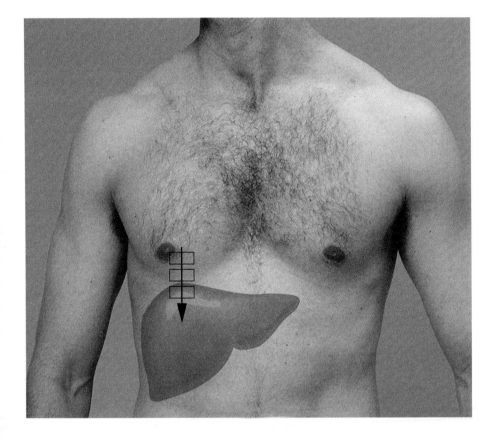

AUSCULTATION

Listen to the chest anteriorly and laterally as the patient breathes with mouth open, somewhat more deeply than normal. Compare symmetric areas of the lungs, using the pattern suggested for percussion and extending it to adjacent areas as indicated.

Listen to the breath sounds, noting their intensity and identifying any variations from normal vesicular breathing. Breath sounds are usually louder in the upper anterior lung fields. Bronchovesicular breath sounds may be heard over the large airways, especially on the right.

Identify any adventitious sounds, time them in the respiratory cycle, and locate them on the chest wall. Do they clear with deep breathing?

See Table 7-6, Adventitious (Added) Lung Sounds: Causes and Qualities (p. 275), and Table 7-7, Physical Findings in Selected Chest Disorders (pp. 276–277).

If indicated, *listen for transmitted voice sounds.*

SPECIAL TECHNIQUES

Clinical Assessment of Pulmonary Function. A simple but informative way to assess the complaint of breathlessness in an ambulatory patient is to walk with the patient down the hall or climb one flight of stairs. Observe the rate, effort, and sound of the patient's breathing.

Forced Expiratory Time. This test assesses the expiratory phase of breathing, which is typically slowed in obstructive pulmonary disease. Ask the patient to take a deep breath in and then breathe out as quickly and completely as possible with mouth open. Listen over the trachea with the diaphragm of a stethoscope and time the audible expiration. Try to get three consistent readings, allowing a short rest between efforts if necessary.

If the patient understands and cooperates in performing the test, a forced expiration time of 6 seconds or more suggests obstructive pulmonary disease.

Identification of a Fractured Rib. Local pain and tenderness of one or more ribs raise the question of fracture. By anteroposterior compression of the chest, you can help to distinguish a fracture from soft-tissue injury. With one hand on the sternum and the other on the thoracic spine, squeeze the chest. Is this painful, and where?

An increase in the local pain (distant from your hands) suggests rib fracture rather than just soft-tissue injury.

RECORDING YOUR FINDINGS

Note that initially you may use sentences to describe your findings; later you will use phrases. The style below contains phrases appropriate for most write-ups.

> ### Recording the Physical Examination— The Thorax and Lungs
>
> "Thorax is symmetric with good expansion. Lungs resonant. Breath sounds vesicular; no rales, wheezes, or rhonchi. Diaphragms descend 4 cm bilaterally."
>
> **OR**
>
> "Thorax symmetric with moderate kyphosis and increased anteroposterior (AP) diameter, decreased expansion. Lungs are hyperresonant. Breath sounds distant with delayed expiratory phase and scattered expiratory wheezes. Fremitus decreased; no bronchophony, egophony, or whispered pectoriloquy. Diaphragms descend 2 cm bilaterally."

Suggests chronic obstructive lung disease

Bibliography

CITATIONS

1. Centers for Disease Control and Prevention (CDC). At a glance. Targeting tobacco use: the nation's leading cause of death, 2004. Available at: http://www.cdc.gov/nccdphp/aag/pdf/aag_osh2004.pdf. Accessed October 29, 2004. [See also Centers for Disease Control Tobacco Information and Prevention Source (TIPS). Available at: http://www.cdc.gov/tobacco/issue.htm. Accessed October 29, 2004.]
2. Rigotti NA. Putting the research into practice. BMJ 327(7428):1395–1396, 2003.

ADDITIONAL REFERENCES

Examination of the Lungs

Badgett RG, et al. Can moderate obstructive pulmonary disease be diagnosed by historical and physical findings alone? Am J Med 94:188, 1993.

Bettancourt PE, DelBono EA, Speigelman D, et al. Clinical utility of chest auscultation in common pulmonary disease. Am J Resp Crit Care Med 150:1921, 1994.

Cugell DW. Lung sound nomenclature. Am Rev Respir Dis 136:1016, 1987.

Epler GR, Carrington CB, Gaensler EA. Crackles (rales) in the interstitial pulmonary diseases. Chest 73:333, 1978.

Holleman DR, Simel DL. Does the clinical examination predict airflow limitation? JAMA 273:313, 1995.

Koster MEY, Baughmann RP, Loudon RG. Continuous adventitious lung sounds. J Asthma 27:237, 1990.

Kraman SS. Lung sounds for the clinician. Arch Intern Med 146:1411, 1986.

Lehrer S. Understanding Lung Sounds, 3rd ed. Philadelphia, WB Saunders, 2002.

Lichtenstein D, Goldstein I, Mourgeon E, et al. Comparative diagnostic performances of auscultation, chest radiography, and lung ultrasonography in acute respiratory distress syndrome. Anesthesiology 100(1):9–15, 2004.

Loudon RG. The lung exam. Clin Chest Med 8:265, 1987.

Metlay JP, Kapoor WN, Fine MJ. Does this patient have community-acquired pneumonia? Diagnosing pneumonia by history and physical examination. JAMA 278(17):1440, 1997.

Nath AR, Carpel LH. Inspiratory crackles—early and late. Thorax 29:223, 1974.

Nath AR, Carpel LH. Lung crackles in bronchiectasis. Thorax 35:694, 1980.

Schapira RM, et al. The value of the forced expiratory time in the physical diagnosis of obstructive airways disease. JAMA 270:731, 1993.

Straus SE, Finaly AM, Sackett DL, et al, for the CARE-COAD1 Group. The accuracy of patient history, wheezing, and laryngeal measurements in diagnosing obstructive airway disease. JAMA 283(14):1853–1857, 2000.

Pulmonary Conditions

American Thoracic Society and Centers for Disease Control and Prevention. Diagnostic standards and classification of tuberculosis in adults and children. Am J Respir Crit Care Med 161(4 Pt 1):1376–1395, 2000.

Baum GL, Crapo JD, et al (eds). Baum's Textbook of Pulmonary Diseases, 7th ed. Philadelphia, Lippincott Williams & Wilkins, 2004.

Chunilal SD, Eikelboom JW, Attia J, et al. Does this patient have pulmonary embolism? JAMA 290(20):2849–2858, 2003.

Fiore MC, Bailey WC, Cohen SJ, et al. Treating Tobacco Use and Dependence. Quick Reference Guide for Clinicians. Rockville, MD, U.S. Department of Health and Human Services, Public Health Service, 2000. Available at: http://www.surgeongeneral.gov/tobacco/tobaqrg.pdf. Accessed May 22, 2005.

Global Initiative for Chronic Obstructive Lung Disease (GOLD), World Health Organization (WHO), National Heart, Lung and Blood Institute (NHLBI). Global Strategy for the Diagnosis, Management, and Prevention of Chronic Obstructive Pulmonary Disease. Bethesda, MD, Global Initiative for Chronic Obstructive Lung Disease, World Health Organization, National Heart, Lung and Blood Institute, 2004. Available at: http://www.guideline.gov. Accessed May 22, 2005.

Irwin RS, Madison JM. The diagnosis and treatment of cough. N Engl J Med 343(23):1715–1721, 2000.

Treatment of tuberculosis. MMWR Recomm Rep 52(RR–11):1–77, 2003.

Weinberger S. Principles of Pulmonary Medicine, 4th ed. Philadelphia, WB Saunders, 2004.

Williams SG, Schmidt DK, Redd SC, Storms W. Key clinical activities for quality asthma care: recommendations of the National Asthma Education and Prevention Program. MMWR Recomm Rep 52(RR–6):1–8, 2003.

Woodruff PG, Fahy JV. Asthma: prevalence, pathogenesis, and prospects for novel therapies. JAMA 286(4):395–398, 2001.

TABLE 7-1   **Chest Pain**

Problem	Process	Location	Quality	Severity
Cardiovascular				
Angina Pectoris	Temporary myocardial ischemia, usually secondary to coronary atherosclerosis	Retrosternal or across the anterior chest, sometimes radiating to the shoulders, arms, neck, lower jaw, or upper abdomen	Pressing, squeezing, tight, heavy, occasionally burning	Mild to moderate, sometimes perceived as discomfort rather than pain
Myocardial Infarction	Prolonged myocardial ischemia, resulting in irreversible muscle damage or necrosis	Same as in angina	Same as in angina	Often but not always a severe pain
Pericarditis	▪ Irritation of parietal pleura adjacent to the pericardium	Precordial, may radiate to the tip of the shoulder and to the neck	Sharp, knifelike	Often severe
	▪ Mechanism unclear	Retrosternal	Crushing	Severe
Dissecting Aortic Aneurysm	A splitting within the layers of the aortic wall, allowing passage of blood to dissect a channel	Anterior chest, radiating to the neck, back, or abdomen	Ripping, tearing	Very severe
Pulmonary				
Tracheobronchitis	Inflammation of trachea and large bronchi	Upper sternal or on either side of the sternum	Burning	Mild to moderate
Pleural Pain	Inflammation of the parietal pleura, as in pleurisy, pneumonia, pulmonary infarction, or neoplasm	Chest wall overlying the process	Sharp, knifelike	Often severe
Gastrointestinal and Other				
Reflex Esophagitis	Inflammation of the esophageal mucosa by reflux of gastric acid	Retrosternal, may radiate to the back	Burning, may be squeezing	Mild to severe
Diffuse Esophageal Spasm	Motor dysfunction of the esophageal muscle	Retrosternal, may radiate to the back, arms, and jaw	Usually squeezing	Mild to severe
Chest Wall Pain	Variable, often unclear	Often below the left breast or along the costal cartilages; also elsewhere	Stabbing, sticking, or dull, aching	Variable
Anxiety	Unclear	Precordial, below the left breast, or across the anterior chest	Stabbing, sticking, or dull, aching	Variable

Note: Remember that chest pain may be referred from extrathoracic structures such as the neck (arthritis) and abdomen (biliary colic, acute cholecystitis). Pleural pain may be due to abdominal conditions such as subdiaphragmatic abscess.

Timing	Factors That Aggravate	Factors That Relieve	Associated Symptoms
Usually 1–3 min but up to 10 min. Prolonged episodes up to 20 min	Exertion, especially in the cold; meals; emotional stress. May occur at rest	Rest, nitroglycerin	Sometimes dyspnea, nausea, sweating
20 min to several hours			Nausea, vomiting, sweating, weakness
Persistent	Breathing, changing position, coughing, lying down, sometimes swallowing	Sitting forward may relieve it.	Of the underlying illness
Persistent			Of the underlying illness
Abrupt onset, early peak, persistent for hours or more	Hypertension		Syncope, hemiplegia, paraplegia
Variable	Coughing	Lying on the involved side may relieve it.	Cough
Persistent	Breathing, coughing, movements of the trunk		Of the underlying illness
Variable	Large meal; bending over, lying down	Antacids, sometimes belching	Sometimes regurgitation, dysphagia
Variable	Swallowing of food or cold liquid; emotional stress	Sometimes nitroglycerin	Dysphagia
Fleeting to hours or days	Movement of chest, trunk, arms		Often local tenderness
Fleeting to hours or days	May follow effort, emotional stress		Breathlessness, palpitations, weakness, anxiety

TABLE 7-2   Dyspnea

Problem	Process	Timing
Left-Sided Heart Failure *(left ventricular failure or mitral stenosis)*	Elevated pressure in pulmonary capillary bed with transudation of fluid into interstitial spaces and alveoli, decreased compliance (increased stiffness) of the lungs, increased work of breathing	Dyspnea may progress slowly, or suddenly as in acute pulmonary edema.
Chronic Bronchitis*	Excessive mucus production in bronchi, followed by chronic obstruction of airways	Chronic productive cough followed by slowly progressive dyspnea
Chronic Obstructive Pulmonary Disease (COPD)*	Overdistention of air spaces distal to terminal bronchioles, with destruction of alveolar septa and chronic obstruction of the airways	Slowly progressive dyspnea; relatively mild cough later
Asthma	Bronchial hyperresponsiveness involving release of inflammatory mediators, increased airway secretions, and bronchoconstriction	Acute episodes, separated by symptom-free periods. Nocturnal episodes common
Diffuse Interstitial Lung Diseases *(such as sarcoidosis, widespread neoplasms, asbestosis, and idiopathic pulmonary fibrosis)*	Abnormal and widespread infiltration of cells, fluid, and collagen into interstitial spaces between alveoli. Many causes	Progressive dyspnea, which varies in its rate of development with the cause
Pneumonia	Inflammation of lung parenchyma from the respiratory bronchioles to the alveoli	An acute illness, timing varies with the causative agent
Spontaneous Pneumothorax	Leakage of air into pleural space through blebs on visceral pleura, with resulting partial or complete collapse of the lung	Sudden onset of dyspnea
Acute Pulmonary Embolism	Sudden occlusion of all or part of pulmonary arterial tree by a blood clot that usually originates in deep veins of legs or pelvis	Sudden onset of dyspnea
Anxiety With Hyperventilation	Overbreathing, with resultant respiratory alkalosis and fall in the partial pressure of carbon dioxide in the blood	Episodic, often recurrent

---

*Chronic bronchitis and *chronic obstructive pulmonary disease (COPD)* may coexist.

Factors That Aggravate	Factors That Relieve	Associated Symptoms	Setting
Exertion, lying down	Rest, sitting up, though dyspnea may become persistent	Often cough, orthopnea, paroxysmal nocturnal dyspnea; sometimes wheezing	History of heart disease or its predisposing factors
Exertion, inhaled irritants, respiratory infections	Expectoration; rest, though dyspnea may become persistent	Chronic productive cough, recurrent respiratory infections; wheezing may develop	History of smoking, air pollutants, recurrent respiratory infections
Exertion	Rest, though dyspnea may become persistent	Cough, with scant mucoid sputum	History of smoking, air pollutants, sometimes a familial deficiency in alpha$_1$-antitrypsin
Variable, including allergens, irritants, respiratory infections, exercise, and emotion	Separation from aggravating factors	Wheezing, cough, tightness in chest	Environmental and emotional conditions
Exertion	Rest, though dyspnea may become persistent	Often weakness, fatigue. Cough less common than in other lung diseases	Varied. Exposure to one of many substances may be causative.
		Pleuritic pain, cough, sputum, fever, though not necessarily present	Varied
		Pleuritic pain, cough	Often a previously healthy young adult
		Often none. Retrosternal oppressive pain if the occlusion is massive. Pleuritic pain, cough, and hemoptysis may follow an embolism if pulmonary infarction ensues. Symptoms of anxiety (see below).	Postpartum or postoperative periods; prolonged bed rest; congestive heart failure, chronic lung disease, and fractures of hip or leg; deep venous thrombosis (often not clinically apparent)
More often occurs at rest than after exercise. An upsetting event may not be evident.	Breathing in and out of a paper or plastic bag sometimes helps the associated symptoms.	Sighing, lightheadedness, numbness or tingling of the hands and feet, palpitations, chest pain	Other manifestations of anxiety may be present.

TABLE 7-3   Cough and Hemoptysis*

Problem	Cough and Sputum	Associated Symptoms and Setting
Acute Inflammation		
Laryngitis	Dry cough (without sputum), may become productive of variable amounts of sputum	An acute, fairly minor illness with hoarseness. Often associated with viral nasopharyngitis
Tracheobronchitis	Dry cough, may become productive (as above)	An acute, often viral illness, with burning retrosternal discomfort
Mycoplasma and Viral Pneumonias	Dry hacking cough, often becoming productive of mucoid sputum	An acute febrile illness, often with malaise, headache, and possibly dyspnea
Bacterial Pneumonias	Pneumococcal: sputum mucoid or purulent; may be blood-streaked, diffusely pinkish, or rusty	An acute illness with chills, high fever, dyspnea, and chest pain. Often preceded by acute upper respiratory infection
	Klebsiella: similar; or sticky, red, and jellylike	Typically occurs in older alcoholic men
Chronic Inflammation		
Postnasal Drip	Chronic cough; sputum mucoid or mucopurulent	Repeated attempts to clear the throat. Postnasal discharge may be sensed by patient or seen in posterior pharynx. Associated with chronic rhinitis, with or without sinusitis
Chronic Bronchitis	Chronic cough; sputum mucoid to purulent, may be blood-streaked or even bloody	Often long-standing cigarette smoking. Recurrent superimposed infections. Wheezing and dyspnea may develop.
Bronchiectasis	Chronic cough; sputum purulent, often copious and foul-smelling; may be blood-streaked or bloody	Recurrent bronchopulmonary infections common; sinusitis may coexist.
Pulmonary Tuberculosis	Cough dry or sputum that is mucoid or purulent; may be blood-streaked or bloody	Early, no symptoms. Later, anorexia, weight loss, fatigue, fever, and night sweats
Lung Abscess	Sputum purulent and foul-smelling; may be bloody	A febrile illness. Often poor dental hygiene and a prior episode of impaired consciousness
Asthma	Cough, with thick mucoid sputum, especially near end of an attack	Episodic wheezing and dyspnea, but cough may occur alone. Often a history of allergy
Gastroesophageal Reflux	Chronic cough, especially at night or early in the morning	Wheezing, especially at night (often mistaken for asthma), early morning hoarseness, and repeated attempts to clear the throat. Often a history of heartburn and regurgitation
Neoplasm		
Cancer of the Lung	Cough dry to productive; sputum may be blood-streaked or bloody	Usually a long history of cigarette smoking. Associated manifestations are numerous.
Cardiovascular Disorders		
Left Ventricular Failure or Mitral Stenosis	Often dry, especially on exertion or at night; may progress to the pink frothy sputum of pulmonary edema or to frank hemoptysis	Dyspnea, orthopnea, paroxysmal nocturnal dyspnea
Pulmonary Emboli	Dry to productive; may be dark, bright red, or mixed with blood	Dyspnea, anxiety, chest pain, fever; factors that predispose to deep venous thrombosis
Irritating Particles, Chemicals, or Gases	Variable. There may be a latent period between exposure and symptoms.	Exposure to irritants. Eyes, nose, and throat may be affected.

---

*Characteristics of hemoptysis are printed in red.

TABLE 7-4   **Deformities of the Thorax**

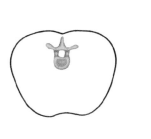
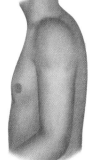

Normal Adult

The thorax in the normal adult is wider than it is deep. Its lateral diameter is larger than its anteroposterior diameter.

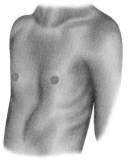
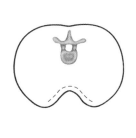

Funnel Chest (*Pectus Excavatum*)

Note depression in the lower portion of the sternum. Compression of the heart and great vessels may cause murmurs.

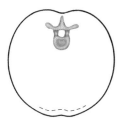
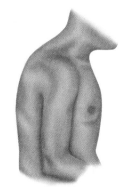

Barrel Chest

There is an increased anteroposterior diameter. This shape is normal during infancy, and often accompanies normal aging and chronic obstructive pulmonary disease.

Depressed costal cartilages

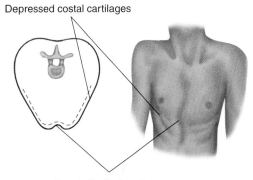

Anteriorly displaced sternum

Pigeon Chest (*Pectus Carinatum*)

The sternum is displaced anteriorly, increasing the anteroposterior diameter. The costal cartilages adjacent to the protruding sternum are depressed.

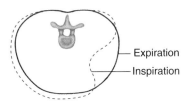

Expiration

Inspiration

Traumatic Flail Chest

Multiple rib fractures may result in paradoxical movements of the thorax. As descent of the diaphragm decreases intrathoracic pressure, on inspiration the injured area caves inward; on expiration, it moves outward.

Spinal convexity to the right
(patient bending forward)

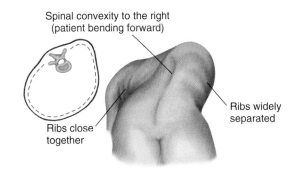

Ribs widely separated

Ribs close together

Thoracic Kyphoscoliosis

Abnormal spinal curvatures and vertebral rotation deform the chest. Distortion of the underlying lungs may make interpretation of lung findings very difficult.

TABLE 7-5   **Normal and Altered Breath and Voice Sounds**

The origins of breath sounds are still unclear. According to leading theories, turbulent air flow in the central airways produces the tracheal and bronchial breath sounds. As these sounds pass through the lungs to the periphery, lung tissue filters out their higher-pitched components, and only the soft and lower-pitched components reach the chest wall, where they are heard as vesicular breath sounds. Normally, tracheal and bronchial sounds may be heard over the trachea and mainstem bronchi; vesicular breath sounds predominate throughout most of the lungs.

When lung tissue loses its air, it transmits high-pitched sounds much better. If the tracheobronchial tree is open, bronchial breath sounds may replace the normal vesicular sounds over airless areas of the lung. This change is seen in lobar pneumonia when the alveoli fill with fluid, red cells, and white cells—a process called *consolidation*. Other causes include pulmonary edema or hemorrhage. Bronchial breath sounds usually correlate with an increase in tactile fremitus and transmitted voice sounds. These findings are summarized below.

	Normal Air-Filled Lung	**Airless Lung, as in Lobar Pneumonia**
Breath Sounds	Predominantly vesicular	Bronchial or bronchovesicular over the involved area
Transmitted Voice Sounds	Spoken words muffled and indistinct Spoken "ee" heard as "ee" Whispered words faint and indistinct, if heard at all	Spoken words louder, clearer (*bronchophony*) Spoken "ee" heard as "ay" (*egophony*) Whispered words louder, clearer (*whispered pectoriloquy*)
Tactile Fremitus	Normal	Increased

Crackles

Crackles have two leading explanations. (1) They result from a series of tiny explosions when small airways, deflated during expiration, pop open during inspiration. This mechanism probably explains the late inspiratory crackles of interstitial lung disease and early congestive heart failure. (2) Crackles result from air bubbles flowing through secretions or lightly closed airways during respiration. This mechanism probably explains at least some coarse crackles.

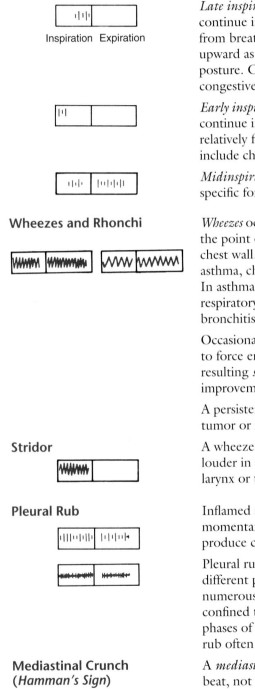

Inspiration Expiration

Late inspiratory crackles may begin in the first half of inspiration but must continue into late inspiration. They are usually fine and fairly profuse, and persist from breath to breath. These crackles appear first at the bases of the lungs, spread upward as the condition worsens, and shift to dependent regions with changes in posture. Causes include interstitial lung disease (such as fibrosis) and early congestive heart failure.

Early inspiratory crackles appear soon after the start of inspiration and do not continue into late inspiration. They are often but not always coarse and are relatively few in number. Expiratory crackles are sometimes associated. Causes include chronic bronchitis and asthma.

Midinspiratory and expiratory crackles are heard in bronchiectasis but are not specific for this diagnosis. Wheezes and rhonchi may be associated.

Wheezes and Rhonchi

Wheezes occur when air flows rapidly through bronchi that are narrowed nearly to the point of closure. They are often audible at the mouth as well as through the chest wall. Causes of wheezes that are generalized throughout the chest include asthma, chronic bronchitis, COPD, and congestive heart failure (cardiac asthma). In asthma, wheezes may be heard only in expiration or in both phases of the respiratory cycle. Rhonchi suggest secretions in the larger airways. In chronic bronchitis, wheezes and rhonchi often clear with coughing.

Occasionally in severe obstructive pulmonary disease, the patient is no longer able to force enough air through the narrowed bronchi to produce wheezing. The resulting *silent chest* should raise immediate concern and not be mistaken for improvement.

A persistent localized wheeze suggests a partial obstruction of a bronchus, as by a tumor or foreign body. It may be inspiratory, expiratory, or both.

Stridor

A wheeze that is entirely or predominantly inspiratory is called *stridor*. It is often louder in the neck than over the chest wall. It indicates a partial obstruction of the larynx or trachea, and demands immediate attention.

Pleural Rub

Inflamed and roughened pleural surfaces grate against each other as they are momentarily and repeatedly delayed by increased friction. These movements produce creaking sounds known as a *pleural rub* (or pleural friction rub).

Pleural rubs resemble crackles acoustically, although they are produced by different pathologic processes. The sounds may be discrete, but sometimes are so numerous that they merge into a seemingly continuous sound. A rub is usually confined to a relatively small area of the chest wall, and typically is heard in both phases of respiration. When inflamed pleural surfaces are separated by fluid, the rub often disappears.

Mediastinal Crunch (*Hamman's Sign*)

A *mediastinal crunch* is a series of precordial crackles synchronous with the heart beat, not with respiration. Best heard in the left lateral position, it is due to mediastinal emphysema (pneumomediastinum).

TABLE 7-7   **Physical Findings in Selected Chest Disorders**

The black boxes in this table suggest a framework for clinical assessment. Start with the three boxes under Percussion Note: resonant, dull, and hyperresonant. Then move from each of these to other boxes that emphasize some of the key differences among various conditions. The changes described vary with the extent and severity of the disorder. Abnormalities deep in the chest usually produce fewer signs than superficial ones, and may cause no signs at all. Use the table for the direction of typical changes, not for absolute distinctions.

Condition	Percussion Note	Trachea	Breath Sounds	Adventitious Sounds	Tactile Fremitus and Transmitted Voice Sounds
Normal The tracheobronchial tree and alveoli are clear; pleurae are thin and close together; mobility of the chest wall is unimpaired.	**Resonant**	Midline	Vesicular, except perhaps bronchovesicular and bronchial sounds over the large bronchi and trachea, respectively	None, except perhaps a few transient inspiratory crackles at the bases of the lungs	Normal
Chronic Bronchitis The bronchi are chronically inflamed and a productive cough is present. Airway obstruction may develop.	**Resonant**	Midline	Vesicular (normal)	None; or scattered coarse *crackles* in early inspiration and perhaps expiration; or *wheezes* or *rhonchi*	Normal
Left-Sided Heart Failure (*Early*) Increased pressure in the pulmonary veins causes congestion and interstitial edema (around the alveoli); bronchial mucosa may become edematous.	**Resonant**	Midline	Vesicular	*Late inspiratory crackles* in the dependent portions of the lungs; possibly *wheezes*	Normal
Consolidation Alveoli fill with fluid or blood cells, as in pneumonia, pulmonary edema, or pulmonary hemorrhage.	**Dull** over the airless area	Midline	*Bronchial* over the involved area	*Late inspiratory crackles* over the involved area	*Increased* over the involved area, with *bronchophony, egophony,* and *whispered pectoriloquy*
Atelectasis (*Lobar Obstruction*) When a plug in a mainstem bronchus (as from mucus or a foreign object) obstructs air flow, affected lung tissue collapses into an airless state.	**Dull** over the airless area	May be *shifted toward involved side*	*Usually absent* when bronchial plug persists. Exceptions include right upper lobe atelectasis, where adjacent tracheal sounds may be transmitted.	None	*Usually absent* when the bronchial plug persists. In exceptions (e.g., right upper lobe atelectasis) may be increased

(table continues next page)

TABLE 7-7   **Physical Findings in Selected Chest Disorders** (Continued)

Condition	Percussion Note	Trachea	Breath Sounds	Adventitious Sounds	Tactile Fremitus and Transmitted Voice Sounds
Pleural Effusion Fluid accumulates in the pleural space, separates air-filled lung from the chest wall, blocking the transmission of sound.	**Dull** to flat over the fluid	*Shifted toward opposite side* in a large effusion	*Decreased to absent,* but bronchial breath sounds may be heard near top of large effusion.	None, except a *possible pleural* rub	*Decreased to absent, but may be increased* toward the top of a large effusion
Pneumothorax When air leaks into the pleural space, usually unilaterally, the lung recoils from the chest wall. Pleural air blocks transmission of sound.	**Hyperresonant** or tympanitic over the pleural air	*Shifted toward opposite side* if much air	*Decreased to absent* over the pleural air	None, except a *possible pleural* rub	*Decreased to absent* over the pleural air
Chronic Obstructive Pulmonary Disease (COPD) Slowly progressive disorder in which the distal air spaces enlarge and lungs become hyperinflated. Chronic bronchitis is often associated.	Diffusely **hyperresonant**	Midline	*Decreased to absent*	None, or the crackles, wheezes, and rhonchi of associated chronic bronchitis	*Decreased*
Asthma Widespread narrowing of the tracheobronchial tree diminishes air flow to a fluctuating degree. During attacks, air flow decreases further, and lungs hyperinflate.	**Resonant** to diffusely **hyperresonant**	Midline	*Often obscured by wheezes*	*Wheezes, possibly crackles*	*Decreased*

The Cardiovascular System

ANATOMY AND PHYSIOLOGY

■ SURFACE PROJECTIONS OF THE HEART
■ AND GREAT VESSELS

Understanding cardiac anatomy and physiology is particularly important in the examination of the cardiovascular system. Learn to visualize the underlying structures of the heart as you examine the anterior chest.

Note that the *right ventricle* occupies most of the anterior cardiac surface. This chamber and the pulmonary artery form a wedgelike structure behind and to the left of the sternum, outlined in red.

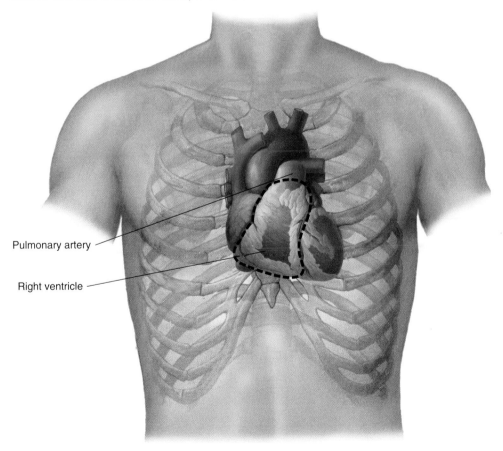

Pulmonary artery

Right ventricle

The inferior border of the right ventricle lies below the junction of the sternum and the xiphoid process. The right ventricle narrows superiorly and meets the pulmonary artery at the level of the sternum or "base of the heart"—a clinical term that refers to the proximal surface of the heart at the right and left 2nd interspaces close to the sternum.

The *left ventricle,* behind the right ventricle and to the left, as outlined, forms the left lateral margin of the heart. Its tapered inferior tip is often termed the cardiac "apex." It is clinically important because it produces the *apical impulse,* sometimes called the *point of maximal impulse,* or *PMI.* This impulse locates the left border of the heart and is usually found in the 5th interspace 7 cm to 9 cm lateral to the midsternal line. It is approximately the size of a quarter, roughly 1 to 2.5 cm in diameter. Because the most prominent cardiac impulse may not be apical, some authorities discourage use of the term PMI.

The right heart border is formed by the *right atrium,* a chamber not usually identifiable on physical examination. The *left atrium* is mostly posterior and cannot be examined directly, although its small atrial appendage may make up a segment of the left heart border between the pulmonary artery and the left ventricle.

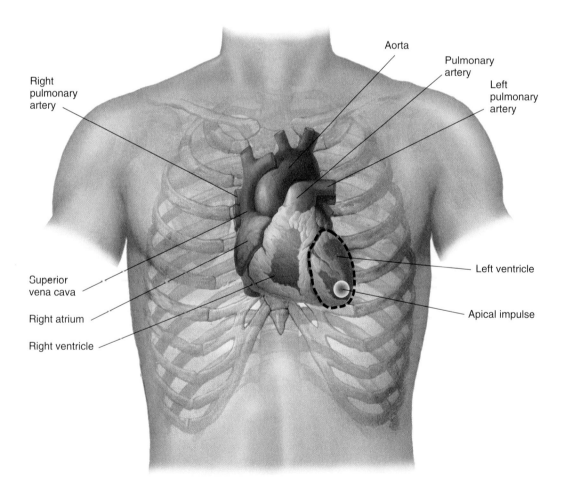

Above the heart lie the great vessels. The *pulmonary artery,* already mentioned, bifurcates quickly into its left and right branches. The *aorta* curves upward from the left ventricle to the level of the sternal angle, where it arches backward to the left and then down. On the right, the superior vena cava empties into the right atrium.

Although not illustrated, the inferior vena cava also empties into the right atrium. The *superior* and *inferior venae cavae* carry venous blood to the heart from the upper and lower portions of the body.

CARDIAC CHAMBERS, VALVES, AND CIRCULATION

Circulation through the heart is shown in the diagram below, which identifies the cardiac chambers, valves, and direction of blood flow. Because of their positions, the *tricuspid* and *mitral valves* are often called *atrioventricular valves.* The *aortic* and *pulmonic valves* are called *semilunar valves* because each of their leaflets is shaped like a half moon. Although this diagram shows all valves in an open position, they do not open simultaneously in the living heart.

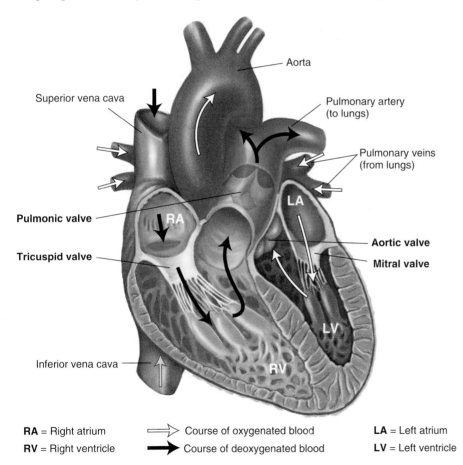

RA = Right atrium   ⇨ Course of oxygenated blood   **LA** = Left atrium
RV = Right ventricle   ➡ Course of deoxygenated blood   **LV** = Left ventricle

As the heart valves close, the heart sounds arise from vibrations emanating from the leaflets, the adjacent cardiac structures, and the flow of blood. It is essential to understand the positions and movements of the valves in relation to events in the cardiac cycle.

EVENTS IN THE CARDIAC CYCLE

The heart serves as a pump that generates varying pressures as its chambers contract and relax. *Systole is the period of ventricular contraction.* In the diagram below, pressure in the left ventricle rises from less than 5 mm Hg in its resting state to a normal peak of 120 mm Hg. After the ventricle ejects much of its blood into the aorta, the pressure levels off and starts to fall. *Diastole is the period of ventricular relaxation.* Ventricular pressure falls further to below 5 mm Hg, and blood flows from atrium to ventricle. Late in diastole, ventricular pressure rises slightly during inflow of blood from atrial contraction.

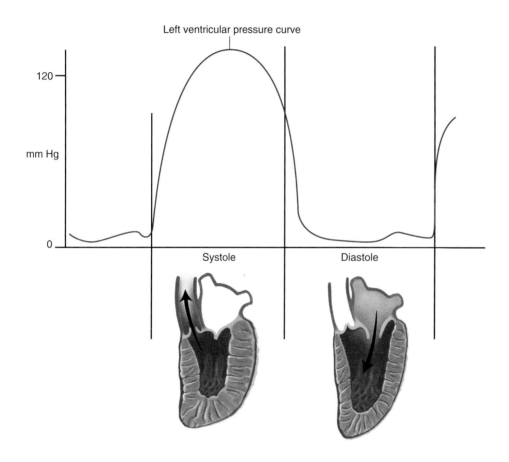

Note that during *systole* the aortic valve is open, allowing ejection of blood from the left ventricle into the aorta. The mitral valve is closed, preventing blood from regurgitating back into the left atrium. In contrast, during *diastole* the aortic valve is closed, preventing regurgitation of blood from the aorta back into the left ventricle. The mitral valve is open, allowing blood to flow from the left atrium into the relaxed left ventricle.

Understanding the interrelationships of the *pressure gradients* in these three chambers—left atrium, left ventricle, and aorta—together with the position and movement of the valves is fundamental to understanding heart sounds. Trace these changing pressures and sounds through one cardiac cycle. Note that during auscultation the first and second heart sounds define the duration of *systole* and *diastole*. An extensive literature deals with the exact causes of heart sounds. Possible explanations include actual closure of valve leaflets, tensing of related structures, leaflet positions and pressure gradients at the time of atrial and ventricular systole, and the effects of columns of blood. The explanations given here are oversimplified but retain clinical usefulness.

During *diastole,* pressure in the blood-filled left atrium slightly exceeds that in the relaxed left ventricle, and blood flows from left atrium to left ventricle across the open mitral valve. Just before the onset of ventricular systole, atrial contraction produces a slight pressure rise in both chambers.

During *systole,* the left ventricle starts to contract and ventricular pressure rapidly exceeds left atrial pressure, thus shutting the mitral valve. *Closure of the mitral valve produces the first heart sound, S_1.*

As left ventricular pressure continues to rise, it quickly exceeds the pressure in the aorta and forces the aortic valve open. In some pathologic conditions, opening of the aortic valve is accompanied by an early systolic ejection sound (Ej). *Normally, maximal left ventricular pressure corresponds to systolic blood pressure.*

As the left ventricle ejects most of its blood, ventricular pressure begins to fall. When left ventricular pressure drops below aortic pressure, the aortic valve shuts. *Aortic valve closure produces the second heart sound, S_2,* and another diastole begins.

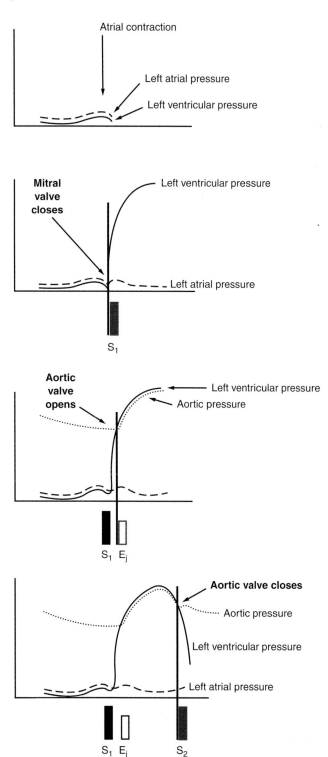

In *diastole,* left ventricular pressure continues to drop and falls below left atrial pressure. The mitral valve opens. This is usually a silent event, but may be audible as a pathologic opening snap (OS) if valve leaflet motion is restricted, as in mitral stenosis.

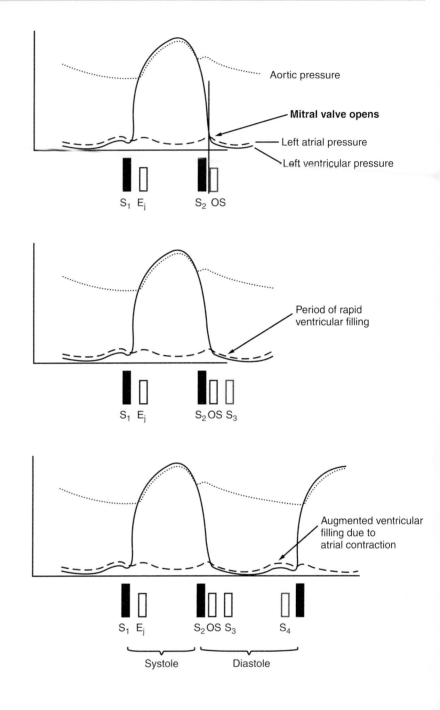

After the mitral valve opens, there is a period of rapid ventricular filling as blood flows early in diastole from left atrium to left ventricle. In children and young adults, a third heart sound, S_3, may arise from rapid deceleration of the column of blood against the ventricular wall. In older adults, an S_3, sometimes termed "an S_3 gallop," usually indicates a pathologic change in ventricular compliance.

Finally, although not often heard in normal adults, a fourth heart sound, S_4, marks atrial contraction. It immediately precedes S_1 of the next beat, and also reflects a pathologic change in ventricular compliance.

THE SPLITTING OF HEART SOUNDS

While these events are occurring on the left side of the heart, similar changes are occurring on the right, involving the right atrium, right ventricle, tricuspid valve, pulmonic valve, and pulmonary artery. Right ventricular and pulmonary arterial pressures are significantly lower than corresponding pressures on the left side. Furthermore, right-sided events usually occur slightly later than those on the left. Instead of a single heart sound, you may hear two discernible components, the first from left-sided aortic valve closure, or A_2, and the second from right-sided closure of the pulmonic valve, or P_2.

Consider the second heart sound and its two components, A_2 and P_2, which come from closure of the aortic and pulmonic valves, respectively. During inspiration A_2 and P_2 separate slightly, and may split S_2 into its two audible components. During expiration, these two components are fused into a single sound, S_2.

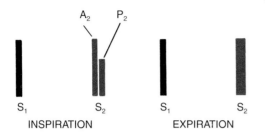

Current explanations of inspiratory splitting cite increased capacitance in the pulmonary vascular bed during inspiration, which prolongs ejection of blood from the right ventricle, delaying closure of the pulmonic valve, or P_2. Ejection of blood from the left ventricle is comparatively shorter, so A_2 occurs slightly earlier.

Of the two components of the second heart sound, A_2 is normally louder, reflecting the high pressure in the aorta. It is heard throughout the precordium. P_2, in contrast, is relatively soft, reflecting the lower pressure in the pulmonary artery. It is heard best in its own area—the 2nd and 3rd left interspaces close to the sternum. It is here that you should search for splitting of the second heart sound.

S_1 also has two components, an earlier mitral and a later tricuspid sound. The mitral sound, its principal component, is much louder, again reflecting the high pressures on the left side of the heart. It can be heard throughout the precordium and is loudest at the cardiac apex. The softer tricuspid component is heard best at the lower left sternal border, and it is here that you may hear a split S_1. The earlier louder mitral component may mask the tricuspid sound, however, and splitting is not always detectable. Splitting of S_1 does not vary with respiration.

HEART MURMURS

Heart murmurs are distinguishable from heart sounds by their longer duration. They are attributed to turbulent blood flow and may be "innocent," as with flow murmurs of young adults, or diagnostic of valvular heart disease. A *stenotic valve* has an abnormally narrowed valvular orifice that obstructs blood flow, as in *aortic stenosis,* and causes a characteristic murmur. So does a valve that fails to fully close, as in *aortic regurgitation* or *insufficiency.* Such a valve allows blood to leak backward in a retrograde direction and produces a *regurgitant* murmur.

To identify murmurs accurately, you must learn to assess the chest wall location where they are best heard, their timing in systole or diastole, and their qualities. In the section on Techniques of Examination, you will learn to integrate several characteristics, including murmur intensity, pitch, duration, and direction of radiation (see pp. 316–319).

RELATION OF AUSCULTATORY FINDINGS TO THE CHEST WALL

The locations on the chest wall where you hear heart sounds and murmurs help to identify the valve or chamber where they originate. Sounds and murmurs arising from the mitral valve are usually heard best at and around the cardiac apex. Those originating in the tricuspid valve are heard best at or near the lower left sternal border. Murmurs arising from the pulmonic valve are usually heard best in the 2nd and 3rd left interspaces close to the sternum, but at times may also be heard at higher or lower levels, and those originating in the aortic valve may be heard anywhere from the right 2nd interspace to the apex. These areas overlap, as illustrated below, and you will need to correlate auscultatory findings with other portions of the cardiac examination to identify sounds and murmurs accurately.

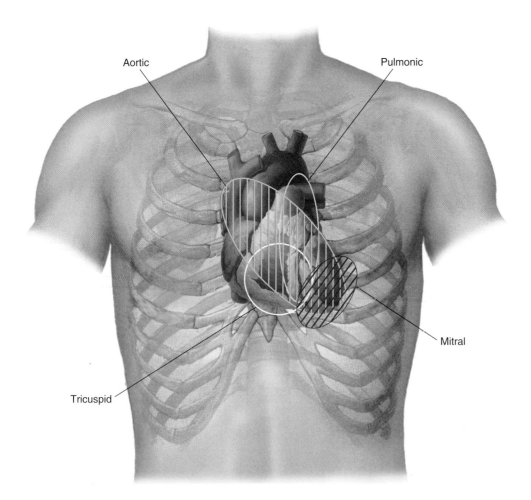

THE CONDUCTION SYSTEM

An electrical conduction system stimulates and coordinates the contraction of cardiac muscle.

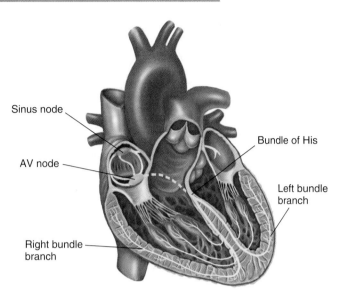

Each normal electrical impulse is initiated in the *sinus node*, a group of specialized cardiac cells located in the right atrium near the junction of the vena cava. The sinus node acts as the cardiac pacemaker and automatically discharges an impulse about 60 to 100 times a minute. This impulse travels through both atria to the *atrioventricular node*, a specialized group of cells located low in the atrial septum. Here the impulse is delayed before passing down the bundle of His and its branches to the ventricular myocardium. Muscular contraction follows: first the atria, then the ventricles. The normal conduction pathway is diagrammed in simplified form above.

The electrocardiogram, or ECG, records these events. Contraction of cardiac smooth muscle produces electrical activity, resulting in a series of waves on the ECG. The components of the *normal ECG* and their duration are briefly summarized here, but you will need further instruction and practice to interpret recordings from actual patients. Note:

- The small *P wave* of atrial depolarization (duration up to 80 milliseconds; *PR interval* 120 to 200 milliseconds)

- The larger *QRS complex* of ventricular depolarization (up to 100 milliseconds), consisting of one or more of the following:

    –the *Q wave*, a downward deflection from septal depolarization
    –the *R wave*, an upward deflection from ventricular depolarization
    –the *S wave*, a downward deflection following an R wave

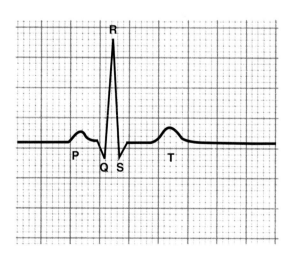

- A *T wave* of ventricular repolarization, or recovery (duration relates to QRS).

The electrical impulse slightly precedes the myocardial contraction that it stimulates. The relation of electrocardiographic waves to the cardiac cycle is shown below.

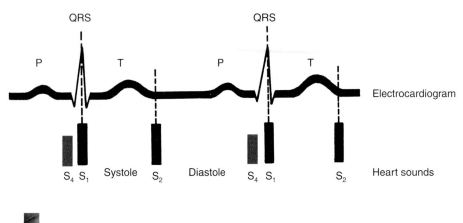

THE HEART AS A PUMP

The left and right ventricles pump blood into the systemic and pulmonary arterial trees, respectively. *Cardiac output,* the volume of blood ejected from each ventricle during 1 minute, is the product of *heart rate* and *stroke volume.* Stroke volume (the volume of blood ejected with each heartbeat) depends in turn on preload, myocardial contractility, and afterload.

Preload refers to the load that stretches the cardiac muscle before contraction. The volume of blood in the right ventricle at the end of diastole, then, constitutes its preload for the next beat. Right ventricular preload is increased by increasing venous return to the right heart. Physiologic causes include inspiration and the increased volume of blood flow from exercising muscles. The increased blood volume in a dilated right ventricle of congestive heart failure also increases preload. Causes of decreased right ventricular preload include exhalation, decreased left ventricular output, and pooling of blood in the capillary bed or the venous system.

Myocardial contractility refers to the ability of the cardiac muscle, when given a load, to shorten. Contractility increases when stimulated by action of the sympathetic nervous system, and decreases when blood flow or oxygen delivery to the myocardium is impaired.

Afterload refers to the degree of vascular resistance to ventricular contraction. Sources of resistance to left ventricular contraction include the tone in the walls of the aorta, the large arteries, and the peripheral vascular tree (primarily the small arteries and arterioles), as well as the volume of blood already in the aorta.

Pathologic increases in preload and afterload, called *volume overload* and *pressure overload,* respectively, produce changes in ventricular function that may be clinically detectable. These changes include alterations in ventricular impulses, detectable by palpation, and in normal heart sounds. Pathologic heart sounds and murmurs may also develop.

ARTERIAL PULSES AND BLOOD PRESSURE

With each contraction, the left ventricle ejects a volume of blood into the aorta and on into the arterial tree. The ensuing pressure wave moves rapidly through the arterial system, where it is felt as the *arterial pulse*. Although the pressure wave travels quickly—many times faster than the blood itself—a palpable delay between ventricular contraction and peripheral pulses makes the pulses in the arms and legs unsuitable for timing events in the cardiac cycle.

Blood pressure in the arterial system varies during the cardiac cycle, peaking in systole and falling to its lowest trough in diastole. These are the levels that are measured with the blood pressure cuff, or sphygmomanometer. The difference between systolic and diastolic pressures is known as the *pulse pressure*.

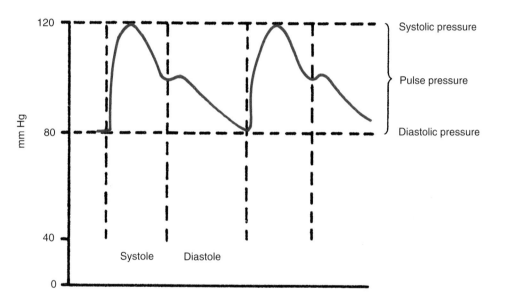

The principal factors influencing arterial pressure are:

■ Left ventricular stroke volume

■ Distensibility of the aorta and the large arteries

■ Peripheral vascular resistance, particularly at the arteriolar level

■ Volume of blood in the arterial system.

Changes in any of these four factors alter systolic pressure, diastolic pressure, or both. Blood pressure levels fluctuate strikingly through any 24-hour period, varying with physical activity; emotional state; pain; noise; environmental temperature; the use of coffee, tobacco, and other drugs; and even the time of day.

JUGULAR VENOUS PRESSURE (JVP)

Systemic venous pressure is much lower than arterial pressure. Although venous pressure ultimately depends on left ventricular contraction, much of this force is dissipated as blood flows through the arterial tree and the capillary bed. Walls of veins contain less smooth muscle than walls of arteries. This reduces venous tone and makes veins more distensible. Other important determinants of venous pressure include blood volume and the capacity of the right heart to eject blood into the pulmonary arterial system. Cardiac disease may alter these variables, producing abnormalities in central venous pressure. For example, venous pressure falls when left ventricular output or blood volume is significantly reduced; it rises when the right heart fails or when increased pressure in the pericardial sac impedes the return of blood to the right atrium. These venous pressure changes are reflected in the height of the venous column of blood in the internal jugular veins, termed the *jugular venous pressure* or *JVP*.

Pressure in the jugular veins reflects right atrial pressure, giving clinicians an important clinical indicator of cardiac function and right heart hemodynamics. Assessing the JVP is an essential, though challenging, clinical skill. The JVP is best estimated from the internal jugular vein, usually on the *right side,* because the right internal jugular vein has a more direct anatomic channel into the right atrium.[1]

The internal jugular veins lie deep to the sternomastoid muscles in the neck and are not directly visible, so the clinician must learn to identify the *pulsations* of the internal jugular vein that are transmitted to the surface of the neck, making sure to carefully distinguish these venous pulsations from pulsations of the carotid artery. If pulsations from the internal jugular vein cannot be identified, those of the external jugular vein can be used, but they are less reliable.

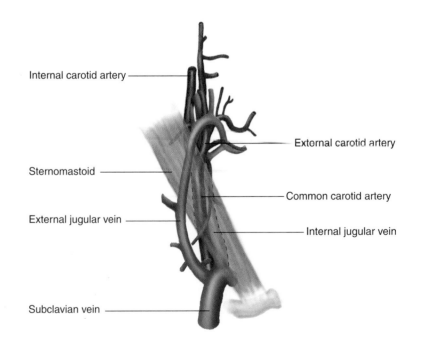

Internal carotid artery

External carotid artery

Sternomastoid

Common carotid artery

External jugular vein

Internal jugular vein

Subclavian vein

To estimate the level of the JVP, you will learn to find the *highest point of oscillation in the internal jugular vein* or, if necessary, the point above which the external jugular vein appears collapsed. The JVP is usually measured in vertical distance above the *sternal angle*, the bony ridge adjacent to the second rib where the manubrium joins the body of the sternum.

Study carefully the illustrations below. Note that regardless of the patient's position, the sternal angle remains roughly 5 cm above the right atrium. In this patient, however, the pressure in the internal jugular vein is somewhat elevated.

■ In *Position A*, the head of the bed is raised to the usual level, about 30°, but the JVP cannot be measured because the meniscus, or level of oscillation, is above the jaw and therefore not visible.

■ In *Position B*, the head of the bed is raised to 60°. The "top" of the internal jugular vein is now easily visible, so the vertical distance from the sternal angle or right atrium can now be measured.

■ In *Position C*, the patient is upright and the veins are barely discernible above the clavicle, making measurement untenable.

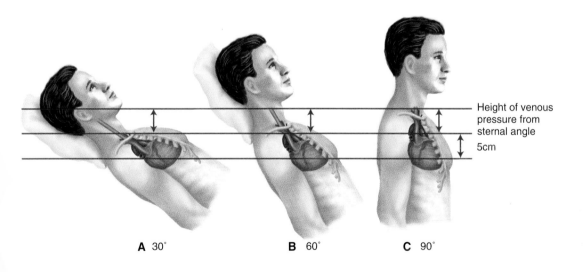

A 30°   B 60°   C 90°

Height of venous pressure from sternal angle

5cm

Note that the height of the venous pressure as measured from the sternal angle is the *same* in all three positions, but your ability to *measure* the height of the column of venous blood, or JVP, differs according to how you position the patient. Jugular venous pressure measured at more than 4 cm above the sternal angle, or more than 9 cm above the right atrium, is considered elevated or abnormal. The techniques for measuring the JVP are fully described in Techniques of Examination on pp. 302–304.

JUGULAR VENOUS PULSATIONS

The oscillations that you see in the internal jugular veins, and often in the externals, reflect changing pressures within the right atrium. The right internal jugular vein empties more directly into the right atrium and reflects these pressure changes best.

Careful observation reveals that the undulating pulsations of the internal jugular veins, and sometimes the externals, are composed of two quick peaks and two troughs.

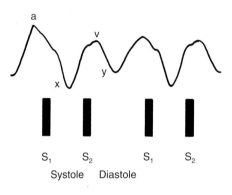

The first elevation, the *a wave*, reflects the slight rise in atrial pressure that accompanies atrial contraction. It occurs just before the first heart sound and before the carotid pulse. The following trough, the *x descent,* starts with atrial relaxation. It continues as the right ventricle, contracting during systole, pulling the floor of the atrium downward. During ventricular systole, blood continues to flow into the right atrium from the venae cavae. The tricuspid valve is closed, the chamber begins to fill, and right atrial pressure begins to rise again, creating the second elevation, the *v wave.* When the tricuspid valve opens early in diastole, blood in the right atrium flows passively into the right ventricle, and right atrial pressure falls again, creating the second trough or *y descent.* To remember these four oscillations in an oversimplified way, think of the following sequence: atrial contraction, atrial relaxation, atrial filling, and atrial emptying. (You can think of the *a* wave as <u>a</u>trial contraction and the *v* wave as <u>v</u>enous filling.)

To the naked eye, the two descents are the most obvious events in the normal jugular pulse. Of the two, the sudden collapse of the *x* descent late in systole is more prominent, occurring just before the second heart sound. The *y* descent follows the second heart sound early in diastole.

CHANGES OVER THE LIFE SPAN

Aging may affect the location of the apical impulse, the pitch of heart sounds and murmurs, the stiffness of the arteries, and blood pressure. For example, the *apical impulse* is usually felt easily in children and young adults; as the chest deepens in its anteroposterior diameter, the impulse gets harder to find. For the same reason, *splitting of the second heart sound* may be harder to hear in older people as its pulmonic component becomes less audible. Further, at some time over the life span, almost everyone has a *heart murmur.* Most murmurs occur without other evidence of cardiovascular abnormality and may therefore be considered innocent normal variants. These common murmurs vary with age, and familiarity with their patterns helps you to distinguish normal from abnormal. Turn to pp. 671–815, Chapter 18, Assessing Children:

Infancy Through Adolescence, and to pp. 817–838, Chapter 19, The Pregnant Woman, for information on how to distinguish these innocent murmurs.

Murmurs may originate in large blood vessels as well as in the heart. The *jugular venous hum*, which is very common in children, may still be heard through young adulthood (see p. 762). A second, more important example is the *cervical systolic murmur* or *bruit*, which may be innocent in children but suspicious for arterial obstruction in adults.

THE HEALTH HISTORY

Common or Concerning Symptoms

- Chest pain
- Palpitations
- Shortness of breath: dyspnea, orthopnea, or paroxysmal nocturnal dyspnea
- Swelling or edema

Chest pain or discomfort is one of the most important symptoms you will assess as a clinician. As you listen to the patient's story, you must always keep serious adverse events in mind, such as *angina pectoris, myocardial infarction,* or even a *dissecting aortic aneurysm.*[2–4] This section approaches chest symptoms from the *cardiac standpoint,* including chest pain, palpitations, orthopnea, paroxysmal nocturnal dyspnea (PND), and edema. For this complaint, however, it is wise to think through the range of possible cardiac, pulmonary, and extrathoracic etiologies. You should review the Health History section of Chapter 7, The Thorax and Lungs, which enumerates the various possible sources of chest pain: the myocardium, the pericardium, the aorta, the trachea and large bronchi, the parietal pleura, the esophagus, the chest wall, and extrathoracic structures such as the neck, gallbladder, and stomach. This review is important, because symptoms such as dyspnea, wheezing, cough, and even hemoptysis (see pp. 248–250) can be cardiac as well as pulmonary in origin.

See Table 7-1, Chest Pain, pp. 268–269.

Your initial questions should be broad . . . "Do you have any pain or discomfort in your chest?" Ask the patient to point to the pain and to describe all seven of its attributes. After listening closely to the patient's description, move on to more specific questions such as "Is the pain related to exertion?" and "What kinds of activities bring on the pain?" Also "How intense is the pain, on a scale of 1 to 10?" . . . "Does it radiate into the neck, shoulder, back, or down your arm?" . . . "Are there any associated symptoms like shortness of breath, sweating, palpitations, or nausea?" . . . "Does it ever wake you up at night?" . . . "What do you do to make it better?"

Exertional chest pain with radiation to the left side of the neck and down the left arm in *angina pectoris;* sharp pain radiating into the back or into the neck in *aortic dissection.*

Palpitations are an unpleasant awareness of the heartbeat. When reporting these sensations, patients use various terms such as skipping, racing, fluttering, pounding, or stopping of the heart. Palpitations may result from an irregular heartbeat, from rapid acceleration or slowing of the heart, or from increased forcefulness of cardiac contraction. Such perceptions, however, also depend on how patients respond to their own body sensations. Palpitations do not necessarily mean heart disease. In contrast, the most serious dysrhythmias, such as ventricular tachycardia, often do not produce palpitations.

See Tables 8-1 and 8-2 for selected heart rates and rhythms (pp. 324–325)

Symptoms or signs of irregular heart action warrant an electrocardiogram. Only *atrial fibrillation*, which is "irregularly irregular," can be reliably identified at the bedside.

You may ask directly about palpitations, but if the patient does not understand your question, reword it. "Are you ever aware of your heartbeat? What is it like?" Ask the patient to tap out the rhythm with a hand or finger. Was it fast or slow? Regular or irregular? How long did it last? If there was an episode of rapid heartbeats, did they start and stop suddenly or gradually? (For this group of symptoms, an electrocardiogram is indicated.)

It is helpful to teach selected patients how to make serial measurements of their pulse rates in case they have further episodes.

Clues in the history include transient skips and flipflops (possible premature contractions); rapid regular beating of sudden onset and offset (possible paroxysmal supraventricular tachycardia); a rapid regular rate of less than 120 beats per minute, especially if starting and stopping more gradually (possible sinus tachycardia).

Shortness of breath is a common patient concern and may represent dyspnea, orthopnea, or paroxysmal nocturnal dyspnea. *Dyspnea* is an uncomfortable awareness of breathing that is inappropriate to a given level of exertion. This complaint is often made by patients with cardiac or pulmonary problems, as discussed in Chapter 7, The Thorax and Lungs, p. 249.

Orthopnea is dyspnea that occurs when the patient is lying down and improves when the patient sits up. Classically, it is quantified according to the number of pillows the patient uses for sleeping, or by the fact that the patient needs to sleep sitting up. Make sure, however, that the reason the patient uses extra pillows or sleeps upright is shortness of breath when supine and not other causes.

Orthopnea suggests *left ventricular heart failure* or *mitral stenosis;* it may also accompany *obstructive lung disease.*

Paroxysmal nocturnal dyspnea, or *PND,* describes episodes of sudden dyspnea and orthopnea that awaken the patient from sleep, usually 1 or 2 hours after going to bed, prompting the patient to sit up, stand up, or go to a window for air. There may be associated wheezing and coughing. The episode usually subsides but may recur at about the same time on subsequent nights.

PND suggests *left ventricular heart failure* or *mitral stenosis* and may be mimicked by *nocturnal asthma* attacks.

Edema refers to the accumulation of excessive fluid in the interstitial tissue spaces and appears as swelling. Questions about edema are typically included in the cardiac history, but edema has many other causes, both local and general. Focus your questions on the location, timing, and setting of the swelling, and on associated symptoms. "Have you had any swelling anywhere? Where? . . . Anywhere else? When does it occur? Is it worse in the morning or at night? Do your shoes get tight?"

Dependent edema appears in the lowest body parts: the feet and lower legs when sitting, or the sacrum when bedridden. Causes may be cardiac (*congestive heart failure*), nutritional (*hypoalbuminemia*), or positional.

Continue with "Are the rings tight on your fingers? Are your eyelids puffy or swollen in the morning? Have you had to let out your belt?" Also, "Have your clothes gotten too tight around the middle?" It is useful to ask patients

Edema occurs in renal and liver disease: periorbital puffiness, tight rings in *nephrotic syndrome;*

who retain fluid to record daily morning weights, because edema may not be obvious until several liters of extra fluid have accumulated.

HEALTH PROMOTION AND COUNSELING

Important Topics for Health Promotion and Counseling

- Preventing hypertension
- Preventing cardiovascular disease and stroke
- Lowering cholesterol and low-density lipoprotein (LDL)
- Lifestyle modification and risk intervention, including healthy eating and counseling about weight and exercise

Despite improvements in risk factor modification, cardiovascular disease remains the leading cause of death for both men and women, accounting for approximately one third of all U.S. deaths. Both *primary prevention,* in those without evidence of cardiovascular disease, and *secondary prevention,* in those with known cardiovascular events such as angina or myocardial infarction, remain important priorities for the office, the hospital, and the nation's public health. Education and counseling will guide your patients to maintain optimal levels of blood pressure, cholesterol, weight, and exercise and reduce risk factors for cardiovascular disease and stroke.

Preventing Hypertension. According to the U.S. Preventive Services Task Force, hypertension accounts for "35% of all myocardial infarctions and strokes, 49% of all episodes of heart failure, and 24% of all premature deaths."[5] The Task Force strongly recommends *screening of adults 18 years and older for high blood pressure.* Recent long-term population-based studies have fueled a dramatic shift in national strategies to prevent and reduce blood pressure (BP). "The Seventh Report of the Joint National Committee on Prevention, Detection, Evaluation, and Treatment of High Blood Pressure," known as JNC 7, the National High Blood Pressure Education Program, and clinical investigators have issued several key messages (see box on next page)[6,7]: These findings underlie the tougher and simpler blood pressure classification of JNC 7 (see table on p. 109)[10]:

- The former six categories of blood pressure have been collapsed to four, with normal blood pressure defined as <120/80 mm Hg.

- Systolic blood pressures of 120 to 139 mm Hg and diastolic blood pressures of 80 to 89 mm Hg are no longer "high normal"; they are "prehypertension."

■ Drug therapy should begin with stage 1 hypertension, namely systolic blood pressure of 140 to 159 mm Hg or diastolic blood pressure of 90 to 99 mm Hg.

■ Adoption of healthy lifestyles by all people is now considered "indispensable."

KEY MESSAGES ABOUT HYPERTENSION

■ "Individuals who are normotensive at 55 years have a 90% lifetime risk for developing hypertension."[6]

■ "More than 1 of every 2 adults older than 60 years of age has hypertension,"[7] and only 34% of those with hypertension have achieved blood pressure goals.[6]

■ "The relationship between pressure and risk of cardiovascular disease (CVD) events is continuous, consistent, and independent of other risk factors. . . . For individuals aged 40 to 70 years, each increment of 20 mm Hg in systolic BP or 10 mm Hg in diastolic BP doubles the risk of CVD across the entire BP range from 115/75 to 185/115 mm Hg."[6,8]

■ Recent large population studies of cardiovascular risk factors reveal two striking findings[9]:
  1. Only approximately 4.8% to 9.9% of the young and middle-aged population is at low risk.
  2. The benefits of low-risk status are enormous: a 72% to 85% reduction in CVD mortality and a 40% to 58% reduction in mortality from all causes, leading to a gain of 5.8 to 9.5 years in life expectancy. This gain "holds for both African Americans and whites, and for those of lower and higher socioeconomic status."[9]

■ Hence, identifying and treating people with risk factors are not enough. *A population-wide strategy is critical to prevent and reduce the magnitude of all the major risk factors* so that people develop favorable behaviors in childhood and *remain* at *low risk for life.*[9]

Risk factors for hypertension include physical inactivity, microalbuminuria or estimated GFR less than 60 mL/min, family history of premature CVD (<55 years for men and <65 years for women), excess intake of dietary sodium, insufficient intake of potassium, and excess consumption of alcohol.[6]

Preventing Cardiovascular Disease and Stroke. The American Heart Association (AHA) in its 2002 update placed the challenge for implementing risk factor reduction squarely on clinicians: "The challenge for health care professionals is to engage greater numbers of patients, at an earlier stage of their disease, in comprehensive cardiovascular risk reduction" to expand the benefits of primary prevention. "The continuing message is that adoption of healthy life habits remains the cornerstone of primary prevention." "The imperative is to prevent the first episode of coronary disease or stroke or the development of aortic aneurysm and peripheral vascular disease because of the still-high rate of first events that are fatal or disabling."[11]

As a first step, clinicians need to identify not only elevated blood pressure but also other well-studied risk factors for coronary heart disease (CHD). In its "Guidelines for Primary Prevention of Cardiovascular Disease and Stroke," the AHA recommends *risk factor screening* for adults beginning at age 20, and *global absolute CHD risk estimation* for all adults 40 years and

---

RISK FACTORS AND SCREENING FREQUENCY FOR ADULTS BEGINNING AT AGE 20

Risk Factor	Frequency
Family history of coronary heart disease (CHD)	Update regularly
Smoking status Diet Alcohol intake Physical activity	At each routine visit
Blood pressure Body mass index Waist circumference Pulse (to detect atrial fibrillation)	At each routine visit (at least every 2 years)
Fasting lipoprotein profile Fasting glucose	At least every 5 years If risk factors for hyperlipidemia or diabetes present, every 2 years

Source: Pearson TA, Blair SN, Daniels SR, et al. AHA guidelines for primary prevention of cardiovascular disease and stroke: 2000 update. Circulation 106:388–391, 2002.

GLOBAL RISK ESTIMATION FOR 10-YEAR RISK FOR CHD FOR ADULTS ≥ AGE 40

Establish multiple risk score for CHD based on:

- Age
- Sex
- Smoking status
- Systolic (and sometimes diastolic) blood pressure
- Total (and sometimes LDL) cholesterol
- HDL cholesterol
- Diabetes

For calculation of global CHD risk, use the risk calculators found at either of the Web sites below (or other equations):

http://www.americanheart.org/presenter.jhtml?identifier=3003499
http://hin.nhlbi.nih.gov/atpiii/calculator.asp?usertype=prof

Source: Pearson TA, Blair SN, Daniels SR, et al. AHA guidelines for primary prevention of cardiovascular disease and stroke: 2000 update. Circulation 106:388–391, 2002.

---

older.[11] The goal of global risk estimation is to help patients keep their risk as low as possible. Note that diabetes, or 10-year risk of more than 20%, is considered equivalent to established CHD risk equivalents.

Lowering Cholesterol and LDL.   In 2001 the National Heart, Lung, and Blood Institute of the National Institutes of Health published the "Third Report of the National Cholesterol Education Program Expert Panel," known as ATP III.[12] Publication of the full NCEP report followed in 2002.[13] These reports provide evidence-based recommendations on the management of high cholesterol and related lipid disorders, and document that "epidemiological surveys have shown that serum cholesterol levels are continuously correlated with CHD risk over a broad range of cholesterol values," in many of the world's populations.[14] Key features of ATP III are as follows:

- Identifying LDL as the primary target of cholesterol-lowering therapy

- Classifying three risk categories:

  - *High risk (10-year risk > 20%):* established CHD and CHD risk equivalents
  - *Moderately high risk (10-year risk 10%–20%):* multiple, or 2+, risk factors
  - *Low risk (10-year risk < 10%):* zero to 1 risk factor

  Risk factors include cigarette smoking, BP >140/90 mm Hg or use of antihypertensive medication, HDL <40 mg/dL, family history of CHD in male first-degree relative <age 55 or female first-degree relative <age 65, and age ≥45 for men or ≥55 for women.

  CHD includes history of myocardial infarction, stable or unstable angina, coronary artery procedures such as angioplasty or bypass surgery, or evidence of significant myocardial ischemia.

  CHD risk equivalents include *noncoronary atherosclerotic disease,* such as peripheral arterial disease, abdominal aortic aneurysm, and carotid artery disease (transient ischemic attacks or stroke of carotid origin or > 50% obstruction of the carotid artery); *diabetes;* and *2+ risk factors with 10-year risk for CHD of > 20%.*

- Defining *high risk* as "all persons with CHD or CHD risk equivalents," with an *LDL goal for high-risk people of ≤ 100 mg/dL*

In July 2004, NCEP updated these reports based on the findings in five major clinical trials.[14] For *high-risk people,* NCEP now recommends an LDL goal of less than 70 mg/dL and intensive lipid therapy as a *therapeutic option.*[15] The NCEP cites data showing that high-risk patients benefit from a further 30% to 40% drop in LDL even when LDL is less than 100 mg/dL.

The U.S. Preventive Services Task Force recommends routine screening of LDL for men 35 years or older and for women 45 years or older.[16] Screening should begin at 20 years for those with risk factors for CHD.[17,18]

Counsel your patients to obtain a *fasting lipid profile* to determine levels of total and LDL cholesterol. Use the risk calculators on p. 297, or consult ATP III, to *establish your patient's 10-year risk category.* Use the 2004 guidelines below, which now have four risk groups, to plan your interventions regarding lifestyle change and lipid-lowering medications.

■ Updated ATP III Guidelines

10-year Risk Category	LDL Goal	Consider Drug Therapy if LDL:
High risk (>20%)	<100 mg/dL *Optional goal:* <70 mg/dL	≥100 mg/dL (<100 mg/dL: consider drug options, including further 30%–40% reduction in LDL)
Moderately high risk (10%–20%)	<130 mg/dL *Optional goal:* <100 mg/dL	≥130 mg/dL (100–129 mg/dL: consider drug options to achieve goal of <100 mg/dL)
Moderate risk (<10%)	<130 mg/dL	≥160 mg/dL
Lower risk (0–1 risk factor)	<160 mg/dL	≥190 mg/dL (160–189 mg/dL: drug therapy *optional*)

(Source: Adapted from Grundy SM, Cleeman JI, Merz NB, et al, for the Coordinating Committee of the National Cholesterol Education Program. Implications of recent clinical trials for the National Cholesterol Education Adult Treatment Panel III guidelines. Circulation 110(2):227–239, 2004.)

Lifestyle Modification and Risk Intervention. JNC VII, the National High Blood Pressure Education Program, and the AHA encourage a series of well-studied effective lifestyle modifications and risk interventions

LIFESTYLE MODIFICATIONS TO PREVENT OR MANAGE HYPERTENSION

- Optimal weight, or BMI of 18.5–24.9 kg/m²
- Salt intake of less than 6 grams of sodium chloride or 2.4 grams of sodium per day
- Regular aerobic exercise such as brisk walking for at least 30 minutes per day, most days of the week
- Moderate alcohol consumption per day of 2 drinks or fewer for men and 1 drink or fewer for women (2 drinks = 1 oz ethanol, 24 oz beer, 10 oz wine, or 2–3 oz whiskey)
- Dietary intake of more than 3,500 mg of potassium
- Diet rich in fruits, vegetables, and low-fat dairy products with reduced content of saturated and total fat

Source: Whelton PK, He J, Appel LJ, et al. Primary prevention of hypertension. Clinical and Public Health Advisory from the National High Blood Pressure Education Program. JAMA 288(15):1882–1888, 2002.

to prevent hypertension, CVD, and stroke. Lifestyle modifications for hypertension can lower systolic blood pressure from 2 to 20 mm Hg.[6] Lifestyle modifications to reduce hypertension overlap with those recommended for reducing risk for CVD and stroke, as seen below.

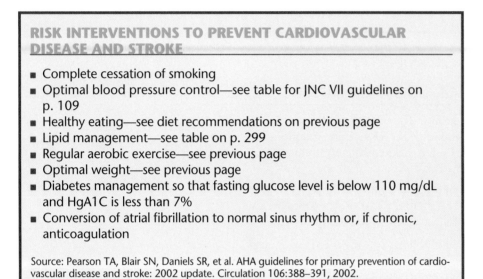

RISK INTERVENTIONS TO PREVENT CARDIOVASCULAR DISEASE AND STROKE

- Complete cessation of smoking
- Optimal blood pressure control—see table for JNC VII guidelines on p. 109
- Healthy eating—see diet recommendations on previous page
- Lipid management—see table on p. 299
- Regular aerobic exercise—see previous page
- Optimal weight—see previous page
- Diabetes management so that fasting glucose level is below 110 mg/dL and HgA1C is less than 7%
- Conversion of atrial fibrillation to normal sinus rhythm or, if chronic, anticoagulation

Source: Pearson TA, Blair SN, Daniels SR, et al. AHA guidelines for primary prevention of cardiovascular disease and stroke: 2002 update. Circulation 106:388–391, 2002.

Healthy Eating. Begin with a dietary history (see pp. 92–93), then target low intake of cholesterol and total fat, especially less saturated and *trans* fat. Foods with monounsaturated fats, polyunsaturated fats, and omega-3 fatty acids in fish oils help to lower blood cholesterol. Review the food sources of these healthy and unhealthy fats.[19]

Sources of Unhealthy Fats

- *Foods high in cholesterol:* dairy products, egg yolks, liver and organ meats, high-fat meat and poultry

- *Foods high in saturated fat:* high-fat dairy products—cream, cheese, ice cream, whole and 2% milk, and sour cream; bacon, butter; chocolate; coconut oil; lard and gravy from meat drippings; high-fat meats like ground beef, bologna, hot dogs, and sausage

- *Foods high in* trans *fat:* snacks and baked goods with hydrogenated or partially hydrogenated oil, stick margarines, shortening, french fries

Sources of Healthy Fats

- *Foods high in monounsaturated fat:* nuts, such as almonds, pecans, and peanuts; sesame seeds; avocados; canola oil; olive and peanut oil; peanut butter

- *Foods high in polyunsaturated fat:* corn, safflower, cottonseed, and soybean oil; walnuts; pumpkin or sunflower seeds; soft (tub) margarine; mayonnaise; salad dressings

■ *Foods high in omega-3 fatty acids:* albacore tuna, herring, mackerel, rainbow trout, salmon, sardines

Counseling About Weight and Exercise.   The January 2004 "Progress Review—Nutrition and Overweight" in Healthy People 2010 reports that "Dietary factors are associated with 4 of the 10 leading causes of death—coronary heart disease, some types of cancer, stroke, and type 2 diabetes—as well as with high blood pressure and osteoporosis. Overall, the data on the three Healthy People 2010 objectives for the weight status of adults and children reflect a trend for the worse."[20] More than 60% of all Americans are now obese or overweight, with a BMI greater than or equal to 25.

Counseling about weight has become a clinician imperative. Assess body mass index (BMI) as described in Chapter 4, pp. 90–92. Discuss the principles of healthy eating—patients with high fat intake are more likely to accumulate body fat than patients with high intake of protein and carbohydrate. Review the patient's eating habits and weight patterns in the family. Set realistic goals that will help the patient maintain healthy eating habits *for life*.

Regular exercise is the number one health indicator for Healthy People 2010. In its April 2004 "Progress Review—Physical Activity and Fitness," Healthy People 2010 states that "in 2000, poor diet coupled with lack of exercise was the second leading actual cause of death. The gap between this risk factor and tobacco use, the leading cause, has narrowed substantially over the past decade."[21] To reduce risk for CHD, counsel patients to pursue aerobic exercise, or exercise that increases muscle oxygen uptake, for at least 30 minutes on most days of the week. Spur motivation by emphasizing the immediate benefits to health and well-being. Deep breathing, sweating in cool temperatures, and pulse rates exceeding 60% of the maximum normal age-adjusted heart rate, or 220 minus the person's age, are markers that help patients recognize onset of aerobic metabolism. Be sure to evaluate any cardiovascular, pulmonary, or musculoskeletal conditions that present risks before selecting an exercise regimen.

TECHNIQUES OF EXAMINATION

As you begin the cardiovascular examination, review the blood pressure and heart rate recorded during the General Survey and Vital Signs at the start of the physical examination. If you need to repeat these measurements, or if they have not already been done, take the time to measure the blood pressure and heart rate using optimal technique (see Chapter 4, Beginning the Physical Examination: General Survey and Vital Signs, especially pp. 106–112).[22–26]

In brief, for *blood pressure*, after letting the patient rest for at least 5 minutes in a quiet setting, choose a correctly sized cuff and position the patient's arm at heart level, either resting on a table if seated or supported at midchest level if standing. Make sure the bladder of the cuff is centered over the brachial artery. Inflate the cuff about 30 mm Hg above the pressure at which the brachial or radial pulse disappears. As you deflate the cuff, listen first for the sounds of at least two consecutive heartbeats—these mark the *systolic* pressure. Then listen for the disappearance point of the heartbeats, which marks the *diastolic* pressure. For *heart rate*, measure the radial pulse using the pads of your index and middle fingers, or assess the apical pulse using your stethoscope (see p. 111).

Now you are ready to systematically assess the components of the cardio-vascular system:

- The jugular venous pressure and pulsations
- The carotid upstrokes and presence or absence of bruits
- The point of maximal impulse (PMI) and any heaves, lifts, or thrills
- The first and second heart sounds, S_1 and S_2
- Presence or absence of extra heart sounds such as S_3 or S_4
- Presence or absence of any cardiac murmurs.

JUGULAR VENOUS PRESSURE AND PULSATIONS

Jugular Venous Pressure (JVP). Estimating the JVP is one of the most important and frequently used skills of physical examination. At first it will seem difficult, but with practice and supervision you will find that the JVP provides valuable information about the patient's volume status and cardiac function. As you have learned, the JVP reflects pressure in the right atrium, or central venous pressure, and is best assessed from pulsations in the right internal jugular vein. Note, however, that the jugular veins and pulsations are difficult to see in children younger than 12 years of age, so they are not useful for evaluating the cardiovascular system in this age group.

To assist you in learning this portion of the cardiac examination, steps for assessing the JVP are outlined on the next page. As you begin your assessment, take a moment to reflect on the patient's volume status and consider how you may need to alter the elevation of the head of the bed or examining table. The usual starting point for assessing the JVP is to elevate the head of the bed to 30°. Identify the external jugular vein on each side, then find the internal jugular venous pulsations transmitted from deep in the neck to the overlying soft tissues. The JVP is the elevation at which the highest oscillation point, or meniscus, of the jugular venous pulsations is usually evident in euvolemic patients. In patients who are *hypovolemic*, you may anticipate that *the JVP will be low*, causing you to subsequently *lower the head of the bed*, sometimes even to 0°, to see the point of oscillation best. Likewise, in volume-overloaded or *hypervolemic* patients, you may anticipate that *the JVP will be high*, causing you to subsequently *raise the head of the bed*.

A hypovolemic patient may have to lie flat before you see the neck veins. In contrast, when jugular venous pressure is increased, an elevation up to 60° or even 90° may be required. In all these positions, the sternal angle usually remains about 5 cm above the right atrium, as diagrammed on p. 291.

STEPS FOR ASSESSING THE JUGULAR VENOUS PRESSURE (JVP)

- Make the patient comfortable. *Raise the head slightly on a pillow to relax the sternomastoid muscles.*
- *Raise the head of the bed or examining table to about 30°. Turn the patient's head slightly away from the side you are inspecting.*
- Use *tangential lighting* and examine both sides of the neck. Identify the external jugular vein on each side, then find the internal jugular venous pulsations.
- *If necessary, raise or lower the head of the bed* until you can see the oscillation point or meniscus of the internal jugular venous pulsations in the lower half of the neck.
- Focus on the *right internal jugular vein.* Look for pulsations in the suprasternal notch, between the attachments of the sternomastoid muscle on the sternum and clavicle, or just posterior to the sternomastoid. The table below helps you distinguish internal jugular pulsations from those of the carotid artery.
- *Identify the highest point of pulsation in the right internal jugular vein.* Extend a long rectangular object or card horizontally from this point and a centimeter ruler vertically from the sternal angle, making an exact right angle. Measure the vertical distance in centimeters above the sternal angle where the horizontal object crosses the ruler. *This distance, measured in centimeters above the sternal angle or the right atrium, is the JVP.*

The following features help to distinguish jugular from carotid artery pulsations:[1]

■ Distinguishing Internal Jugular and Carotid Pulsations

Internal Jugular Pulsations	Carotid Pulsations
Rarely palpable	Palpable
Soft, rapid, undulating quality, usually with two elevations and two troughs per heart beat	A more vigorous thrust with a single outward component
Pulsations eliminated by light pressure on the vein(s) just above the sternal end of the clavicle	Pulsations not eliminated by this pressure
Level of the pulsations changes with position, dropping as the patient becomes more upright.	Level of the pulsations unchanged by position
Level of the pulsations usually descends with inspiration.	Level of the pulsations not affected by inspiration

Establishing the true vertical and horizontal lines to measure the JVP is difficult, much like the problem of hanging a picture straight when you are close to it. Place your ruler on the sternal angle and line it up with something in the room that you know to be vertical. Then place a card or rectangular object at an exact right angle to the ruler. This constitutes your horizontal line. Move it up or down—still horizontal—so that the lower edge rests at the top of the jugular pulsations, and read the vertical distance on the ruler. Round your measurement off to the nearest centimeter.

Increased pressure suggests *right-sided congestive heart failure* or, less commonly, *constrictive pericarditis, tricuspid stenosis,* or *superior vena cava obstruction.*[27–33]

In patients with obstructive lung disease, venous pressure may appear elevated on expiration only; the veins collapse on inspiration. This finding does not indicate congestive heart failure.

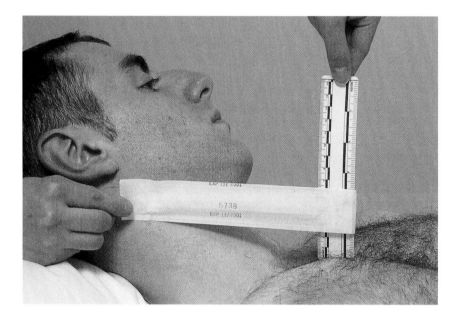

Venous pressure measured at greater than 3 cm or possibly 4 cm above the sternal angle, or more than 8 cm or 9 cm in total distance above the right atrium, is considered elevated *above normal.*

If you are unable to see pulsations in the internal jugular vein, look for them in the external jugular vein. If you see no pulsation, use *the point above which the external jugular veins appear to collapse.* Make this observation on each side of the neck. Measure the vertical distance of this point from the sternal angle.

Unilateral distention of the external jugular vein is usually caused by local kinking or obstruction. Occasionally, even bilateral distention has a local cause.

The highest point of venous pulsations may lie below the level of the sternal angle. Under these circumstances, venous pressure is not elevated and seldom needs to be measured.

Even though students may not see clinicians making these measurements very frequently in clinical settings, practicing exact techniques for measuring the JVP is important. Eventually, with experience, clinicians and cardiologists come to identify the JVP and estimate its height visually.

Jugular Venous Pulsations. *Observe the amplitude and timing of the jugular venous pulsations.* In order to time these pulsations, feel the left carotid artery with your right thumb or listen to the heart simultaneously. The *a* wave just precedes S_1 and the carotid pulse, the *x* descent can be seen

Prominent *a* waves indicate increased resistance to right atrial contraction, as in *tricuspid stenosis,* or, more commonly, the decreased

as a systolic collapse, the *v* wave almost coincides with S_2, and the *y* descent follows early in diastole. Look for absent or unusually prominent waves.

compliance of a hypertrophied right ventricle. The *a* waves disappear in atrial fibrillation. Larger *v* waves characterize tricuspid regurgitation.

Jugular venous pulsations

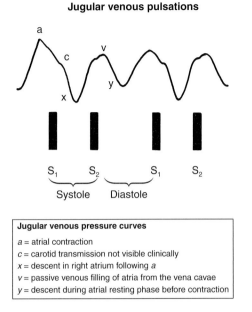

Jugular venous pressure curves

a = atrial contraction
c = carotid transmission not visible clinically
x = descent in right atrium following *a*
v = passive venous filling of atria from the vena cavae
y = descent during atrial resting phase before contraction

Considerable practice and experience are required to master jugular venous pulsations. A beginner is well-advised to concentrate primarily on jugular venous pressure.

THE CAROTID PULSE

After you measure the JVP, move on to assessment of the *carotid pulse*. The carotid pulse provides valuable information about cardiac function and is especially useful for detecting stenosis or insufficiency of the aortic valve. Take the time to assess the quality of the carotid upstroke, its amplitude and contour, and presence or absence of any overlying *thrills* or *bruits*.

For irregular rhythms, see Table 8-1, Selected Heart Rates and Rhythms (p. 324), and Table 8-2, Selected Irregular Rhythms (p. 325).

To assess *amplitude and contour,* the patient should be lying down with the head of the bed still elevated to about 30°. When feeling for the carotid artery, first inspect the neck for carotid pulsations. These may be visible just medial to the sternomastoid muscles. Then place your left index and middle fingers (or left thumb) on the right carotid artery in the lower third of the neck, press posteriorly, and feel for pulsations.

A tortuous and kinked carotid artery may produce a unilateral pulsatile bulge.

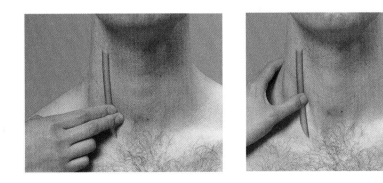

Decreased pulsations may be caused by decreased stroke volume, but may also result from local factors in the artery such as atherosclerotic narrowing or occlusion.

Press just inside the medial border of a well-relaxed sternomastoid muscle, roughly at the level of the cricoid cartilage. Avoid pressing on the *carotid sinus,* which lies at the level of the top of the thyroid cartilage. For the left carotid artery, use your right fingers or thumb. Never press both carotids at the same time. This may decrease blood flow to the brain and induce syncope.

Pressure on the carotid sinus may cause a reflex drop in pulse rate or blood pressure.

Slowly increase pressure until you feel a maximal pulsation, then slowly decrease pressure until you best sense the arterial pressure and contour. Try to assess:

See Table 4-7, Abnormalities of the Arterial Pulse and Pressure Waves (p. 119).

- The *amplitude of the pulse.* This correlates reasonably well with the pulse pressure.

Small, thready, or weak pulse in *cardiogenic shock*; *bounding* pulse in *aortic insufficiency* (see p. 119).

- The *contour of the pulse wave,* namely the speed of the upstroke, the duration of its summit, and the speed of the downstroke. The normal upstroke is *brisk*. It is smooth, rapid, and follows S_1 almost immediately. The summit is smooth, rounded, and roughly midsystolic. The downstroke is less abrupt than the upstroke.

Delayed carotid upstroke in *aortic stenosis*

- Any *variations in amplitude,* either from beat to beat or with respiration.

Pulsus alternans (see p. 119), bigeminal pulse (beat-to-beat variation); paradoxical pulse (respiratory variation)

Thrills and Bruits. During palpation of the carotid artery, you may detect humming vibrations, or *thrills,* that feel like the throat of a purring cat. Routinely, but especially in the presence of a thrill, listen over both carotid arteries with the diaphragm of your stethoscope for a *bruit,* a murmur-like sound of vascular rather than cardiac origin.

You should also listen for carotid bruits if the patient is middle-aged or elderly or if you suspect cerebrovascular disease. Ask the patient to hold breathing for a moment so that breath sounds do not obscure the vascular sound, then listen with the bell.[34] Heart sounds alone do not constitute a bruit.

A carotid bruit with or without a thrill in a middle-aged or older person suggests but does not prove arterial narrowing. An aortic murmur may radiate to the carotid artery and sound like a bruit.

Further examination of arterial pulses is described in Chapter 14, The Peripheral Vascular System.

The Brachial Artery. The carotid arteries reflect aortic pulsations more accurately, but in patients with carotid obstruction, kinking, or thrills, they are unsuitable. If so, assess the pulse in the *brachial artery,* applying the techniques described above for determining amplitude and contour.

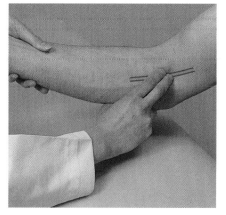

Use the index and middle fingers or thumb of your opposite hand. Cup your hand under the patient's elbow and feel for the pulse just medial to the biceps tendon. The patient's arm should rest with the elbow extended, palm up. With your free hand, you may need to flex the elbow to a varying degree to get optimal muscular relaxation.

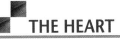

THE HEART

For most of the cardiac examination, the patient should be *supine* with the upper body raised by elevating the head of the bed or table to about 30°. Two other positions are also needed: (1) *turning to the left side,* and (2) *leaning forward.* These positions bring the ventricular apex and left ventricular outflow tract closer to the chest wall, enhancing detection of the point of maximal impulse and aortic insufficiency. *The examiner should stand at the patient's right side.*

The table below summarizes patient positions and a suggested sequence for the examination.

■ *Sequence of the Cardiac Examination*

Patient Position	Examination	Accentuated Findings
Supine, with the head elevated 30°	Inspect and palpate the precordium: the 2nd right and left interspaces; the right ventricle; and the left ventricle, including the apical impulse (diameter, location, amplitude, duration).	
Left lateral decubitus	Palpate the apical impulse if not previously detected. Listen at the apex with the *bell* of the stethoscope.	Low-pitched extra sounds (S$_3$, opening snap, diastolic rumble of mitral stenosis)
Supine, with the head elevated 30°	Listen at the tricuspid area with the *bell.*	
	Listen at all the auscultatory areas with the *diaphragm.*	
Sitting, leaning forward, after full exhalation	Listen along the left sternal border and at the apex with the *diaphragm.*	Soft decrescendo diastolic murmur of aortic insufficiency

During the cardiac examination, remember to correlate your findings with the patient's jugular venous pressure and carotid pulse. It is also important to identify both the anatomical location of your findings and their timing in the cardiac cycle.

■ Note the *anatomical location* of sounds in terms of interspaces and their distance from the midsternal, midclavicular, or axillary lines. The midsternal line offers the most reliable zero point for measurement, but some feel that the midclavicular line accommodates the different sizes and shapes of patients.

■ Identify the *timing of impulses or sounds* in relation to the cardiac cycle. Timing of sounds is often possible through auscultation alone. In most people with normal or slow heart rates, it is easy to identify the paired heart sounds by listening through a stethoscope. S_1 is the first of these sounds, S_2 is the second, and the relatively long diastolic interval separates one pair from the next.

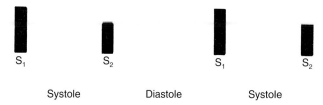

| S_1 | S_2 | S_1 | S_2 |
| Systole | Diastole | Systole | |

The relative intensity of these sounds may also be helpful. S_1 is usually louder than S_2 at the apex; more reliably, S_2 is usually louder than S_1 at the base.

Even experienced clinicians are sometimes uncertain about the timing of heart sounds, especially extra sounds and murmurs. "Inching" can then be helpful. Return to a place on the chest—most often the base—where it is easy to identify S_1 and S_2. Get their rhythm clearly in mind. Then inch your stethoscope down the chest in steps until you hear the new sound.

Auscultation alone, however, can be misleading. The intensities of S_1 and S_2, for example, may be abnormal. At rapid heart rates, moreover, diastole shortens, and at about a rate of 120, the durations of systole and diastole become indistinguishable. *Use palpation of the carotid pulse or of the apical impulse to help determine whether the sound or murmur is systolic or diastolic.* Because both the carotid upstroke and the apical impulse occur in systole, right after S_1, sounds or murmurs coinciding with them are systolic; sounds or murmurs occurring after the carotid upstroke or apical impulse are diastolic.

For example, S_1 is decreased in *first-degree heart block*, and S_2 is decreased in *aortic stenosis*.

INSPECTION AND PALPATION

Overview. Careful *inspection* of the anterior chest may reveal the location of the *apical impulse* or *point of maximal impulse (PMI)*, or less commonly, the ventricular movements of a left-sided S_3 or S_4. Tangential light is best for making these observations. Use *palpation* to confirm the characteristics of the apical impulse. Palpation is also valuable for detecting thrills and the ventricular movements of an S_3 or S_4.

Begin with general palpation of the chest wall. First palpate for heaves, lifts, or thrills using your *fingerpads.* Hold them flat or obliquely on the body surface, using light pressure for an S_3 or S_4, and firmer pressure for S_1 and S_2. Ventricular impulses may heave or lift your fingers. Then check for *thrills* by pressing the *ball of your hand* firmly on the chest. If subsequent auscultation reveals a loud murmur, go back and check for thrills over that area again. Be sure to assess the right ventricle by palpating the right ventricular area at the lower left sternal border and in the subxiphoid area, the pulmonary artery in the left 2nd interspace, and the aortic area in the right 2nd interspace. Review the diagram on the next page. *Note that the "areas" designated for the left and right ventricle, the pulmonary artery, and the aorta pertain to the majority of patients whose hearts are situated in the left chest, with normal anatomy of the great vessels.*

Thrills may accompany loud, harsh, or rumbling murmurs as in *aortic stenosis, patent ductus arteriosus, ventricular septal defect,* and, less commonly, *mitral stenosis.* They are palpated more easily in patient positions that accentuate the murmur.

On rare occasions, a patient has *dextrocardia*—a heart situated on the right side. The apical impulse

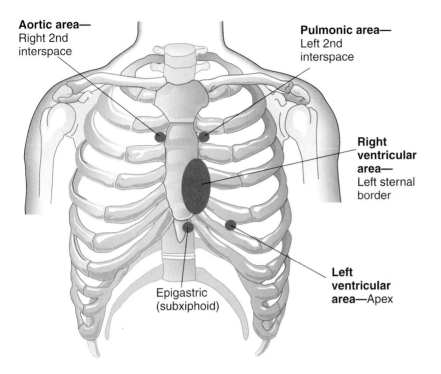

Aortic area— Right 2nd interspace

Pulmonic area— Left 2nd interspace

Right ventricular area— Left sternal border

Left ventricular area—Apex

Epigastric (subxiphoid)

will then be found on the right. If you cannot find an apical impulse, percuss for the dullness of heart and liver and for the tympany of the stomach. In *situs inversus,* all three of these structures are on opposite sides from normal. A right-sided heart with a normally placed liver and stomach is usually associated with congenital heart disease.

Left Ventricular Area—The Apical Impulse or Point of Maximal Impulse (PMI). The apical impulse represents the brief early pulsation of the left ventricle as it moves anteriorly during contraction and touches the chest wall. Note that in most examinations the apical impulse is the point of maximal impulse, or PMI; however, some pathologic conditions may produce a pulsation that is more prominent than the apex beat, such as an enlarged right ventricle, a dilated pulmonary artery, or an aneurysm of the aorta.

If you cannot identify the apical impulse with the patient supine, ask the patient to roll partly onto the left side—this is the *left lateral decubitus* position. Palpate again using the palmar surfaces of several fingers. If you cannot find

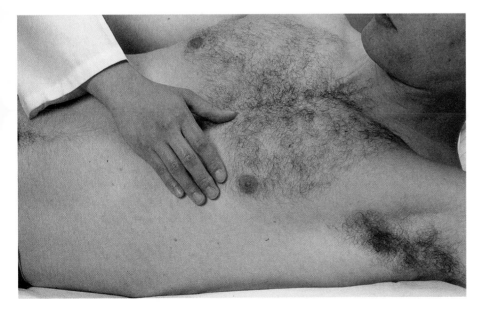

the apical impulse, ask the patient to exhale fully and stop breathing for a few seconds. When examining a woman, it may be helpful to displace the left breast upward or laterally as necessary; alternatively, ask her to do this for you.

Once you have found the apical impulse, make finer assessments with your fingertips, and then with one finger.

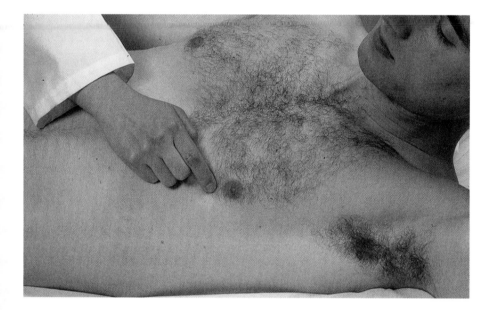

With experience, you will learn to feel the apical impulse in a high percentage of patients. Obesity, a very muscular chest wall, or an increased anteroposterior diameter of the chest, however, may make it undetectable. Some apical impulses hide behind the rib cage, despite positioning.

Now assess the location, diameter, amplitude, and duration of the apical impulse. You may wish to have the patient breathe out and briefly stop breathing to check your findings.

See Table 8-3, Variations and Abnormalities of the Ventricular Impulses (p. 326).

- *Location.* Try to assess location with the patient *supine* because the left lateral decubitus position displaces the apical impulse to the left. Locate two points: the interspaces, usually the 5th or possibly the 4th, which give the vertical location; and the distance in centimeters from the midsternal line, which gives the horizontal location. Note that even though the apical impulse normally falls roughly at the midclavicular line, measurements from this line are less reproducible because clinicians vary in their estimates of the midpoint of the clavicle.

The apical impulse may be displaced upward and to the left by pregnancy or a high left diaphragm.

Lateral displacement from cardiac enlargement in *congestive heart failure, cardiomyopathy, ischemic heart disease.* Displacement in deformities of the thorax and mediastinal shift.

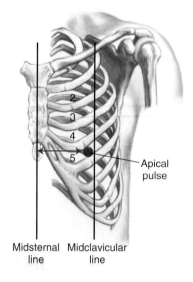

Midsternal line   Midclavicular line

Apical pulse

■ *Diameter.* Palpate the diameter of the apical impulse. In the supine patient, it usually measures less than 2.5 cm and occupies only one interspace. It may feel larger in the left lateral decubitus position.

In the left lateral decubitus position, a diameter greater than 3 cm indicates left ventricular enlargement.

■ *Amplitude.* Estimate the amplitude of the impulse. It is usually small and feels *brisk* and *tapping*. Some young people have an increased amplitude, or hyperkinetic impulse, especially when excited or after exercise; its duration, however, is normal.

Increased amplitude may also reflect *hyperthyroidism, severe anemia,* pressure overload of the left ventricle (e.g., *aortic stenosis*), or volume overload of the left ventricle (e.g., *mitral regurgitation*).

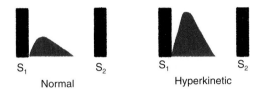

Normal   Hyperkinetic

■ *Duration.* Duration is the most useful characteristic of the apical impulse for identifying hypertrophy of the left ventricle. To assess duration, listen to the heart sounds as you feel the apical impulse, or watch the movement of your stethoscope as you listen at the apex. Estimate the proportion of systole occupied by the apical impulse. Normally it lasts through the first two thirds of systole, and often less, but does not continue to the second heart sound.

A sustained, high-amplitude impulse that is normally located suggests left ventricular hypertrophy from pressure overload (as in hypertension). If such an impulse is displaced laterally, consider volume overload.

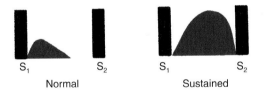

Normal   Sustained

A sustained low-amplitude (hypokinetic) impulse may result from dilated cardiomyopathy.

S₃ and S₄.   By inspection and palpation, you may detect ventricular movements that are synchronous with pathologic third and fourth heart sounds. For the left ventricular impulses, feel the apical beat gently with one finger. The patient should lie partly on the left side, breathe out, and briefly stop breathing. By inking an X on the apex, you may be able to see these movements.

A brief middiastolic impulse indicates an S_3; an impulse just before the systolic apical beat itself indicates an S_4.

Right Ventricular Area—The Left Sternal Border in the 3rd, 4th, and 5th Interspaces.   The patient should rest supine at 30°. Place the tips of your curved fingers in the 3rd, 4th, and 5th interspaces and try to feel the systolic impulse of the right ventricle. Again, asking the patient to breathe out and then briefly stop breathing improves your observation.

If an impulse is palpable, assess its location, amplitude, and duration. A brief systolic tap of low or slightly increased amplitude is sometimes felt in thin or shallow-chested people, especially when stroke volume is increased, as by anxiety.

A marked increase in amplitude with little or no change in duration occurs in chronic volume overload of the right ventricle, as from an *atrial septal defect*.

An impulse with increased amplitude and duration occurs with pressure overload of the right ventricle, as in *pulmonic stenosis* or *pulmonary hypertension*.

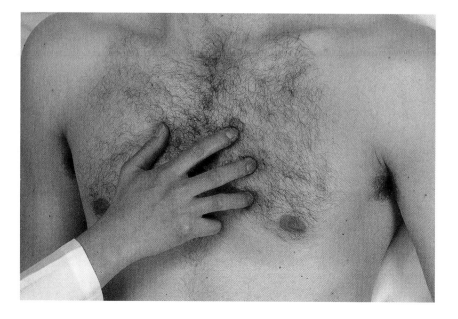

The diastolic movements of *right-sided third and fourth heart sounds* may be felt occasionally. Feel for them in the 4th and 5th left interspaces. Time them by auscultation or carotid palpation.

In patients with an increased anteroposterior (AP) diameter, palpation of the *right ventricle* in the *epigastric* or *subxiphoid area* is also useful. With your hand flattened, press your index finger just under the rib cage and up toward the left shoulder and try to feel right ventricular pulsations.

In obstructive pulmonary disease, hyperinflated lung may prevent palpation of an enlarged right ventricle in the left parasternal area. The impulse is felt easily, however, high in the epigastrium where heart sounds are also often heard best.

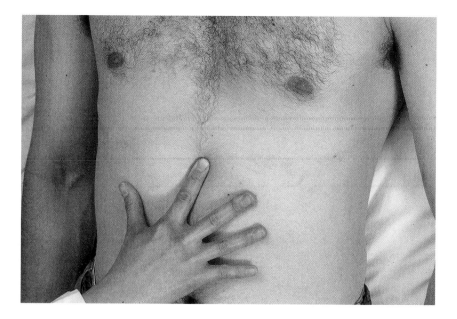

Asking the patient to inhale and briefly stop breathing is helpful. The inspiratory position moves your hand well away from the pulsations of the abdominal aorta, which might otherwise be confusing. The diastolic movements of S_3 and S_4, if present, may also be felt here.

Pulmonic Area—The Left 2nd Interspace.   This interspace overlies the *pulmonary artery.* As the patient holds expiration, look and feel for an impulse and feel for possible heart sounds. In thin or shallow-chested patients, the pulsation of a pulmonary artery may sometimes be felt here, especially after exercise or with excitement.

A prominent pulsation here often accompanies dilatation or increased flow in the pulmonary artery. A palpable S_2 suggests increased pressure in the pulmonary artery (*pulmonary hypertension*).

Aortic Area—The Right 2nd Interspace.   This interspace overlies the aortic outflow tract. Search for pulsations and palpable heart sounds.

A palpable S_2 suggests systemic *hypertension.* A pulsation here suggests a dilated or aneurysmal aorta.

PERCUSSION

In most cases, palpation has replaced percussion in the estimation of cardiac size. When you cannot feel the apical impulse, however, percussion may suggest where to search for it. Occasionally, percussion may be your only tool. Under these circumstances, cardiac dullness often occupies a large area. Starting well to the left on the chest, percuss from resonance toward cardiac dullness in the 3rd, 4th, 5th, and possibly 6th interspaces.

A markedly dilated failing heart may have a hypokinetic apical impulse that is displaced far to the left. A large pericardial effusion may make the impulse undetectable.

AUSCULTATION

Overview.   Auscultation of heart sounds and murmurs is a rewarding and important skill of physical examination that leads directly to several clinical diagnoses. In this section, you will learn the techniques for identifying S_1 and S_2, extra sounds in systole and diastole, and systolic and diastolic murmurs. Review the auscultatory areas on the next page with the following caveats: (1) some authorities discourage use of these names because murmurs of more than one origin may occur in a given area; and (2) these areas may not apply to patients with dextrocardia or anomalies of the great vessels. Also, if the heart is enlarged or displaced, your pattern of auscultation should be altered accordingly.

In a quiet room, listen to the heart with your stethoscope *in the right 2nd interspace* close to the sternum, *along the left sternal border* in each interspace from the 2nd through the 5th, and *at the apex.* Recall that the upper margins of the heart are sometimes termed the "base" of the heart. Some clinicians begin auscultation at the apex, others at the base. Either pattern is satisfactory. You should also listen in any area where you detect an abnormality and in areas adjacent to murmurs to determine where they are loudest and where they radiate.

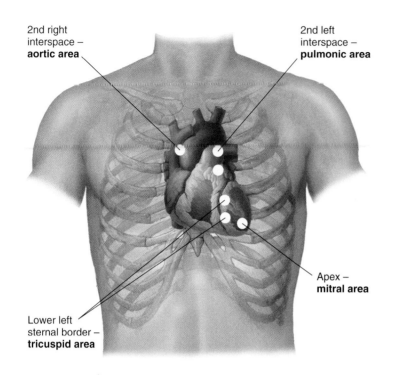

2nd right interspace – **aortic area**

2nd left interspace – **pulmonic area**

Apex – **mitral area**

Lower left sternal border – **tricuspid area**

Heart sounds and murmurs that originate in the four valves are illustrated in the diagram below. Pulmonic sounds are usually heard best in the 2nd and 3rd left interspaces, but may extend further.

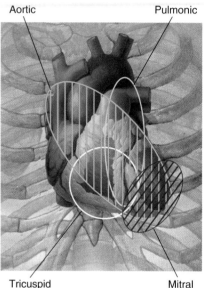

Aortic

Pulmonic

Tricuspid

Mitral

(Redrawn from Leatham A: Introduction to the Examination of the Cardiovascular System, 2nd ed. Oxford, Oxford University Press, 1979)

Know your stethoscope! It is important to understand the uses of both the diaphragm and the bell.

- *The diaphragm.* The diaphragm is better for picking up the relatively high-pitched sounds of S_1 and S_2, the murmurs of aortic and mitral regurgitation, and pericardial friction rubs. *Listen throughout the precordium* with the diaphragm, pressing it firmly against the chest.

- *The bell.* The bell is more sensitive to the low-pitched sounds of S_3 and S_4 and the murmur of mitral stenosis. Apply the bell lightly, with just enough pressure to produce an air seal with its full rim. *Use the bell at the apex, then move medially along the lower sternal border.* Resting the heel of your hand on the chest like a fulcrum may help you to maintain light pressure.

Pressing the bell firmly on the chest makes it function more like the diaphragm by stretching the underlying skin. Low-pitched sounds such as S_3 and S_4 may disappear with this technique—an observation that may help to identify them. In contrast, high-pitched sounds such as a midsystolic click, an ejection sound, or an opening snap, will persist or get louder.

Listen to the entire precordium with the patient supine. For new patients and patients needing a complete cardiac examination, use two other important positions to listen for mitral stenosis and aortic regurgitation.

- Ask the patient to *roll partly onto the left side into the left lateral decubitus position,* bringing the left ventricle close to the chest wall. Place the bell of your stethoscope lightly on the apical impulse.

This position accentuates or brings out a left-sided S_3 and S_4 and mitral murmurs, especially *mitral stenosis.* You may otherwise miss these important findings.

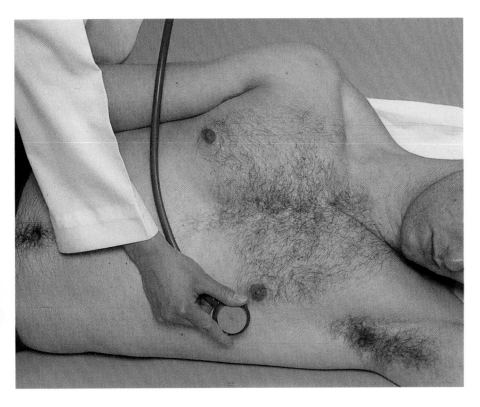

■ Ask the patient to *sit up, lean forward, exhale completely, and stop breathing in expiration*. Pressing the diaphragm of your stethoscope on the chest, listen along the left sternal border and at the apex, pausing periodically so the patient may breathe.

This position accentuates or brings out aortic murmurs. You may easily miss the soft diastolic murmur of *aortic regurgitation* unless you listen at this position.

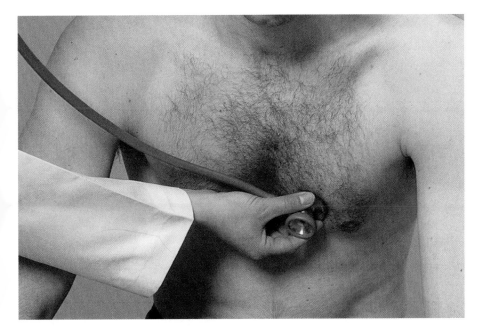

Listening for Heart Sounds. Throughout your examination, take your time at each auscultatory area. Concentrate on each of the events in the cardiac cycle listed on the next page and sounds you may hear in systole and diastole.

■ *Auscultatory Sounds*

Heart Sounds	Guides to Auscultation	
S_1	Note its intensity and any apparent splitting. Normal splitting is detectable along the lower left sternal border.	See Table 8-4, Variations in the First Heart Sound—S_1 (p. 327).
S_2	Note its intensity.	
Split S_2	Listen for splitting of this sound in the 2nd and 3rd left interspaces. Ask the patient to breathe quietly, and then slightly more deeply than normal. Does S_2 split into its two components, as it normally does? If not, ask the patient to (1) breathe a little more deeply, or (2) sit up. Listen again. A thick chest wall may make the pulmonic component of S_1 inaudible.	See Table 8-5, Variations in the Second Heart Sound—S_2 (p. 328). When either A_2 or P_2 is absent, as in disease of the respective valves, S_2 is persistently single.
	Width of split. How wide is the split? It is normally quite narrow.	
	Timing of split. When in the respiratory cycle do you hear the split? It is normally heard late in inspiration.	Expiratory splitting suggests an abnormality (p. 328).
	Does the split disappear as it should, during exhalation? If not, listen again with the patient sitting up.	Persistent splitting results from delayed closure of the pulmonic valve or early closure of the aortic valve.
	Intensity of A_2 and P_2. Compare the intensity of the two components, A_2 and P_2. A_2 is usually louder.	A loud P_2 suggests pulmonary hypertension.
Extra Sounds in Systole	Such as ejection sounds or systolic clicks	The systolic click of mitral valve prolapse is the most common of these sounds. See Table 8-6, Extra Heart Sounds in Systole (p. 329).
	Note their location, timing, intensity, and pitch, and the effects of respiration on the sounds.	
Extra Sounds in Diastole	Such as S_3, S_4, or an opening snap	See Table 8-7, Extra Heart Sounds in Diastole (p. 330).
	Note the location, timing, intensity, and pitch, and the effects of respiration on the sounds. (An S_3 or S_4 in athletes is a normal finding.)	
Systolic and Diastolic Murmurs	Murmurs are differentiated from heart sounds by their longer duration.	See Table 8-8, Pansystolic (Holosystolic) Murmurs (p. 331), Table 8-9, Midsystolic Murmurs (pp. 332–333), and Table 8-10, Diastolic Murmurs (p. 334).

Attributes of Heart Murmurs.   If you detect a heart murmur, you must learn to identify and describe its *timing, shape, location of maximal intensity, radiation* or transmission from this location, *intensity, pitch,* and *quality.*

■ *Timing.* First decide if you are hearing a *systolic murmur,* falling between S_1 and S_2, or a *diastolic murmur,* falling between S_2 and S_1. Palpating the carotid pulse as you listen can help you with timing. *Murmurs that coincide with the carotid upstroke are systolic.*

Systolic murmurs are usually *midsystolic* or *pansystolic.* Late systolic murmurs may also be heard.

Diastolic murmurs usually indicate valvular heart disease. Systolic murmurs may indicate valvular disease, but often occur when the heart valves are entirely normal.

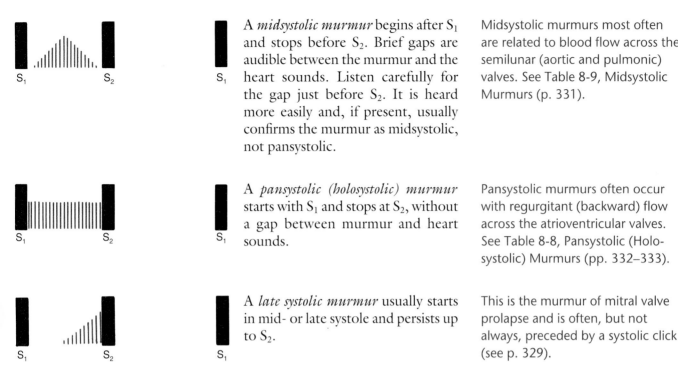

A *midsystolic murmur* begins after S_1 and stops before S_2. Brief gaps are audible between the murmur and the heart sounds. Listen carefully for the gap just before S_2. It is heard more easily and, if present, usually confirms the murmur as midsystolic, not pansystolic.

Midsystolic murmurs most often are related to blood flow across the semilunar (aortic and pulmonic) valves. See Table 8-9, Midsystolic Murmurs (p. 331).

A *pansystolic (holosystolic) murmur* starts with S_1 and stops at S_2, without a gap between murmur and heart sounds.

Pansystolic murmurs often occur with regurgitant (backward) flow across the atrioventricular valves. See Table 8-8, Pansystolic (Holosystolic) Murmurs (pp. 332–333).

A *late systolic murmur* usually starts in mid- or late systole and persists up to S_2.

This is the murmur of mitral valve prolapse and is often, but not always, preceded by a systolic click (see p. 329).

Diastolic murmurs may be *early diastolic, middiastolic,* or *late diastolic.*

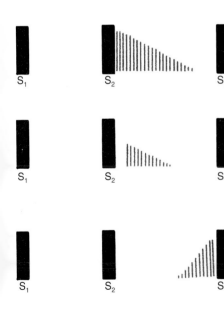

An *early diastolic murmur* starts right after S_2, without a discernible gap, and then usually fades into silence before the next S_1.

Early diastolic murmurs typically accompany regurgitant flow across incompetent semilunar valves.

A *middiastolic murmur* starts a short time after S_2. It may fade away, as illustrated, or merge into a late diastolic murmur.

Middiastolic and presystolic murmurs reflect turbulent flow across the atrioventricular valves. See Table 8-10, Diastolic Murmurs (p. 334).

A *late diastolic (presystolic) murmur* starts late in diastole and typically continues up to S_1.

An occasional murmur, such as the murmur of a patent ductus arteriosus, starts in systole and continues without pause through S_2 into but not necessarily throughout diastole. It is then called a *continuous murmur.* Other cardiovascular sounds, such as pericardial friction rubs or venous hums, have *both systolic and diastolic components.* Observe and describe these sounds according to the characteristics used for systolic and diastolic murmurs.

See Table 8-11, Cardiovascular Sounds With Both Systolic and Diastolic Components (p. 335).

■ *Shape.* The shape or configuration of a murmur is determined by its intensity over time.

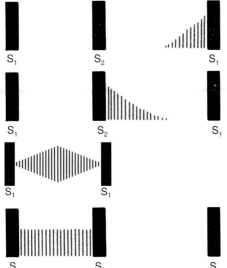

A *crescendo murmur* grows louder.

The presystolic murmur of *mitral stenosis* in normal sinus rhythm

A *decrescendo murmur* grows softer.

The early diastolic murmur of *aortic regurgitation*

A *crescendo–decrescendo murmur* first rises in intensity, then falls.

The midsystolic murmur of *aortic stenosis* and *innocent flow murmurs*

A *plateau murmur* has the same intensity throughout.

The pansystolic murmur of *mitral regurgitation*

■ *Location of Maximal Intensity.* This is determined by the site where the murmur originates. Find the location by exploring the area where you hear the murmur. Describe where you hear it best in terms of the interspace and its relation to the sternum, the apex, or the midsternal, the midclavicular, or one of the axillary lines.

For example, a murmur best heard in the 2nd right interspace (the aortic area) usually originates at or near the aortic valve.

■ *Radiation or Transmission From the Point of Maximal Intensity.* This reflects not only the site of origin but also the intensity of the murmur and the direction of blood flow. Explore the area around a murmur and determine where else you can hear it.

A loud murmur of *aortic stenosis* often radiates into the neck (in the direction of arterial flow).

■ *Intensity.* This is usually graded on a 6-point scale and expressed as a fraction. The numerator describes the intensity of the murmur wherever it is loudest, and the denominator indicates the scale you are using. Intensity is influenced by the thickness of the chest wall and the presence of intervening tissue.

An identical degree of turbulence would cause a louder murmur in a thin person than in a very muscular or obese person. Emphysematous lungs may diminish the intensity of murmurs.

Learn to grade murmurs using the 6-point scale below. Note that grades 4 through 6 require the added presence of a palpable thrill.

■ Gradations of Murmurs

Grade	Description
Grade 1	Very faint, heard only after listener has "tuned in"; may not be heard in all positions
Grade 2	Quiet, but heard immediately after placing the stethoscope on the chest
Grade 3	Moderately loud
Grade 4	Loud, with palpable thrill
Grade 5	Very loud, with thrill. May be heard when the stethoscope is partly off the chest
Grade 6	Very loud, with thrill. May be heard with stethoscope entirely off the chest

- *Pitch.* This is categorized as high, medium, or low.

- *Quality.* This is described in terms such as blowing, harsh, rumbling, and musical.

A fully described murmur might be: a "medium-pitched, grade 2/6, blowing decrescendo diastolic murmur, heard best in the 4th left interspace, with radiation to the apex" (aortic regurgitation).

Other useful characteristics of murmurs—and heart sounds too—include variation with respiration, with the position of the patient, or with other special maneuvers.

Murmurs originating in the right side of the heart tend to change more with respiration than left-sided murmurs.

INTEGRATING CARDIOVASCULAR ASSESSMENT

A good cardiovascular examination requires more than observation. You need to think about the possible meanings of your individual observations, fit them together in a logical pattern, and correlate your cardiac findings with the patient's blood pressure, arterial pulses, venous pulsations, jugular venous pressure, the remainder of your physical examination, and the patient's history.

Evaluating the common systolic murmur illustrates this point. In examining an asymptomatic teenager, for example, you might hear a grade 2/6 midsystolic murmur in the 2nd and 3rd left interspaces. Because this suggests a murmur of pulmonic origin, you should assess the size of the right ventricle by carefully palpating the left parasternal area. Because pulmonic stenosis and atrial septal defects can occasionally cause such murmurs, listen carefully to the splitting of the second heart sound and try to hear any ejection sounds. Listen to the murmur after the patient sits up. Look for evidence of anemia, hyperthyroidism, or pregnancy that could produce such a murmur by increasing the flow across the aortic or the pulmonic valve. If all your findings are normal, your patient probably has an *innocent murmur*—one with no pathologic significance.

In a 60-year-old person with angina, you might hear a harsh 3/6 mid-systolic crescendo–decrescendo murmur in the right 2nd interspace radiating to the neck. These findings suggest *aortic stenosis,* but could arise from *aortic sclerosis* (leaflets sclerotic but not stenotic), a dilated aorta, or increased flow across a normal valve. Assess any delay in the carotid upstroke and the blood pressure for evidence of *aortic stenosis.* Check the apical impulse for left ventricular hypertrophy. Listen for *aortic regurgitation* as the patient leans forward and exhales.

Put all this information together to make a hypothesis about the origin of the murmur.

SPECIAL TECHNIQUES

Aids to Identify Systolic Murmurs.   Elsewhere in this chapter you have learned how to improve your auscultation of heart sounds and murmurs by placing the patient in different positions. Two additional techniques help you distinguish the murmurs of mitral valve prolapse and hypertrophic cardiomyopathy from aortic stenosis.

(1) **Standing and Squatting.**   When a person stands, venous return to the heart decreases, as does peripheral vascular resistance. Arterial blood pressure, stroke volume, and the volume of blood in the left ventricle all decline. When squatting, changes occur in the opposite direction. These changes help (1) to identify a prolapsed mitral valve, and (2) to distinguish hypertrophic cardiomyopathy from aortic stenosis.

Secure the patient's gown so that it will not interfere with your examination, and ready yourself for prompt auscultation. Instruct the patient to squat next to the examining table and hold on to it for balance. Listen to the heart with the patient in the squatting position and again in the standing position.

(2) **Valsalva Maneuver.**   When a person strains down against a closed glottis, venous return to the right heart is decreased, and after a few seconds, left ventricular volume and arterial blood pressure both fall. Release of the effort has the opposite effects. These changes help to distinguish prolapse of the mitral valve and hypertrophic cardiomyopathy from aortic stenosis.

The patient should be lying down. Ask the patient to "bear down," or place one hand on the midabdomen and instruct the patient to strain against it. By adjusting the pressure of your hand you can alter the patient's effort to the desired level. Use your other hand to place your stethoscope on the patient's chest.

■ *Maneuvers to Identify Systolic Murmurs*

		Effect on Systolic Sounds and Murmurs		
Maneuver	**Cardiovascular Effect**	*Mitral Valve Prolapse*	*Hypertrophic Cardiomyopathy*	*Aortic Stenosis*
Standing; Strain Phase of Valsalva	**Decreased left ventricular volume** from ↓ venous return to heart	↑ prolapse of mitral valve	↑ outflow obstruction	↓ blood volume ejected into aorta
	Decreased vascular tone: ↓ arterial blood pressure	*Click moves earlier in systole* and *murmur lengthens*	↑ **intensity of murmur**	↓ **intensity of murmur**
Squatting; Release of Valsalva	**Increased left ventricular volume** from ↑ venous return to heart	↓ prolapse of mitral valve	↓ outflow obstruction	↑ blood volume ejected into aorta
	Increased vascular tone: ↑ arterial blood pressure; ↑ peripheral vascular resistance	*Delay of click* and *murmur shortens*	↓ **intensity of murmur**	↑ **intensity of murmur**

Pulsus Alternans.   In *pulsus alternans,* the rhythm of the pulse remains regular, but the *force* of the arterial pulse alternates because of alternating strong and weak ventricular contractions. *Pulsus alternans* almost always indicates severe left-sided heart failure and is usually best felt by applying light pressure on the radial or femoral arteries.[35] Use a blood pressure cuff to confirm your finding. After raising the cuff pressure, lower it slowly to the systolic level—the initial Korotkoff sounds are the strong beats. As you lower the cuff, you will hear the softer sounds of the alternating weak beats.

Alternately loud and soft Korotkoff sounds or a sudden doubling of the apparent heart rate as the cuff pressure declines indicates a *pulsus alternans* (see p. 119).

The upright position may accentuate the alternation.

Paradoxical Pulse.   If you have noted that the pulse varies in amplitude with respiration or if you suspect pericardial tamponade (because of increased jugular venous pressure, a rapid and diminished pulse, and dyspnea, for example), use a blood-pressure cuff to check for a *paradoxical pulse.* This is a greater than normal drop in systolic pressure during inspiration. As the

The level identified by first hearing Korotkoff sounds is the highest systolic pressure during the respiratory cycle. The level identified by hearing sounds throughout the cycle is the

patient breathes, quietly if possible, lower the cuff pressure slowly to the systolic level. Note the pressure level at which the first sounds can be heard. Then drop the pressure very slowly until sounds can be heard throughout the respiratory cycle. Again note the pressure level. The difference between these two levels is normally no greater than 3 or 4 mm Hg.

lowest systolic pressure. A difference between these levels of more than 10 mm Hg indicates a paradoxical pulse and suggests *pericardial tamponade,* possible *constrictive pericarditis,* but most commonly *obstructive airway disease* (see p. 119).

RECORDING YOUR FINDINGS

Note that initially you may use sentences to describe your findings; later you will use phrases. The style below contains phrases appropriate for most write-ups.

Recording the Physical Examination— The Cardiovascular Examination

"The jugular venous pulse (JVP) is 3 cm above the sternal angle with the head of bed elevated to 30°. Carotid upstrokes are brisk, without bruits. The point of maximal impulse (PMI) is tapping, 7 cm lateral to the midsternal line in the 5th intercostal space. Good S_1 and S_2. No murmurs or extra sounds."

OR

"The JVP is 5 cm above the sternal angle with the head of bed elevated to 50°. Carotid upstrokes are brisk; a bruit is heard over the left carotid artery. The PMI is diffuse, 3 cm in diameter, palpated at the anterior axillary line in the 5th and 6th intercostal spaces. S_1 and S_2 are soft. S_3 present. Harsh 2/6 holosystolic murmur best heard at the apex, radiating to the lower left sternal border (LLSB). No S_4 or diastolic murmurs."

Suggests *congestive heart failure* with possible *left carotid occlusion* and *mitral regurgitation.*[36–38]

Bibliography

CITATIONS

1. Cook DJ, Simel DL. Does this patient have abnormal central venous pressure? JAMA 275(8):630–634, 1996.
2. Lee TH, Goldman L. Evaluation of the patient with acute chest pain. N Engl J Med 342(16):1187–1195, 2000.
3. Goldman L, Kirtane AJ. Triage of patient with acute chest syndrome and possible cardiac ischemia: the elusive search for diagnostic perfection. Ann Intern Med 139(12):987–995, 2003.
4. Snow V, Barry P, Fihn SD, et al. Evaluation of primary care patients with chronic stable angina: guidelines from the American College of Physicians. Ann Intern Med 141(1):57–64, 2004.
5. U.S. Preventive Services Task Force. Screening for high blood pressure: recommendations and rationale. Rockville, MD, Agency for Healthcare Research and Quality, July 2003. Available at: http://www.ahrq.gov/clinic/3rduspstf/hibloodrr.htm. Accessed March 6, 2005.
6. Chobanion AV, Bakris GL, Black HR, et al. The seventh report of the Joint National Committee on Preventions, Detection,

Evaluation, and Treatment of High Blood Pressure—the JNC 7 report. JAMA 289(19):2560–2572, 2003. Available at: www.nhlbi.nih.gov/guidelines/hypertension/jncintro.htm.
7. Whelton PK, He J, Appel LJ, et al. Primary prevention of hypertension. Clinical and Public Health Advisory from the National High Blood Pressure Education Program. JAMA 288(15):1882–1888, 2002.
8. Vasan RS, Larson MG, Leip EP, et al. Impact of high-normal blood pressure on the risk of cardiovascular disease. N Engl J Med 345(18):1291–1297, 2001.
9. Stamler J, Stamler R, Neaton JD, et al. Low risk-factor profile and long-term cardiovascular and noncardiovascular mortality and life expectancy—findings for 5 large cohorts of young adult and middle-aged men and women. JAMA 282(21):2012–2018, 1999.
10. Vidt DG, Borazanian RA. Treat high blood pressure sooner: tougher, simpler JNC 7 guidelines. Cleve Clin J Med 70(8): 721–728, 2003.
11. Pearson TA, Blair SN, Daniels SR, et al. AHA guidelines for primary prevention of cardiovascular disease and stroke: 2002 update. Circulation 106:388–391, 2002.

BIBLIOGRAPHY

12. Third Report of the National Cholesterol Education Program (NCEP) Expert Panel. Detection, evaluation, and treatment of high blood cholesterol in adults—executive summary. National Cholesterol Education Program, National Heart, Lung, and Blood Institute, National Institutes of Health. NIH Publication No. 01-3670. May 2001. Available at: www.nhlbi.nih.gov/guidelines/cholesterol/index.htm. Accessed August 31, 2004.

13. National Cholesterol Education Panel. Third report of the National Cholesterol Education Program (NCEP) Expert Panel on detection, evaluation, and treatment of high blood cholesterol in adults (Adult Treatment Panel III) final report. Circulation 106:3143–3421, 2002.

14. Grundy SM, Cleeman JI, Merz NB, et al, for the Coordinating Committee of the National Cholesterol Education Program. Implications of recent clinical trials for the National Cholesterol Education Program Adult Treatment Panel III guidelines. Circulation 110:227–239, 2004.

15. Heart Protection Study Collaborative Group. MRC/BHF Heart Protection Study of cholesterol lowering with simvastatin in 20,356 high risk individuals: a randomized placebo-controlled trial. Lancet 360(9326):7–22, 2002.

16. Screening for lipid disorders: recommendations and rationale. Am J Prev Med 20(3S):73–76, 2001. Agency for Healthcare Research and Quality, Rockville, MD. Available at: http://www.ahrq.gov/clinic/ajpmsuppl/lipidrr.htm. Accessed January 15, 2005.

17. Pignone MP, Phillips CJ, Atkins D, et al. Summary of the evidence. Screening and treating adults for lipid disorders. Agency for Healthcare Research and Quality, Rockville, MD. Available at: http://www.ahrq.gov/clinic/ajpmsuppl/pignone1.htm. Accessed January 15, 2005.

18. Walsh JME, Pignone M. Drug treatment of hyperlipidemia in women. JAMA 291(18):2243–2252, 2004.

19. American Diabetes Association. Toolkit No. 7—protect your heart: choose fats wisely. March 2004. Available at: http://www.diabetes.org/type-1-diabetes/well-being/Choose-Fats.jsp. Accessed March 17, 2005.

20. Healthy People 2010. Progress review—nutrition and overweight. U.S. Department of Health and Human Services—Public Health Service. January 21, 2004. Available at: http://www.healthypeople.gov/data/2010prog/focus19/default.htm. Accessed March 17, 2005.

21. Healthy People 2010. Progress review—physical activity and fitness. U.S. Department of Health and Human Services—Public Health Service. April 14, 2004. Available at: http://www.healthypeople.gov/data/2010prog/focus22/. Accessed March 17, 2005.

22. Beevers G, Lip GY, O'Brien E. ABC of hypertension. Blood pressure measurement. Part I. Sphygmomanometry: factors common in all techniques. BMJ 322:981–985, 2001.

23. Beevers G, Lip GY, O'Brien E. ABC of hypertension. Blood pressure measurement. Part II. Conventional sphygmomanometry: technique of auscultatory blood pressure measurement. BMJ 322:1043–1047, 2001.

24. McAlister FA, Straus SE. Evidence-based treatment of hypertension. measurement of blood pressure: an evidence based review. BMJ 322:098–911, 2001.

25. Tholl U, Forstner K, Anlauf M. Measuring blood pressure: pitfalls and recommendations. Nephrol Dial Transplant 19:766, 2004.

26. Edmonds ZV, Mower WR, Lovato LM, et al. The reliability of vital sign measurements. Ann Emerg Med 39(3):233–237, 2002.

27. Lange RA, Hillis LD. Acute pericarditis. N Engl J Med 351(21):2195–2202, 2004.

28. Spodick D. Acute pericarditis: current concepts and practice. JAMA 289(9): 1150–1153, 2003.

29. Drazner MH, Rame E, Stevenson LW, et al. Prognostic importance of elevated jugular venous pressure and a third heart sound in patients with heart failure. N Engl J Med 345(8):574–581, 2001.

30. Khot UN. Prognostic importance of physical examination for heart failure in non-ST elevation acute coronary syndromes. The enduring value of Killip classification. JAMA 290(16): 2174–2181, 2003.

31. Jessup M, Brozena S. Medical progress: heart failure. N Engl J Med 348(20):2007–2017, 2003.

32. Aurigemma GP, Gaasch WH. Diastolic heart failure. N Engl J Med 351(11):1097–1104, 2004.

33. Badgett RG, Lucey CR, Muirow CD. Can the clinical examination diagnose left-sided heart failure in adults? JAMA 277(21):1712–1719, 1997.

34. Sauve JS, Laupacis A, Ostbye T, et al. Does this patient have a clinically important carotid bruit? JAMA 270(23): 2843–2845, 1993.

35. Cha K, Falk RH. Images in clinical medicine: pulsus alternans. N Engl J Med 334(13):834, 1996.

36. Halder AW, Larson MG, Franklin SS, et al. Systolic blood pressure, diastolic blood pressure, and pulse pressure as predictors of risk for congestive heart failure in the Framingham Heart Study. Ann Intern Med 138(1):10–16, 2003.

37. Thomas JT, Kelly RF, Thomas SJ, et al. Utility of history, physical examination, electrocardiogram, and chest radiograph for differentiating normal from decreased systolic function in patients with heart failure. Am J Med 112(6): 437–445, 2002.

38. Fonarow GC, Adams KF, Abraham WT, et al. Risk stratification for in-hospital mortality in acutely decompensated heart failure. Classification and regression tree analysis. JAMA 293(5):572–580, 2005.

39. Etchells E, Bell C, Robb K. Does this patient have an abnormal systolic murmur? JAMA 277(7):564–571, 1997.

40. Lembo NJ, Dell'Italia LJ, Crawford MH, et al. Bedside diagnosis of systolic murmurs. N Engl J Med 318:1572–1578, 1988.

41. Etchells E, Glenns, Shadowitz S, et al. A bedside clinical prediction rule for detecting moderate or severe aortic stenosis. J Gen Intern Med 13:699–704, 1998.

42. Picrard LA, Lancellotti P. The role of ischemic mitral regurgitation in the pathogenesis of acute pulmonary edema. N Engl J Med 351(16):1627–1634, 2004.

43. Enriquez-Serano M, Tajik AJ. Aortic regurgitation. N Engl J Med 351(15):1539–1546, 2004.

44. Babu AN, Kymes SM, Fryer SMC. Eponyms and the diagnosis of aortic regurgitation: what says the evidence? Ann Intern Med 138(9):736–742, 2003.

BIBLIOGRAPHY

ADDITIONAL REFERENCES

Beckman JA, Creager MA, Libby P. Diabetes and atherosclerosis: epidemiology, pathophysiology, and management. JAMA 287(19):2570–2581, 2002.

Cohn JN, Hoke L, Whitwam W, et al. Screening for early detection of cardiovascular disease in asymptomatic individuals. Am Heart J 146(4):679–685, 2003.

Dosh SA. The diagnosis of essential and secondary hypertension in adults. J Fam Pract 50(8):707–712, 2001.

Drezner JA. Sudden cardiac death in young athletes: causes, athlete's heart, and screening guidelines. Postgrad Med 108(5):37–44, 47–50, 2000.

Fletcher GF, Balady GJ, Amsterdam EA, et al. Exercise standards for testing and training: a statement for healthcare professionals from the American Heart Association. Circulation 104(14):1694–1740, 2001.

Fuster V, Alexander RW, O'Rourke RA, et al. Hurst's the Heart, 11th ed. New York, McGraw-Hill, Medical Pub Division, 2004.

Hansson GK. Inflammation, atherosclerosis, and coronary artery disease. N Engl J Med 352(16):1685–1695, 2005.

Kuperstein R, Feinberg MS, Eldar M, Schwammenthal E. Physical determinants of systolic murmur intensity in aortic stenosis. Am J Cardiol 95(6):774–776, 2005.

Lee AJ, Price JF, Russell MJ, et al. Improved prediction of fatal myocardial infarction using the ankle brachial index in addition to conventional risk factors: the Edinburgh Artery Study. Circulation 110(19):3075–3080, 2004.

Oparil S, Saman MA, Calhoun DA. Pathogenesis of hypertension. Ann Intern Med 139(9):761–776, 2003.

Perloff, JK. Physical Examination of the Heart and Circulation, 3rd ed. Philadelphia, WB Saunders, 2000.

Pryor DB, Shaw L, McCants CB. Value of the history and physical in identifying patients at increased risk for coronary artery disease. Ann Intern Med 118(2):81–90, 1993.

Selvanayagam J, De Pasquale C, Arnolda L. Usefulness of clinical assessment of the carotid pulse in the diagnosis of aortic stenosis. Am J Cardiol 93(4):493–495, 2004.

Selvin E, Erlinger TP. Prevalence of and risk factors for peripheral arterial disease in the United States: results from the National Health and Nutrition Examination Survey. Circulation 110(6):738–743, 2004.

Smulyan H, Safar ME. The diastolic blood pressure in systolic hypertension. Ann Intern Med 132(3):233–237, 2000.

Stein RA, Zusman R. Management of sexual dysfunction in patients with cardiovascular disease: recommendations of the Princeton Consensus Panel. Am J Cardiol 86(2A):62F–68F, 2000.

Taylor HA Jr. Sexual activity and the cardiovascular patient: guidelines. Am J Cardiol 84(5B):6N–10N, 1999.

Thomas JT, Kelly RF, Thomas SJ, et al. Utility of history, physical examination, electrocardiogram, and chest radiograph for differentiating normal from decreased systolic function in patients with heart failure. Am J Med 112(6):437–445, 2002.

Zipes DP, Braunwald E (eds). Braunwald's Heart Disease: A Textbook of Cardiovascular Medicine, 7th ed. Philadelphia, Elsevier Saunders, 2005.

TABLE 8-1   **Selected Heart Rates and Rhythms**

Cardiac rhythms may be classified as *regular* or *irregular*. When rhythms are irregular or rates are fast or slow, obtain an ECG to identify the origin of the beats (sinus node, AV node, atrium, or ventricle) and the pattern of conduction. Note that with AV (atrioventricular) block, arrhythmias may have a fast, normal, or slow ventricular rate.

ECG Pattern		Usual Resting Rate
WHAT IS THE RATE?		
FAST (>100)	Sinus tachycardia	100–180
	Supraventricular (atrial or nodal) tachycardia	150–250
	Atrial flutter with a regular ventricular response	100–175
	Ventricular tachycardia	110–250
OR		
NORMAL (60–100)	Normal sinus rhythm	60–100
	Second-degree AV block	60–100
	Atrial flutter with a regular ventricular response	75–100
OR		
SLOW (<60)	Sinus bradycardia	<60
	Second-degree AV block	30–60
	Complete heart block	<40
RHYTHMIC OR SPORADIC	With early beats, atrial or nodal (supraventricular) premature contraction OR ventricular premature contractions	
	Sinus arrhythmia	See Table 8-2
OR		
TOTAL	Atrial fibrillation	
	Atrial flutter with varying block	

IS THE RHYTHM REGULAR OR IRREGULAR?

REGULAR

IRREGULAR

WHAT IS THE PATTERN OF IRREGULARITY?

TABLE 8-2	Selected Irregular Rhythms

Type of Rhythm	ECG Waves and Heart Sounds	
Atrial or Nodal Premature Contractions (*Supraventricular*)	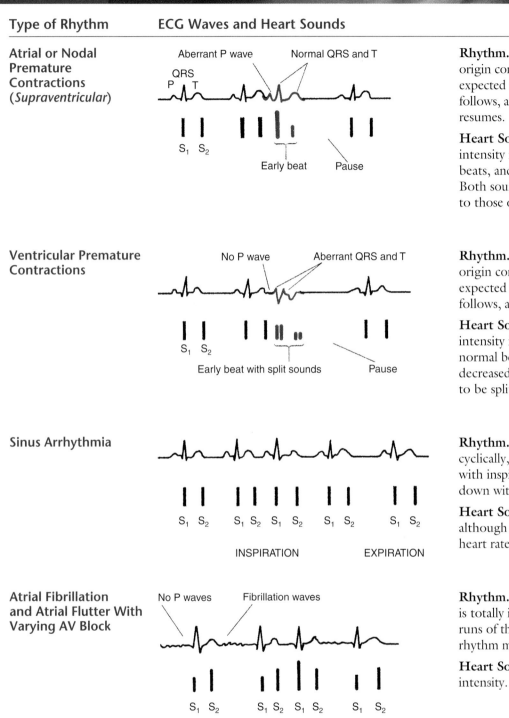	**Rhythm.** A beat of atrial or nodal origin comes earlier than the next expected normal beat. A pause follows, and then the rhythm resumes. **Heart Sounds.** S_1 may differ in intensity from the S_1 of normal beats, and S_2 may be decreased. Both sounds are otherwise similar to those of normal beats.
Ventricular Premature Contractions		**Rhythm.** A beat of ventricular origin comes earlier than the next expected normal beat. A pause follows, and the rhythm resumes. **Heart Sounds.** S_1 may differ in intensity from the S_1 of the normal beats, and S_2 may be decreased. Both sounds are likely to be split.
Sinus Arrhythmia		**Rhythm.** The heart varies cyclically, usually speeding up with inspiration and slowing down with expiration. **Heart Sounds.** Normal, although S_1 may vary with the heart rate.
Atrial Fibrillation and Atrial Flutter With Varying AV Block		**Rhythm.** The ventricular rhythm is totally irregular, although short runs of the irregular ventricular rhythm may seem regular. **Heart Sounds.** S_1 varies in intensity.

TABLE 8-3   **Variations and Abnormalities of the Ventricular Impulses**

In the healthy heart, the *left ventricular impulse* is usually the *point of maximal impulse,* or *PMI.* This brief impulse is generated by the movement of the ventricular apex against the chest wall during contraction. The *right ventricular impulse* is normally not palpable beyond infancy, and its characteristics are indeterminate. In contrast, learn the classical descriptors of the left ventricular PMI:

- *Location:* in the 4th or 5th interspace, ~7–10 cm lateral to the midsternal line, depending on the diameter of the chest
- *Diameter: discrete,* or ≤2 cm
- *Amplitude: brisk* and *tapping*
- *Duration:* ≤2/3 of systole

Careful examination of the ventricular impulse gives you important clues about underlying cardiovascular hemodynamics. The quality of the ventricular impulse changes as the left and right ventricles adapt to high-output states (anxiety, hyperthyroidism, and severe anemia) and to the more pathologic conditions of chronic pressure or volume overload. Note below the distinguishing features of three types of ventricular impulses: the *hyperkinetic ventricular impulse* from transiently increased stroke volume—this change does not necessarily indicate heart disease; the *sustained* ventricular impulse of ventricular hypertrophy from chronic pressure load, known as *increased afterload* (see p. 311); and the *diffuse* ventricular impulse of ventricular dilation from chronic volume overload, or *increased preload.*

| | Left Ventricular Impulse | | | Right Ventricular Impulse | | |
	Hyperkinetic	*Pressure Overload*	*Volume Overload*	*Hyperkinetic*	*Pressure Overload*	*Volume Overload*
Examples of Causes	Anxiety, hyperthyroidism, severe anemia	Aortic stenosis, hypertension	Aortic or mitral regurgitation	Anxiety, hyperthyroidism, severe anemia	Pulmonic stenosis, pulmonary hypertension	Atrial septal defect
Location	Normal	Normal	Displaced to the left and possibly downward	3rd, 4th, or 5th left interspaces	3rd, 4th, or 5th left interspaces, also subxiphoid	Left sternal border, extending toward the left cardiac border, also subxiphoid
Diameter	~2 cm, though increased amplitude may make it seem larger	>2 cm	>2 cm	Not useful	Not useful	Not useful
Amplitude	More forceful tapping	More forceful tapping	*Diffuse*	Slightly more forceful	More forceful	Slightly to markedly more forceful
Duration	<2/3 systole	*Sustained* (up to S_2)	Often slightly sustained	Normal	Sustained	Normal to slightly sustained

TABLE 8-4   Variations in the First Heart Sound—S_1

Normal Variations

S_1 S_2

S_1 is softer than S_2 at the *base* (right and left 2nd interspaces).

S_1 S_2

S_1 is often but not always louder than S_2 at the *apex*.

Accentuated S_1

S_1 S_2

S_1 is accentuated in (1) tachycardia, rhythms with a short PR interval, and high cardiac output states (e.g., exercise, anemia, hyperthyroidism), and (2) mitral stenosis. In these conditions, the mitral valve is still open wide at the onset of ventricular systole, and then closes quickly.

Diminished S_1

S_1 S_2

S_1 is diminished in first-degree heart block (delayed conduction from atria to ventricles). Here the mitral valve has had time after atrial contraction to float back into an almost closed position before ventricular contraction shuts it. It closes less loudly. S_1 is also diminished (1) when the mitral valve is calcified and relatively immobile, as in mitral regurgitation, and (2) when left ventricular contractility is markedly reduced, as in congestive heart failure or coronary heart disease.

Varying S_1

S_1 S_2 S_1 S_2

S_1 varies in intensity (1) in complete heart block, when atria and ventricles are beating independently of each other, and (2) in any totally irregular rhythm (e.g., atrial fibrillation). In these situations, the mitral valve is in varying positions before being shut by ventricular contraction. Its closure sound, therefore, varies in loudness.

Split S_1

S_1 S_2

S_1 may be split normally along the lower left sternal border where the tricuspid component, often too faint to be heard, becomes audible. This split may sometimes be heard at the apex, but consider also an S_4, an aortic ejection sound, and an early systolic click. Abnormal splitting of both heart sounds may be heard in right bundle branch block and in premature ventricular contractions.

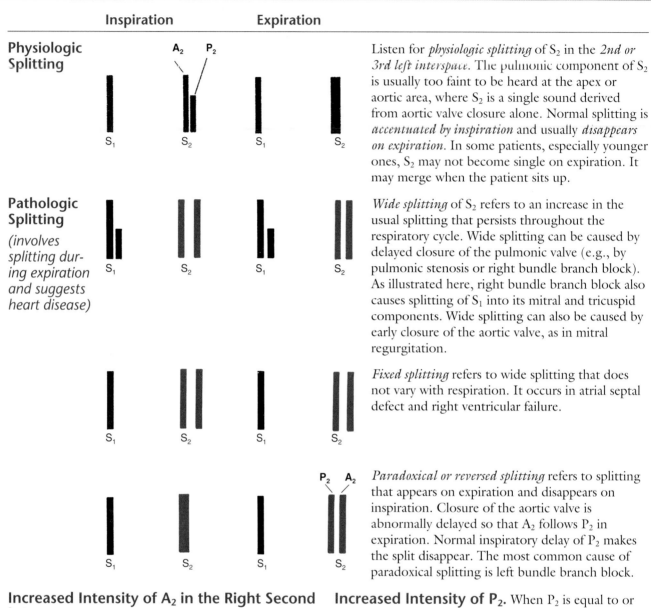

	Inspiration	Expiration	

Physiologic Splitting

Listen for *physiologic splitting* of S_2 in the *2nd or 3rd left interspace*. The pulmonic component of S_2 is usually too faint to be heard at the apex or aortic area, where S_2 is a single sound derived from aortic valve closure alone. Normal splitting is *accentuated by inspiration* and usually *disappears on expiration*. In some patients, especially younger ones, S_2 may not become single on expiration. It may merge when the patient sits up.

Pathologic Splitting

(involves splitting during expiration and suggests heart disease)

Wide splitting of S_2 refers to an increase in the usual splitting that persists throughout the respiratory cycle. Wide splitting can be caused by delayed closure of the pulmonic valve (e.g., by pulmonic stenosis or right bundle branch block). As illustrated here, right bundle branch block also causes splitting of S_1 into its mitral and tricuspid components. Wide splitting can also be caused by early closure of the aortic valve, as in mitral regurgitation.

Fixed splitting refers to wide splitting that does not vary with respiration. It occurs in atrial septal defect and right ventricular failure.

Paradoxical or reversed splitting refers to splitting that appears on expiration and disappears on inspiration. Closure of the aortic valve is abnormally delayed so that A_2 follows P_2 in expiration. Normal inspiratory delay of P_2 makes the split disappear. The most common cause of paradoxical splitting is left bundle branch block.

Increased Intensity of A_2 in the Right Second Interspace (where only A_2 can usually be heard) occurs in systemic hypertension because of the increased pressure load. It also occurs when the aortic root is dilated, probably because the aortic valve is then closer to the chest wall.

Decreased or Absent A_2 in the Right Second Interspace is noted in calcific aortic stenosis because of valve immobility. If A_2 is inaudible, no splitting is heard.

Increased Intensity of P_2. When P_2 is equal to or louder than A_2, suspect pulmonary hypertension. Other causes include a dilated pulmonary artery and an atrial septal defect. When a split S_2 is heard widely, even at the apex and the right base, P_2 is accentuated.

Decreased or Absent P_2 is usually due to the increased anteroposterior diameter of the chest associated with aging. It can also result from pulmonic stenosis. If P_2 is inaudible, no splitting is heard.

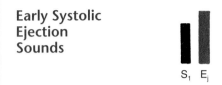

TABLE 8-6   **Extra Heart Sounds in Systole**

There are two kinds of extra heart sounds in systole: (1) early ejection sounds, and (2) clicks, commonly heard in mid- and late systole.

Early Systolic Ejection Sounds

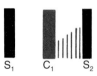

S_1 E_j S_2

Early systolic ejection sounds occur shortly after S_1, coincident with opening of the aortic and pulmonic valves. They are relatively high in pitch, have a sharp, clicking quality, and are heard better with the diaphragm of the stethoscope. An ejection sound indicates cardiovascular disease.

Listen for an *aortic ejection sound* at both the base and apex. It may be louder at the apex and usually does not vary with respiration. An aortic ejection sound may accompany a dilated aorta, or aortic valve disease from congenital stenosis or a bicuspid valve.

A *pulmonic ejection sound* is heard best in the 2nd and 3rd left interspaces. When S_1, usually relatively soft in this area, appears to be loud, you may be hearing a pulmonic ejection sound. Its intensity often *decreases with inspiration*. Causes include dilatation of the pulmonary artery, pulmonary hypertension, and pulmonic stenosis.

Systolic Clicks

S_1 C_1 S_2

Systolic clicks are usually due to *mitral valve prolapse*—an abnormal systolic ballooning of part of the mitral valve into the left atrium. The clicks are usually mid- or late systolic. Prolapse of the mitral valve is a common cardiac condition, affecting about 5% of the general population. There is equal prevalence in men and women.

The click is usually single, but you may hear more than one, usually *at or medial to the apex*, but also *at the lower left sternal border*. It is high-pitched, so listen with the diaphragm. The click is often followed by a late systolic murmur from mitral regurgitation—a flow of blood from left ventricle to left atrium. The murmur usually crescendos up to S_2. Auscultatory findings are notably variable. Most patients have only a click, some have only a murmur, and some have both. Systolic clicks may also be of extracardial or mediastinal origin.

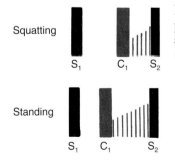

Squatting

S_1 C_1 S_2

Standing

S_1 C_1 S_2

Findings vary from time to time and often change with body position. Several positions are recommended to identify the syndrome: supine, seated, squatting, and standing. *Squatting delays the click and murmur; standing moves them closer to S_1.*

TABLE 8-7   **Extra Heart Sounds in Diastole**

Opening Snap

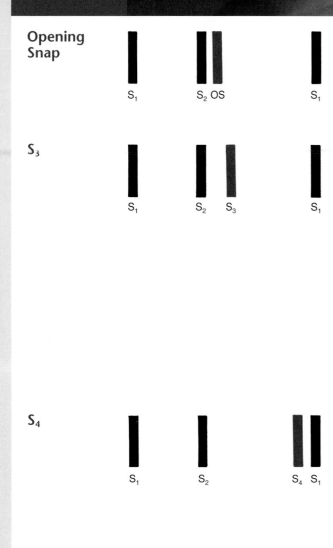

The *opening snap* is a very early diastolic sound usually produced by the opening of a *stenotic mitral valve*. It is heard best just medial to the apex and along the lower left sternal border. When it is loud, an opening snap radiates to the apex and to the pulmonic area, where it may be mistaken for the pulmonic component of a split S_2. Its high pitch and snapping quality help to distinguish it from an S_2. It is heard better with the diaphragm.

S_3

You will detect *physiologic* S_3 frequently in children and in young adults to the age of 35 or 40. It is common during the last trimester of pregnancy. Occurring early in diastole during rapid ventricular filling, it is later than an opening snap, dull and low in pitch, and heard best at the apex in the left lateral decubitus position. Use the bell of the stethoscope should be used with very light pressure.

A *pathologic* S_3 or *ventricular gallop* sounds just like a physiologic S_3. An S_3 in a person over age 40 (possibly a little older in women) is almost certainly pathologic. Causes include decreased myocardial contractility, congestive heart failure, and volume overloading of a ventricle, as in mitral or tricuspid regurgitation. A *left-sided* S_3 is heard typically at the apex in the left lateral decubitus position. A *right-sided* S_3 is usually heard along the lower left sternal border or below the xiphoid with the patient supine, and is louder on inspiration. The term *gallop* comes from the cadence of three heart sounds, especially at rapid heart rates, and sounds like "Kentucky."

S_4

An S_4 (*atrial sound* or *atrial gallop*) occurs just before S_1. It is dull, low in pitch, and heard better with the bell. An S_4 is heard occasionally in an apparently normal person, especially in trained athletes and older age groups. More commonly, it is due to increased resistance to ventricular filling following atrial contraction. This increased resistance is related to decreased compliance (increased stiffness) of the ventricular myocardium.

Causes of a left-sided S_4 include hypertensive heart disease, coronary artery disease, aortic stenosis, and cardiomyopathy. A *left-sided* S_4 is heard best at the apex in the left lateral position; it may sound like "Tennessee." The less common *right-sided* S_4 is heard along the lower left sternal border or below the xiphoid. It often gets louder with inspiration. Causes of a right-sided S_4 include pulmonary hypertension and pulmonic stenosis.

An S_4 may also be associated with delayed conduction between atria and ventricles. This delay separates the normally faint atrial sound from the louder S_1 and makes it audible. An S_4 is never heard in the absence of atrial contraction, which occurs with atrial fibrillation.

Occasionally, a patient has both an S_3 and an S_4, producing a *quadruple rhythm* of four heart sounds. At rapid heart rates, the S_3 and S_4 may merge into one loud extra heart sound, called a *summation gallop*.

TABLE 8-8 — Pansystolic (Holosystolic) Murmurs

Pansystolic (holosystolic) murmurs are pathologic, arising from blood flow from a chamber with high pressure to one of lower pressure, through a valve or other structure that should be closed. The murmur begins immediately with S_1 and continues up to S_2.

	Mitral Regurgitation	Tricuspid Regurgitation	Ventricular Septal Defect
Murmur	*Location.* Apex	*Location.* Lower left sternal border	*Location.* 3rd, 4th, and 5th left interspaces
	Radiation. To the left axilla, less often to the left sternal border	*Radiation.* To the right of the sternum, to the xiphoid area, and perhaps to the left midclavicular line, but not into the axilla	*Radiation.* Often wide
	Intensity. Soft to loud; if loud, associated with an apical thrill	*Intensity.* Variable	*Intensity.* Often very loud, with a thrill
	Pitch. Medium to high	*Pitch.* Medium	*Pitch.* High, holosystolic
	Quality. Harsh, holosystolic	*Quality.* Blowing, holosystolic	*Quality.* Often harsh
	Aids. Unlike tricuspid regurgitation, it does not become louder in inspiration.	*Aids.* Unlike mitral regurgitation, the intensity may increase slightly with inspiration.	
Associated Findings	S_1 is often decreased. An apical S_3 reflects volume overload on the left ventricle. The apical impulse is increased in amplitude and may be *sustained*.	The right ventricular impulse is increased in amplitude and may be *sustained*. An S_3 may be audible along the lower left sternal border. The jugular venous pressure is often elevated, and large *v* waves may be seen in the jugular veins.	A_2 may be obscured by the loud murmur. Findings vary with the severity of the defect and with associated lesions.
Mechanism	When the *mitral valve fails to close fully in systole*, blood regurgitates from left ventricle to left atrium, causing a murmur. This leakage creates volume overload on the left ventricle, with subsequent dilatation and hypertrophy. Several structural abnormalities cause this condition, and findings may vary accordingly.	When the *tricuspid valve fails to close fully in systole*, blood regurgitates from right ventricle to right atrium, producing a murmur. The most common cause is right ventricular failure and dilatation, with resulting enlargement of the tricuspid orifice. Either pulmonary hypertension or left ventricular failure is the usual initiating cause.	A ventricular septal defect is a congenital abnormality in which *blood flows from the relatively high-pressure left ventricle into the low-pressure right ventricle through a hole*. The defect may be accompanied by other abnormalities, but an uncomplicated lesion is described here.

TABLE 8-9   Midsystolic Murmurs

Midsystolic ejection murmurs are the most common kind of heart murmur. They may be (1) *innocent*—without any detectable physiologic or structural abnormality; (2) *physiologic*—from physiologic changes in body metabolism; or (3) *pathologic*—arising from a structural abnormality in the heart or great vessels.[39,40] Midsystolic murmurs tend to peak near midsystole and usually stop before S_2. The crescendo–decrescendo or "diamond" shape is not always audible, but the gap between the murmur and S_2 helps to distinguish midsystolic from pansystolic murmurs.

	Innocent Murmurs	**Physiologic Murmurs**
	S_1 S_2	S_1 S_2
Murmur	*Location.* 2nd to 4th left interspaces between the left sternal border and the apex *Radiation.* Little *Intensity.* Grade 1 to 2, possibly 3 *Pitch.* Soft to medium *Quality.* Variable *Aids.* Usually decreases or disappears on sitting	Similar to innocent murmurs
Associated Findings	None: normal splitting, no ejection sounds, no diastolic murmurs, and no palpable evidence of ventricular enlargement. Occasionally, both an innocent murmur and another kind of murmur are present.	Possible signs of a likely cause
Mechanism	Innocent murmurs result from turbulent blood flow, probably generated by ventricular ejection of blood into the aorta from the left and occasionally the right ventricle. Very common in children and young adults—may also be heard in older people. There is no underlying cardiovascular disease.	Turbulence due to a temporary increase in blood flow in predisposing conditions such as anemia, pregnancy, fever, and hyperthyroidism.

Pathologic Murmurs

Aortic Stenosis[41]	*Hypertrophic Cardiomyopathy*	*Pulmonic Stenosis*

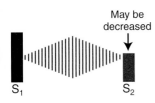

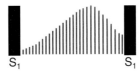

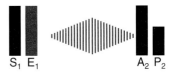

Location. Right 2nd interspace

Radiation. Often to the carotids, down the left sternal border, even to the apex

Intensity. Sometimes soft but often loud, with a thrill

Pitch. Medium, harsh; crescendo–decrescendo may be higher at the apex

Quality. Often harsh; may be more musical at the apex

Aids. Heard best with the patient sitting and leaning forward

A_2 decreases as aortic stenosis worsens. A_2 may be delayed and merge with $P_2 \rightarrow$ single S_2 on expiration or paradoxical S_2 split. Carotid upstroke may be *delayed* with slow rise and small amplitude. Hypertrophied left ventricle may $\rightarrow$ *sustained* apical impulse and an S_4 from decreased compliance.

Significant aortic valve stenosis impairs blood flow across the valve, causing turbulence, and increases left ventricular afterload. Causes are congenital, rheumatic, and degenerative; findings may differ with each cause. Other conditions mimic aortic stenosis without obstructing flow: *aortic sclerosis,* a stiffening of aortic valve leaflets associated with aging; a *bicuspid aortic valve,* a congenital condition that may not be recognized until adulthood; a *dilated aorta,* as in arteriosclerosis, syphilis, or Marfan's syndrome; *pathologically increased flow across the aortic valve* during systole, as in aortic regurgitation.

Location. 3rd and 4th left interspaces

Radiation. Down the left sternal border to the apex, possibly to the base, but not to the neck

Intensity. Variable

Pitch. Medium

Quality. Harsh

Aids. Decreases with squatting, increases with straining down from Valsalva

An S_3 may be present. An S_4 is often present at the apex (unlike mitral regurgitation). The apical impulse may be *sustained* and have two palpable components. The carotid pulse rises *quickly,* unlike the pulse in aortic stenosis.

Massive ventricular hypertrophy is associated with unusually rapid ejection of blood from the left ventricle during systole. Outflow tract obstruction to flow may coexist. Accompanying distortion of the mitral valve may cause mitral regurgitation.

Location. 2nd and 3rd left interspaces

Radiation. If loud, toward the left shoulder and neck

Intensity. Soft to loud; if loud, associated with a thrill

Pitch. Medium; crescendo–decrescendo

Quality. Often harsh

In severe stenosis, S_2 is widely split, and P_2 is diminished or inaudible. An early pulmonic ejection sound is common. May hear a right-sided S_4. Right ventricular impulse often increased in amplitude and *sustained.*

Pulmonic valve stenosis impairs flow across the valve, increasing right ventricular afterload. Congenital and usually found in children. In an *atrial septal defect,* the systolic murmur from pathologically increased flow across the pulmonic valve may mimic pulmonic stenosis.

TABLE 8-10   Diastolic Murmurs

Diastolic murmurs almost always indicate heart disease. There are two basic types. *Early decrescendo diastolic murmurs* signify regurgitant flow through an incompetent semilunar valve, more commonly the aortic. *Rumbling diastolic murmurs in mid- or late diastole* suggest stenosis of an atrioventricular valve, usually the mitral.

	Aortic Regurgitation[43,44]	**Mitral Stenosis**
Murmur	*Location.* 2nd to 4th left interspaces	*Location.* Usually limited to the apex
	Radiation. If loud, to the apex, perhaps to the right sternal border	*Radiation.* Little or none
	Intensity. Grade 1 to 3	*Intensity.* Grade 1 to 4
	Pitch. High. *Use the diaphragm.*	*Pitch.* Decrescendo low-pitched rumble. *Use the bell.*
	Quality. Blowing decrescendo; may be mistaken for breath sounds	
	Aids. The murmur is heard best with the *patient sitting, leaning forward*, with breath held after exhalation.	*Aids.* Placing the bell exactly on the apical impulse, turning the patient into a *left lateral position*, and mild exercise all help to make the murmur audible. It is heard better in exhalation.
Associated Findings	An ejection sound may be present.	S_1 is accentuated and may be palpable at the apex.
	An S_3 or S_4, if present, suggests severe regurgitation.	An opening snap (OS) often follows S_2 and initiates the murmur.
	Progressive changes in the apical impulse include increased amplitude, displacement laterally and downward, widened diameter, and increased duration.	If pulmonary hypertension develops, P_2 is accentuated, and the right ventricular impulse becomes palpable.
	The pulse pressure increases, and *arterial pulses are often large and bounding.* A midsystolic flow murmur or an Austin Flint murmur suggests large regurgitant flow.	Mitral regurgitation and aortic valve disease may be associated with mitral stenosis.
Mechanism	The leaflets of the aortic valve fail to close completely during diastole, and blood regurgitates from the aorta back into the left ventricle. Volume overload on the left ventricle results. Two other murmurs may be associated: (1) a midsystolic murmur from the resulting increased forward flow across the aortic valve, and (2) a mitral diastolic (*Austin Flint*) murmur, attributed to diastolic impingement of the regurgitant flow on the anterior leaflet of the mitral valve.	When the leaflets of the mitral valve thicken, stiffen, and become distorted from the effects of rheumatic fever, the *mitral valve fails to open sufficiently in diastole.* The resulting murmur has two components: (1) middiastolic (during rapid ventricular filling), and (2) presystolic (during atrial contraction). The latter disappears if atrial fibrillation develops, leaving only a middiastolic rumble.

Some cardiovascular sounds extend beyond one phase of the cardiac cycle. Three examples, further described below, are: (1) a *venous hum*, a benign sound produced by turbulence of blood in the jugular veins—common in children; (2) a *pericardial friction rub*, produced by inflammation of the pericardial sac; and (3) *patent ductus arteriosus*, a congenital abnormality in which an open channel persists between aorta and pulmonary artery. *Continuous murmurs* begin in systole and extend through S_2 into all or part of diastole, as in *patent ductus arteriosus*.

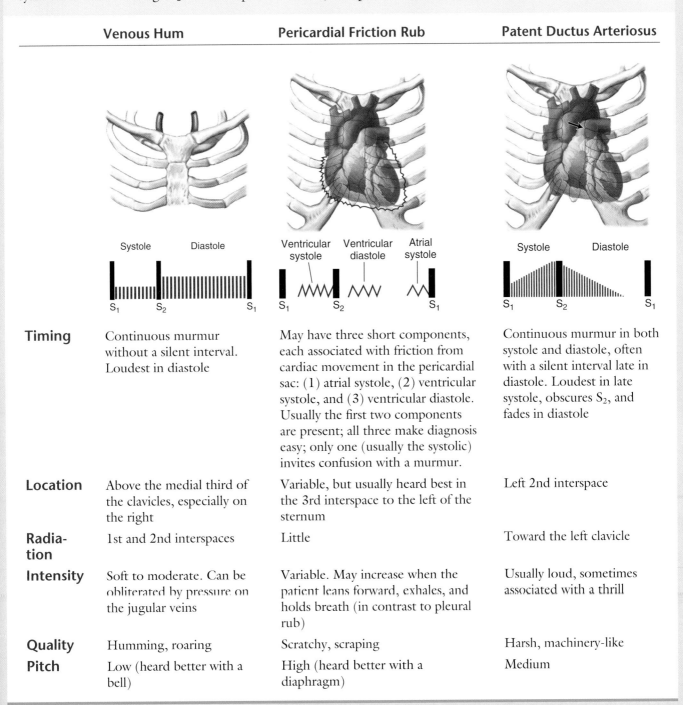

	Venous Hum	**Pericardial Friction Rub**	**Patent Ductus Arteriosus**
Timing	Continuous murmur without a silent interval. Loudest in diastole	May have three short components, each associated with friction from cardiac movement in the pericardial sac: (1) atrial systole, (2) ventricular systole, and (3) ventricular diastole. Usually the first two components are present; all three make diagnosis easy; only one (usually the systolic) invites confusion with a murmur.	Continuous murmur in both systole and diastole, often with a silent interval late in diastole. Loudest in late systole, obscures S_2, and fades in diastole
Location	Above the medial third of the clavicles, especially on the right	Variable, but usually heard best in the 3rd interspace to the left of the sternum	Left 2nd interspace
Radiation	1st and 2nd interspaces	Little	Toward the left clavicle
Intensity	Soft to moderate. Can be obliterated by pressure on the jugular veins	Variable. May increase when the patient leans forward, exhales, and holds breath (in contrast to pleural rub)	Usually loud, sometimes associated with a thrill
Quality	Humming, roaring	Scratchy, scraping	Harsh, machinery-like
Pitch	Low (heard better with a bell)	High (heard better with a diaphragm)	Medium

The Breasts and Axillae

ANATOMY AND PHYSIOLOGY

The Female Breast

The female breast lies against the anterior thoracic wall, extending from the clavicle and 2nd rib down to the 6th rib, and from the sternum across to the midaxillary line. Its surface area is generally rectangular rather than round.

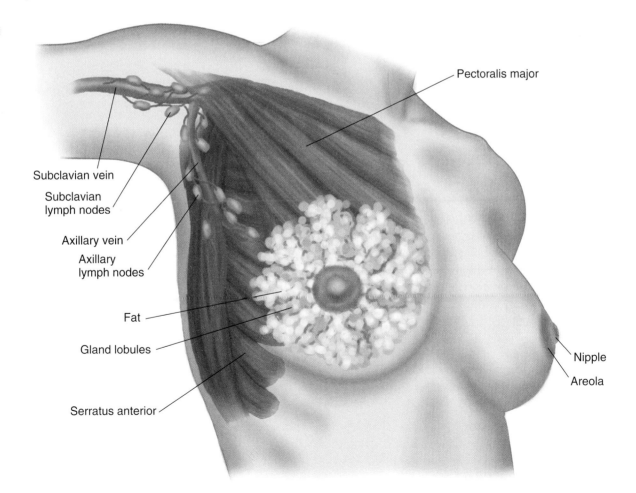

Pectoralis major

Subclavian vein

Subclavian lymph nodes

Axillary vein

Axillary lymph nodes

Fat

Gland lobules

Serratus anterior

Nipple

Areola

The breast overlies the pectoralis major and at its inferior margin, the serratus anterior.

To describe clinical findings, the breast is often divided into four quadrants based on horizontal and vertical lines crossing at the nipple. An axillary tail of breast tissue extends toward the anterior axillary fold. Alternatively, findings can be localized as the time on the face of a clock (e.g., 3 o'clock) and the distance in centimeters from the nipple.

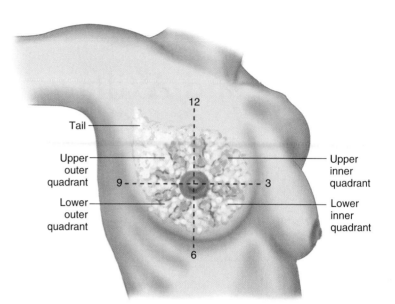

The breast is hormonally sensitive tissue, responsive to the changes of monthly cycling and aging. *Glandular tissue*, namely secretory tubuloalveolar glands and ducts, forms 15 to 20 septated *lobes* radiating around the nipple. Within each lobe are many smaller *lobules*. These drain into milk-producing ducts and sinuses that open onto the surface of the *areola*, or nipple. *Fibrous connective tissue* provides structural support in the form of fibrous bands or suspensory ligaments connected to both the skin and the underlying fascia. *Adipose tissue*, or fat, surrounds the breast, predominantly in the superficial and peripheral areas. The proportions of these components vary with age, the general state of nutrition, pregnancy, exogenous hormone use, and other factors.

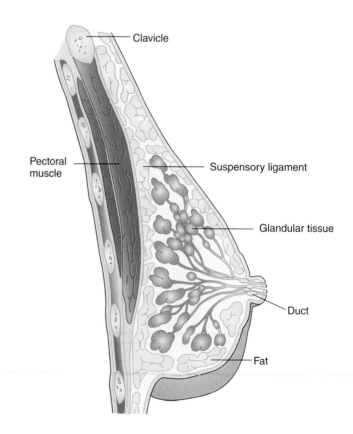

The surface of the areola has small, rounded elevations formed by sebaceous glands, sweat glands, and accessory areolar glands. A few hairs are often seen on the areola.

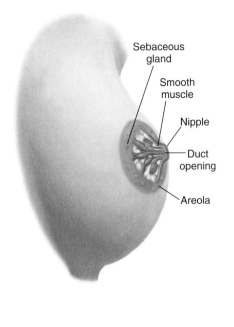

Both the nipple and the areola are well supplied with smooth muscle that contracts to express milk from the ductal system during breast-feeding. Rich sensory innervation, especially in the nipple, triggers "milk letdown" following neurohormonal stimulation from infant sucking. Tactile stimulation of the area, including the breast examination, makes the nipple smaller, firmer, and more erect, whereas the areola puckers and wrinkles. These smooth muscle reflexes are normal and should not be mistaken for signs of breast disease.

The adult breast may be soft, but it often feels granular, nodular, or lumpy. This uneven texture is normal and may be termed *physiologic nodularity*. It is often bilateral. It may be evident throughout the breast or only in parts of it. The nodularity may increase before menses—a time when breasts often enlarge and become tender or even painful. For breast changes during adolescence and pregnancy, see pp. 778–779 and p. 818.

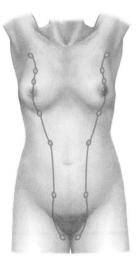

Occasionally, one or more extra or supernumerary nipples are located along the "milk line," illustrated on the right. Only a small nipple and areola are usually present, often mistaken for a common mole. There may be underlying glandular tissue. An extra nipple has no pathologic significance.

■ THE MALE BREAST

The *male breast* consists chiefly of a small nipple and areola. These overlie a thin disc of undeveloped breast tissue that may not be distinguishable clinically from the surrounding tissues. A firm button of breast tissue 2 cm or more in diameter has been described in roughly one of three adult men. The limits of normal have not yet been clearly established.

■ LYMPHATICS

Lymphatics from most of the breast drain toward the axilla. Of the axillary lymph nodes, the *central nodes* are palpable most frequently. They lie along the chest wall, usually high in the axilla and midway between the anterior and posterior axillary folds. Into them drain channels from three other groups of lymph nodes, which are seldom palpable:

- *Pectoral nodes—anterior,* located along the lower border of the pectoralis major inside the anterior axillary fold. These nodes drain the anterior chest wall and much of the breast.

- *Subscapular nodes—posterior,* located along the lateral border of the scapula; palpated deep in the posterior axillary fold. They drain the posterior chest wall and a portion of the arm.

- *Lateral nodes—*located *along the upper humerus.* They drain most of the arm.

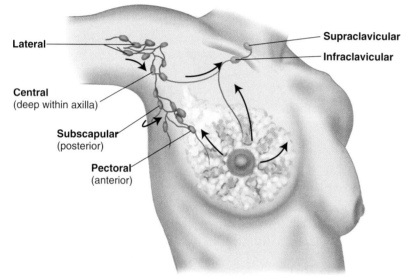

ARROWS INDICATE DIRECTION OF LYMPH FLOW

Lymph drains from the central axillary nodes to the *infraclavicular* and *supraclavicular* nodes.

Not all the lymphatics of the breast drain into the axilla. Malignant cells from a breast cancer may spread directly to the infraclavicular nodes or into deep channels within the chest.

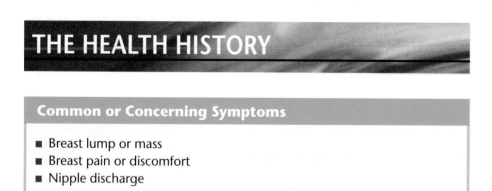

THE HEALTH HISTORY

Common or Concerning Symptoms

- Breast lump or mass
- Breast pain or discomfort
- Nipple discharge

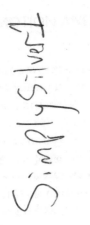

Simply Silver

...uded in the history or deferred
...mine your breasts?" ... "How
...he examines the breast during
...ne when estrogen stimulation
...et of menses. Ask whether she
...sts. About 50% of women have
...al enlargement and tenderness
...mass, ask about the precise lo-
...change in size or variation with

Lumps may be physiologic or pathologic, ranging from cysts and fibroadenomas to breast cancer. See Table 9-1, Visible Signs of Breast Cancer (p. 356), and Table 9-2, Common Breast Masses, (p. 357).

Also ask about any *discharge from the nipples* and when it occurs. If it appears only after squeezing the nipple, it is considered physiologic. If the discharge is spontaneous and seen on the underwear or nightclothes without local stimulation, ask about its color, consistency, and quantity. Is it unilateral or bilateral?

A milky bilateral discharge, or *galactorrhea,* may reflect pregnancy or prolactin or other hormonal imbalance.

Spontaneous persistent nonlactational discharge that is bloody or unilateral suggests local breast disease from *papilloma* or, rarely, possible *breast cancer.*

HEALTH PROMOTION AND COUNSELING

Important Topics for Health Promotion and Counseling

- Risk factors for breast cancer
- Breast cancer screening
- Breast self-examination (BSE)

Women may experience a wide range of changes in breast tissue and sensation, from cyclic swelling and nodularity to a distinct lump or mass. The examination of the breast provides a meaningful opportunity for the clinician and the female patient to explore concerns important to women's health—what to do if a lump or mass is detected, risk factors for breast cancer, and screening measures such as breast self-examination, the clinical breast examination (CBE) by a skilled clinician, and mammography.

Breast masses show marked variation in etiology, from fibroadenomas and cysts seen in younger women, to abscess or mastitis, to primary breast cancer. All breast masses warrant careful evaluation. On initial assessment, the woman's age and physical characteristics of the mass provide clues to its origin, but definitive diagnostic measures should be pursued.

■ Palpable Masses of the Breast

Age	Common Lesion	Characteristics
15–25	Fibroadenoma	Usually fine, round, mobile, nontender
25–50	Cysts	Usually soft to firm, round, mobile; often tender
	Fibrocystic changes	Nodular, ropelike
	Cancer	Irregular, stellate, firm, not clearly delineated from surrounding tissue
Over 50	Cancer until proven otherwise	As above
Pregnancy/lactation	Lactating adenomas, cysts, mastitis, and cancer	As above

Adapted from Schultz MZ, Ward BA, Reiss M. Breast diseases. In Noble J, Greene HL, Levinson W, et al. (eds). Primary Care Medicine, 2nd ed. St. Louis, Mosby, 1996. See also Venet L, Strax P, Venet W, et al. Adequacies and inadequacies of breast examinations by physicians in mass screenings. Cancer 28(6):1546–1551, 1971.

Risk Factors for Breast Cancer. Breast cancer is the most common cause of cancer in women worldwide, accounting for more than 10% of all female malignancies. In the United States, a woman born now has a 13% lifetime risk for developing breast cancer. The probability of diagnosis increases by decade: from age 30 to 40, ≤0.5%; from age 40 to 50, 1.49%; from age 50 to 60, 2.79%; and from age 60 to 70, 3.38%.[1] Breast cancer is the second leading cause of cancer death in women, with highest mortality rates in women younger than 35 and older than 75. Mortality rates have declined for white women younger than 55, probably as a result of more widespread use of mammography and more aggressive treatment regimens, but have increased for African American women.[2]

Women with *breast symptoms* merit active investigation. Breast cancer may occur in up to 4% of women with breast complaints and in up to 11% of women complaining specifically of a breast lump or mass.[3] Also pursue complaints of nipple discharge. Although most nipple discharge is benign, approximately 5% of women may have associated breast cancer, especially in older age groups.[4]

Rarely, men report concerns about a breast mass. Breast cancer in men is ≤1% of all breast cancers and is usually diagnosed between the ages of 60 and 70. Risk factors include estrogen exposure, including excess estrogen stimulation in Klinefelter's syndrome or cirrhosis; radiation exposure; and positive family history in female relatives.

For *screening of asymptomatic women*, target risk factors, including family history. Risk factors for breast cancer are present in up to 55% of cases, and a positive family history is present in an additional 10%.[2] The clinician and individual patient should review age and demographic data, family history, reproductive history, and any prior history of proliferative breast disease, especially if a biopsy has shown atypical hyperplasia or lobular carcinoma in situ. Several models help establish the woman patient's risk of breast cancer. The Breast Cancer Risk Assessment Tool of the National Cancer Institute (http://bcra.nci.nih.gov/brc/) and the Gail model are among the most widely used.[5,6]

■ Summary of Breast Cancer Risk Factors

Factor	Relative Risk (%)
Family History	
First-degree relative with breast cancer	1.2–3.0
Premenopausal	3.1
Premenopausal and bilateral	8.5–9.0
Postmenopausal	1.5
Postmenopausal and bilateral	4.0–5.4
BRCA1/BRCA2 genes	3.0–7.0
Menstrual History	
Age at menarche <12	1.3
Age at menopause >55	1.5–2.0
Pregnancy	
First live birth from ages 25–29	1.5
First live birth after age 30	1.9
First live birth after age 35	2.0–3.0
Nulliparous	3.0
Breast Conditions and Diseases	
Nonproliferative disease	1.0
Proliferative disease	1.9
Proliferative with atypical hyperplasia	4.4
Lobular carcinoma in situ	6.9–12.0
Breast density on mammography	1.8–6.0

Adapted from Bilmoria MM, Morrow M. The woman at increased risk for breast cancer: evaluation and management strategies. CA Cancer J Clin 45(5):263, 1995, and from Clemons M, Goss P. Estrogen and the risk of breast cancer. N Engl J Med 344(4):276–285, 2001.

Demographic Factors—Age, Education and Income, Location, Ethnicity.[2] Currently, the cumulative lifetime risk for breast cancer is approximately one in seven, and approximately one in nine for invasive breast cancer, reflecting earlier diagnosis of in situ cancers on mammography. More than three fourths of breast cancer cases occur in women older than age 50, and more than half in women older than age 65. Higher education and income levels appear to double the risk for breast cancer, possibly because of differences in age at first birth and parity. Risk is highest in urban areas and varies by region (highest in Hawaii and lowest in Utah) and ethnicity. Rates are highest among Caucasian women, then fall successively for African Americans, Latinas, and Asian Americans.

Family History. The relative risk for breast cancer, or risk relative to an individual without a given risk factor, associated with menarche and menopause, age of first pregnancy, and breast conditions and diseases is summarized in the table above. Risk for familial breast cancer falls into two patterns: family history of breast cancer and genetic predisposition. First-degree relatives, namely a mother or sister with breast cancer, establish a "positive family history." Within this group, menopausal status and extent of disease play key roles. Having a first-degree relative with breast cancer who is premenopausal confers highest risk. Even when a mother or sister has bilateral breast cancer, however, the probability of breast cancer is only 25%.[7]

Inherited disease in women carrying the breast cancer susceptibility genes *BRCA1* and *BRCA2* accounts for 5% to 10% of breast cancers.[8] These genes are autosomal dominant, and, when present, risk for cancer is 50% in women younger than age 50 and 80% in women older than age 65. Red flags for these mutations include multiple relatives with breast cancer, ovarian cancer, or both; a woman with more than one primary cancer (e.g., bilateral disease or combined breast and ovarian); and vertical transmission through two or more generations.

Menstrual History and Pregnancy. Early menarche, delayed menopause, and first live birth after age 35 each raise the risk for breast cancer twofold to threefold. These factors, especially when combined, relate to duration of breast tissue exposure to stimulation from unopposed estrogen.[9]

Breast Conditions and Diseases. Benign breast disease with biopsy findings of atypical hyperplasia or lobular carcinoma in situ carries significantly increased relative risks—4.4 and 6.9 to 12.0, respectively.

Breast Cancer Screening. Although not validated as a method for detecting breast cancer, recent guidelines support *breast self-examination* (BSE) as a means of promoting health awareness. Women choosing to do BSE should be instructed about technique and encouraged to report any new breast symptoms. For women at average risk for breast cancer, the American Cancer Society recommends *clinical breast examination* (CBE) by a health professional every 3 years for women between ages 20 and 39 then annually after age 40 and annual *mammography* beginning at age 40.[10, 11] Intervals for mammography between ages 40 and 50, however, are still subject to controversy. Mammography is less accurate in breasts that are glandular and dense, especially when stimulated by higher estrogen levels before menopause, contributing to varying estimates of benefit. For women at increased risk, many clinicians advise initiating screening mammograms between ages 30 and 40, then every 2 to 3 years until age 50. For women between the ages of 50 and 69, annual CBE and mammography are widely recommended.[7]

After age 70, the benefits of mammography are less well defined. The American Geriatrics Society recommends mammography every 1 to 3 years after age 75 for women with a life expectancy of 4 years or more, particularly in the presence of risk factors or long-term exposure to hormone replacement therapy. If comorbid conditions limit life expectancy, including dementia, clinicians should discuss the decision of mammography with the patient and her family because the benefit of screening will be reduced.[12]

TECHNIQUES OF EXAMINATION

■ THE FEMALE BREAST

The clinical breast examination is an important component of women's health care: it enhances detection of breast cancers that mammography may miss and provides an opportunity to demonstrate techniques for self-examination to the patient. Clinical investigation has shown, however, that variations in examiner experience and technique affect the value of the clinical breast examination. Clinicians are advised to adopt a more standardized approach, especially for palpation, and to use a systemic and thorough search pattern, varying palpation pressure, and a circular motion with the fingerpads.[13] These techniques will be discussed in more detail in the following pages. Inspection is routinely recommended, but its value in breast cancer detection is less well studied.

As you begin the examination of the breasts, be aware that women and girls may feel apprehensive. Be reassuring and adopt a courteous and gentle approach. Before you begin, let the patient know that you are about to examine her breasts. This may be a good time to ask if she has noticed any lumps or other problems and if she performs a monthly breast self-examination. If she does not, teach her good technique and watch as she repeats the steps of examination after you, giving helpful correction as needed.

An adequate inspection requires full exposure of the chest, but later in the examination, cover one breast while you are palpating the other. Because breasts tend to swell and become more nodular before menses as a result of increasing estrogen stimulation, the best time for examination is 5 to 7 days *after* the onset of menstruation. Nodules appearing during the premenstrual phase should be reevaluated at this later time.

INSPECTION

Inspect the breasts and nipples with the patient in the sitting position and disrobed to the waist. A thorough examination of the breast includes careful inspection for skin changes, symmetry, contours, and retraction in four views—arms at sides, arms over head, arms pressed against hips, and leaning forward. When examining an adolescent girl, assess her breast development according to Tanner's sex maturity ratings described on page 779.

Arms at Sides.   Note the clinical features listed below.

■ The *appearance of the skin,* including

   Color

   Thickening of the skin and unusually prominent pores, which may accompany lymphatic obstruction

Side notes (Examples of Abnormalities):

Risk factors for breast cancer include previous breast cancer, an affected mother or sister, biopsy showing atypical hyperplasia, increasing age, early menarche, late menopause, late or no pregnancies, and previous radiation to the chest wall.

See Patient Instructions for the Breast Self-Examination, p. 353.

Redness may be from local infection or inflammatory carcinoma.

Thickening and prominent pores suggest breast cancer.

■ The *size and symmetry of the breasts.* Some difference in the size of the breasts, including the areolae, is common and is usually normal, as shown in the photograph below.

■ The *contour of the breasts.* Look for changes such as masses, dimpling, or flattening. Compare one side with the other.

Flattening of the normally convex breast suggests cancer. See Table 9-1, Visible Signs of Breast Cancer (p. 356).

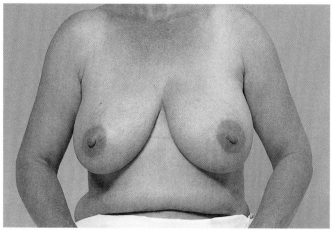

ARMS AT SIDES

■ The *characteristics of the nipples,* including *size and shape, direction* in which they point, any *rashes* or *ulceration,* or any *discharge.*

Asymmetry of directions in which nipples point suggests an underlying cancer. Rash or ulceration in Paget's disease of the breast (see p. 356).

Occasionally, the shape of the nipple is *inverted,* or depressed below the areolar surface. It may be enveloped by folds of areolar skin, as illustrated. Long-standing inversion is usually a normal variant of no clinical consequence, except for possible difficulty when breast-feeding.

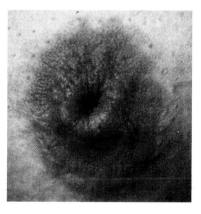

Recent or fixed flattening or depression of the nipple suggests nipple retraction. A retracted nipple may also be broadened and thickened, suggesting an underlying cancer.

Arms Over Head; Hands Pressed Against Hips; Leaning Forward. To bring out dimpling or retraction that may otherwise be invisible, ask the patient to raise her arms over her head, then press her hands against her hips to contract the pectoral muscles. Inspect the breast contours carefully in each position. If the breasts are large or pendulous, it may be useful to have the patient stand and lean forward, supported by the back of the chair or the examiner's hands.

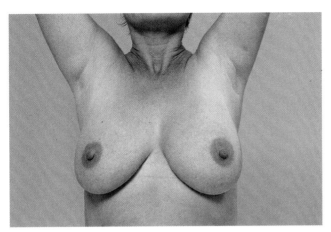

ARMS OVER HEAD

Dimpling or retraction of the breasts in these positions suggests an underlying cancer. When a cancer or its associated fibrous strands are attached to both the skin and the fascia overlying the pectoral muscles, pectoral contraction can draw the skin inward, causing dimpling.

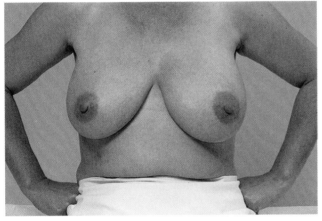

HANDS PRESSED AGAINST HIPS

Occasionally, these signs may be associated with benign lesions such as posttraumatic fat necrosis or mammary duct ectasia, but they must always be further evaluated.

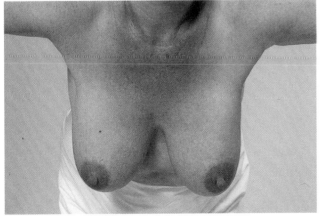

LEANING FORWARD

This position may reveal an asymmetry of the breast or nipple not otherwise visible. Retraction of the nipple and areola suggests an underlying cancer. See Table 9-1, Visible Signs of Breast Cancer (p. 356).

PALPATION

The Breast.   Palpation is best performed when the breast tissue is flattened. The patient should be supine. Plan to palpate a rectangular area extending from the clavicle to the inframammary fold or bra line, and from the midsternal line to the posterior axillary line and well into the axilla for the tail of the breast.

A thorough examination will take 3 minutes for each breast. Use the *finger-pads* of the 2nd, 3rd, and 4th fingers, keeping the fingers slightly flexed. It is important to be *systematic*. Although a circular or wedge pattern can be used, the *vertical strip pattern* is currently the best validated technique for detecting breast masses. Palpate in *small, concentric circles* at each examining point, if possible applying light, medium, and deep pressure. You will need to press more firmly to reach the deeper tissues of a large breast. Your examination should cover the entire breast, including the periphery, tail, and axilla.

When pressing deeply on the breast, you may mistake a normal rib for a hard breast mass.

■ To examine *the lateral portion of the breast,* ask the patient to roll onto the opposite hip, placing her hand on her forehead but keeping the shoulders pressed against the bed or examining table. This flattens the lateral breast tissue. Begin palpation in the axilla, moving in a straight line down to the bra line, then move the fingers medially and palpate in a vertical strip up the chest to the clavicle. Continue in vertical overlapping strips until you reach the nipple, then reposition the patient to flatten the medial portion of the breast.

Nodules in the tail of the breast are sometimes mistaken for enlarged axillary lymph nodes (and vice versa).

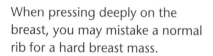

■ To examine *the medial portion of the breast,* ask the patient to lie with her shoulders flat against the bed or examining table, placing her hand at her neck and lifting up her elbow until it is even with her shoulder. Palpate in a straight line down from the nipple to the bra line, then back to the clavicle, continuing in vertical overlapping strips to the midsternum.

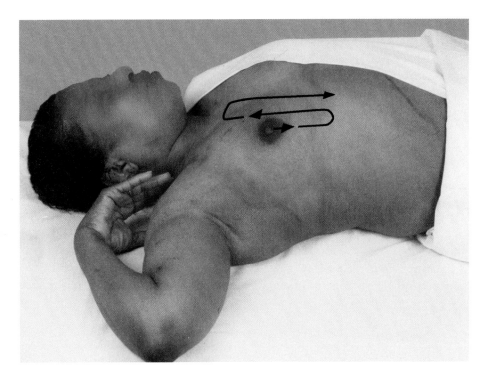

Examine the breast tissue carefully for:

- *Consistency* of the tissues. Normal consistency varies widely, depending in part on the relative proportions of firmer glandular tissue and soft fat. Physiologic nodularity may be present, increasing before menses. There may be a firm transverse ridge of compressed tissue along the lower margin of the breast, especially in large breasts. This is the normal inframammary ridge, not a tumor.

- *Tenderness*, as in premenstrual fullness

- *Nodules.* Palpate carefully for any lump or mass that is qualitatively different from or larger than the rest of the breast tissue. This is sometimes called a dominant mass and may reflect a pathologic change that requires evaluation by mammogram, aspiration, or biopsy. Assess and describe the characteristics of any nodule:

    Location—by quadrant or clock, with centimeters from the nipple

    Size—in centimeters

    Shape—round or cystic, disclike, or irregular in contour

    Consistency—soft, firm, or hard

    Delimitation—well circumscribed or not

    Tenderness

    Mobility—in relation to the skin, pectoral fascia, and chest wall. Gently move the breast near the mass and watch for dimpling.

Tender cords suggest *mammary duct ectasia,* a benign but sometimes painful condition of dilated ducts with surrounding inflammation, sometimes with associated masses.

See Table 9-2, Common Breast Masses (p. 357).

Hard, irregular, poorly circumscribed nodules, fixed to the skin or underlying tissues, strongly suggest cancer.

Cysts, inflamed areas; some cancers may be tender.

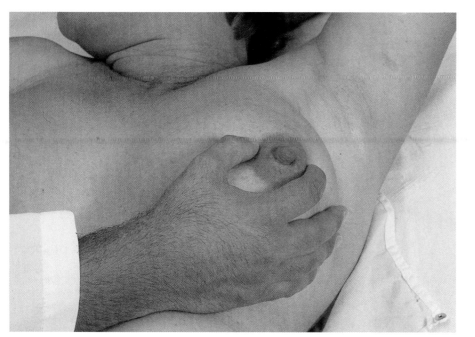

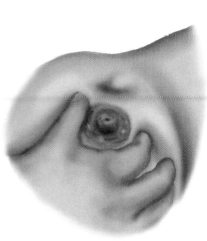

Next, try to move the mass itself while the patient relaxes her arm and then while she presses her hand against her hip.

A mobile mass that becomes fixed when the arm relaxes is attached to the ribs and intercostal muscles; if fixed when the hand is pressed against the hip, it is attached to the pectoral fascia.

The Nipple. Palpate each nipple, noting its elasticity.

Thickening of the nipple and loss of elasticity suggest an underlying cancer.

◢ THE MALE BREAST

Examination of the male breast may be brief but is important. *Inspect the nipple and areola* for nodules, swelling, or ulceration. *Palpate the areola and breast tissue* for nodules. If the breast appears enlarged, distinguish between the soft fatty enlargement of obesity and the firm disc of glandular enlargement, called *gynecomastia.*

Gynecomastia is attributed to an imbalance of estrogens and androgens, sometimes drug related. A hard, irregular, eccentric, or ulcerating nodule is not gynecomastia and suggests breast cancer.

◢ THE AXILLAE

Although the axillae may be examined with the patient lying down, a sitting position is preferable.

INSPECTION

Inspect the skin of each axilla, noting evidence of:

- Rash

- Infection

- Unusual pigmentation

Deodorant and other rashes

Sweat gland infection (*hidradenitis suppurativa*)

Deeply pigmented, velvety axillary skin suggests *acanthosis nigricans*—one form is associated with internal malignancy.

PALPATION

To examine the left axilla, ask the patient to relax with the left arm down. Help by supporting the left wrist or hand with your left hand. Cup together the fingers of your right hand and reach as high as you can toward the apex of the axilla. Warn the patient that this may feel uncomfortable. Your fingers should lie directly behind the pectoral muscles, pointing toward the midclavicle. Now press your fingers in toward the chest wall and slide them downward, trying to feel the central nodes against the chest wall. Of the axillary nodes, these are the most often palpable. One or more soft, small (<1 cm), nontender nodes are frequently felt.

Enlarged axillary nodes from infection of the hand or arm, recent immunizations or skin tests in the arm, or part of a generalized lymphadenopathy. Check the epitrochlear nodes and other groups of lymph nodes.

Nodes that are large (≥1 cm) and firm or hard, matted together, or fixed to the skin or to underlying tissues suggest malignant involvement.

Use your left hand to examine the right axilla.

If the central nodes feel large, hard, or tender, or if there is a suspicious lesion in the drainage areas for the axillary nodes, feel for the other groups of axillary lymph nodes:

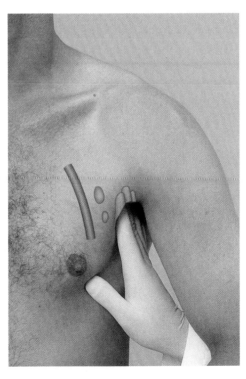

- *Pectoral nodes*—grasp the anterior axillary fold between your thumb and fingers, and with your fingers, palpate inside the border of the pectoral muscle.

- *Lateral nodes*—from high in the axilla, feel along the upper humerus.

- *Subscapular nodes*—step behind the patient and, with your fingers, feel inside the muscle of the posterior axillary fold.

Also, feel for infraclavicular nodes and re-examine the supraclavicular nodes.

■ SPECIAL TECHNIQUES

Assessment of Spontaneous Nipple Discharge. If there is a history of spontaneous nipple discharge, try to determine its origin by compressing the areola with your index finger, placed in radial positions around the nipple. Watch for discharge appearing through one of the duct openings on the nipple's surface. Note the color, consistency, and quantity of any discharge and the exact location where it appears.

Milky discharge unrelated to a prior pregnancy and lactation is called *nonpuerperal galactorrhea.* Leading causes are hormonal and pharmacologic.

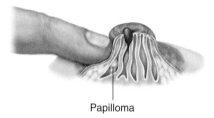
Papilloma

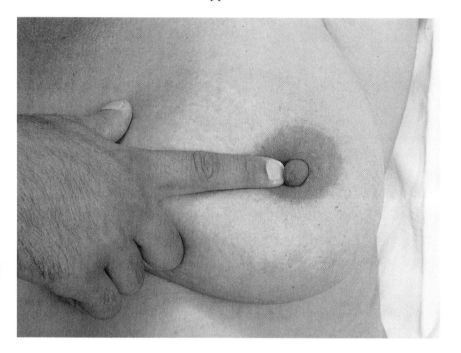

A nonmilky unilateral discharge suggests local breast disease. The causative lesion is usually benign, but may be malignant, especially in elderly women. A benign intraductal papilloma is shown above in its usual subareolar location. Note the drop of blood exuding from a duct opening.

Examination of the Mastectomy Patient. The woman with a mastectomy warrants special care on examination. Inspect the mastectomy scar and axilla carefully for any masses or unusual nodularity. Note any change in color or signs of inflammation. Lymphedema may be present in the axilla and upper arm from impaired lymph drainage after surgery. Palpate gently along the scar—these tissues may be unusually sensitive. Use a circular motion with two or three fingers. Pay special attention to the upper outer quadrant and axilla. Note any enlargement of the lymph nodes or signs of inflammation or infection.

Masses, nodularity, and change in color or inflammation, especially in the incision line, suggest recurrence of breast cancer.

It is especially important to carefully palpate the breast tissue and incision lines of women with breast augmentation or reconstruction.

Instructions for the Breast Self-Examination. The office or hospital visit is an important time to teach the patient how to perform the breast self-examination (BSE). A high proportion of breast masses are detected by women examining their own breasts. Although BSE has not been shown to reduce breast cancer mortality, monthly BSE is inexpensive and may promote stronger health awareness and more active self-care. For early detection of breast cancer, the BSE is most useful when coupled with regular breast examination by an experienced clinician and mammography. The BSE is best timed just after menses, when hormonal stimulation of breast tissue is low.

PATIENT INSTRUCTIONS FOR THE BREAST SELF-EXAMINATION (BSE)

Lying Supine

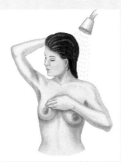

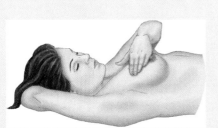

1. Lie down with a pillow under your right shoulder. Place your right arm behind your head.
2. Use the finger pads of the three middle fingers on your left hand to feel for lumps in the right breast. The finger pads are the top third of each finger.
3. Press firmly enough to know how your breast feels. A firm ridge in the lower curve of each breast is normal. If you're not sure how hard to press, talk with your health care provider, or try to copy the way the doctor or nurse does it.

4. Press firmly on the breast in an up-and-down or "strip" pattern. You can also use a circular or wedge pattern, but be sure to use the same pattern every time. Check the entire breast area, and remember how your breast feels from month to month.
5. Repeat the examination on your left breast, using the finger pads of the right hand.
6. If you find any masses, lumps, or skin changes, see your doctor right away.

Standing

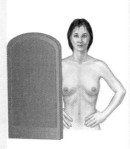

1. Repeat the examination of both breasts while standing, with one arm behind your head. The upright position makes it easier to check the upper outer part of the breasts (toward your armpit). This is where about half of breast cancers are found. You may want to do the upright part of the BSE while you are in the shower. Your soapy hands will make it easy to check how your breasts feel as they glide over the wet skin.

2. For added safety, you might want to check your breasts by standing in front of a mirror right after your BSE each month. See If there are any changes in the way your breasts look, such as dimpling of the skin, changes in the nipple, redness, or swelling.
3. If you find any masses, lumps, or skin changes, see your doctor right away.

Adapted from the American Cancer Society. Available at: www.cancer.org. Accessed November 17, 2004.

RECORDING YOUR FINDINGS

Note that initially you may use sentences to describe your findings; later you will use phrases. The style below contains phrases appropriate for most write-ups.

Recording the Physical Examination—Breasts and Axillae

"Breasts symmetric and without masses. Nipples without discharge." (Axillary adenopathy usually included after Neck in section on Lymph Nodes, see p. 203.)

OR

"Breasts pendulous with diffuse fibrocystic changes. Single firm 1 × 1 cm mass, mobile and nontender, with overlying peau d'orange appearance in right breast, upper outer quadrant at 11 o'clock."

Suggests possible breast cancer

Bibliography

CITATIONS

1. National Cancer Institute. Cancer Facts. Available at: http://cis.nci.nih.gov/fact/5_6.htm. Accessed November 4, 2004.
2. Costanza ME. Epidemiology and risk factors for breast cancer. Available at: www.utdol.com. Accessed November 4, 2004.
3. Barton MB, Elmore JG, Fletcher SW. Breast symptoms among women enrolled in a health maintenance organization: frequency, evaluation, and outcome. Ann Intern Med 130(8): 651–657, 1999.
4. Murad TM, Contesso G, Mouriesse H. Nipple discharge from the breast. Ann Surg 195(3):259–264, 1982.
5. Gail MH, Brinton LA, Byar DP, et al. Projecting individualized probabilities of developing breast cancer for white females who are being examined annually. J Natl Cancer Inst 81: 1879–1886, 1989.
6. Gail MH, Benichou J. Validation studies on a model for breast cancer risk (editorial). J Natl Cancer Inst 86:573–575, 1994.
7. U.S. Preventive Services Task Force. Screening for breast cancer. In: Guide to Clinical Preventive Services, 2nd ed. Baltimore, Williams & Wilkins, 73–87, 1996.
8. Peshkin BN, Isaacs C. Risk assessment in women with an inherited predisposition to cancer. Available at: http://www.utdol.com. Accessed November 4, 2004.
9. Clemons M, Goss P. Estrogen and the risk of breast cancer. N Engl J Med 344(4):276–285, 2001.
10. Smith RA, Saslow D, Sawyer KA, et al. American Cancer Society guidelines for breast cancer screening: update 2003. CA Cancer J Clin 53(3):141–169, 2003.
11. American Cancer Society. How to perform a breast self exam. Available at: www.cancer.org. Accessed November 4, 2004.
12. American Geriatrics Society Clinical Practice Committee. Position statement: breast cancer screening in older women. Available at: http://www.americangeriatrics.org. Accessed November 4, 2004.
13. Barton MB, Harris R, Fletcher S. Does this patient have breast cancer? The screening clinical breast examination: should it be done? How? JAMA 282(13):1270–1280, 1999.

ADDITIONAL REFERENCES

American Geriatrics Society Clinical Practice Committee. Position Statement: Breast Cancer Screening in Older Women. Available at: http://www.americangeriatrics.org. Accessed November 4, 2004.

Bland KI, Vezerdis MP, Copeland EM. Breast (Chapter 16). In Brunicardi FC, Schwartz SI (eds). Schwartz's Principles of Surgery, 8th ed. New York: McGraw-Hill Medical, 2005.

Armstrong K, Eisen A, Weber B. Assessing the risk of breast cancer. N Engl J Med 342(8):564–571, 2000.

Chlebowski RT, Hentrix SL, Langer RD, et al. Influence of estrogen plus progestin on breast cancer and mammography in healthy postmenopausal women: The Women's Health Initiative Randomized Trial. JAMA 289(24):3243–3253, 2003.

Chlebowski RT. Reducing the risk of breast cancer. N Engl J Med 343(3):191–198, 2000.

Fletcher SW, Barton MD. Evaluation of breast lumps. Available at: http://www.utdol.com. Accessed November 4, 2004.

Giordano SH, Cohen DS, Buzdar AU. Breast carcinoma in men: a population-based study. Cancer 101(1):51–57, 2004.

Harris JR, Morrow M, Bonadonna G. Cancer of the breast. In DeVita VT, Hellman S, Rosenberg (eds). Cancer: Principles & Practice of Oncology, 7th ed. Philadelphia, Lippincott Williams & Wilkins, 2004.

BIBLIOGRAPHY

Hollerman DR, Simel DL. Does the clinical examination predict airflow limitation? JAMA 273(4):313–319, 1995.

Kudva YC, Reynolds C, O'Brien TO, et al. "Diabetic mastopathy," or sclerosing lymphocytic lobulitis, is strongly associated with type 1 diabetes. Diabetes Care 25(1):121–126, 2002.

Lannin DR, Mathews HF, Mitchell J, et al. Impacting cultural attitudes in African-American women to decrease breast cancer mortality. Am J Surg 184(5):418–423, 2002.

Mandalblatt J, Saha S, Teusch S, et al. The cost-effectiveness of screening mammography beyond age 65 years: a systematic review for the U.S. Preventive Services Task Force. Ann Intern Med 139(10):835–842, 2003.

U.S. Preventive Services Task Force. Screening for breast cancer: recommendations and rationale. Ann Intern Med 137(5, Part 1): 344–346, 2002.

TABLE 9-1	Visible Signs of Breast Cancer

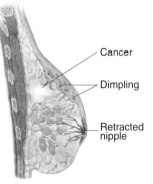

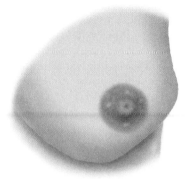

Retraction Signs

As breast cancer advances, it causes fibrosis (scar tissue). Shortening of this tissue produces dimpling, changes in contour, and retraction or deviation of the nipple. Other causes of retraction include fat necrosis and mammary duct ectasia.

Abnormal Contours

Look for any variation in the normal convexity of each breast, and compare one side with the other. Special positioning may again be useful. Shown here is marked flattening of the lower outer quadrant of the left breast.

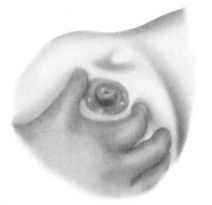

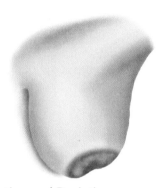

Skin Dimpling

Look for this sign with the patient's arm at rest, during special positioning, and on moving or compressing the breast, as illustrated here.

Nipple Retraction and Deviation

A retracted nipple is flattened or pulled inward, as illustrated here. It may also be broadened, and feels thickened. When involvement is radially asymmetric, the nipple may deviate or point in a different direction from its normal counterpart, typically toward the underlying cancer.

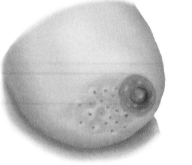

Edema of the Skin

Edema of the skin is produced by lymphatic blockade. It appears as thickened skin with enlarged pores—the so-called *peau d'orange* (orange peel) *sign*. It is often seen first in the lower portion of the breast or areola.

Paget's Disease of the Nipple

This is an uncommon form of breast cancer that usually starts as a scaly, eczemalike lesion. The skin may also weep, crust, or erode. A breast mass may be present. Suspect Paget's disease in any persisting dermatitis of the nipple and areola.

TABLE 9-2 **Common Breast Masses**

The three most common kinds of breast masses are *fibroadenoma* (a benign tumor), *cysts,* and *breast cancer.* The clinical characteristics of these masses are listed below. However, any breast mass should be carefully evaluated and usually warrants further investigation by ultrasound, aspiration, mammography, or biopsy. The masses depicted below are rather large, for purposes of illustration. Ideally, breast cancer should be identified early, when the mass is small. *Fibrocystic changes,* not illustrated, are also commonly palpable as nodular, ropelike densities in women ages 25–50. They may be tender or painful. They are considered benign and are not viewed as a risk factor for breast cancer.

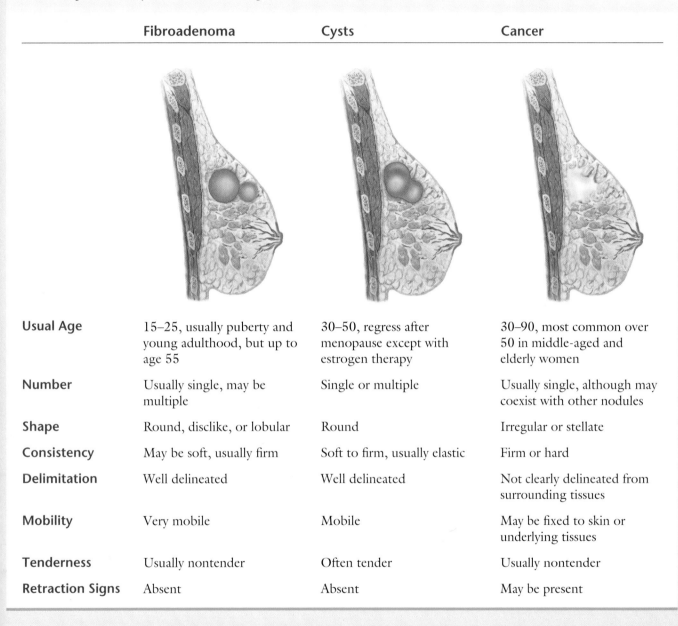

	Fibroadenoma	Cysts	Cancer
Usual Age	15–25, usually puberty and young adulthood, but up to age 55	30–50, regress after menopause except with estrogen therapy	30–90, most common over 50 in middle-aged and elderly women
Number	Usually single, may be multiple	Single or multiple	Usually single, although may coexist with other nodules
Shape	Round, disclike, or lobular	Round	Irregular or stellate
Consistency	May be soft, usually firm	Soft to firm, usually elastic	Firm or hard
Delimitation	Well delineated	Well delineated	Not clearly delineated from surrounding tissues
Mobility	Very mobile	Mobile	May be fixed to skin or underlying tissues
Tenderness	Usually nontender	Often tender	Usually nontender
Retraction Signs	Absent	Absent	May be present

The Abdomen

ANATOMY AND PHYSIOLOGY

Visualize or palpate the landmarks of the abdominal wall and pelvis, as illustrated. The rectus abdominis muscles become more prominent when the patient raises the head and shoulders from the supine position.

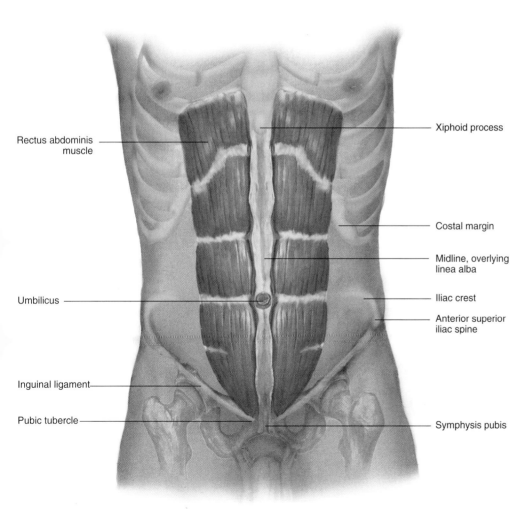

Rectus abdominis muscle

Xiphoid process

Costal margin

Midline, overlying linea alba

Umbilicus

Iliac crest

Anterior superior iliac spine

Inguinal ligament

Pubic tubercle

Symphysis pubis

For descriptive purposes, the abdomen is often divided by imaginary lines crossing at the umbilicus, forming the right upper, right lower, left upper, and left lower quadrants. Another system divides the abdomen into nine sections. Terms for three of them are commonly used: epigastric, umbilical, and hypogastric, or suprapubic.

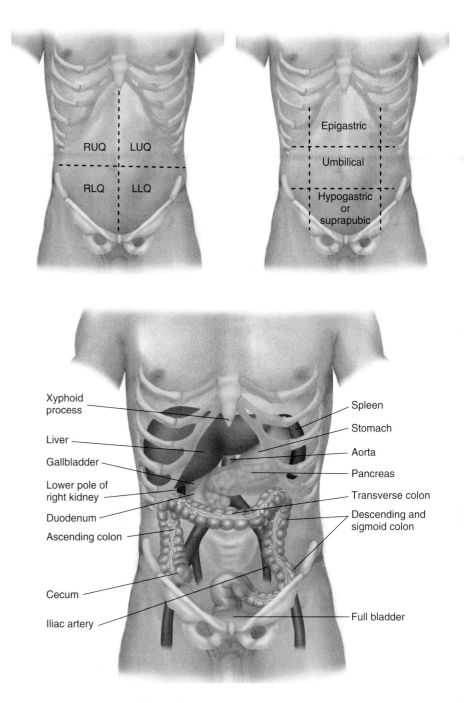

When examining the abdomen, you may be able to feel several normal structures. The sigmoid *colon* is frequently palpable as a firm, narrow tube in the left lower quadrant, whereas the cecum and part of the ascending colon form a softer, wider tube in the right lower quadrant. Portions of the transverse and descending colon may also be palpable. None of these structures should be mistaken for a tumor. Although the normal *liver* often extends down just below the right costal margin, its soft consistency makes it difficult to feel through the abdominal wall. The lower margin of the liver, the liver edge, is often palpable. Also in the right upper quadrant, but usually at a deeper level, lies the lower pole of the right kidney. It is occasionally palpable, especially in thin people with relaxed abdominal muscles. Pulsations of the *abdominal aorta* are frequently visible and usually palpable in the upper abdomen, whereas the pulsations of the *iliac arteries* may sometimes be felt in the lower quadrants.

The abdominal cavity extends up under the rib cage to the dome of the diaphragm. In this protected location, beyond the reach of the palpating hand, are much of the liver and *stomach* and all of the usual normal spleen. The *spleen* lies against the diaphragm at the level of the 9th, 10th, and 11th ribs, mostly posterior to the left midaxillary line. It is lateral to and behind the stomach, and just above the left kidney. The tip of a normal spleen is palpable below the left costal margin in a small percentage of adults.

Most of the normal *gallbladder* lies deep to the liver and cannot be distinguished from it clinically. The *duodenum* and *pancreas* lie deep in the upper abdomen, where they are not normally palpable.

A distended *bladder* may be palpable above the symphysis pubis. The bladder accommodates roughly 300 ml of urine filtered by the kidneys into the renal pelvis and the ureters. Bladder expansion stimulates contraction of bladder smooth muscle, the *detrusor muscle,* at relatively low pressures. Rising pressure in the bladder triggers the conscious urge to void.

Increased intraurethral pressure can overcome rising pressures in the bladder and prevent incontinence. Intraurethral pressure is related to such factors as smooth muscle tone in the internal urethral sphincter, the thickness of the urethral mucosa, and in women, sufficient support to the bladder and proximal urethra from pelvic muscles and ligaments to maintain proper anatomical relationships. Striated muscle around the urethra can also contract voluntarily to interrupt voiding.

Neuroregulatory control of the bladder functions at several levels. In infants, the bladder empties by reflex mechanisms in the sacral spinal cord. Voluntary control of the bladder depends on higher centers in the brain and on motor and sensory pathways between the brain and the reflex arcs of the sacral spinal cord. When voiding is inconvenient, higher centers in the brain can inhibit detrusor contractions until the capacity of the bladder, approximately 400 to 500 ml, is exceeded. The integrity of the sacral nerves that innervate the bladder can be tested by assessing perirectal and perineal sensation in the S2, S3, and S4 dermatomes (see p. 606).

Other structures sometimes palpable in the lower abdomen include the *uterus* enlarged by pregnancy or fibroids, which may also rise above the symphysis pubis, and the *sacral promontory,* the anterior edge of the first sacral vertebra. Until you are familiar with this normal structure, you may mistake its stony hard outlines for a tumor. Another stony hard lump that can sometimes mislead you, and may occasionally alarm a patient, is a normal *xiphoid process.*

The *kidneys* are posterior organs. The ribs protect their upper portionss. The *costovertebral angle*—the angle formed by the lower border of the 12th rib and the transverse processes of the upper lumbar vertebrae—defines the region to assess for kidney tenderness.

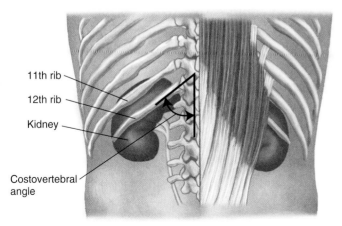

11th rib

12th rib

Kidney

Costovertebral angle

POSTERIOR VIEW

THE HEALTH HISTORY

Common or Concerning Symptoms

Gastrointestinal Disorders
- Indigestion or anorexia
- Nausea, vomiting, or hematemesis
- Abdominal pain
- Dysphagia and/or odynophagia
- Change in bowel function
- Constipation or diarrhea
- Jaundice

Urinary and Renal Disorders
- Suprapubic pain
- Dysuria, urgency, or frequency
- Hesitancy, decreased stream in males
- Polyuria or nocturia
- Urinary incontinence
- Hematuria
- Kidney or flank pain
- Ureteral colic

You will encounter a wide variety of gastrointestinal and urinary complaints in clinical practice. Careful interviewing will often lead you to the underlying disorder. This section addresses such gastrointestinal concerns as *indigestion, anorexia, nausea* or *vomiting, hematemesis, abdominal pain, dysphagia* or *odynophagia, change in bowel function, constipation* and *diarrhea*, and *jaundice*. There is also health history information on disorders of the urinary tract, including complaints of *suprapubic pain, dysuria, urgency, frequency, hesitancy* or *decreased stream* in males, *polyuria, nocturia, incontinence, hematuria, kidney pain*, and *ureteral colic*.

THE GASTROINTESTINAL TRACT

Indigestion, Anorexia, Nausea, Vomiting, Hematemesis. "How is your *appetite*?" is a good starting question and may lead into other important areas such as *indigestion, nausea, vomiting,* and *anorexia*. Patients often complain of *indigestion*, a common complaint that refers to distress associated with eating, but patients use the term for many different symptoms. Find out just what your patient means.

Anorexia, nausea, vomiting in many gastrointestinal disorders; also in pregnancy, diabetic ketoacidosis, adrenal insufficiency, hypercalcemia, uremia, liver disease, emotional states, adverse drug reactions, and other conditions. Induced but without nausea in anorexia/bulimia.

Possible causes include the following:

- *Heartburn,* or a sense of burning or warmth that is retrosternal and may radiate from the epigastrium to the neck. It usually originates in the esophagus. If persistent, especially in the epigastric area, it may raise the question of heart disease. Some patients with coronary artery disease describe their pain as burning, "like indigestion." Pay special attention to what brings on

Heartburn suggests gastric acid reflux into the esophagus; often precipitated by a heavy meal, lying down, or bending forward, also by ingesting alcohol, citrus juices, or

and relieves the discomfort. Is it precipitated by exertion and relieved by rest, suggesting angina, or is it related to meals and made worse during or after eating, suggesting gastroesophageal reflux?

aspirin. If chronic, consider reflux esophagitis. See Table 7-1, Chest Pain, pp. 268–269.

■ *Excessive gas*, especially with frequent belching, abdominal bloating or distention, or *flatus*, the passage of gas by rectum, normally about 600 ml per day. Find out if these symptoms are associated with eating specific foods. Ask if symptoms are related to ingestion of milk or milk products.

Belching, but not bloating or excess flatus, is normally seen in *aerophagia*, or swallowing air. Also consider legumes and other gas-producing foods, intestinal lactase deficiency, and irritable bowel syndrome.

■ Unpleasant *abdominal fullness* after meals of normal size, or *early satiety*, the inability to eat a full meal.

Consider diabetic gastroparesis, anticholinergic drugs, gastric outlet obstruction, gastric cancer; early satiety in hepatitis.

■ *Nausea and vomiting*

■ *Abdominal pain*

Anorexia is a loss or lack of appetite. Find out if it arises from intolerance to certain foods or reluctance to eat because of anticipated discomfort. *Nausea*, often described as "feeling sick to my stomach," may progress to retching or vomiting. *Retching* describes the spasmodic movements of the chest and diaphragm that precede and culminate in *vomiting*, the forceful expulsion of gastric contents out through the mouth.

Anorexia, nausea, vomiting in many gastrointestinal disorders; also in pregnancy, diabetic ketoacidosis, adrenal insufficiency, hypercalcemia, uremia, liver disease, emotional states, adverse drug reactions. Induced but without nausea in anorexia/bulimia nervosa.

Some patients may not actually vomit but raise esophageal or gastric contents without nausea or retching, called *regurgitation*.

Regurgitation in esophageal narrowing from stricture or cancer; also in incompetent gastroesophageal sphincter

Ask about any vomitus or regurgitated material and inspect it yourself if possible. What color is it? What does the vomitus smell like? How much has there been? Ask specifically if it contains any blood and try to determine how much. You may have to help the patient with the amount . . . a teaspoon? Two teaspoons? A cupful?

Fecal odor in small bowel obstruction or gastrocolic fistula

Gastric juice is clear or mucoid. Small amounts of yellowish or greenish bile are common and have no special significance. Brownish or blackish vomitus with a "coffee-grounds" appearance suggests blood altered by gastric acid. Coffee-grounds emesis or red blood is termed *hematemesis*.

Hematemesis in duodenal or peptic ulcer, esophageal or gastric varices, gastritis

Do the patient's symptoms suggest any complications of vomiting such as *aspiration* into the lungs, seen in elderly, debilitated, or obtunded patients? Is there dehydration or electrolyte imbalance from prolonged vomiting, or significant loss of blood?

Symptoms of blood loss such as lightheadedness or syncope depend on the rate and volume of bleeding and rarely appear until blood loss exceeds 500 ml.

Abdominal Pain. *Abdominal pain* has several possible mechanisms and clinical patterns and warrants careful clinical assessment. Be familiar with three broad categories of abdominal pain:

- *Visceral pain* occurs when hollow abdominal organs such as the intestine or biliary tree contract unusually forcefully or are distended or stretched. Solid organs such as the liver can also become painful when their capsules are stretched. Visceral pain may be difficult to localize. It is typically palpable near the midline at levels that vary according to the structure involved, as illustrated on the next page.

  Visceral pain varies in quality and may be gnawing, burning, cramping, or aching. When it becomes severe, it may be associated with sweating, pallor, nausea, vomiting, and restlessness.

See Table 10-1, Abdominal Pain (pp. 394–395).

Visceral pain in the right upper quadrant from liver distention against its capsule in alcoholic hepatitis

Visceral periumbilical pain in early acute appendicitis from distention of inflamed appendix, gradually changing to parietal pain in the right lower quadrant from inflammation of the adjacent parietal peritoneum

Right upper quadrant or epigastric pain from the biliary tree and liver

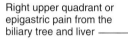

Epigastric pain from the stomach, duodenum, or pancreas

Periumbilical pain from the small intestine, appendix, or proximal colon

Hypogastric pain from the colon, bladder, or uterus. Colonic pain may be more diffuse than illustrated.

Suprapubic or sacral pain from the rectum

TYPES OF VISCERAL PAIN

- *Parietal pain* originates in the parietal peritoneum and is caused by inflammation. It is a steady aching pain that is usually more severe than visceral pain and more precisely localized over the involved structure. It is typically aggravated by movement or coughing. Patients with this type of pain usually prefer to lie still.

- *Referred pain* is felt in more distant sites, which are innervated at approximately the same spinal levels as the disordered structure. Referred pain often develops as the initial pain becomes more intense and thus

Pain of duodenal or pancreatic origin may be referred to the back; pain from the biliary tree, to the

seems to radiate or travel from the initial site. It may be felt superficially or deeply but is usually well localized.

Pain may also be referred to the abdomen from the chest, spine, or pelvis, thus complicating the assessment of abdominal pain.

right shoulder or the right posterior chest.

Pain from *pleurisy* or *acute myocardial infarction* may be referred to the upper abdomen.

Ask patients to *describe the abdominal pain in their own words,* then ask them to *point to the pain.* If clothes interfere, repeat the question during the physical examination. You may need to pursue important details: "Where does the pain start?" "Does it radiate or travel anywhere?" "What is the pain like?" If the patient has trouble describing the pain, try a multiple-choice question such as "Is it aching, burning, gnawing, or what?"

Cramping colicky pain often is related to peristalsis.

You need to ask "How severe is the pain?" "How about on a scale of 1 to 10?" Find out if it is bearable and if it interferes with the patient's usual activities. Does it make the patient lie down?

The description of the *severity of the pain* may tell you something about the patient's responses to pain and its effects on the patient's life, but it is not consistently helpful in assessing the pain's cause. Sensitivity to abdominal pain varies widely and tends to diminish over the later years, masking acute abdominal problems in older people, especially those in or beyond their 70s.

Careful *timing of the pain,* on the other hand, is particularly helpful. Did it start suddenly or gradually? When did the pain begin? How long does it last? What is its pattern over a 24-hour period? Over weeks and months? Are you dealing with an acute illness or a chronic or recurring one?

Determine *what factors aggravate or relieve the pain,* with special reference to meals, antacids, alcohol, medications (including aspirin and aspirinlike drugs and any over-the-counter drugs), emotional factors, and body position. Also, is the pain related to defecation, urination, or menstruation? You also need to elicit any *symptoms associated with the pain,* such as fever or chills, and their sequence.

Citrus fruits may aggravate the pain of *reflux esophagitis;* lactase deficiency is possible if abdominal discomfort is linked to milk ingestion.

Dysphagia and/or Odynophagia.   Less commonly, patients may report difficulty swallowing, or *dysphagia,* the sense that food or liquid is sticking, hesitating, or "won't go down right." Dysphagia may result from esophageal disorders or from difficulty transferring food from the mouth to the esophagus. The sensation of a lump in the throat or in the retrosternal area, unassociated with swallowing, is not true dysphagia.

For types of dysphagia, see Table 10-2, Dysphagia, p. 396.

Ask the patient to point to where the dysphagia occurs and describe with what types of food it occurs. Does it occur with relatively solid foods such as meat, with softer foods such as ground meat and mashed potatoes, or with hot or cold liquids? Has the pattern changed?

Pointing to the throat suggests a transfer or esophageal disorder; pointing to the chest suggests an esophageal disorder.

Establish the timing. When did it start? Is it intermittent or persistent? Is it progressing? If so, over what period? What are the associated symptoms and medical conditions?

Dysphagia with solid food in mechanical narrowing of the esophagus; dysphagia related to both solids and liquids suggests a disorder of esophageal motility.

Odynophagia, or pain on swallowing, may occur in two forms. A sharp, burning pain suggests mucosal inflammation, whereas a squeezing, cramping pain suggests a muscular cause. Odynophagia may accompany dysphagia, but either symptom may occur independently.

Mucosal inflammation in reflux esophagitis or infection from *Candida*, herpes virus, or cytomegalovirus.

Change in Bowel Function.

With respect to the lower gastrointestinal tract, you will frequently need to assess *bowel function*. Start with open-ended questions: "How are your bowel movements?" "How frequent are they?" "Do you have any difficulties?" "Have you noticed any change in your bowel habits?" Frequency of bowel movements normally ranges from about three times a day to twice a week. A change in pattern within these limits, however, may be significant for an individual patient.

Constipation or Diarrhea.

Patients vary widely in their views of constipation and diarrhea. Be sure to clarify what the patient means by these terms. For example, is *constipation* . . . a decrease in frequency of bowel movements? . . . The passage of hard and perhaps painful stools? . . . The need to strain unusually hard? . . . A sense of incomplete defecation or pressure in the rectum? Ask if the patient actually looks at the stool. If yes, what does the stool look like in terms of color and bulk? What remedies has the patient tried? Do medications, stress, unrealistic ideas about normal bowel habits, or time and setting allotted for defecation play a role? Occasionally there is complete constipation with no passage of either feces or gas, or *obstipation*.

See Table 10-3, Constipation (p. 397) and Table 10-4, Diarrhea (pp. 398–399).

Thin pencil-like stool in an obstructing "apple-core" lesion of the sigmoid colon

Obstipation in *intestinal obstruction*

Inquire about the color of the stools and ask about any *black tarry stools*, suggesting *melena*, or *red blood in the stools*, known as *hematochezia*. If either condition is present, find out how long and how often. If the blood is red, how much is there? Is it pure blood mixed in with stool or on the surface of the stool? Is there blood on the toilet paper?

See Table 10-5, Black and Bloody Stools, p. 400.

Blood on the stool surface and on toilet paper in *hemorrhoids*

Diarrhea is an excessive frequency in the passage of stools that are usually unformed or watery. Ask about size, frequency, and volume. Are the stools bulky or small? How many episodes of diarrhea occur each day?

Consistently large diarrheal stools often in small bowel or proximal colon disorders; small frequent stools with urgency of defecation in left colon or rectal disorders

Ask for descriptive terms. Are the stools greasy or oily? Frothy? Foul smelling? Floating on the surface because of excessive gas, making them difficult to flush? Accompanied by mucus, pus, or blood?

Large yellowish or gray greasy foul-smelling stools, sometimes frothy or floating, in *steatorrhea*, or fatty stools—seen in malabsorption

Assess the course of diarrhea over time. Is it acute, chronic, or recurrent? Or is your patient experiencing the first acute episode of a chronic or recurrent illness?

Look into other factors as well. Does the diarrhea awaken the patient at night? What seem to be the aggravating or relieving factors? Does the patient get relief from a bowel movement, or is there an intense urge with

Nocturnal diarrhea suggests a pathophysiologic cause.

straining but little or no result, known as *tenesmus*. What is the setting? Does it entail travel, stress, or a new medication? Do family members or companions have similar symptoms? Are there associated symptoms?

Relief after passing feces or gas suggests left colon or rectal disorders; *tenesmus* in rectal conditions near the anal sphincter

Jaundice.   In some patients, you will be struck by *jaundice* or *icterus*, the yellowish discoloration of the skin and sclerae from increased levels of bilirubin, a bile pigment derived chiefly from the breakdown of hemoglobin. Normally the hepatocytes conjugate, or combine, unconjugated bilirubin with other substances, making the bile water soluble, and then excrete it into the bile. The bile passes through the cystic duct into the common bile duct, which also drains the extrahepatic ducts from the liver. More distally the common bile duct and the pancreatic ducts empty into the duodenum at the ampulla of Vater. Mechanisms of jaundice include the following:

■ Increased production of bilirubin

■ Decreased uptake of bilirubin by the hepatocytes

■ Decreased ability of the liver to conjugate bilirubin

Predominantly unconjugated bilirubin from the first three mechanisms, as in *hemolytic anemia* (increased production) and *Gilbert's syndrome*

■ Decreased excretion of bilirubin into the bile, resulting in absorption of *conjugated* bilirubin back into the blood.

Impaired excretion of conjugated bilirubin in *viral hepatitis, cirrhosis, primary biliary cirrhosis,* drug-induced cholestasis, as from oral contraceptives, methyl testosterone, chlorpromazine

Intrahepatic jaundice can be *hepatocellular,* from damage to the hepatocytes, or *cholestatic,* from impaired excretion as a result of damaged hepatocytes or intrahepatic bile ducts. *Extrahepatic* jaundice arises from obstruction of the extrahepatic bile ducts, most commonly the cystic and common bile ducts.

Obstruction of the common bile duct by gallstones or *pancreatic carcinoma*

As you assess the patient with jaundice, pay special attention to the associated symptoms and the setting in which the illness occurred. What was the *color of the urine* as the patient became ill? When the level of conjugated bilirubin increases in the blood, it may be excreted into the urine, turning the urine a dark yellowish brown or tea color. Unconjugated bilirubin is not water-soluble, so it is not excreted into urine.

Dark urine from bilirubin indicates impaired excretion of bilirubin into the gastrointestinal tract.

Ask also about the *color of the stools.* When excretion of bile into the intestine is completely obstructed, the stools become gray or light colored, or *acholic,* without bile.

Acholic stools briefly in *viral hepatitis,* common in obstructive jaundice

Does the skin itch without other obvious explanation? Is there associated pain? What is its pattern? Has it been recurrent in the past?

Itching in cholestatic or obstructive jaundice; pain from a distended liver capsule, *biliary cholic, pancreatic cancer*

Ask about risk factors for liver diseases, such as:

- *Hepatitis:* Travel or meals in areas of poor sanitation, ingestion of contaminated water or foodstuffs (hepatitis A); parenteral or mucous membrane exposure to infectious body fluids such as blood, serum, semen, and saliva, especially through sexual contact with an infected partner or use of shared needles for injection drug use (hepatitis B); intravenous illicit drug use or blood transfusion (hepatitis C)

- *Alcoholic hepatitis* or *alcoholic cirrhosis* (interview the patient carefully about alcohol use)

- *Toxic liver damage* from medications, industrial solvents, or environmental toxins

- *Gallbladder disease* or *surgery* that may result in extrahepatic biliary obstruction

- *Hereditary disorders* in the Family History

THE URINARY TRACT

General questions for a urinary history include: "Do you have any difficulty passing your urine?" "How often do you go?" "Do you have to get up at night? How often?" "How much urine do you pass at a time?" "Is there any pain or burning?" "Do you ever have trouble getting to the toilet in time?" "Do you ever leak any urine? Or wet yourself involuntarily?" Does the patient sense when the bladder is full and when voiding occurs?

See Table 10-6, Frequency, Nocturia, and Polyuria (p. 401).

Involuntary voiding or lack of awareness suggests cognitive or neurosensory deficits.

Ask women if sudden coughing, sneezing, or laughing makes them lose urine. Roughly half of young women report this experience even before bearing children. Occasional leakage is not necessarily significant. Ask older men, "Do you have trouble starting your stream?" "Do you have to stand close to the toilet to void?" "Is there a change in the force or size of your stream, or straining to void?" "Do you hesitate or stop in the middle of voiding?" "Is there dribbling when you're through?"

Stress incontinence from decreased intraurethral pressure (see pp. 402–403).

Common in men with partial bladder outlet obstruction from *benign prostatic hyperplasia*; also seen with *urethral stricture*

Suprapubic Pain. Disorders in the urinary tract may cause pain in either the abdomen or the back. Bladder disorders may cause *suprapubic pain.* In *bladder infection*, pain in the lower abdomen is typically dull and pressure-like. In sudden overdistention of the bladder, pain is often agonizing; in contrast, chronic bladder distention is usually painless.

Pain of sudden overdistention in acute urinary retention

Dysuria, Urgency, or Frequency. Infection or irritation of either the bladder or urethra often provokes several symptoms. Frequently there is *pain on urination*, usually felt as a burning sensation. Some clinicians refer to this as *dysuria*, whereas others reserve the term dysuria for difficulty voiding. Women may report internal urethral discomfort, sometimes described as a pressure, or an external burning from the flow of urine across irritated

Painful urination with cystitis or urethritis

Also consider bladder stones, foreign bodies, tumors; also *acute prostatitis.* In women, internal

or inflamed labia. Men typically feel a burning sensation proximal to the glans penis. In contrast, *prostatic pain* is felt in the perineum and occasionally in the rectum.

burning in urethritis, external burning in *vulvovaginitis*

Other associated symptoms are common. Urinary *urgency* is an unusually intense and immediate desire to void, sometimes leading to involuntary voiding or *urge incontinence*. Urinary *frequency*, or abnormally frequent voiding, may occur. Ask about any related fever or chills, blood in the urine, or any pain in the abdomen, flank, or back (see illustration on next page). Men with partial obstruction to urinary outflow often report *hesitancy* in starting the urine stream, *straining to void, reduced caliber and force of the urinary stream,* or *dribbling* as voiding is completed.

Urgency in bladder infection or irritation. In men, painful urination without frequency or urgency suggests urethritis.

Polyuria or Nocturia.　Three additional terms describe important alterations in the pattern of urination. *Polyuria* refers to a significant increase in 24-hour urine volume, roughly defined as exceeding 3 liters. It should be distinguished from urinary frequency, which can involve voiding in high amounts, seen in polyuria, or in small amounts, as in infection. *Nocturia* refers to urinary frequency at night, sometimes defined as awakening the patient more than once; urine volumes may be large or small. Clarify any change in nocturnal voiding patterns and the number of trips to the bathroom.

Abnormally high renal production of urine in polyuria. Frequency without polyuria during the day or night in bladder disorder or impairment to flow at or below the bladder neck

Urinary Incontinence.　Up to 30% of older patients are concerned about *urinary incontinence*, an involuntary loss of urine that may become socially embarrassing or cause problems with hygiene. If the patient reports incontinence, ask when it happens and how often. Find out if the patient has leaking of small amounts of urine with increased intra-abdominal pressure from coughing, sneezing, laughing, or lifting. Or, is it difficult for the patient to hold the urine once there is an urge to void, and loss of large amounts of urine? Is there a sensation of bladder fullness, frequent leakage or voiding of small amounts but difficulty emptying the bladder?

See Table 10-7, Urinary Incontinence (pp. 402–403).

Stress incontinence with increased intra-abdominal pressure from decreased contractility of urethral sphincter or poor support of bladder neck; *urge incontinence* if unable to hold the urine, from detrusor overactivity; *overflow incontinence* when the bladder cannot be emptied until bladder pressure exceeds urethral pressure, from anatomical obstruction by prostatic hypertrophy or stricture, also neurogenic abnormalities

As described earlier, bladder control involves complex neuroregulatory and motor mechanisms (see p. 361). A number of central or peripheral nerve lesions may affect normal voiding. Can the patient sense when the bladder is full? And when voiding occurs? Although there are four broad categories of incontinence, a patient may have a combination of causes.

In addition, the patient's functional status may significantly affect voiding behaviors even when the urinary tract is intact. Is the patient mobile? Alert? Able to respond to voiding cues and reach the bathroom? Is alertness or voiding affected by medications?

Functional incontinence from impaired cognition, musculoskeletal problems, immobility

Hematuria.　Blood in the urine, or *hematuria*, is an important cause for concern. When visible to the naked eye, it is called *gross hematuria*. The urine may appear frankly bloody. Blood may be detected only during microscopic urinalysis, known as *microscopic hematuria*. Smaller amounts of blood may tinge the urine with a pinkish or brownish cast. In women, be sure to distinguish menstrual blood from hematuria. If the urine is reddish,

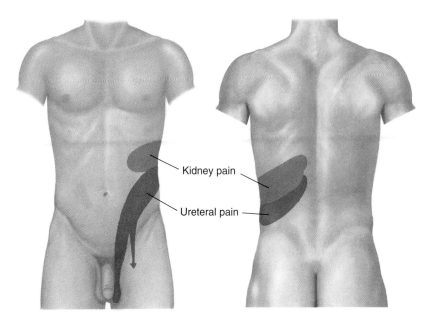

Kidney pain

Ureteral pain

ask about ingestion of beets or medications that might discolor the urine. Test the urine with a dipstick and microscopic examination before you settle on the term hematuria.

Kidney or Flank Pain; Ureteral Colic. Disorders of the urinary tract may also cause *kidney pain*, often reported as *flank pain* at or below the posterior costal margin near the costovertebral angle. It may radiate anteriorly toward the umbilicus. Kidney pain is a visceral pain usually produced by distention of the renal capsule and typically dull, aching, and steady. *Ureteral pain* is dramatically different. It is usually severe and colicky, originating at the costovertebral angle and radiating around the trunk into the lower quadrant of the abdomen, or possibly into the upper thigh and testicle or labium. Ureteral pain results from sudden distention of the ureter and associated distention of the renal pelvis. Ask about any associated fever or chills, or hematuria.

Kidney pain occurs in *acute pyelonephritis*.

Renal or ureteral colic is caused by sudden obstruction of a ureter, as by urinary stones or blood clots.

HEALTH PROMOTION AND COUNSELING

Important Topics for Health Promotion and Counseling

- Screening for alcohol and substance abuse
- Risk factors for hepatitis A, B, and C
- Screening for colon cancer

Health promotion and counseling relevant to the abdomen include screening for alcoholism, for risk of infectious hepatitis, and for risk of colon cancer.

Clues from social patterns and behavioral problems in the history and findings of liver enlargement or tenderness on physical examination often alert the clinician to possible alcoholism or risk for infectious hepatitis. Past medical history and family history are important when assessing risk for colon cancer.

The effects of addiction to *alcohol* on public health may be even greater than those of addiction to illicit drugs. More than 10 million Americans currently abuse alcohol. Lifetime prevalence of alcohol abuse or dependence is approximately 13.5%.[1] Alcohol abuse is highly correlated with fatal car accidents, suicide and other comorbid mental health disorders, hypertension, family disruption, violence, and malignancies of the upper gastrointestinal tract and liver, to name but a few of its sequelae.

Assessing patients for use of alcohol and other substances is a prime clinical responsibility. The clinician should focus on detection, counseling, and, for significant impairment, specific recommendations for treatment. When asking about alcohol use, recall current definitions of risky or hazardous drinking and harmful drinking.[2]

- *Risky or hazardous drinking:* For *women*—more than 7 drinks per week or more than 3 drinks per occasion; for *men*—more than 14 drinks per week or more than 4 drinks per occasion

- *Harmful drinking*—drinking that causes physical, social, or psychological harm from alcohol use but does not meet the criteria for dependence

Use the four CAGE questions, validated across many studies, to screen for alcohol dependence or abuse[2,3] (see Chapter 2, Interviewing and the Health History, pp. 50–51). Effective interventions about misuse can be brief. Initial counseling of approximately 15 minutes, with intermittent follow-up by trained office staff for feedback, advice, and goal setting, reduces consumption by 13%–34% over 6 to 12 months.[2,4-6] Motivational interviewing has also been successful in promoting abstinence.[7] One model for brief interventions is FRAMES: **F**eedback based on thorough assessment; **R**esponsibility; **A**dvice on behavior change; a **M**enu of options for making change; **E**mpathy about the difficulty of changing; and support for **S**elf-efficacy in achieving change.[8] Tailor recommendations for treatment to the severity of the problem, ranging from support groups to inpatient detoxification to more extended rehabilitation.

Protective measures against infectious hepatitis include counseling about how the viruses are spread and the need for immunization. Transmission of hepatitis A is fecal–oral: fecal shedding in food handlers leads to contamination of water and foods. Illness occurs approximately 30 days after exposure. Hepatitis A vaccine is recommended for travelers to endemic areas, food handlers, military personnel, caretakers of children, Native Americans and Alaskan natives, and selected health care, sanitation, and laboratory workers. Vaccination is also recommended for homosexual contacts and injection drug users. For immediate protection and prophylaxis for household contacts and travelers, consider administering immune serum globulin.

Hepatitis B poses more serious threats to patients' health, including risk for fulminant hepatitis as well as chronic infection and subsequent cirrhosis and hepatocellular carcinoma. Transmission occurs during contact with infected body fluids, such as blood, semen, saliva, and vaginal secretions. Adults between the ages of 20 and 39 are most affected, especially injection drug users and sex workers. Up to one tenth of infected adults become chronically infected asymptomatic carriers. Behavioral counseling and serologic screening are advised for patients at risk. Because up to 30% of patients have no identifiable risk factors, hepatitis B vaccine is recommended for all young adults not previously immunized, injection drug users and their sexual partners, people at risk for sexually transmitted diseases, travelers to endemic areas, recipients of blood products as in hemodialysis, and health care workers with frequent exposure to blood products. Many of these groups should also be screened for HIV infection. The U.S. Preventive Services Task Force currently recommends screening for only pregnant women at their first prenatal visit because 30%–40% of infected individuals have no identifiable risk factors.[9]

Hepatitis C is transmitted by repeated percutaneous exposures to blood and is present in approximately 2% of U.S. adults. Infected patients are often asymptomatic; some experience fatigue, malaise, anorexia, nausea, and reduced quality of life. More than 70% develop chronic liver disease. Because of its low prevalence and low rate of progression to cirrhosis, routine screening of the general or even high-risk populations is currently not recommended.[10] Risk factors include injection drug use, transfusion before 1990, an HCV-infected mother, and unsafe sex.

It is also important to screen patients for *colorectal cancer*, the fourth most common U.S. malignancy and the second leading cause of death from cancer.[11] Lifetime risk for diagnosis at age 50 is approximately 5%. Roughly 80% of colorectal cancers originate from adenomatous polyps, usually those larger than 1 cm. Prevalence increases from approximately 20% at age 50 to 50% at age 75.[12] For men and women at average risk, the American Cancer Society recommends one of the following tests beginning at age 50:[13]

- Fecal occult blood test (FOBT) annually

- Flexible sigmoidoscopy every 5 years

- Annual FOBT plus flexible sigmoidoscopy every 5 years

- Double-contrast barium enema every 5 years

- Colonoscopy every 10 years

The U.S. Preventive Services Task Force finds strong evidence in support of screening beginning at age 50.

Most colorectal cancers are sporadic, but approximately 20% occur in patients with specific risk factors: prior adenomatous polyps or colorectal cancer; ulcerative colitis; colorectal cancer in a first-degree relative; and family history of adenomatous polyps before age 60. Familial adenomatous polyposis or hereditary nonpolyposis colorectal cancer accounts for approximately 6% of colorectal malignancies. Screening in these groups should begin at age 40 or earlier. Note that the FOBT has a highly variable sensitivity (26%–92%), but good specificity (90%–99%).[14] It produces many false-positive results related to diet, selected medications, and gastrointestinal conditions such as ulcer disease, diverticulosis, and hemorrhoids. The benefits of sigmoidoscopy are linked to the length of the sigmoidoscope and its depth of insertion. Detection rates for colorectal cancer and insertion depths are roughly as follows: 25%–30% at 20 cm; 50%–55% at 35 cm; 40%–65% at 40–50 cm. Full colonoscopy or air contrast barium enema detects 80%–95% of colorectal cancers, but these procedures are more uncomfortable, and colonoscopy is more expensive. When counseling patients about prevention, there is preliminary but inconsistent evidence that diets high in fiber may reduce risk for colorectal malignancy.

TECHNIQUES OF EXAMINATION

For a skilled abdominal examination, you need good light, a relaxed patient, and full exposure of the abdomen from above the xiphoid process to the symphysis pubis. The groin should be visible. The genitalia should remain draped. The abdominal muscles should be relaxed to enhance all aspects of the examination, but especially palpation.

Tips for Enhancing Examination of the Abdomen

- Check that the patient has an empty bladder.
- Make the patient comfortable in the supine position, with a pillow for under the head and perhaps another for under the knees. Slide your hand under the low back to see if the patient is relaxed and lying flat on the table.
- Ask the patient to keep the arms at the sides or folded across the chest. If the arms are above the head, the abdominal wall stretches and tightens, making palpation difficult.
- Before you begin palpation, ask the patient to point to any areas of pain and examine these areas last.
- Warm your hands and stethoscope. To warm your hands, rub them together or place them under hot water. You can also palpate through the patient's gown to absorb warmth from the patient's body before exposing the abdomen.
- Approach the patient calmly and avoid quick unexpected movements. *Watch the patient's face for any signs of pain or discomfort.* Make sure you avoid long fingernails.
- Distract the patient if necessary with conversation or questions. If the patient is frightened or ticklish, begin palpation with the patient's hand under yours. After a few moments, slip your hand underneath to palpate directly.

An arched back thrusts the abdomen forward and tightens the abdominal muscles.

Visualize each organ in the region you are examining. Stand at the patient's right side and proceed in an orderly fashion with inspection, auscultation, percussion, and palpation. Assess the liver, spleen, kidneys, and aorta.

THE ABDOMEN

INSPECTION

Starting from your usual standing position at the right side of the bed, inspect the abdomen. As you look at the contour of the abdomen, watch for peristalsis. It is helpful to sit or bend down so that you can view the abdomen tangentially.

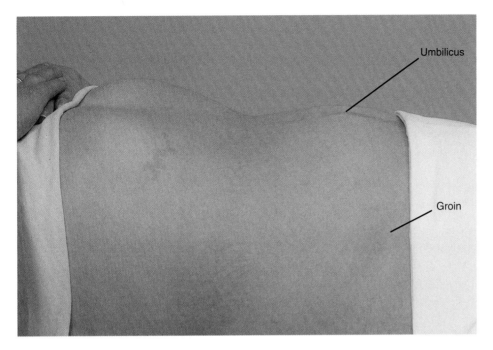

Inspect the surface, contours, and movements of the abdomen, including the following:

- *The skin,* note:

  Scars. Describe or diagram their location.

  Striae. Old silver striae or stretch marks are normal.

  Pink–purple striae of *Cushing's syndrome*

  Dilated veins. A few small veins may be visible normally.

  Dilated veins of *hepatic cirrhosis* or of *inferior vena cava obstruction*

  Rashes and lesions

- *The umbilicus.* Observe its contour and location and any inflammation or bulges suggesting a hernia.

  See Table 10-8, Localized Bulges in the Abdominal Wall (p. 404).

- *The contour of the abdomen*

  Is it flat, rounded, protuberant, or scaphoid (markedly concave or hollowed)?

  See Table 10-9, Protuberant Abdomens (p. 405).

  Do the flanks bulge, or are there any local bulges? Also survey the inguinal and femoral areas.

  Bulging flanks of *ascites;* suprapubic bulge of a distended bladder or pregnant uterus; hernias

  Is the abdomen symmetric?

  Asymmetry from an enlarged organ or mass

  Are there visible organs or masses? Look for an enlarged liver or spleen that has descended below the rib cage.

  Lower abdominal mass of an ovarian or a uterine tumor

- *Peristalsis.* Observe for several minutes if you suspect intestinal obstruction. Peristalsis may be visible normally in very thin people.

  Increased peristaltic waves of *intestinal obstruction*

■ *Pulsations.* The normal aortic pulsation is frequently visible in the epigastrium.

Increased pulsation of an *aortic aneurysm* or of *increased pulse pressure*

AUSCULTATION

Auscultation provides important information about bowel motility. *Listen to the abdomen before performing percussion or palpation because these maneuvers may alter the frequency of bowel sounds.* Practice auscultation until you are thoroughly familiar with variations in normal bowel sounds and can detect changes suggestive of inflammation or obstruction. Auscultation may also reveal *bruits,* or vascular sounds resembling heart murmurs, over the aorta or other arteries in the abdomen. Bruits suggest vascular occlusive disease.

Place the diaphragm of your stethoscope gently on the abdomen. Listen for bowel sounds and note their frequency and character. Normal sounds consist of clicks and gurgles, occurring at an estimated frequency of 5 to 34 per minute. Occasionally you may hear *borborygmi*—long prolonged gurgles of hyperperistalsis—the familiar "stomach growling." Because bowel sounds are widely transmitted through the abdomen, listening in one spot, such as the right lower quadrant, is usually sufficient.

Bowel sounds may be altered in diarrhea, intestinal obstruction, *paralytic ileus,* and *peritonitis.* See Table 10-10, Sounds in the Abdomen (p. 406).

If the patient has high blood pressure, listen in the epigastrium and in each upper quadrant for *bruits.* Later in the examination, when the patient sits up, listen also in the costovertebral angles. Epigastric bruits confined to systole may be heard normally.

A bruit in one of these areas that has both systolic and diastolic components strongly suggests *renal artery stenosis* as the cause of hypertension.

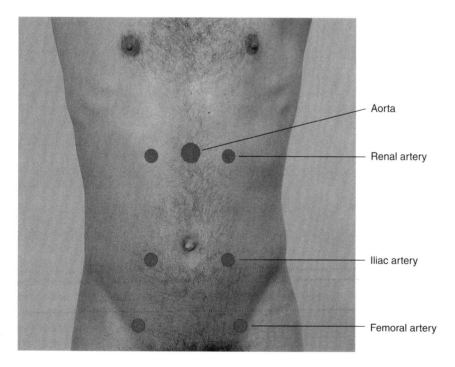

- Aorta
- Renal artery
- Iliac artery
- Femoral artery

Listen for bruits over the aorta, the iliac arteries, and the femoral arteries. Bruits confined to systole are relatively common, however, and do not necessarily signify occlusive disease.

Bruits with both systolic and diastolic components suggest the turbulent blood flow of *partial arterial occlusion* or *arterial insufficiency.* See Table 10-10, Sounds in the Abdomen (p. 406).

Listening points for bruits in these vessels are illustrated above.

Listen over the liver and spleen for *friction rubs*.

See Table 10-10, Sounds in the Abdomen (p. 406).

Friction rubs in liver tumor, gonococcal infection around the liver, splenic infarction

PERCUSSION

Percussion helps you to assess the amount and distribution of gas in the abdomen and to identify possible masses that are solid or fluid filled. Its use in estimating the size of the liver and spleen will be described in later sections.

Percuss the abdomen lightly in all four quadrants to assess the distribution of *tympany* and *dullness*. Tympany usually predominates because of gas in the gastrointestinal tract, but scattered areas of dullness from fluid and feces there are also typical.

A protuberant abdomen that is tympanitic throughout suggests *intestinal obstruction*. See Table 10-9, Protuberant Abdomens (p. 405).

■ Note any large dull areas that might indicate an underlying mass or enlarged organ. This observation will guide your palpation.

Pregnant uterus, ovarian tumor, distended bladder, large liver or spleen

■ On each side of a protuberant abdomen, note where abdominal tympany changes to the dullness of solid posterior structures.

Dullness in both flanks indicates further assessment for ascites (see pp. 387–389).

Briefly percuss the lower anterior chest, between lungs above and costal margins below. On the right, you will usually find the dullness of liver; on the left, the tympany that overlies the gastric air bubble and the splenic flexure of the colon.

In *situs inversus* (rare), organs are reversed: air bubble on the right, liver dullness on the left.

PALPATION

Light Palpation.   Feeling the abdomen gently is especially helpful for identifying abdominal tenderness, muscular resistance, and some superficial organs and masses. It also serves to reassure and relax the patient.

Keeping your hand and forearm on a horizontal plane, with fingers together and flat on the abdominal surface, palpate the abdomen with a light, gentle, dipping motion. When moving your hand from place to place, raise it just off the skin. Moving smoothly, feel in all quadrants.

Identify any superficial organs or masses and any area of tenderness or increased resistance to your hand. If resistance is present, try to distinguish voluntary guarding from involuntary muscular spasm. To do this:

■ Try all the relaxing methods you know (see p. 374).

Involuntary rigidity (muscular spasm) typically persists despite these maneuvers. It indicates *peritoneal inflammation.*

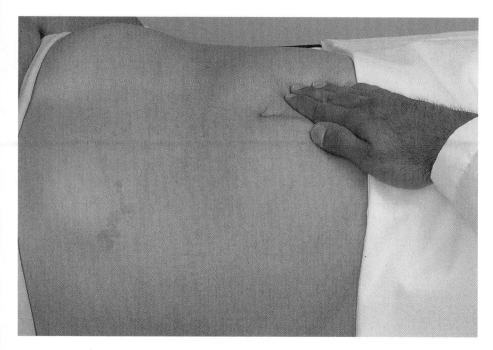

- Feel for the relaxation of abdominal muscles that normally accompanies exhalation.

- Ask the patient to mouth-breathe with jaw dropped open.

Voluntary guarding usually decreases with these maneuvers.

Deep Palpation. This is usually required to delineate abdominal masses. Again using the palmar surfaces of your fingers, feel in all four quadrants. Identify any masses and note their location, size, shape, consistency, tenderness, pulsations, and any mobility with respiration or with the examining hand. Correlate your palpable findings with their percussion notes.

Abdominal masses may be categorized in several ways: physiologic (pregnant uterus), inflammatory (diverticulitis of the colon), vascular (an aneurysm of the abdominal aorta), neoplastic (carcinoma of the colon), or obstructive (a distended bladder or dilated loop of bowel).

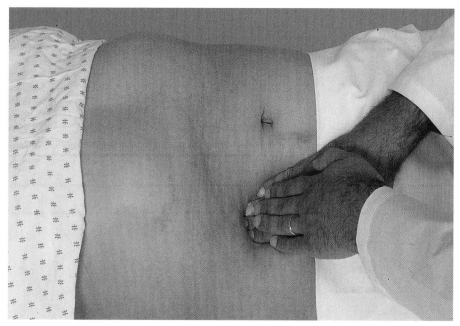

TWO-HANDED DEEP PALPATION

Assessment for Peritoneal Inflammation. Abdominal pain and tenderness, especially when associated with muscular spasm, suggest inflammation of the parietal peritoneum. Localize the pain as accurately as possible. First, even before palpation, *ask the patient to cough* and determine where the cough produced pain. Then, *palpate gently with one finger* to map the tender area. Pain produced by light percussion has similar localizing value. These gentle maneuvers may be all you need to establish an area of peritoneal inflammation.

Abdominal pain when coughing or with light percussion suggests peritoneal inflammation. See Table 10-11, Tender Abdomens (pp. 407–408).

If not, look for *rebound tenderness.* Press down with your fingers firmly and slowly, then withdraw them quickly. Watch and listen to the patient for signs of pain. Ask the patient "Which hurts more, when I press or let go?" Have the patient locate the pain exactly. Pain induced or increased by quick withdrawal constitutes *rebound tenderness* caused by rapid movement of an inflamed peritoneum.

Rebound tenderness suggests peritoneal inflammation. If tenderness is felt elsewhere than where you were trying to elicit rebound, that area may be the real source of the problem.

THE LIVER

Because the rib cage shelters most of the liver, assessment is difficult. Liver size and shape can be estimated by percussion and perhaps palpation, however, and the palpating hand helps you to evaluate its surface, consistency, and tenderness.

PERCUSSION

Measure the vertical span of liver dullness in the right midclavicular line. Starting at a level below the umbilicus (in an area of tympany, not dullness), lightly percuss upward toward the liver. Ascertain the *lower border of liver dullness* in the midclavicular line.

Next, identify the *upper border of liver dullness* in the midclavicular line. Lightly percuss from lung resonance down toward liver dullness. Gently displace a woman's breast as necessary to be sure that you start in a resonant area. The course of percussion is shown below.

The span of liver dullness is *increased* when the liver is enlarged.

The span of liver dullness is *decreased* when the liver is small, or when free air is present below the diaphragm, as from a *perforated hollow viscus.* Serial observations may show a decreasing span of dullness with resolution of *hepatitis* or *congestive heart failure* or, less commonly, with progression of *fulminant hepatitis.*

Liver dullness may be displaced downward by the low diaphragm of *chronic obstructive pulmonary disease.* Span, however, remains normal.

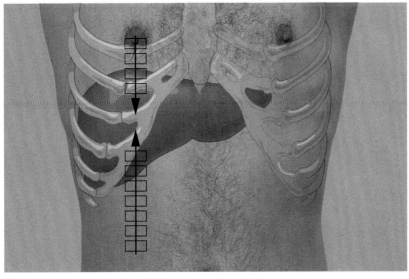

PERCUSSING LIVER SPAN

Now measure in centimeters the distance between your two points—the vertical span of liver dullness. Normal liver spans, shown below, are generally greater in men than in women, in tall people than in short. If the liver seems to be enlarged, outline the lower edge by percussing in other areas.

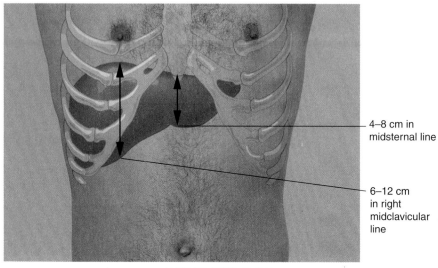

4–8 cm in midsternal line

6–12 cm in right midclavicular line

NORMAL LIVER SPANS

Dullness of a right pleural effusion or consolidated lung, if adjacent to liver dullness, may falsely *increase* the estimate of liver size.

Gas in the colon may produce tympany in the right upper quadrant, obscure liver dullness, and falsely *decrease* the estimate of liver size.

Although percussion is probably the most accurate clinical method for estimating the vertical size of the liver, it typically leads to underestimation.

PALPATION

Place your left hand behind the patient, parallel to and supporting the right 11th and 12th ribs and adjacent soft tissues below. Remind the patient to relax on your hand if necessary. By pressing your left hand forward, the patient's liver may be felt more easily by your other hand.

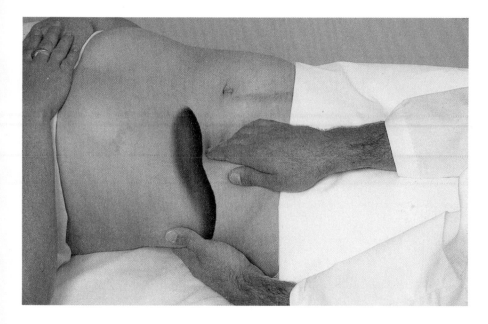

Place your right hand on the patient's right abdomen lateral to the rectus muscle, with your fingertips well below the lower border of liver dullness. Some examiners like to point their fingers up toward the patient's head, whereas others prefer a somewhat more oblique position, as shown below. In either case, press gently in and up.

Ask the patient to take a deep breath. Try to feel the liver edge as it comes down to meet your fingertips. If you feel it, lighten the pressure of your palpating hand slightly so that the liver can slip under your finger pads and you can feel its anterior surface. Note any tenderness. If palpable at all, the normal liver edge is soft, sharp, and regular, with a smooth surface. The normal liver may be slightly tender.

Firmness or hardness of the liver, bluntness or rounding of its edge, and irregularity of its contour suggest an abnormality of the liver.

On inspiration, the liver is palpable about 3 cm below the right costal margin in the midclavicular line. Some people breathe more with their chests than with their diaphragms. It may be helpful to train such a patient to "breathe with the abdomen," thus bringing the liver, as well as the spleen and kidneys, into a palpable position during inspiration.

An obstructed, distended gallbladder may form an oval mass below the edge of the liver and merging with it. It is dull to percussion.

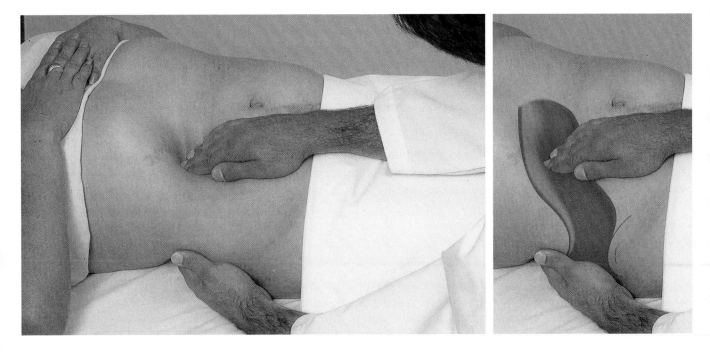

In order to feel the liver, you may have to alter your pressure according to the thickness and resistance of the abdominal wall. If you cannot feel it, move your palpating hand closer to the costal margin and try again.

The edge of an enlarged liver may be missed by starting palpation too high in the abdomen.

Try to trace the liver edge both laterally and medially. Palpation through the rectus muscles, however, is especially difficult. Describe or sketch the liver edge, and measure its distance from the right costal margin in the midclavicular line.

See Table 10-12, Liver Enlargement: Apparent and Real (p. 409).

The "hooking technique" may be helpful, especially when the patient is obese. Stand to the right of the patient's chest. Place both hands, side by side, on the right abdomen below the border of liver dullness. Press in with your fingers and up toward the costal margin. Ask the patient to take a deep breath. The liver edge shown below is palpable with the fingerpads of both hands.

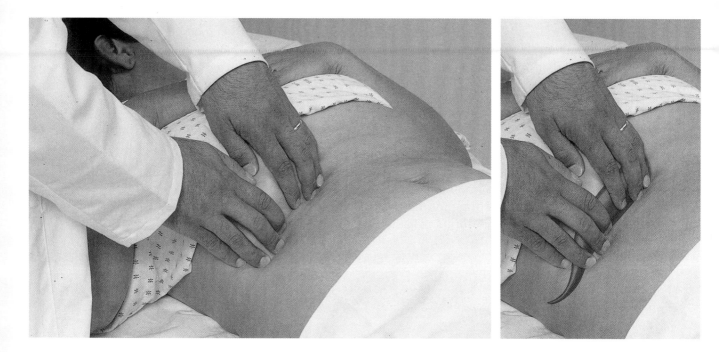

Assessing Tenderness of a Nonpalpable Liver. Place your left hand flat on the lower right rib cage and then gently strike your hand with the ulnar surface of your right fist. Ask the patient to compare the sensation with that produced by a similar strike on the left side.

Tenderness over the liver suggests inflammation, as in *hepatitis*, or congestion, as in *heart failure*.

THE SPLEEN

When a spleen enlarges, it expands anteriorly, downward, and medially, often replacing the tympany of stomach and colon with the dullness of a solid organ. It then becomes palpable below the costal margin. Percussion cannot confirm splenic enlargement but can raise your suspicions of it. Palpation can confirm the enlargement, but often misses large spleens that do not descend below the costal margin.

PERCUSSION

Two techniques may help you to detect *splenomegaly,* an enlarged spleen:

- *Percuss the left lower anterior chest wall* between lung resonance above and the costal margin, an area termed *Traube's space.* As you percuss along the routes suggested by the arrows in the following figures, note the lateral extent of tympany.

Dullness, as shown on the following page, raises the question of splenomegaly.

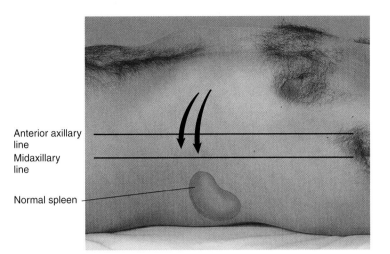

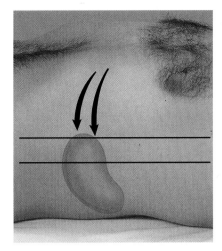

This is variable, but if tympany is prominent, especially laterally, splenomegaly is not likely. The dullness of a normal spleen is usually hidden within the dullness of other posterior tissues.

- *Check for a splenic percussion sign.* Percuss the lowest interspace in the left anterior axillary line, as shown below. This area is usually tympanitic. Then ask the patient to take a deep breath, and percuss again. When spleen size is normal, the percussion note usually remains tympanitic.

Fluid or solids in the stomach or colon may also cause dullness in Traube's space.

A change in percussion note from tympany to dullness on inspiration suggests splenic enlargement. This is a *positive splenic percussion sign.*

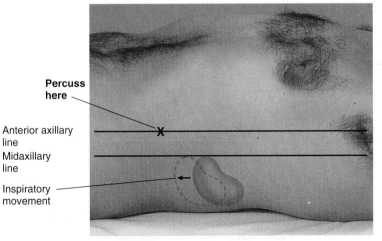

NEGATIVE SPLENIC PERCUSSION SIGN

POSITIVE SPLENIC PERCUSSION SIGN

If either or both of these tests is positive, pay extra attention to palpation of the spleen.

The splenic percussion sign may also be positive when spleen size is normal.

PALPATION

With your left hand, reach over and around the patient to support and press forward the lower left rib cage and adjacent soft tissue. With your right hand below the left costal margin, press in toward the spleen. Begin palpation low

An enlarged spleen may be missed if the examiner starts too high in the abdomen to feel the lower edge.

enough so that you are below a possibly enlarged spleen. (If your hand is close to the costal margin, moreover, it is not sufficiently mobile to reach up under the rib cage.) Ask the patient to take a deep breath. Try to feel the tip or edge of the spleen as it comes down to meet your fingertips. Note any tenderness, assess the splenic contour, and measure the distance between the spleen's lowest point and the left costal margin. In a small percentage of normal adults, the tip of the spleen is palpable. Causes include a low, flat diaphragm, as in chronic obstructive pulmonary disease, and a deep inspiratory descent of the diaphragm.

A palpable spleen tip, though not necessarily abnormal, may indicate splenic enlargement. The spleen tip below is just palpable deep to the left costal margin.

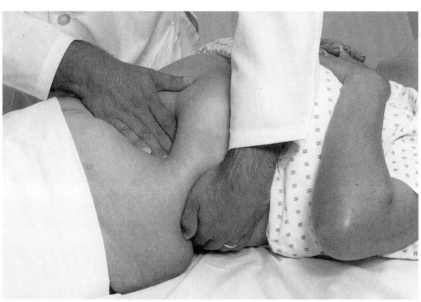

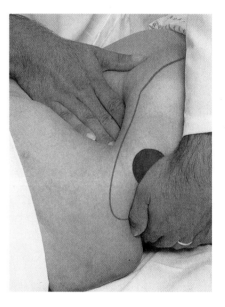

Repeat with the patient lying on the right side with legs somewhat flexed at hips and knees. In this position, gravity may bring the spleen forward and to the right into a palpable location.

The enlarged spleen is palpable about 2 cm below the left costal margin on deep inspiration.

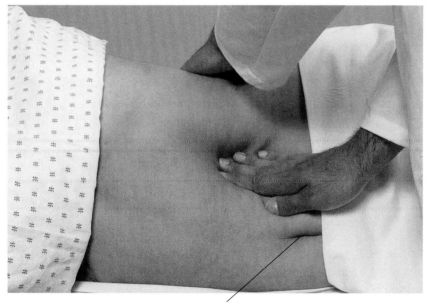

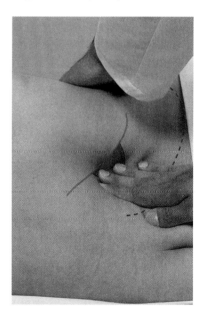

Umbilicus

PALPATING THE SPLEEN—PATIENT LYING ON RIGHT SIDE

■ THE KIDNEYS

PALPATION

Although kidneys are not usually palpable, you should learn and practice the techniques for examination. Detecting an enlarged kidney may prove to be very important.

Palpation of the Left Kidney.   Move to the patient's left side. Place your right hand behind the patient just below and parallel to the 12th rib, with your fingertips just reaching the costovertebral angle. Lift, trying to displace the kidney anteriorly. Place your left hand gently in the left upper quadrant, lateral and parallel to the rectus muscle. Ask the patient to take a deep breath. At the peak of inspiration, press your left hand firmly and deeply into the left upper quadrant, just below the costal margin, and try to "capture" the kidney between your two hands. Ask the patient to breathe out and then to stop breathing briefly. Slowly release the pressure of your left hand, feeling at the same time for the kidney to slide back into its expiratory position. If the kidney is palpable, describe its size, contour, and any tenderness.

Alternatively, try to feel for the left kidney by a method similar to feeling for the spleen. With your left hand, reach over and around the patient to lift the left loin, and with your right hand feel deep in the left upper quadrant. Ask the patient to take a deep breath, and feel for a mass. A normal left kidney is rarely palpable.

Palpation of the Right Kidney.   To capture the right kidney, return to the patient's right side. Use your left hand to lift from in back, and your right hand to feel deep in the left upper quadrant. Proceed as before.

A normal right kidney may be palpable, especially in thin, well-relaxed women. It may or may not be slightly tender. The patient is usually aware of a capture

A left flank mass (see the solid line on photo on previous page) may represent marked *splenomegaly* or an enlarged left kidney. Suspect *splenomegaly* if notch is palpated on medial border, edge extends beyond the midline, percussion is dull, and your fingers can probe deep to the medial and lateral borders but not between the mass and the costal margin. Confirm findings with further evaluation.

Attributes favoring an *enlarged kidney* over an enlarged spleen include preservation of normal tympany in the left upper quadrant and the ability to probe with your fingers between the mass and the costal margin, but not deep to its medial and lower borders.

Causes of kidney enlargement include hydronephrosis, cysts, and tumors. Bilateral enlargement suggests *polycystic kidney disease.*

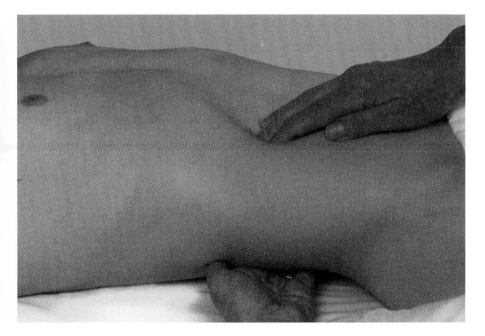

and release. Occasionally, a right kidney is located more anteriorly than usual and then must be distinguished from the liver. The edge of the liver, if palpable, tends to be sharper and to extend farther medially and laterally. It cannot be captured. The lower pole of the kidney is rounded.

Assessing Kidney Tenderness.
You may note tenderness when examining the abdomen, but also search for it at each costovertebral angle. Pressure from your fingertips may be enough to elicit tenderness, but if not, use fist percussion. Place the ball of one hand in the costovertebral angle and strike it with the ulnar surface of your fist. Use enough force to cause a perceptible but painless jar or thud in a normal person.

To save the patient needless exertion, integrate this assessment with your examination of the back (see p. 10).

Pain with pressure or fist percussion suggests *pyelonephritis* but may also have a musculoskeletal cause.

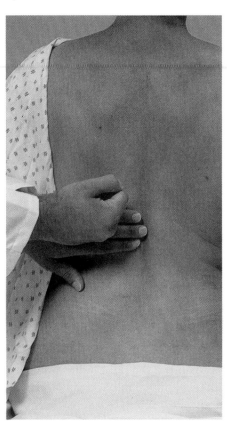

**ASSESSING COSTOVERTEBRAL
ANGLE TENDERNESS**

THE BLADDER

The bladder normally cannot be examined unless it is distended above the symphysis pubis. On palpation, the dome of the distended bladder feels smooth and round. Check for tenderness. Use percussion to check for dullness and to determine how high the bladder rises above the symphysis pubis.

Bladder distention from outlet obstruction due to *urethral stricture, prostatic hyperplasia;* also from medications and neurologic disorders such as *stroke, multiple sclerosis.*

Suprapubic tenderness in *bladder infection*

THE AORTA

Press firmly deep in the upper abdomen, slightly to the left of the midline, and identify the aortic pulsations. In people older than age 50, try to assess the width of the aorta by pressing deeply in the upper abdomen with one hand on each side of the aorta, as illustrated. In this age group, a normal aorta is not more than 3.0 cm wide (average 2.5 cm). This measurement does not include the thickness of the abdominal wall. The ease of feeling

In an older person, a periumbilical or upper abdominal mass with expansile pulsations suggests an *aortic aneurysm.*

aortic pulsations varies greatly with the thickness of the abdominal wall and with the anteroposterior diameter of the abdomen.

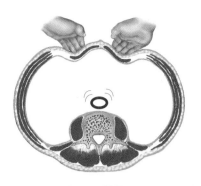

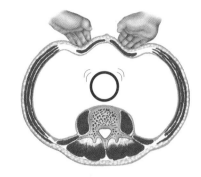

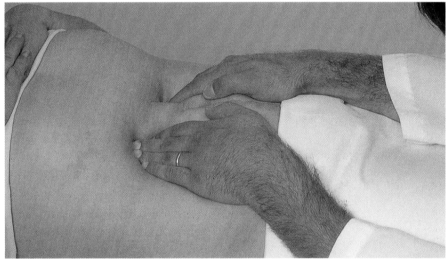

An *aortic aneurysm* is a pathologic dilatation of the aorta, usually due to arteriosclerosis. A merely tortuous abdominal aorta, however, may be difficult to distinguish from an aneurysm on clinical grounds.

Although an aneurysm is usually painless, pain may herald its most dreaded and frequent complication—rupture of the aorta.

Apparent enlargement of the aorta indicates assessment by ultrasound.

SPECIAL TECHNIQUES

Assessment Techniques for:

- Ascites
- Appendicitis
- Acute cholecystitis
- Ventral hernia
- Mass in abdominal wall

ASSESSING POSSIBLE ASCITES

A protuberant abdomen with bulging flanks suggests the possibility of ascitic fluid. Because ascitic fluid characteristically sinks with gravity, whereas gas-filled loops of bowel float to the top, percussion gives a dull note in dependent areas of the abdomen. Look for such a pattern by percussing outward in several directions from the central area of tympany. Map the border between tympany and dullness.

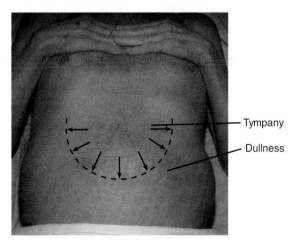

Tympany

Dullness

Two further techniques help to confirm ascites, although both signs may be misleading.

- *Test for shifting dullness.* After mapping the borders of tympany and dullness, ask the patient to turn onto one side. Percuss and mark the borders again. In a person without ascites, the borders between tympany and dullness usually stay relatively constant.

In ascites, dullness shifts to the more dependent side, whereas tympany shifts to the top.

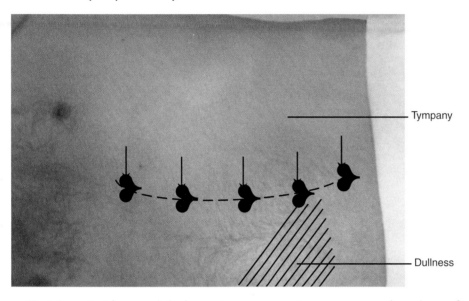

Tympany

Dullness

- *Test for a fluid wave.* Ask the patient or an assistant to press the edges of both hands firmly down the midline of the abdomen. This pressure helps to stop the transmission of a wave through fat. While you tap one flank sharply with your fingertips, feel on the opposite flank for an impulse trans-

An easily palpable impulse suggests ascites.

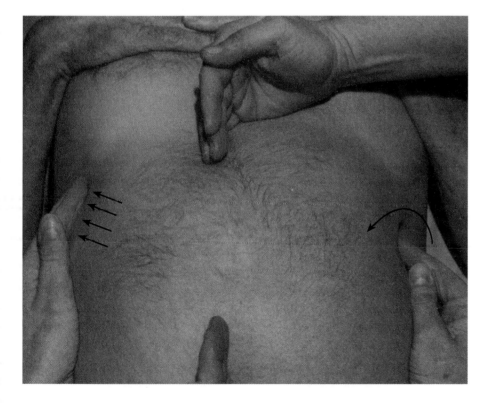

mitted through the fluid. Unfortunately, this sign is often negative until ascites is obvious, and it is sometimes positive in people without ascites.

Identifying an Organ or a Mass in an Ascitic Abdomen. Try to *ballotte* the organ or mass, exemplified here by an enlarged liver. Straighten and stiffen the fingers of one hand together, place them on the abdominal surface, and make a brief jabbing movement directly toward the anticipated structure. This quick movement often displaces the fluid so that your fingertips can briefly touch the surface of the structure through the abdominal wall.

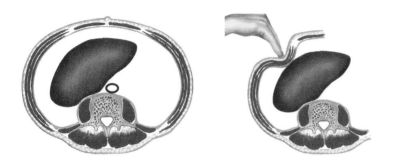

ASSESSING POSSIBLE APPENDICITIS

- Ask the patient to point to where the pain began and where it is now. Ask the patient to cough. Determine whether and where pain results.

  The pain of appendicitis classically begins near the umbilicus, then shifts to the right lower quadrant, where coughing increases it. Older patients report this pattern less frequently than younger ones.

- Search carefully for an area of local tenderness.

  Localized tenderness anywhere in the right lower quadrant, even in the right flank, may indicate appendicitis.

- Feel for muscular rigidity.

  Early voluntary guarding may be replaced by involuntary muscular rigidity.

- *Perform a rectal examination and, in women, a pelvic examination.* These maneuvers may not help you to discriminate between a normal and an inflamed appendix, but they may help to identify an inflamed appendix atypically located within the pelvic cavity. They may also suggest other causes of the abdominal pain.

  Right-sided rectal tenderness may be caused by, for example, inflamed adnexa or an inflamed seminal vesicle, as well as by an inflamed appendix.

Additional techniques are sometimes helpful:

- Check the tender area for rebound tenderness. (If other signs are typically positive, you can save the patient unnecessary pain by omitting this test.)

  Rebound tenderness suggests peritoneal inflammation, as from appendicitis.

- Check for *Rovsing's sign* and for referred rebound tenderness. Press deeply and evenly in the *left* lower quadrant. Then quickly withdraw your fingers.

  Pain in the *right* lower quadrant during *left*-sided pressure suggests appendicitis (a positive Rovsing's sign). So does right lower quadrant pain on quick withdrawal (*referred rebound tenderness*).

- Look for a *psoas sign*. Place your hand just above the patient's right knee and ask the patient to raise that thigh against your hand. Alternatively, ask the patient to turn onto the left side. Then extend the patient's right leg at the hip. Flexion of the leg at the hip makes the psoas muscle contract; extension stretches it.

  Increased abdominal pain on either maneuver constitutes a *positive psoas* sign, suggesting irritation of the psoas muscle by an inflamed appendix.

- Look for an *obturator sign*. Flex the patient's right thigh at the hip, with the knee bent, and rotate the leg internally at the hip. This maneuver stretches the internal obturator muscle. (Internal rotation of the hip is described on p. 542.)

  Right hypogastric pain constitutes a positive obturator sign, suggesting irritation of the obturator muscle by an inflamed appendix.

- Test for *cutaneous hyperesthesia*. At a series of points down the abdominal wall, gently pick up a fold of skin between your thumb and index finger, without pinching it. This maneuver should not normally be painful.

  Localized pain with this maneuver, in all or part of the right lower quadrant, may accompany appendicitis.

ASSESSING POSSIBLE ACUTE CHOLECYSTITIS

When right upper quadrant pain and tenderness suggest acute cholecystitis, look for *Murphy's sign*. Hook your left thumb or the fingers of your right hand under the costal margin at the point where the lateral border of the rectus muscle intersects with the costal margin. Alternatively, if the liver is enlarged, hook your thumb or fingers under the liver edge at a comparable point below. Ask the patient to take a deep breath. Watch the patient's breathing and note the degree of tenderness.

A sharp increase in tenderness with a sudden stop in inspiratory effort constitutes a *positive Murphy's sign* of *acute cholecystitis*. Hepatic tenderness may also increase with this maneuver, but is usually less well localized.

ASSESSING VENTRAL HERNIAS

Ventral hernias are hernias in the abdominal wall exclusive of groin hernias. If you suspect but do not see an umbilical or incisional hernia, ask the patient to raise both head and shoulders off the table.

The bulge of a hernia will usually appear with this action (see p. 419).

Inguinal and femoral hernias are discussed in the next chapter. They can give rise to important abdominal problems and must not be overlooked.

The cause of intestinal obstruction or peritonitis may be missed by overlooking a strangulated femoral hernia.

MASS IN THE ABDOMINAL WALL

To Distinguish an Abdominal Mass From a Mass in the Abdominal Wall. An occasional mass is in the abdominal wall rather than inside the abdominal cavity. Ask the patient either to raise the head and shoulders or to strain down, thus tightening the abdominal muscles. Feel for the mass again.

A mass in the abdominal wall remains palpable; an intra-abdominal mass is obscured by muscular contraction.

RECORDING YOUR FINDINGS

Note that initially you may use sentences to describe your findings; later you will use phrases. The style below contains phrases appropriate for most write-ups.

Recording the Physical Examination—The Abdomen

"Abdomen is protuberant with active bowel sounds. It is soft and non-tender; no masses or hepatosplenomegaly. Liver span is 7 cm in the right midclavicular line; edge is smooth and palpable 1 cm below the right costal margin. Spleen and kidneys not felt. No costovertebral angle (CVA) tenderness."

OR

"Abdomen is flat. No bowel sounds heard. It is firm and boardlike, with increased tenderness, guarding, and rebound in the right midquadrant. Liver percusses to 7 cm in the midclavicular line; edge not felt. Spleen and kidneys not felt. No CVA tenderness.

Suggests peritonitis from possible appendicitis (see pp. 389–400 and pp. 387–388)

Bibliography

CITATIONS

1. Regier DA, Farmer ME, Rae DS, et al. Comorbidity of mental disorders with alcohol and other drug abuse. Results from the Epidemiologic Catchment Area (ECA) Study. JAMA 264(19): 2511–2518, 1990.
2. U.S. Preventive Services Task Force. Screening and Behavioral Counseling Interventions in Primary Care to Reduce Alcohol Misuse: Recommendation Statement. Rockville, MD, Agency for Healthcare Research and Quality, April 2004. Available at: http://www.ahrq.gov/clinic/3rduspstf/alcohol/alcomisrs. htm. Accessed December 4, 2004.
3. Ewing JA. Detecting alcoholism: the CAGE questionnaire. JAMA 252(14):1905–1907, 1984.
4. Whitlock EP, Green CA, Polen MR. Behavioral Counseling Interventions in Primary Care to Reduce Risky/Harmful Alcohol Use, Systematic Evidence Review. No. 30. (Prepared by the Oregon Evidence-based Practice Center under Contract No. 290-97-0018). Rockville, MD, Agency for Healthcare Research and Quality, April 2004. Available at www.ahrq/gov/clinic/serfiles.htm.
5. Whitlock EP, Orleans CT, Pender N., Allan J. Evaluating primary care behavioral counseling interventions. An evidence-based approach. Am J Prev Med 22(4):267–284, 2002.
6. Fiellin DA, Reid MC, O'Connor PG. Screening for alcohol problems in primary care: a systematic review. Arch Intern Med 160(13):1977–1989, 2000.
7. Miller WR, Rollnick S, Con K. Motivational Interviewing: Preparing People for Change, 2nd ed. New York, Guilford Press, 2002.
8. Miller WR, Sanchez VC. Motivating Young Alcoholics for Treatment and Lifestyle Changes. In Howard G (ed): Issues in Alcohol Use and Misuse by Young Adults. Notre Dame, IN, University of Notre Dame Press, 1993.
9. U.S. Preventive Services Task Force. Screening for Hepatitis B Infection: Recommendation Statement. Rockville, MD, Agency for Healthcare Research and Quality, February 2004. Available at: http://www.ahrq.gov/clinic/3rduspstf/hepbscr/ hepbrs.htm. Accessed December 4, 2004.
10. U.S. Preventive Services Task Force. Screening for Hepatitis C Infection: Recommendation Statement. Rockville, MD, Agency for Healthcare Research and Quality, March 2004. Available at: http://www.ahrq.gov/clinic/uspstf/uspshepc.htm. Accessed December 4, 2004.
11. U.S. Preventive Services Task Force Screening for Colorectal Cancer: Recommendations and Rationale. Rockville, MD, Agency for Healthcare Research and Quality, July 2002. Available at: http://www.ahrq.gov/clinic/3rduspstf/colorectal/ colorr.htm. Accessed December 4, 2004.
12. Winawer SJ, Shike M. Prevention and control of colorectal cancer. In Greenwald P, Kramer BS, Weed DL, eds. Cancer Prevention and Control. New York, Marcel-Dekker, 537–560, 1995.
13. American Cancer Society. ACS cancer detection guidelines. Available at: www.cancer.org. Accessed November 18, 2004.
14. U.S. Preventive Services Task Force. Screening for colorectal cancer. In Guide to Clinical Preventive Services, 2nd ed. Baltimore, Williams & Wilkins, 89–103, 1996.

ADDITIONAL REFERENCES

Examination of the Abdomen

Fink HA, Lederle FA, Rptj CS. The accuracy of physical examination to detect abdominal aortic aneurysm. Arch Intern Med 160(6):833–836, 2000.

Lederle FA, Simel DL. Does the patient have abdominal aortic aneurysm? JAMA 281(1):77–82, 1999.

McGee SR. Percussion and physical diagnosis: separating myth from science. Dis Mon 41(10):641–688, 1995.

Silen W, Cope Z. Cope's Early Diagnosis of the Acute Abdomen, 21st ed. Oxford, UK, and New York, Oxford University Press, 2005.

Sleisenger MH, Feldman M, Griedman LS, et al (eds). Sleisenger and Fortran's Gastrointestinal and Liver Disease: Pathophysiology, Diagnosis, Management, 8th ed. Philadelphia, WB Saunders, 2006.

Turnbull JM. Is listening for abdominal bruits useful in the evaluation of hypertension? JAMA 274(16):1299–1301, 1995.

Yamamoto W, Kono H, Maekawa H, et al. The relationship between abdominal pain regions and specific diseases: an epidemiologic approach to clinical practice. J Epidemiol 7(1):27–32, 1997.

Examination of the Liver

Meidl EJ, Ende J. Evaluation of liver size by physical examination. J Gen Intern Med 8(11):635–637, 1993.

Naylor CD. Physical examination of the liver. JAMA 271(23): 1859–1865, 1994.

Williams JW, Simel DL. Does this patient have ascites? How to divine fluid in the abdomen. JAMA 267(19):2645–2648, 1992.

Zoli M, Magliotti D, Drimaldi M, et al. Physical examination of the liver: is it still worth it? Am J Gastroenterol 90(9):1428–1432, 1995.

BIBLIOGRAPHY

Examination of the Spleen

Barkun ANB, Camus M, Green L, et al. The bedside assessment of splenic enlargement. Am J Med 91(5):512–518, 1991.

Barkun AN, Camus M, Meagher T, et al. Splenic enlargement and Traube's space: how useful is percussion? Am J Med 87(5): 562–566, 1989.

Grover SA, Barkun AN, Sackett DL. Does this patient have splenomegaly? JAMA 270(18):2218–1121, 1993.

Tamayo SG, Rickman LS, Matthews WC, et al. Examiner dependence on physical diagnostic tests of splenomegaly: a prospective study with multiple observers. J Gen Intern Med 8(2):69–75, 1993.

Gastrointestinal Conditions

Craig AS, Schaffner W. Prevention of hepatitis A with the hepatitis A vaccine. N Engl J Med 350(5):476–480, 2004.

Lembo A, Camilleri M. Chronic constipation. N Engl J Med 349(14):1360–1368, 2003.

Mertz HR. Irritable bowel syndrome. N Engl J Med 349(22): 2136–2146, 2003.

Thielman NM, Guerrant RL. Acute infectious diarrhea. N Engl J Med 350(1):38–47, 2004.

| TABLE 10-1 | Abdominal Pain |

Problem	Process	Location	Quality
Peptic Ulcer and Dyspepsia (*These disorders cannot be reliably differentiated by symptoms and signs.*)	Peptic ulcer refers to a demonstrable ulcer, usually in the duodenum or stomach. Dyspepsia causes similar symptoms but no ulceration. Infection by *Helicobacter pylori* is often present.	Epigastric, may radiate to the back	Variable: gnawing burning, boring, aching, pressing, or hungerlike
Cancer of the Stomach	A malignant neoplasm	Epigastric	Variable
Acute Pancreatitis	An acute inflammation of the pancreas	Epigastric, may radiate to the back or other parts of the abdomen; may be poorly localized	Usually steady
Chronic Pancreatitis	Fibrosis of the pancreas secondary to recurrent inflammation	Epigastric, radiating through to the back	Steady, deep
Cancer of the Pancreas	A malignant neoplasm	Epigastric and in either upper quadrant; often radiates to the back	Steady, deep
Biliary Colic	Sudden obstruction of the cystic duct or common bile duct by a gallstone	Epigastric or right upper quadrant; may radiate to the right scapula and shoulder	Steady, aching; *not* colicky
Acute Cholecystitis	Inflammation of the gallbladder, usually from obstruction of the cystic duct by a gallstone	Right upper quadrant or upper abdominal; may radiate to the right scapular area	Steady, aching
Acute Diverticulitis	Acute inflammation of a colonic diverticulum, a saclike mucosal outpouching through the colonic muscle	Left lower quadrant	May be cramping at first, but becomes steady
Acute Appendicitis	Acute inflammation of the appendix with distention or obstruction	■ Poorly localized *periumbilical pain,* followed usually by ■ *Right lower quadrant pain*	■ Mild but increasing, possibly cramping ■ Steady and more severe
Acute Mechanical Intestinal Obstruction	Obstruction of the bowel lumen, most commonly caused by (1) adhesions or hernias (small bowel), or (2) cancer or diverticulitis (colon)	■ *Small bowel:* periumbilical or upper abdominal ■ *Colon:* lower abdominal or generalized	■ Cramping ■ Cramping
Mesenteric Ischemia	Blood supply to the bowel and mesentery blocked from thrombosis or embolus (acute arterial occlusion), or reduced from hypoperfusion	May be periumbilical at first, then diffuse	Cramping at first, then steady

Timing	Factors That May Aggravate	Factors That May Relieve	Associated Symptoms and Setting
Intermittent. Duodenal ulcer is more likely than gastric ulcer or dyspepsia to cause pain that (1) wakes the patient at night, and (2) occurs intermittently over a few weeks, then disappears for months, and then recurs.	Variable	Food and antacids may bring relief, but not necessarily in any of these disorders and least commonly in gastric ulcer.	Nausea, vomiting, belching, bloating; heartburn (more common in duodenal ulcer); weight loss (more common in gastric ulcer). Dyspepsia is more common in the young (20–29 yrs), gastric ulcer in those over 50 yrs, and duodenal ulcer in those from 30–60 yrs.
The history of pain is typically shorter than in peptic ulcer. The pain is persistent and slowly progressive.	Often food	*Not* relieved by food or antacids	Anorexia, nausea, early satiety, weight loss, and sometimes bleeding. Most common in ages 50–70
Acute onset, persistent pain	Lying supine	Leaning forward with trunk flexed	Nausea, vomiting, abdominal distention, fever. Often a history of previous attacks and alcohol abuse or gallstones
Chronic or recurrent course	Alcohol, heavy or fatty meals	Possibly leaning forward with trunk flexed; often intractable	Symptoms of decreased pancreatic function may appear: diarrhea with fatty stools (steatorrhea) and diabetes mellitus.
Persistent pain; relentlessly progressive illness		Possibly leaning forward with trunk flexed; often intractable	Anorexia, nausea, vomiting, weight loss, and jaundice. Emotional symptoms, including depression
Rapid onset over a few minutes, lasts one to several hours and subsides gradually. Often recurrent			Anorexia, nausea, vomiting, restlessness
Gradual onset; course longer than in biliary colic	Jarring, deep breathing		Anorexia, nausea, vomiting, fever
Often a gradual onset			Fever, constipation. There may be initial brief diarrhea.
▪ Lasts roughly 4–6 hr			Anorexia, nausea, possibly vomiting, which typically follow the onset of pain; low fever
▪ Depends on intervention	▪ Movement or cough	▪ If it subsides temporarily, suspect perforation of the appendix.	
▪ Paroxysmal; may decrease as bowel mobility is impaired			▪ Vomiting of bile and mucus (high obstruction) or fecal material (low obstruction). Obstipation develops
▪ Paroxysmal, though typically milder			▪ Obstipation early. Vomiting late if at all. Prior symptoms of underlying cause.
Usually abrupt in onset, then persistent			Vomiting, diarrhea (sometimes bloody), constipation, shock

TABLE 10-2   Dysphagia

Process and Problem	Timing	Factors That Aggravate	Factors That Relieve	Associated Symptoms and Conditions
Transfer Dysphagia, *due to motor disorders affecting the pharyngeal muscles*	Acute or gradual onset and a variable course, depending on the underlying disorder	Attempts to start the swallowing process		Aspiration into the lungs or regurgitation into the nose with attempts to swallow. Neurologic evidence of stroke, bulbar palsy, or other neuro-muscular conditions
Esophageal Dysphagia				
Mechanical Narrowing				
■ Mucosal rings and webs	Intermittent	Solid foods	Regurgitation of the bolus of food	Usually none
■ Esophageal stricture	Intermittent, may become slowly progressive	Solid foods	Regurgitation of the bolus of food	A long history of heartburn and regurgitation
■ Esophageal cancer	May be intermittent at first; progressive over months	Solid foods, with progression to liquids	Regurgitation of the bolus of food	Pain in the chest and back and weight loss, especially late in the course of illness
Motor Disorders				
■ Diffuse esophageal spasm	Intermittent	Solids or liquids	Maneuvers described below; sometimes nitroglycerin	Chest pain that mimics angina pectoris or myocardial infarction and lasts minutes to hours; possibly heartburn
■ Scleroderma	Intermittent, may progress slowly	Solids or liquids	Repeated swallowing, movements such as straightening the back, raising the arms, or a Valsalva maneuver (straining down against a closed glottis)	Heartburn. Other manifestations of scleroderma
■ Achalasia	Intermittent, may progress	Solids or liquids		Regurgitation, often at night when lying down, with nocturnal cough; possibly chest pain precipitated by eating

TABLE 10-3 Constipation

Problem	Process	Associated Symptoms and Setting
Life Activities and Habits		
Inadequate Time or Setting for the Defecation Reflex	Ignoring the sensation of a full rectum inhibits the defecation reflex.	Hectic schedules, unfamiliar surroundings, bed rest
False Expectations of Bowel Habits	Expectations of "regularity" or more frequent stools than a person's norm	Beliefs, treatments, and advertisements that promote the use of laxatives
Diet Deficient in Fiber	Decreased fecal bulk	Other factors such as debilitation and constipating drugs may contribute.
Irritable Bowel Syndrome	A common disorder of bowel motility	Small, hard stools, often with mucus. Periods of diarrhea. Cramping abdominal pain. Stress may aggravate.
Mechanical Obstruction		
Cancer of the Rectum or Sigmoid Colon	Progressive narrowing of the bowel lumen	Change in bowel habits; often diarrhea, abdominal pain, and bleeding. In rectal cancer, tenesmus and pencil-shaped stools
Fecal Impaction	A large, firm, immovable fecal mass, most often in the rectum	Rectal fullness, abdominal pain, and diarrhea around the impaction. Common in debilitated, bedridden, and often elderly patients
Other Obstructing Lesions (such as diverticulitis, volvulus, intussusception, or hernia)	Narrowing or complete obstruction of the bowel	Colicky abdominal pain, abdominal distention, and in intussusception, often "currant jelly" stools (red blood and mucus)
Painful Anal Lesions	Pain may cause spasm of the external sphincter and voluntary inhibition of the defecation reflex.	Anal fissures, painful hemorrhoids, perirectal abscesses
Drugs	A variety of mechanisms	Opiates, anticholinergics, antacids containing calcium or aluminum, and many others
Depression	A disorder of mood. See Table 16-1, Disorders of Mood.	Fatigue, feelings of depression, and other somatic symptoms
Neurologic Disorders	Interference with the autonomic innervation of the bowel	Spinal cord injuries, multiple sclerosis, Hirschsprung's disease, and other conditions
Metabolic Conditions	Interference with bowel motility	Pregnancy, hypothyroidism, hypercalcemia

TABLE 10-4   Diarrhea

Problem	Process	Characteristics of Stool
Acute Diarrhea		
Secretory Infections	Infection by viruses, preformed bacterial toxins (such as *Staphylococcus aureus, Clostridium perfringens*, toxigenic *Escherichia coli, Vibrio cholerae*), cryptosporidium, *Giardia lamblia*	Watery, without blood, pus, or mucus
Inflammatory Infections	Colonization or invasion of intestinal mucosa (nontyphoid *Salmonella, Shigella, Yersinia, Campylobacter*, enteropathic *E. coli, Entamoeba histolytica*)	Loose to watery, often with blood, pus, or mucus
Drug-Induced Diarrhea	Action of many drugs, such as magnesium-containing antacids, antibiotics, antineoplastic agents, and laxatives	Loose to watery
Chronic Diarrhea		
Diarrheal Syndromes		
■ Irritable bowel syndrome	A disorder of bowel motility with alternating diarrhea and constipation	Loose; may show mucus but no blood. Small, hard stools with constipation
■ Cancer of the sigmoid colon	Partial obstruction by a malignant neoplasm	May be blood-streaked
Inflammatory Bowel Disease		
■ Ulcerative colitis	Inflammation of the mucosa and submucosa of the rectum and colon with ulceration; cause unknown	Soft to watery, often containing blood
■ Crohn's disease of the small bowel (regional enteritis) or colon (granulomatous colitis)	Chronic inflammation of the bowel wall, typically involving the terminal ileum and/or proximal colon	Small, soft to loose or watery, usually free of gross blood (enteritis) or with less bleeding than ulcerative colitis (colitis)
Voluminous Diarrheas		
■ Malabsorption syndromes	Defective absorption of fat, including fat-soluble vitamins, with steatorrhea (excessive excretion of fat) as in pancreatic insufficiency, bile salt deficiency, bacterial overgrowth	Typically bulky, soft, light yellow to gray, mushy, greasy or oily, and sometimes frothy; particularly foul-smelling; usually floats in the toilet
■ Osmotic diarrheas		
Lactose intolerance	Deficiency in intestinal lactase	Watery diarrhea of large volume
Abuse of osmotic purgatives	Laxative habit, often surreptitious	Watery diarrhea of large volume
■ Secretory diarrheas from bacterial infection, secreting villous adenoma, fat or bile salt malabsorption, hormone-mediated conditions (gastrin in Zollinger–Ellison syndrome, vasoactive intestinal peptide [VIP])	Variable	Watery diarrhea of large volume

Timing	Associated Symptoms	Setting, Persons at Risk
Duration of a few days, possibly longer. Lactase deficiency may lead to a longer course.	Nausea, vomiting, periumbilical cramping pain. Temperature normal or slightly elevated	Often travel, a common food source, or an epidemic
An acute illness of varying duration	Lower abdominal cramping pain and often rectal urgency, tenesmus; fever	Travel, contaminated food or water. Men and women who have had frequent anal intercourse.
Acute, recurrent, or chronic	Possibly nausea; usually little if any pain	Prescribed or over-the-counter medications
Often worse in the morning. Diarrhea rarely wakes the patient at night.	Crampy lower abdominal pain, abdominal distention, flatulence, nausea, constipation	Young and middle-aged adults, especially women
Variable	Change in usual bowel habits, crampy lower abdominal pain, constipation	Middle-aged and older adults, especially older than 55 yrs
Onset ranges from insidious to acute. Typically recurrent, may be persistent. Diarrhea may wake the patient at night.	Crampy lower or generalized abdominal pain, anorexia, weakness, fever	Often young people
Insidious onset, chronic or recurrent. Diarrhea may wake the patient at night.	Crampy periumbilical or right lower quadrant (enteritis) or diffuse (colitis) pain, with anorexia, low fever, and/or weight loss. Perianal or perirectal abscesses and fistulas	Often young people, especially in the late teens, but also in the middle years. More common in people of Jewish descent
Onset of illness typically insidious	Anorexia, weight loss, fatigue, abdominal distention, often crampy lower abdominal pain. Symptoms of nutritional deficiencies such as bleeding (vitamin K), bone pain and fractures (vitamin D), glossitis (vitamin B), and edema (protein)	Variable, depending on cause
Follows the ingestion of milk and milk products; is relieved by fasting	Crampy abdominal pain, abdominal distention, flatulence	African Americans, Asians, Native Americans
Variable	Often none	Persons with anorexia nervosa or bulimia nervosa
Variable	Weight loss, dehydration, nausea, vomiting, and cramping abdominal pain	Variable depending on cause

TABLE 10-5   Black and Bloody Stools

Problem	Selected Causes	Associated Symptoms and Setting
Melena Melena refers to the passage of black, tarry (sticky and shiny) stools. Tests for occult blood are positive. Melena signifies the loss of at least 60 ml of blood into the gastrointestinal tract (less in infants and children), usually from the esophagus, stomach, or duodenum. Less commonly, when intestinal transit is slow, the blood may originate in the jejunum, ileum, or ascending colon. In infants, melena may result from swallowing blood during the birth process.	Peptic ulcer Gastritis or stress ulcers Esophageal or gastric varices Reflux esophagitis Mallory-Weiss tear, a mucosal tear in the esophagus due to retching and vomiting	Often, but not necessarily, a history of epigastric pain Recent ingestion of alcohol, aspirin, or other anti-inflammatory drugs; recent bodily trauma, severe burns, surgery, or increased intracranial pressure Cirrhosis of the liver or other cause of portal hypertension History of heartburn Retching, vomiting, often recent ingestion of alcohol
Black, Nonsticky Stools Black stools may result from other causes and then usually give negative results when tested for occult blood. (Ingestion of iron or other substances, however, may cause a positive test result in the absence of blood.) These stools have no pathologic significance.	Ingestion of iron, bismuth salts as in Pepto-Bismol, licorice, or even commercial chocolate cookies	

Red Blood in the Stools
 	
Red blood usually originates in the colon, rectum, or anus, and much less frequently in the jejunum or ileum. Upper gastrointestinal hemorrhage, however, may also cause red stools. The amount of blood lost is then usually large (more than a liter). Transit time through the intestinal tract is accordingly rapid, giving insufficient time for the blood to turn black.
	Cancer of the colon
	Benign polyps of the colon
	Diverticula of the colon
	Inflammatory conditions of the colon and rectum
	  ■ Ulcerative colitis, Crohn's disease
	  ■ Infectious dysenteries
	  ■ Proctitis (various causes) in men or women who have had frequent anal intercourse
	Ischemic colitis
	
	Hemorrhoids
	
	Anal fissure
		Often a change in bowel habits
		Often no other symptoms
		
		Often no other symptoms
		
		See Table 10-4, Diarrhea.
		
		See Table 10-4, Diarrhea.
		Rectal urgency, tenesmus
		
		Lower abdominal pain and sometimes fever or shock in persons older than age 50 yrs
		Blood on the toilet paper, on the surface of the stool, or dripping into the toilet
		Blood on the toilet paper or on the surface of the stool; anal pain

Reddish but Nonbloody Stools	Ingestion of beets	Pink urine, which usually precedes the reddish stool

TABLE 10-6   Frequency, Nocturia, and Polyuria

Problem	Mechanisms	Selected Causes	Associated Symptoms
Frequency	Decreased capacity of the bladder		
	■ Increased bladder sensitivity to stretch because of inflammation	*Infection*, stones, tumor, or foreign body in the bladder	Burning on urination, urinary urgency, sometimes gross hematuria
	■ Decreased elasticity of the bladder wall	Infiltration by scar tissue or tumor	Symptoms of associated inflammation (see above) are common.
	■ Decreased cortical inhibition of bladder contractions	Motor disorders of the central nervous system, such as a stroke	Urinary urgency; neurologic symptoms such as weakness and paralysis
	Impaired emptying of the bladder, with residual urine in the bladder		
	■ Partial mechanical obstruction of the bladder neck or proximal urethra	Most commonly, benign prostatic hyperplasia; also urethral stricture and other obstructive lesions of the bladder or prostate	Prior obstructive symptoms: hesitancy in starting the urinary stream, straining to void, reduced size and force of the stream, and dribbling during or at the end of urination
	■ Loss of peripheral nerve supply to the bladder	Neurologic disease affecting the sacral nerves or nerve roots, e.g., diabetic neuropathy	Weakness or sensory defects
Nocturia *With High Volumes*	Most types of polyuria (see p. 369)		
	Decreased concentrating ability of the kidney with loss of the normal decrease in nocturnal urinary output	Chronic renal insufficiency due to a number of diseases	Possibly other symptoms of renal insufficiency
	Excessive fluid intake before bedtime	Habit, especially involving alcohol and coffee	
	Fluid-retaining, edematous states. Dependent edema accumulates during the day and is excreted when the patient lies down at night.	Congestive heart failure, nephrotic syndrome, hepatic cirrhosis with ascites, chronic venous insufficiency	Edema and other symptoms of the underlying disorder. Urinary output during the day may be reduced as fluid reaccumulates in the body. See Table 14-4, Some Peripheral Causes of Edema.
With Low Volumes	Frequency Voiding while up at night without a real urge, a "pseudo-frequency"	Insomnia	Variable
Polyuria	Deficiency of antidiuretic hormone (diabetes insipidus)	A disorder of the posterior pituitary and hypothalamus	Thirst and polydipsia, often severe and persistent; nocturia
	Renal unresponsiveness to antidiuretic hormone (nephrogenic diabetes insipidus)	A number of kidney diseases, including hypercalcemic and hypokalemic nephropathy; drug toxicity, e.g., from lithium	Thirst and polydipsia, often severe and persistent; nocturia
	Solute diuresis		
	■ Electrolytes, such as sodium salts	Large saline infusions, potent diuretics, certain kidney diseases	Variable
	■ Nonelectrolytes, such as glucose	Uncontrolled diabetes mellitus	Thirst, polydipsia, and nocturia
	Excessive water intake	Primary polydipsia	Polydipsia tends to be episodic. Thirst may not be present. Nocturia is usually absent.

TABLE 10-7   Urinary Incontinence*

Problem	Mechanisms
Stress Incontinence The urethral sphincter is weakened so that transient increases in intra-abdominal pressure raise the bladder pressure to levels that exceed urethral resistance.	In women, most often a weakness of the pelvic floor with inadequate muscular support of the bladder and proximal urethra and a change in the angle between the bladder and the urethra. Suggested causes include childbirth and surgery. Local conditions affecting the internal urethral sphincter, such as postmenopausal atrophy of the mucosa and urethral infection, may also contribute. In men, stress incontinence may follow prostatic surgery.
Urge Incontinence Detrusor contractions are stronger than normal and overcome the normal urethral resistance. The bladder is typically *small*.	▪ Decreased cortical inhibition of detrusor contractions, as by strokes, brain tumors, dementia, and lesions of the spinal cord above the sacral level ▪ Hyperexcitability of sensory pathways, as in bladder infections, tumors, and fecal impaction ▪ Deconditioning of voiding reflexes, as in frequent voluntary voiding at low bladder volumes
Overflow Incontinence Detrusor contractions are insufficient to overcome urethral resistance. The bladder is typically *large*, even after an effort to void.	▪ Obstruction of the bladder outlet, as by benign prostatic hyperplasia or tumor ▪ Weakness of the detrusor muscle associated with peripheral nerve disease at the sacral level ▪ Impaired bladder sensation that interrupts the reflex arc, as from diabetic neuropathy
Functional Incontinence This is a functional inability to get to the toilet in time because of impaired health or environmental conditions.	Problems in mobility resulting from weakness, arthritis, poor vision, or other conditions. Environmental factors such as an unfamiliar setting, distant bathroom facilities, bed rails, or physical restraints
Incontinence Secondary to Medications Drugs may contribute to any type of incontinence listed.	Sedatives, tranquilizers, anticholinergics, sympathetic blockers, and potent diuretics

*Patients may have more than one kind of incontinence.

Symptoms	Physical Signs
Momentary leakage of small amounts of urine concurrent with stresses such as coughing, laughing, and sneezing while the person is in an upright position. A desire to urinate is not associated with pure stress incontinence.	The bladder is not detected on abdominal examination. Stress incontinence may be demonstrable, especially if the patient is examined before voiding and in a standing position. Atrophic vaginitis may be evident.
Incontinence preceded by an urge to void. The volume tends to be moderate. Urgency Frequency and nocturia with small to moderate volumes If acute inflammation is present, pain on urination Possibly "pseudo-stress incontinence"—voiding 10–20 sec after stresses such as a change of position, going up or down stairs, and possibly coughing, laughing, or sneezing	The bladder is not detectable on abdominal examination. When cortical inhibition is decreased, mental deficits or motor signs of central nervous system disease are often, though not necessarily, present. When sensory pathways are hyperexcitable, signs of local pelvic problems or a fecal impaction may be present.
A continuous dripping or dribbling incontinence Decreased force of the urinary stream Prior symptoms of partial urinary obstruction or other symptoms of peripheral nerve disease may be present.	An enlarged bladder is often found on abdominal examination and may be tender. Other possible signs include prostatic enlargement, motor signs of peripheral nerve disease, a decrease in sensation including perineal sensation, and diminished to absent reflexes.
Incontinence on the way to the toilet or only in the early morning	The bladder is not detectable on physical examination. Look for physical or environmental clues to the likely cause.
Variable. A careful history and chart review are important.	Variable

TABLE 10-8 | Localized Bulges in the Abdominal Wall

Localized bulges in the abdominal wall include *ventral hernias* (defects in the wall through which tissue protrudes) and subcutaneous tumors such as *lipomas*. The more common ventral hernias are umbilical, incisional, and epigastric. Hernias and a rectus diastasis usually become more evident when the patient raises head and shoulders from a supine position.

Umbilical Hernia

A protrusion through a defective umbilical ring is most common in infants but also occurs in adults. In infants, but not in adults, it usually closes spontaneously within 1 to 2 years.

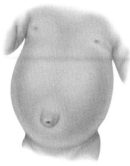

INFANT

Diastasis Recti

Separation of the two rectus abdominis muscles, through which abdominal contents form a midline ridge when the patient raises head and shoulders. Often is seen in repeated pregnancies, obesity, and chronic lung disease. It has no clinical consequences.

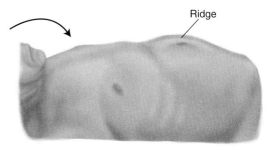

Ridge

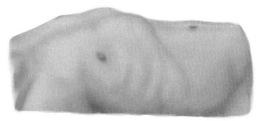

Incisional Hernia

This is a protrusion through an operative scar. Palpate to detect the length and width of the defect in the abdominal wall. A small defect, through which a large hernia has passed, has a greater risk for complications than a large defect.

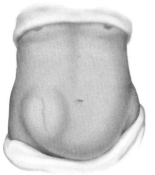

Epigastric Hernia

A small midline protrusion through a defect in the linea alba occurs between the xiphoid process and the umbilicus. With the patient's head and shoulders raised (or with the patient standing), run your fingerpad down the linea alba to feel it.

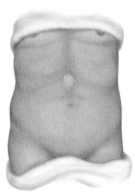

Lipoma

Common, benign, fatty tumors usually occur in the subcutaneous tissues almost anywhere in the body, including the abdominal wall. Small or large, they are usually soft and often lobulated. Press your finger down on the edge of a lipoma. The tumor typically slips out from under it.

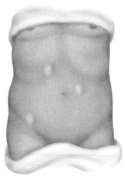

TABLE 10-9   Protuberant Abdomens

Fat

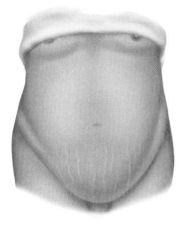

Fat is the most common cause of a protuberant abdomen. Fat thickens the abdominal wall, the mesentery, and omentum. The umbilicus may appear sunken. A *pannus*, or apron of fatty tissue, may extend below the inguinal ligaments. Lift it to look for inflammation in the skin folds or even for a hidden hernia.

Gas

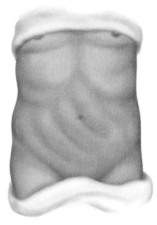

Gaseous distention may be localized or generalized. It causes a tympanitic percussion note. Increased intestinal gas production from certain foods may cause mild distention. More serious are intestinal obstruction and adynamic (paralytic) ileus. Note the location of the distention. Distention becomes more marked in colonic than in small bowel obstruction.

Tumor

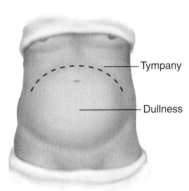

A large, solid tumor, usually rising out of the pelvis, is dull to percussion. Air-filled bowel is displaced to the periphery. Causes include ovarian tumors and uterine myomata. Occasionally a markedly distended bladder may be mistaken for such a tumor.

Pregnancy

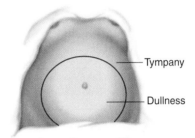

Pregnancy is a common cause of a pelvic "mass." Listen for the fetal heart (see pp. 830–831).

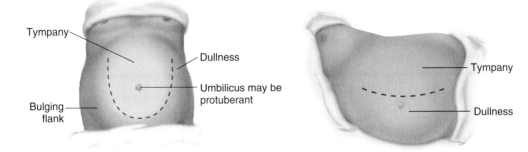

Ascitic Fluid

Ascitic fluid seeks the lowest point in the abdomen, producing bulging flanks that are dull to percussion. The umbilicus may protrude. Turn the patient onto one side to detect the shift in position of the fluid level (shifting dullness). (See pp. 387–389 for the assessment of ascites.)

TABLE 10-10	Sounds in the Abdomen

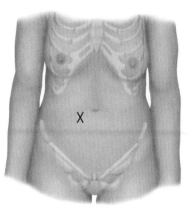

Bowel Sounds

Bowel sounds may be:

- *Increased*, as from diarrhea or *early intestinal obstruction*
- *Decreased*, then absent, as in *adynamic ileus and peritonitis.* Before deciding that bowel sounds are absent, sit down and listen where shown for 2 min or even longer.

High-pitched tinkling sounds suggest intestinal fluid and air under tension in a dilated bowel. *Rushes of high-pitched sounds* coinciding with an abdominal cramp indicate intestinal obstruction.

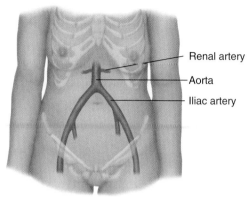

Bruits

A *hepatic bruit* suggests carcinoma of the liver or alcoholic hepatitis. *Arterial bruits* with both systolic and diastolic components suggest partial occlusion of the aorta or large arteries. Partial occlusion of a renal artery may explain hypertension.

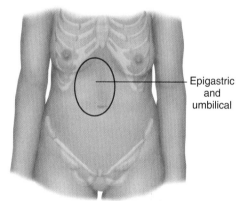

Venous Hum

A venous hum is rare. It is a soft humming noise with both systolic and diastolic components. It indicates increased collateral circulation between portal and systemic venous systems, as in hepatic cirrhosis.

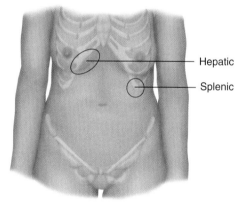

Friction Rubs

Friction rubs are rare. They are grating sounds with respiratory variation. They indicate inflammation of the peritoneal surface of an organ, as from a liver tumor, chlamydial or gonococcal perihepatitis, recent liver biopsy, or splenic infarct. When a systolic bruit accompanies a hepatic friction rub, suspect carcinoma of the liver.

TABLE 10-11 Tender Abdomens

Abdominal Wall Tenderness

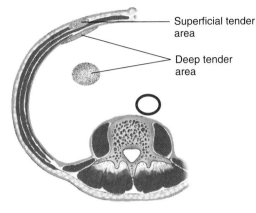

Superficial tender area

Deep tender area

Tenderness may originate in the abdominal wall. When the patient raises head and shoulders, this tenderness persists, whereas tenderness from a deeper lesion (protected by the tightened muscles) decreases.

Visceral Tenderness

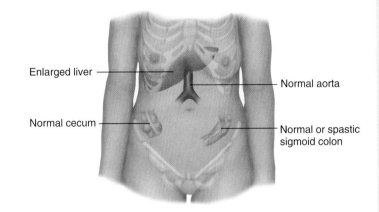

Enlarged liver

Normal aorta

Normal cecum

Normal or spastic sigmoid colon

The structures shown may be tender to deep palpation. Usually the discomfort is dull with no muscular rigidity or rebound tenderness. A reassuring explanation to the patient may prove quite helpful.

Tenderness From Disease in the Chest and Pelvis

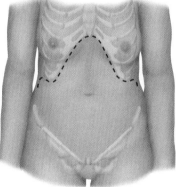

Unilateral or bilateral, upper or lower abdomen

Acute Pleurisy

Abdominal pain and tenderness may result from acute pleural inflammation. When unilateral, it may mimic acute cholecystitis or appendicitis. Rebound tenderness and rigidity are less common; chest signs are usually present.

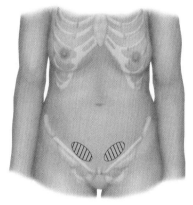

Acute Salpingitis

Frequently bilateral, the tenderness of acute salpingitis (inflammation of the fallopian tubes) is usually maximal just above the inguinal ligaments. Rebound tenderness and rigidity may be present. On pelvic examination, motion of the uterus causes pain.

(table continues next page)

TABLE 10-11   **Tender Abdomens** *(Continued)*

Tenderness of Peritoneal Inflammation

Tenderness associated with peritoneal inflammation is more severe than visceral tenderness. Muscular rigidity and rebound tenderness are frequently but not necessarily present. Generalized peritonitis causes exquisite tenderness throughout the abdomen, together with boardlike muscular rigidity. Local causes of peritoneal inflammation include:

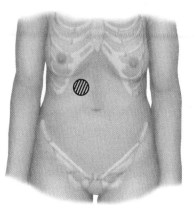

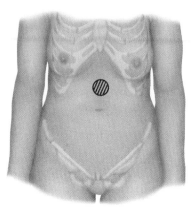

Acute Cholecystitis

Signs are maximal in the right upper quadrant. Check for Murphy's sign (see p. 400).

Acute Pancreatitis

In acute pancreatitis, epigastric tenderness and rebound tenderness are usually present, but the abdominal wall may be soft.

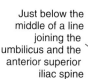
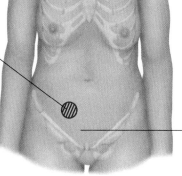

Just below the middle of a line joining the umbilicus and the anterior superior iliac spine

Right rectal tenderness

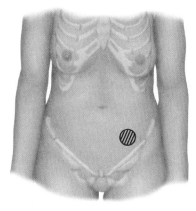

Acute Appendicitis

Right lower quadrant signs are typical of acute appendicitis, but may be absent early in the course. The typical area of tenderness is illustrated. Explore other portions of the right lower quadrant as well as the right flank.

Acute Diverticulitis

Acute diverticulitis most often involves the sigmoid colon and then resembles a left-sided appendicitis.

TABLE 10-12   Liver Enlargement: Apparent and Real

A palpable liver does not necessarily indicate hepatomegaly (an enlarged liver), but more often results from a change in consistency—from the normal softness to an abnormal firmness or hardness, as in cirrhosis. Clinical estimates of liver size should be based on both percussion and palpation, although even these techniques are far from perfect.

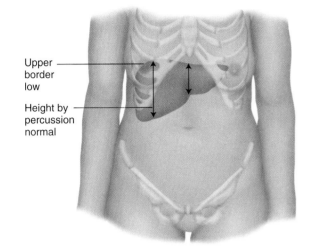

Upper border low

Height by percussion normal

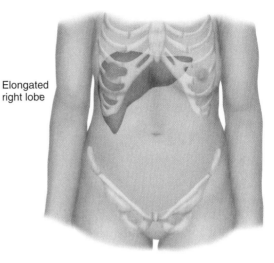

Elongated right lobe

Downward Displacement of the Liver by a Low Diaphragm

This finding is common when the diaphragm is low (e.g., in emphysema). The liver edge may be readily palpable well below the costal margin. Percussion, however, reveals a low upper edge also, and the vertical span of the liver is normal.

Normal Variations in Liver Shape

In some people, especially those with a lanky build, the liver tends to be elongated so that its right lobe is easily palpable as it projects downward toward the iliac crest. Such an elongation, sometimes called *Riedel's lobe*, represents a variation in shape, not an increase in liver volume or size. Examiners can only estimate the upper and lower borders of an organ with three dimensions and differing shapes. Some error is unavoidable.

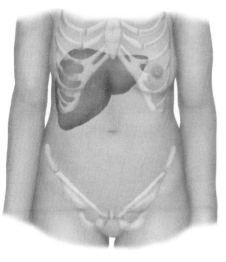

Smooth Large Liver

Cirrhosis may produce an enlarged liver with a firm *nontender* edge. The liver is not always enlarged in this condition, however, and many other diseases may produce similar findings. An enlarged liver with a smooth *tender* edge suggests inflammation, as in hepatitis, or venous congestion, as in right-sided heart failure.

Irregular Large Liver

An enlarged liver that is firm or hard and has an irregular edge or surface suggests malignancy. There may be one or more nodules. The liver may or may not be tender.

Male Genitalia and Hernias

ANATOMY AND PHYSIOLOGY

Review the anatomy of the male genitalia.

The *shaft of the penis* is formed by three columns of vascular erectile tissue: the *corpus spongiosum,* containing the urethra, and two *corpora cavernosa.* The corpus spongiosum forms the bulb of the penis, ending in the cone-

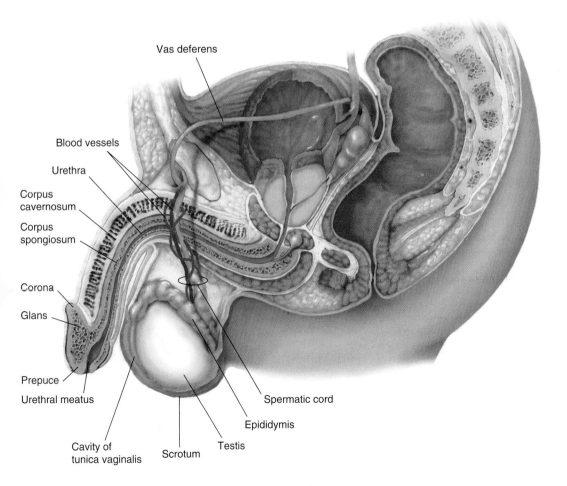

shaped *glans* with its expanded base, or *corona*. In uncircumsized men, the glans is covered by a loose, hoodlike fold of skin called the *prepuce* or *foreskin* where *smegma,* or secretions of the glans, may collect. The urethra is located ventrally in the shaft of the penis; urethral abnormalities may sometimes be felt there. The urethra opens into the vertical, slitlike *urethral meatus,* located somewhat ventrally at the tip of the glans.

The *testes* are ovoid, somewhat rubbery structures approximately 4.5 cm long, although their size ranges from 3.5 cm to 5.5 cm. The left testis usually lies somewhat lower than the right. The testes produce spermatozoa and testosterone. Testosterone stimulates the pubertal growth of the male genitalia, prostate, and seminal vesicles. It also stimulates the development of masculine secondary sex characteristics, including facial hair, body hair, musculoskeletal growth, and enlargement of the larynx, with its associated low-pitched voice.

Surrounding or appended to the testes are several structures. The *scrotum* is a loose wrinkled pouch divided into two compartments, each containing a testis or testicle. Covering the testis, except posteriorly, is the serous membrane of the *tunica vaginalis.* On the posterolateral surface of each testis is the softer comma-shaped *epididymis,* consisting of tightly coiled spermatic ducts that provide a reservoir for storage, maturation, and transport of sperm from the testis to the *vas deferens.*

The *vas deferens,* a cordlike structure, begins at the tail of the epididymis, ascends within the scrotal sac, and passes through the external inguinal ring on its way to the abdomen and pelvis. Behind the bladder, it is joined by the duct from the seminal vesicle and enters the urethra within the prostate gland. Sperm thus passes from the testis and the epididymis through the vas deferens into the urethra. Secretions from the vasa deferentia, the seminal vesicles, and the prostate all contribute to the semen. Within the scrotum, each vas is closely associated with blood vessels, nerves, and muscle fibers. These structures make up the *spermatic cord.*

Male sexual function depends on normal levels of testosterone, adequate arterial blood flow to the inferior epigastric artery and its cremasteric and pubic branches, and intact neural innervation from α-adrenergic and cholinergic pathways. Erection from venous engorgement of the corpora cavernosa results from two types of stimuli. Visual, auditory, or erotic cues trigger sympathetic outflow from higher brain centers to the T11 through L2 levels of the spinal cord. Tactile stimulation initiates sensory impulses from the genitalia to S_2 to S_4 reflex arcs and parasympathetic pathways through the pudendal nerve. Both sets of stimuli appear to increase levels of nitric oxide and cyclic GMP, resulting in local vasodilation.

Lymphatics. Lymphatics from the penile and scrotal surfaces drain into the inguinal nodes. *When you find an inflammatory or possibly malignant lesion* on these surfaces, *assess the inguinal nodes especially carefully* for enlargement or tenderness. The lymphatics of the testes, however, drain into the abdomen, where enlarged nodes are clinically undetectable. See page 477 for further discussion of the inguinal nodes.

Anatomy of the Groin. Because hernias are relatively common, it is important to understand the anatomy of the groin. The basic landmarks are the anterior superior iliac spine, the pubic tubercle, and the inguinal ligament that runs between them. Find these on yourself or a colleague.

The *inguinal canal,* which lies above and approximately parallel to the inguinal ligament, forms a tunnel for the vas deferens as it passes through the abdominal muscles. The exterior opening of the tunnel—the *external inguinal ring*—is a triangular, slitlike structure palpable just above and lateral to the pubic tubercle. The internal opening of the canal—or *internal inguinal ring*—is approximately 1 cm above the midpoint of the inguinal ligament. Neither canal nor internal ring is palpable through the abdominal wall. When loops of bowel force their way through weak areas of the inguinal canal, they produce *inguinal hernias,* as illustrated on pp. 426–427.

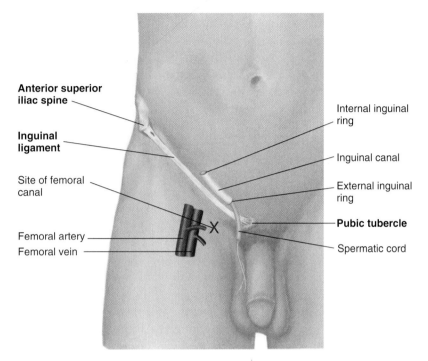

Another potential route for a herniating mass is the *femoral canal.* This lies below the inguinal ligament. Although you cannot see it, you can estimate its location by placing your right index finger, from below, on the right femoral artery. Your middle finger will then overlie the femoral vein; your ring finger, the femoral canal. Femoral hernias protrude here.

THE HEALTH HISTORY

Common or Concerning Symptoms

- Changes in sexual function and response
- Penile discharge or lesions
- Scrotal pain, swelling, or lesions

For men, questions about the genitalia follow naturally after those dealing with the urinary system. You will need to review sexual function and screen for symptoms of infection. Begin with general questions such as "How is sexual function for you?" "Are you satisfied with your sexual life?" "What about your ability to perform sexually?" If the patient reports a sexual problem, ask him to tell you about it. Ask if there has been any change in desire or level of sexual activity recently. What does he think has caused it, what has he tried to do about it, and what are his hopes? Identify the patient's sexual preference as to partners (male, female, or both). Find out if the patient's partner has any concerns.

Direct questions help you to assess each phase of the sexual response. To assess *libido*, or desire, ask "Have you maintained interest in sex?" For the *arousal phase*, ask "Can you achieve and maintain an erection?" Explore the timing, severity, setting, and any other factors that may be contributing to problems. Have any changes in the relationship with his partner or in his life circumstances coincided with onset of a problem? Are there circumstances when erection is normal? On awakening in the early morning or during the night? With other partners? With masturbation?

Lack of libido may arise from psychogenic causes such as depression, endocrine dysfunction, or side effects of medications.

Erectile dysfunction may be from psychogenic causes, especially if early morning erection is preserved; also from decreased testosterone, decreased blood flow in the hypogastric arterial system, or impaired neural innervation.

Other questions relate to the phase of *orgasm* and *ejaculation* of semen. If ejaculation is premature, or early and out of control, ask "About how long does intercourse last?" "Do you climax too soon?" "Do you feel like you have any control over climaxing?" "Do you think your partner would like intercourse to last longer?" For reduced or absent ejaculation, "Do you find that you cannot have orgasm even though you can have an erection?" Try to determine whether the problem involves the pleasurable sensation of orgasm, the ejaculation of seminal fluid, or both. Review the frequency and setting of the problem, medications, surgery, and neurologic symptoms.

Premature ejaculation is common, especially in young men. Less common is reduced or absent ejaculation affecting middle-aged or older men. Possible causes are medications, surgery, neurologic deficits, or lack of androgen. Lack of orgasm with ejaculation is usually psychogenic.

To assess the possibility of genital infection from sexually transmitted diseases (STDs), ask about any *discharge from the penis,* dripping, or staining of underwear. If penile discharge is present, assess the amount, its color and consistency, and any fever, chills, rash, or associated symptoms.

Penile discharge may accompany gonococcal (usually yellow) and nongonococcal urethritis (may be clear or white).

Inquire about *sores or growths on the penis,* and any *pain or swelling in the scrotum*. Ask about previous genital symptoms or a past history of infections from herpes, gonorrhea, or syphilis. A patient who has multiple partners, is homosexual, uses illicit drugs, or has a prior history of STDs is at increased risk for subsequent STDs.

See Table 11-1, Abnormalities of the Penis (p. 422), Table 11-2, Abnormalities of the Scrotal Sac (p. 423), and Table 11-3, Abnormalities of the Testis (p. 424). In addition to STDs, many skin conditions affect the genitalia; likewise, some STDs have minimal symptoms or signs.

Because STDs may involve other parts of the body, additional questions are often indicated. An introductory explanation may be useful. "Sexually transmitted diseases can involve any body opening where you have sex. It's important for you to tell me which openings you use." And further, as needed, "Do you have oral sex? Anal sex?" If the patient's answers are affirmative, ask about symptoms such as sore throat, diarrhea, rectal bleeding, and anal itching or pain.

Infections from oral–penile transmission include gonorrhea, *Chlamydia*, syphilis, and herpes. Symptomatic or asymptomatic proctitis may follow anal intercourse.

For the many patients without symptoms or known risk factors, it is wise to ask, "Do you have any concerns about HIV infection?" as an important screening question and to continue with the more general questions suggested on pp. 48–49.

HEALTH PROMOTION AND COUNSELING

Important Topics for Health Promotion and Counseling

- Prevention of STDs and HIV
- Testicular self-examination

Each clinician must address the high burden of *STDs* on the U.S. population that warrants direct engagement with patients in disease prevention, especially adolescents and young adults. The U.S. Preventive Services Task Force registers an estimated 12 million new infections each year from *Chlamydia* (approximately 4 million cases), gonorrhea (approximately 800,000 cases), and *Trichomas* vaginitis and nonspecific urethritis ("several million cases" annually).[1] More than 1 million Americans are currently infected with HIV, with approximately 40,000 new infections annually. Additional infections that can be transmitted sexually include syphilis, human papillomavirus (HPV), hepatitis B, and genital herpes. Clinicians should educate patients about STD infections and HIV, practice early detection during history-taking and physical examination, and identify and treat infected patients and their partners.

Health promotion and counseling should address patient education about STDs and HIV, early detection of infection during history taking and physical examination, and identification and treatment of infected partners. Discussion of risk factors for STDs and HIV is especially important for adolescents and younger patients, the age groups most adversely affected. Clinicians must be comfortable with eliciting the sexual history and with asking frank but tactful questions about sexual practices. A minimal history includes identifying the patient's sexual orientation, the number of sexual partners in the past month, and any history of STDs (see Chap. 2, p. 48). Questions should be clear and nonjudgmental. You should also identify use of alcohol and drugs, particularly injection drugs. Counsel patients at risk about limiting the number of partners, using condoms, and establishing regular medical care for treatment of STDs and HIV. It is important for men to seek prompt attention for any genital lesions or penile discharge.

The U.S. Preventive Services Task Force recommends counseling and testing for HIV infection in the following groups: all persons at increased risk for infection with HIV, STDs, or both; men with male partners; past or present injection drug users; any past or present partners of people with HIV infection, bisexual practices, or injection drug use; and patients with a history of transfusion between 1978 and 1985.

In addition, encourage men, especially those between the ages of 15 and 35, to perform monthly *testicular self-examinations* and to seek physician evaluation for the following findings: any painless lump, swelling, or enlargement in either testicle; pain or discomfort in a testicle or the scrotum; a feeling of heaviness or a sudden fluid collection in the scrotum; or a dull ache in the lower abdomen or the groin. (See p. 420 for instructions to patients.)[2]

TECHNIQUES OF EXAMINATION

Many students feel uneasy about examining a man's genitalia. "How will the patient react?" "Will he have an erection?" "Will he let me examine him?" It may be reassuring to explain each step of the examination so that the patient knows what to expect. Requesting an assistant to accompany you is common practice. Occasionally, male patients have erections during the examination. If this happens, you should explain to the patient that this is a normal response, finish your examination, and proceed with an unruffled demeanor. If the man refuses to be examined, you should respect his wishes.

A good genital examination can be done with the patient either standing or supine. To check for hernias or varicoceles, however, the patient should stand, and you should sit comfortably on a chair or stool. A gown conveniently covers the patient's chest and abdomen. Wear *gloves* throughout the examination. Expose the genitalia and inguinal areas. For younger patients, review the sexual maturity ratings on page 781.

THE PENIS

INSPECTION

Inspect the penis, including:

- The *skin*

See Table 11-1, Abnormalities of the Penis (p. 422).

- The *prepuce* (foreskin). If it is present, retract it or ask the patient to retract it. This step is essential for the detection of many chancres and carcinomas. Smegma, a cheesy, whitish material, may accumulate normally under the foreskin.

Phimosis is a tight prepuce that cannot be retracted over the glans. *Paraphimosis* is a tight prepuce that, once retracted, cannot be returned. Edema ensues.

■ The *glans.* Look for any ulcers, scars, nodules, or signs of inflammation.

Balanitis (inflammation of the glans); *balanoposthitis* (inflammation of the glans and prepuce)

Check the skin around the base of the penis for excoriations or inflammation. Look for nits or lice at the bases of the pubic hairs.

Pubic or genital excoriations suggest the possibility of lice (crabs) or sometimes scabies.

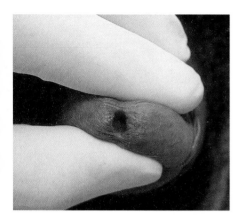

Note the location of the urethral meatus.

Hypospadias is a congenital, ventral displacement of the meatus on the penis (p. 422).

Compress the glans gently between your index finger above and your thumb below. This maneuver should open the urethral meatus and allow you to inspect it for discharge. Normally there is none.

Profuse yellow discharge in gonococcal urethritis; scanty white or clear discharge in non-gonococcal urethritis. Definitive diagnosis requires Gram stain and culture.

If the patient has reported a discharge that you are unable to see, ask him to strip, or milk, the shaft of the penis from its base to the glans. Alternatively, do it yourself. This maneuver may bring some discharge out of the urethral meatus for appropriate examination. Have a glass slide and culture materials ready.

PALPATION

Palpate any abnormality of the penis, noting any tenderness or induration. Palpate the shaft of the penis between your thumb and first two fingers, noting any induration. Palpation of the shaft may be omitted in a young, asymptomatic male patient.

If you retract the foreskin, replace it before proceeding on to examine the scrotum.

Induration along the ventral surface of the penis suggests a urethral stricture or possibly a carcinoma. Tenderness of such an indurated area suggests periurethral inflammation secondary to a urethral stricture.

◤ THE SCROTUM AND ITS CONTENTS

INSPECTION

Inspect the scrotum, including:

See Table 11-2, Abnormalities of the Scrotal Sac (p. 423).

■ The *skin.* Lift up the scrotum so that you can see its posterior surface.

Rashes, epidermoid cysts, rarely skin cancer

■ The *scrotal contours.* Note any swelling, lumps, or veins.

A poorly developed scrotum on one or both sides suggests *cryptorchidism* (an undescended testicle). Common scrotal swellings include indirect inguinal hernias, hydroceles, and scrotal edema. Tender, painful scrotal swelling in acute epididymitis, acute orchitis, torsion of the spermatic cord, or a strangulated inguinal hernia.

See Table 11-3, Abnormalities of the Testis (p. 425) and Table 11-4, Abnormalities of the Epididymis and Spermatic Cord (p. 425).

PALPATION

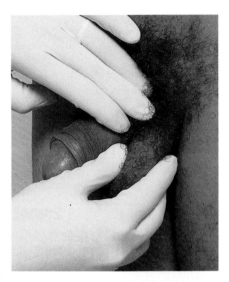

Palpate each testis and epididymis between your thumb and first two fingers. Locate the epididymis on the superior posterior surface of each testicle. It feels nodular and cordlike and should not be confused with an abnormal lump.

Note size, shape, consistency, and tenderness; feel for any nodules. Pressure on the testis normally produces a deep visceral pain.

Any painless nodule in the testis must raise the possibility of *testicular cancer,* a potentially curable cancer with a peak incidence between the ages of 15 and 35 years.

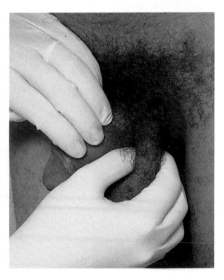

Palpate each spermatic cord, including the vas deferens, between your thumb and fingers from the epididymis to the superficial inguinal ring.

Note any nodules or swellings.

Multiple tortuous veins in this area, usually on the left, may be palpable and even visible. They indicate a *varicocele* (p. 425).

The vas deferens, if chronically infected, may feel thickened or beaded. A cystic structure in the spermatic cord suggests a hydrocele of the cord.

Swelling in the scrotum other than the testicles can be evaluated by transillumination. After darkening the room, shine the beam of a strong flashlight from behind the scrotum through the mass. Look for transmission of the light as a red glow.

Swellings containing serous fluid, as in hydroceles, light up with a red glow, or transilluminate. Those containing blood or tissue, such as a normal testis, a tumor, or most hernias, do not.

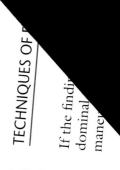

▪▪ HERNIAS

INSPECTION

Inspect the inguinal and femoral areas carefully for bulges. While you continue your observation, ask the patient to strain and bear down, as if having a bowel movement (the Valsalva maneuver) to enhance detection of hernias.

A bul
sugg

PALPATION

Palpate for an inguinal hernia. With the patient still standing, and using in turn your right hand for the patient's right side and your left hand for the patient's left side, invaginate loose scrotal skin with your index finger. Start at a point low enough to be sure that your finger will have enough mobility to reach as far as the internal inguinal ring if this proves possible. Follow the spermatic cord upward to above the inguinal ligament and find the triangular, slitlike opening of the external inguinal ring. This is just above and lateral to the pubic tubercle. If the ring is somewhat enlarged, it may admit your index finger. If possible, gently follow the inguinal canal laterally in its oblique course. With your finger located either at the external ring or within the canal, ask the patient to strain down or cough. Note any palpable herniating mass as it touches your finger.

See Table 11-5, Course and Presentation of Hernias in the Groin (p. 426).

See Table 11-6, Differentiation of Hernias in the Groin (p. 427).

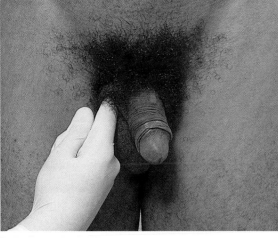

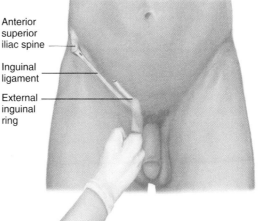

Anterior superior iliac spine —

Inguinal ligament —

External inguinal ring —

Palpate for a femoral hernia by placing your fingers on the anterior thigh in the region of the femoral canal. Ask the patient to strain down again or cough. Note any swelling or tenderness.

Evaluating a Possible Scrotal Hernia. If you find a large scrotal mass and suspect that it may be a hernia, ask the patient to lie down. The mass may return to the abdomen by itself. If so, it is a hernia. If not:

▪ Can you get your fingers above the mass in the scrotum?

If you can, suspect a hydrocele.

▪ Listen to the mass with a stethoscope for bowel sounds.

Bowel sounds may be heard over a hernia, but not over a hydrocele.

ngs suggest a hernia, gently try to reduce it (return it to the abdominal cavity) by sustained pressure with your fingers. Do not attempt this ...ver if the mass is tender or the patient reports nausea and vomiting.

...story may be helpful here. The patient can usually tell you what happens to his swelling on lying down and may be able to demonstrate how he reduces it himself. Remember to ask him.

A hernia is *incarcerated* when its contents cannot be returned to the abdominal cavity. A hernia is *strangulated* when the blood supply to the entrapped contents is compromised. Suspect strangulation in the presence of tenderness, nausea, and vomiting and consider surgical intervention.

SPECIAL TECHNIQUES

THE TESTICULAR SELF-EXAMINATION

The incidence of testicular cancer is low, about 4 per 100,000 men, but it is the most common cancer of young men between ages 15 and 35. Although the testicular self-examination (TSE) has not been formally endorsed as a screen for testicular carcinoma, you may wish to teach your patient the TSE to enhance health awareness and self-care. When detected early, testicular carcinoma has an excellent prognosis. Risk factors include cryptorchidism, which confers a high risk for testicular carcinoma in the undescended testicle; a history of carcinoma in the contralateral testicle; mumps orchitis; an inguinal hernia; and a hydrocele in childhood.

PATIENT INSTRUCTIONS FOR THE TESTICULAR SELF-EXAMINATION*

This examination is best performed after a warm bath or shower. The heat relaxes the scrotum and makes it easier to find anything unusual.

- Standing in front of a mirror, check for any swelling on the skin of the scrotum.
- Examine each testicle with both hands. Cup the index and middle fingers under the testicle and place the thumbs on top.
- Roll the testicle gently between the thumbs and fingers. One testicle may be larger than the other . . . that's normal, but be concerned about any lump or area of pain.
- Find the epididymis. This is a soft, tubelike structure at the back of the testicle that collects and carries sperm, not an abnormal lump.
- If you find any lump, don't wait. See your doctor. The lump may just be an infection, but if it is cancer, it will spread unless stopped by treatment.

* Medline Plus. U.S. National Library of Medicine and National Cancer Institute. Medical Encyclopedia—Testicular self-examination. Available at: www.nlm.nih.gov/medlineplus/ency/article/003909.htm. Accessed October 31, 2004.

RECORDING YOUR FINDINGS

Note that initially you may use sentences to describe your findings; later you will use phrases. The style below contains phrases appropriate for most write-ups.

Recording the Physical Examination— Male Genitalia and Hernias

"Circumsized male. No penile discharge or lesions. No scrotal swelling or discoloration. Testes descended bilaterally, smooth, without masses. Epididymis nontender. No inguinal or femoral hernias."

OR

"Uncircumsized male; prepuce easily retractible. No penile discharge or lesions. No scrotal swelling or discoloration. Testes descended bilaterally; right testicle smooth; 1 × 1 cm firm nodule on left lateral testicle. It is fixed and nontender. Epididymis nontender. No inguinal or femoral hernias."

Suspicious for testicular carcinoma, the most common form of cancer in men between the ages of 15 and 35

Bibliography

CITATIONS

1. Agency for Healthcare Research and Quality. Electronic Archive. Guide to Clinical Preventive Services, 2nd ed. 1996. Available at: www.ahrq.gov/clinic/cpsix.htm#counseling. Accessed October 31, 2004. (For the *Guide to Clinical Preventive Services*, 3rd ed., periodic updates, see www.ahrq/gov/clinic/cps3dix.htm. Accessed October 31, 2004.)
2. National Cancer Institute. Cancer Facts. Available at: http://cis.nih.gov/fact/6_34.htm. Accessed October 31, 2004.

ADDITIONAL REFERENCES

Barry MJ. Prostate-specific antigen testing for early diagnosis of prostate cancer. N Engl J Med 344(18):1373–1377, 2001.

Campbell MF, Walsh PC, Patrick C, Retik AB (eds). Campbell's Urology, 8th ed. Philadelphia, WB Saunders, 2002.

DeBusk RF. Sexual activity in patients with angina. JAMA 290(23):3129–3132, 2003.

Delancey JOL, Ashton-Miller JA. Pathophysiology of adult urinary incontinence. Gastroenterology 126(Suppl 1):S23–S32, 2004.

Eubanks S. Hernias (Chapter 42). In Townsend CM, Sabiston DC (eds). Sabiston Textbook of Surgery: The Biological Basis of Modern Surgical Practice, 17th ed. Philadelphia, Elsevier Saunders, 2004.

Fitzgibbons RJ, Filipi CJ, Quinn TH. Inguinal hernias (Chapter 36). In Brunicardi FC, Andersen DK, Billiar TR, et al (eds). Schwartz's Principles of Surgery, 8th ed. New York, McGraw-Hill, 2005.

Gillenwater JY. Adult and Pediatric Urology, 4th ed. Philadelphia, Lippincott Williams & Wilkins, 2002.

Handsfield HH. Color Atlas and Synopsis of Sexually Transmitted Diseases, 2nd ed. New York, McGraw-Hill, 2001.

Laumann EO, Paik A, Rosen RC. Sexual function in the United States: prevalence and predictors. JAMA 281(6):537–544, 1999.

Tanagho EA, McAninch JW (eds). Smith's General Urology, 16th ed. New York, Lange Medical Books, McGraw-Hill, 2004.

Teunissen TAM, de Jonge A, van Weel C, et al. Treating urinary incontinence in the elderly—conservative measures that work: a systematic review. J Fam Pract 53(1):25–30, 2004.

TABLE 11-1   **Abnormalities of the Penis**

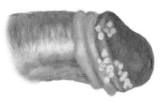

Venereal Wart
(Condyloma acuminatum)
Venereal warts are rapidly growing excrescences that are moist and often malodorous. They result from infection by human papillomavirus.

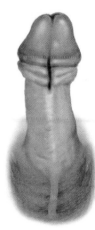

Hypospadias
Hypospadias is a congenital displacement of the urethral meatus to the inferior surface of the penis. A groove extends from the actual urethral meatus to its normal location on the tip of the glans.

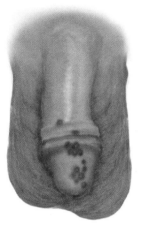

Genital Herpes
A cluster of small vesicles, followed by shallow, painful, nonindurated ulcers on red bases, suggests a herpes simplex infection. The lesions may occur anywhere on the penis. Usually there are fewer lesions when the infection recurs.

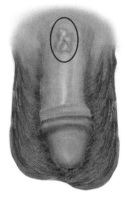

Peyronie's Disease
In Peyronie's disease, palpable nontender hard plaques are found just beneath the skin, usually along the dorsum of the penis. The patient complains of crooked, painful erections.

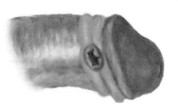

Syphilitic Chancre
A syphilitic chancre usually appears as an oval or round, dark red, painless erosion or ulcer with an indurated base. Nontender enlarged inguinal lymph nodes are typically associated. Chancres may be multiple and, when secondarily infected, may be painful. They may then be mistaken for the lesions of herpes. Chancres are infectious.

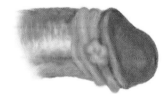

Carcinoma of the Penis
Carcinoma may appear as an indurated nodule or ulcer that is usually nontender. Limited almost completely to men who are not circumcised in childhood, it may be masked by the prepuce. Any persistent penile sore must be considered suspicious.

TABLE 11-2   Abnormalities of the Scrotal Sac

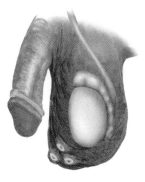

Epidermoid Cysts

These are firm, yellowish, nontender, cutaneous cysts up to about 1 cm in diameter. They are common and frequently multiple.

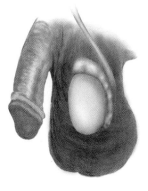

Scrotal Edema

Pitting edema may make the scrotal skin taut. This may accompany the generalized edema of congestive heart failure or nephrotic syndrome.

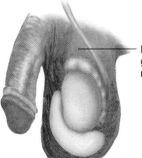

Fingers can get above mass

Hydrocele

A hydrocele is a nontender, fluid-filled mass within the tunica vaginalis. It transilluminates, and the examining fingers can get above the mass within the scrotum.

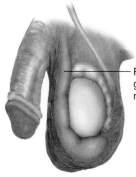

Fingers cannot get above mass

Scrotal Hernia

A hernia within the scrotum is usually an *indirect inguinal hernia*. It comes through the external inguinal ring, so the examining fingers cannot get above it within the scrotum.

TABLE 11-3   **Abnormalities of the Testis**

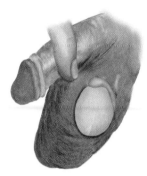

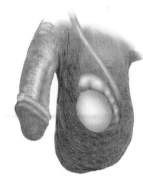

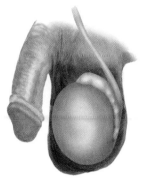

Cryptorchidism

In cryptorchidism, the testis is atrophied and may lie in the inguinal canal or the abdomen, resulting in an undeveloped scrotum, as above. There is no palpable left testis or epididymis. Cryptorchidism markedly raises the risk for testicular cancer.

Small Testis

In adults, the length is usually ≤ 3.5 cm. Small firm testes in *Klinefelter's syndrome*, usually ≤ 2 cm. Small soft testes suggesting atrophy seen in cirrhosis, myotonic dystrophy, use of estrogens, and hypopituitarism; may also follow orchitis.

Acute Orchitis

The testis is acutely inflamed, painful, tender, and swollen. It may be difficult to distinguish from the epididymis. The scrotum may be reddened. Seen in mumps and other viral infections; usually unilateral.

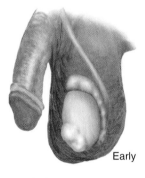

Early

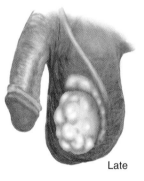

Late

Tumor of the Testis

Usually appears as a painless nodule. Any nodule within the testis warrants investigation for malignancy.

As a testicular neoplasm grows and spreads, it may seem to replace the entire organ. The testicle characteristically feels heavier than normal.

TABLE 11-4   **Abnormalities of the Epididymis and Spermatic Cord**

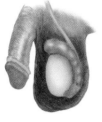

Acute Epididymitis

An acutely inflamed epididymis is tender and swollen and may be difficult to distinguish from the testis. The scrotum may be reddened and the vas deferens inflamed. It occurs chiefly in adults. Coexisting urinary tract infection or prostatitis supports the diagnosis.

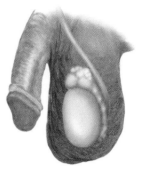

Spermatocele and Cyst of the Epididymis

A painless, movable cystic mass just above the testis suggests a spermatocele or an epididymal cyst. Both transilluminate. The former contains sperm, and the latter does not, but they are clinically indistinguishable.

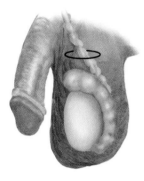

Tuberculous Epididymitis

The chronic inflammation of tuberculosis produces a firm enlargement of the epididymis, which is sometimes tender, with thickening or beading of the vas deferens.

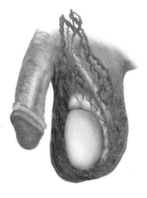

Varicocele

Varicocele refers to varicose veins of the spermatic cord, usually found on the left. It feels like a soft " bag of worms" separate from the testis, and slowly collapses when the scrotum is elevated in the supine patient. Infertility may be associated.

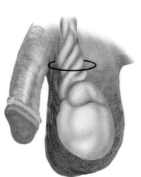

Torsion of the Spermatic Cord

Torsion, or twisting, of the testicle on its spermatic cord produces an acutely painful, tender, and swollen organ that is retracted upward in the scrotum. The scrotum becomes red and edematous. There is no associated urinary infection. Torsion, most common in adolescents, is a surgical emergency because of obstructed circulation.

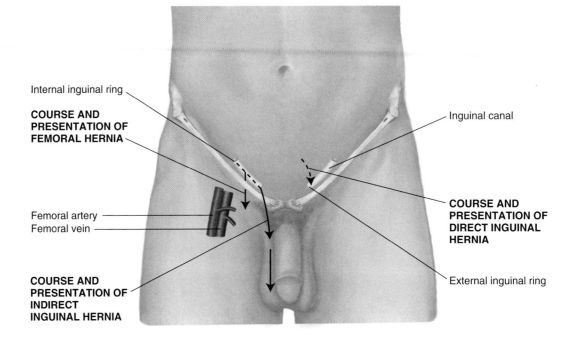

Internal inguinal ring

COURSE AND PRESENTATION OF FEMORAL HERNIA

Femoral artery

Femoral vein

COURSE AND PRESENTATION OF INDIRECT INGUINAL HERNIA

Inguinal canal

COURSE AND PRESENTATION OF DIRECT INGUINAL HERNIA

External inguinal ring

TABLE 11-6   Differentiation of Hernias in the Groin

Differentiation among these hernias is not always clinically possible. Understanding their features, however, improves your observation.

	Inguinal		Femoral
	Indirect	*Direct*	**Femoral**
Frequency	Most common, all ages, both sexes	Less common	Least common
Age and Sex	Often in children, may be in adults	Usually in men older than 40, rare in women	More common in women than in men
Point of Origin	Above inguinal ligament, near its midpoint (the internal inguinal ring)	Above inguinal ligament, close to the pubic tubercle (near the external inguinal ring)	Below the inguinal ligament; appears more lateral than an inguinal hernia and may be hard to differentiate from lymph nodes
Course	Often into the scrotum	Rarely into the scrotum	Never into the scrotum
With the examining finger in the inguinal canal during straining or cough	The hernia comes down the inguinal canal and touches the fingertip.	The hernia bulges anteriorly and pushes the side of the finger forward.	The inguinal canal is empty.

Female Genitalia

ANATOMY AND PHYSIOLOGY

Review the anatomy of the external female genitalia, or *vulva*, including the *mons pubis,* a hair-covered fat pad overlying the symphysis pubis; the *labia majora,* rounded folds of adipose tissue; the *labia minora,* thinner pinkish red folds that extend anteriorly to form the *prepuce;* and the *clitoris.* The *vestibule* is the boat-shaped fossa between the labia minora. In its posterior portion lies the vaginal opening, the *introitus,* which in virgins may be hidden by the *hymen.* The term *perineum,* as commonly used clinically, refers to the tissue between the introitus and the anus.

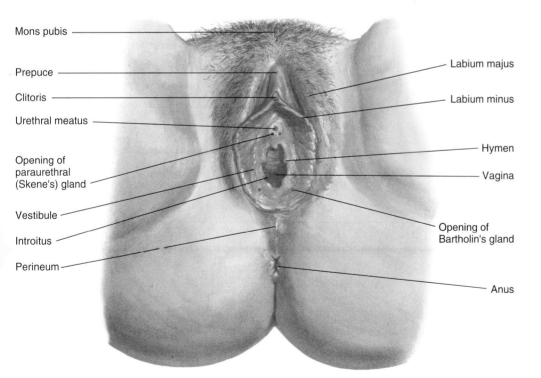

The *urethral meatus* opens into the vestibule between the clitoris and the vagina. Just posterior to it on either side lie the openings of the *paraurethral* (Skene's) *glands.*

The openings of *Bartholin's glands* are located posteriorly on either side of the vaginal opening, but are not usually visible. Bartholin's glands themselves are situated more deeply.

The *vagina* is a musculomembranous tube extending upward and posteriorly between the urethra and the rectum. Its upper third takes a horizontal plane and terminates in the cup-shaped *fornix.* The vaginal mucosa lies in transverse folds, or rugae.

At almost right angles to the vagina lies the *uterus,* a flattened fibromuscular structure shaped like an inverted pear. The uterus has two parts: the body (corpus) and the cervix, which are joined together by the isthmus. The convex upper surface of the body is called the *fundus* of the uterus. The lower part of the uterus, the *cervix,* protrudes into the vagina, dividing the fornix into anterior, posterior, and lateral fornices.

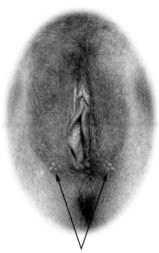

Location of
Bartholin's glands

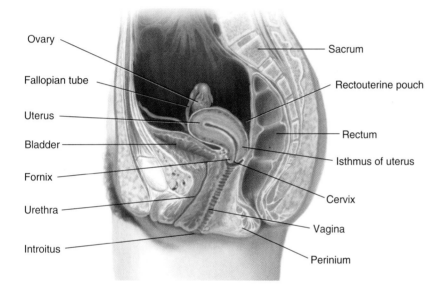

Ovary

Fallopian tube

Uterus

Bladder

Fornix

Urethra

Introitus

Sacrum

Rectouterine pouch

Rectum

Isthmus of uterus

Cervix

Vagina

Perinium

The vaginal surface of the cervix, the *ectocervix,* is seen easily with the help of a speculum. At its center is a round, oval, or slitlike depression, the *external os* of the cervix, which marks the opening into the endocervical canal. The ectocervix is covered by epithelium of two possible types: a plushy, red columnar epithelium surrounding the os, which resembles the lining of the endocervical canal; and a shiny pink squamous epithelium continuous with the vaginal lining. The *squamocolumnar junction* forms the boundary between these two types of epithelium. During puberty, the broad band of columnar epithelium encircling the os, called *ectropion,* is gradually replaced by columnar epithelium. The squamocolumnar junction migrates toward the os, creating the *transformation zone.* This is the area at risk for later dysplasia, which is sampled by the Papanicolaou, or Pap, smear.

A *fallopian tube* with a fanlike tip extends from each side of the uterus toward the ovary. The two ovaries are almond-shaped structures that vary con-

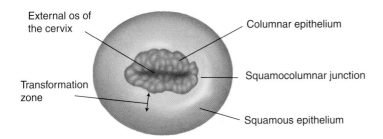

siderably in size but average about 3.5 × 2 × 1.5 cm from adulthood through menopause. The ovaries are palpable on pelvic examination in roughly half of women during the reproductive years. Normally, fallopian tubes cannot be felt. The term *adnexa*, a plural Latin word meaning appendages, refers to the ovaries, tubes, and supporting tissues.

The ovaries have two primary functions: the production of ova and the secretion of hormones, including estrogen, progesterone, and testosterone. Increased hormonal secretions during puberty stimulate the growth of the uterus and its endometrial lining. They stimulate enlargement of the vagina and thicken its epithelium. They also stimulate the development of secondary sex characteristics, including the breasts and pubic hair.

The parietal peritoneum extends downward behind the uterus into a cul de sac called the *rectouterine pouch* (pouch of Douglas). You can just reach this area on rectovaginal examination.

The pelvic organs are supported by a sling of tissues composed of muscle, ligaments, and fascia, through which the urethra, vagina, and rectum all pass.

Assessment of sexual maturity in girls, as classified by Tanner, depends not on internal examination, but on the growth of pubic hair and the development of breasts. Tanner's stages, or sexual maturity ratings, as they relate to pubic hair and breasts are shown in Chapter 18, Assessing Children: Infancy Through Adolescence.

In most women, pubic hair spreads downward in a triangular pattern, pointing toward the vagina. In 10% of women, it may form an inverted triangle, pointing toward the umbilicus. This growth is usually not completed until the middle 20s or later.

Just before menarche, there is a physiologic increase in vaginal secretions—a normal change that sometimes worries a girl or her mother. As menses become established, increased secretions (*leukorrhea*) coincide with ovulation. They also accompany sexual arousal. These normal kinds of discharges must be differentiated from those of infectious processes.

Lymphatics.   Lymph from the vulva and the lower vagina drains into the inguinal nodes. Lymph from the internal genitalia, including the upper vagina, flows into the pelvic and abdominal lymph nodes, which are not palpable.

THE HEALTH HISTORY

Common Concerns

- Menarche, menstruation, menopause, postmenopausal bleeding
- Pregnancy
- Vulvovaginal symptoms
- Sexual activity

Questions in this section focus on menstruation, pregnancy and related topics, vulvovaginal symptoms, and sexual function.

Menarche, Menstruation, Menopause.   For the menstrual history, ask the patient how old she was when her monthly, or menstrual, periods began, or age at *menarche*. When did her last period start, and, if possible, the one before that? How often does she have periods, as measured by the interval between the first days of successive periods? How regular or irregular are they? How long do they last? How heavy is the flow? What color is it? Flow can be assessed roughly by the number of pads or tampons used daily. Because women vary in their practices for sanitary measures, however, ask the patient whether she usually soaks a pad or tampon, spots it lightly, etc. Further, does she use more than one at a time? Does she have any bleeding between periods? Any bleeding after intercourse?

Does the patient have any discomfort or pain before or during her periods? If so, what is it like, how long does it last, and does it interfere with her usual activities? Are there other associated symptoms? Ask a middle-aged or older woman if she has stopped menstruating. When? Did any symptoms accompany her change? Has she had any bleeding since?

Questions about *menarche, menstruation,* and *menopause* often give you an opportunity to explore the patient's need for information and her attitude toward her body. When talking with an adolescent girl, for example, opening questions might include: "How did you first learn about monthly periods? How did you feel when they started? Many girls worry when their periods aren't regular or come late. Has anything like that bothered you?" You can explain that girls in the United States usually begin to menstruate between the ages of 9 and 16 years, and often take 1 year or more before they settle into a reasonable, regular pattern. Age at menarche is variable, depending on genetic endowment, socioeconomic status, and nutrition. The interval between periods ranges roughly from 24 to 32 days; the flow lasts from 3 to 7 days.

Menopause, the absence of menses for 12 consecutive months, usually occurs between the ages of 48 and 55 years.[1] Associated symptoms include hot flashes, flushing, sweating, and disturbances of sleep. Often you will ask, "How do (did) you feel about not having your periods anymore? Has it af-

The dates of previous periods signal possible pregnancy or menstrual irregularities.

Unlike the normal dark red menstrual discharge, excessive flow tends to be bright red and may include "clots" (not true fibrin clots).

Postmenopausal bleeding raises the question of endometrial cancer, although it also has other causes.

fected your life in any way?" *Postmenopausal bleeding* is defined as bleeding that occurs after 6 months without periods and warrants further investigation.

Amenorrhea refers to the absence of periods. Failure to initiate periods is called *primary amenorrhea*, whereas the cessation of periods after they have been established is termed *secondary amenorrhea*. Pregnancy, lactation, and menopause are physiologic forms of the secondary type. *Oligomenorrhea* refers to infrequent periods, which may also be irregular. This pattern is common for as long as 2 years after menarche, and it also occurs before menopause.

Other causes of *secondary amenorrhea* include low body weight from any cause, including malnutrition and anorexia nervosa, stress, chronic illness, and hypothalamic–pituitary–ovarian dysfunction.

Dysmenorrhea is pain with menstruation and is usually felt as a bearing down, aching, or cramping sensation in the lower abdomen and pelvis. Women may report *premenstrual syndrome (PMS)*, a complex of symptoms occurring 4 to 10 days before a period. PMS symptoms include tension, nervousness, irritability, depression, and mood swings; weight gain, abdominal bloating, edema, and tenderness of the breasts; and headaches. Though usually mild, PMS symptoms may be severe and disabling.

Polymenorrhea means abnormally frequent periods, and *menorrhagia* refers to an increased amount or duration of flow. Bleeding may also occur between periods, termed *metrorrhagia* or *intermenstrual bleeding*, after intercourse (*postcoital bleeding*), or after other vaginal contact from practices such as douching.

Increased frequency, increased flow, or bleeding between periods may have systemic causes or may be dysfunctional. *Postcoital bleeding* suggests cervical disease (e.g., polyps, cancer) or, in an older woman, atrophic vaginitis.

Pregnancy. Questions relating to pregnancy include "Have you ever been pregnant? How many times? . . . How many living children do you have? . . . Have you ever had a miscarriage or an abortion? How many times?" Ask about any difficulties during pregnancy and the timing and circumstances of any abortion, whether spontaneous or induced. How did the woman experience these losses? Obstetricians commonly record the pregnancy history using the "gravida-para" system, with the following abbreviations:

■ G = gravida, or total number of pregnancies

■ P = para, or outcomes of pregnancies. After P, you will often see the notations F (full-term), P (premature), A (abortion), and L (living child).

Inquire about methods of contraception used by the patient and her partner. Is the patient satisfied with the method chosen? Are there any questions about the options available?

If amenorrhea suggests a *current pregnancy*, inquire about the history of intercourse and *common early symptoms*: tenderness, tingling, or increased size of the breasts; urinary frequency; nausea and vomiting; easy fatigability; and feelings that the baby is moving, usually noted at about 20 weeks. Be considerate of the patient's feelings in discussing all these topics and explore them as seems indicated. (See also Chapter 19, The Pregnant Woman).

Amenorrhea followed by heavy bleeding suggests a *threatened abortion* or *dysfunctional uterine bleeding* related to lack of ovulation.

Vulvovaginal Symptoms.   The most common vulvovaginal symptoms are *vaginal discharge* and local *itching*. Follow your usual approach. If the patient reports a discharge, inquire about its amount, color, consistency, and odor. Ask about any local *sores* or *lumps* in the vulvar area. Are they painful or not? Because patients vary in their understanding of anatomic terms, be prepared to try alternative phrasing such as "Any itching (or other symptoms) near your vagina? . . . between your legs? . . . where you urinate?"

Sexual Activity.   Start with general questions such as "How is sex for you?" Or "Are you having any problems with sex?" You can also ask, "Are you satisfied with your sex life as it is now? Has there been any significant change in the last few years? Are you satisfied with you ability to perform sexually? How satisfied do you think your partner is? Do you feel that your partner is satisfied with the frequency of sexual activity?"

If the patient has concerns about sexual activity, ask her to tell you about it. Direct questions help you assess each phase of the sexual response: desire, arousal, and orgasm. "Do you have an interest in (appetite for) sex?" inquires about the desire phase. For the orgasmic phase, "Are you able to reach climax (reach an orgasm or 'come')?" "Is it important for you to reach climax?" For arousal, "Do you get sexually aroused? Do you lubricate easily (get wet or slippery)? Do you stay too dry?"

Ask also about *dyspareunia,* or discomfort or pain during intercourse. If present, try to localize the symptom. Is it near the outside, occurring at the start of intercourse, or does she feel it farther in, when her partner is pushing deeper? *Vaginismus* refers to an involuntary spasm of the muscles surrounding the vaginal orifice that makes penetration during intercourse painful or impossible.

In addition to ascertaining the nature of a sexual problem, ask about its onset, severity (persistent or sporadic), setting, and factors, if any, that make it better or worse. What does the patient think is the cause of the problem, what has she tried to do about it, and what does she hope for? The setting of sexual dysfunction is an important but complicated topic, involving the patient's general health; medications and drugs, including use of alcohol; her partner's and her own knowledge of sexual practices and techniques; her attitudes, values, and fears; the relationship and communication between partners; and the setting in which sexual activity takes place.

Local symptoms or findings on physical examination may raise the possibility of *sexually transmitted diseases* (STDs). After establishing the usual attributes of any symptoms, identify the sexual preference as to partners (male, female, or both). Inquire about sexual contacts and establish the number of sexual partners in the prior month. Ask if the patient has concerns about HIV infection, desires HIV testing, or has current or past partners at risk. Also ask

See Table 12-1, Lesions of the Vulva, p. 450; also Table 12-6, Vaginal Discharge, p. 454.

Sexual dysfunctions are classified by the phase of sexual response. A woman may lack desire, she may fail to become aroused and to attain adequate vaginal lubrication, or, despite adequate arousal, she may be unable to reach orgasm much or all of the time. Causes include lack of estrogen, medical illness, and psychiatric conditions.

Superficial pain suggests local inflammation, atrophic vaginitis, or inadequate lubrication; deeper pain may be from pelvic disorders or pressure on a normal ovary. The cause of *vaginismus* may be physical or psychological.

More commonly, however, a sexual problem is related to situational or psychosocial factors.

about oral and anal sex and, if indicated, about symptoms involving the mouth, throat, anus, and rectum. Review the past history of venereal disease. "Have you ever had herpes? . . . any other problems such as gonorrhea? . . . syphilis? . . . pelvic infections?" Continue with the more general questions suggested on pp. 48–49.

HEALTH PROMOTION AND COUNSELING

Important Topics for Health Promotion and Counseling

- The Pap smear
- Options for family planning
- Sexually transmitted diseases and HIV
- Changes in menopause

The Pap Smear.   Widespread screening by Papanicolaou (Pap) smear has contributed to a significant decline in the incidence and mortality of cervical cancer. The U.S. Preventive Services Task Force notes that "the goal of cytologic screening is to sample the transformation zone, the area where physiologic transformation from columnar endocervical epithelium to squamous (ectocervical) epithelium takes place and where dysplasia and cancer arise."[2] There are two primary types of cervical cancer. Approximately 80% to 90% are squamous cell carcinomas; the remaining 10% to 20% are adenocarcinomas in glandular cells.

Risk factors for cervical cancer are both viral and behavioral. The most important risk factor is infection with the high-risk strains of human papillomavirus (HPV), present in 95% to 100% of squamous cell cancers. Most HPV infections are transient and resolve spontaneously within 5 years. Those that persist "progress . . . in an orderly fashion from less severe to more severe lesions."[2] Other risk factors include early sexual activity; multiple sexual partners; a history of STDs; failure to receive screening; age, nutrition, and smoking; immune status; and genetic polymorphisms affecting the entry of HPV DNA into cervical cells.

The American College of Obstetricians and Gynecologists, the American Cancer Society, and the U.S. Preventive Services Task Force have all recently issued new recommendations related to screening frequency in different age groups.[2-5] These recommendations reflect advances in understanding of the progression from low-grade to high-grade cervical lesions and in the technology of Pap smear testing. Cervical intraepithelial neoplasia is the preinvasive pathologic precursor to cervical cancer. It progresses slowly and is readily detected on Pap smear and treated. Moreover, new technologies such as liquid-based cytology, computerized rescreening, and algorithm-based screening, may improve detection of abnormal cervical cells, although the U.S. Preventive Services Task Force concluded in 2003 that evidence comparing the accuracy of these new techniques with conventional Pap smears was still insufficient.[2,6]

Recommendations of the American College of Obstetricians and Gynecologists are summarized below.[4] These are in close agreement with the American Cancer Society and the U.S. Preventive Services Task Force (USPSTF); however, reviewing the three sets of guidelines is useful and informative.

■ **First Screen:** Screen approximately 3 years after first sexual intercourse or by age 21, whichever comes first

■ **Women up to age 30:** Screen annually

■ **Women age 30 or older:**

● Screen every 2 to 3 years if three consecutive annual cervical cytology results are negative or if combined cervical cytology testing and high-risk HPV testing are negative

● Screen more frequently in patients with positive Pap or positive high-risk HPV test; HIV infection; immunosuppression; DES exposure *in utero;* prior history of cervical cancer

■ **Women with hysterectomy:** Discontinue routine screening *if* the cervix was removed for benign reasons and there is no history of abnormal or cancerous cell growth. If the woman has a history of abnormal cell growth, screen annually; in such patients, discontinue screening if three consecutive vaginal cytology tests are negative.

■ **Older women:** ACOG recommends basing continued screening on clinical assessment of individual health and ability to monitor the patient. The USPSTF found low utility of screening *after age 65* but recommends continued screening in older women without prior screening or without information about past screening results. The American Cancer Society recommends discontinuing screening in women *after age 70* if three consecutive Pap tests are negative and Pap smears results in the prior 10 years have been negative. The Society states that testing should continue in healthy women if they have a history of cervical cancer, DES exposure in utero, HIV infection, or a weakened immune system.

Take the time to understand how Pap smear results are reported. Current classifications and management guidelines are based on the *Bethesda System of the National Cancer Institute, revised in 2001.*[7,8] The principal categories are as follows:

■ *Negative for intraepithelial lesion or malignancy:* No cellular evidence of neoplasia is present, although other organisms like *Trichomonas, Can-*

dida, or *Actinomyces* may be reported in this category. Shifts in flora consistent with bacterial vaginosis or cellular changes from herpes simplex may also be reported.

■ *Epithelial cell abnormalities:* These include precancerous or cancerous lesions:

● *Squamous cells,* including *atypical squamous cells* (ASC), which may be of undetermined significance (ASC-US); *low-grade squamous intraepithelial lesions* (LSIL), including mild dysplasia; *high-grade squamous intraepithelial lesions* (HSIL), including moderate and severe dysplasia with features suspicious for invasion; and invasive *squamous cell carcinoma.*

● *Glandular cells,* including *atypical endocervical cells* or *atypical endometrial cells,* specified or not otherwise specified (NOS); *atypical endocervical cells* or *atypical glandular cells, favor neoplastic; endocervical adenocarcinoma in situ;* and *adenocarcinoma*

● *Other malignant neoplasms,* such as sarcomas or lymphomas, both rare

Options for Family Planning.   It is important to counsel women, particularly adolescents, about the timing of ovulation in the menstrual cycle and how to plan or prevent pregnancy. Survey data indicate that more than half of U.S. pregnancies are unintended, affecting up to 80% of the 1 million teen pregnancies each year.[9] Clinicians should be familiar with the numerous options for contraception and their effectiveness. These include natural methods (periodic abstinence, withdrawal, lactation); barrier methods (condom, diaphragm, cervical cap); implantable methods (intrauterine device, subdermal implant); pharmacologic interventions (spermicide, birth control pill, subdermal implant of levonorgestrel, estrogen/progesterone injectables and patch, vaginal ring); and surgery (tubal ligation). The clinician must take the time to understand the patient or couple's concerns and preferences and respect these preferences whenever possible. Continued use of a preferred method is superior to a more effective method that is abandoned. For teenagers, providing a confidential setting eases discussion of topics that may seem private and difficult to explore.

STDs and HIV.   As with men, the clinician should assess risk factors for infection with STDs and HIV by taking a careful sexual history and by counseling patients about spread of disease and ways to reduce high-risk practices (see Chap. 2, Interviewing and the Health History, pp. 48–49). Women with STDs are at higher risk for asymptomatic infection and loss of fertility. Learn to assess women for genital and pelvic infections through careful examination and collection of appropriate cultures and to apply recommended guidelines for serologic testing for infection with HIV (see Chap. 11, Male Genitalia and Hernias, pp. 415–416).

Changes in Menopause.   Be familiar with the psychological and physiologic changes of menopause—mood shifts and changes in self-concept, vasomotor changes ("hot flashes"), accelerated bone loss, increases in total and

LDL cholesterol, and vulvovaginal atrophy leading to symptoms of vaginal drying, dysuria, and sometimes dyspareunia. The clinician must be knowledgeable about estrogen and progesterone replacement therapy and help the patient to weigh the benefits and risks of treatment, taking into account the personal and family history of osteoporosis (risk decreases with hormone treatment) and of breast cancer and endometrial cancer (treatment increases risk). Counseling patients about these decisions may extend over several visits. (See also Chap. 20, The Older Adult, pp. 839–873.)[10,11]

TECHNIQUES OF EXAMINATION

Important Areas of Examination

External Examination	Internal Examination
■ Mons pubis	■ Vagina, vaginal walls
■ Labia majora and minora	■ Cervix
■ Urethral meatus, clitoris	■ Uterus, ovaries
■ Vaginal introitus	■ Pelvic muscles
■ Perineum	■ Rectovaginal wall

Many students feel anxious or uncomfortable when first examining the genitalia of another person. At the same time, patients have their own concerns. Some women have had painful, embarrassing, or even demeaning experiences during previous pelvic examinations, whereas others may be facing their first examination. Patients may fear what the clinician will find and how these findings may affect their lives.

The woman's reactions and behavior give important clues to her feelings and to attitudes toward sexuality. If she adducts her thighs, pulls away, or expresses negative feelings during the examination, you can gently confront her as you would during the interview. "I notice you are having some trouble relaxing. Is it just being here, or are you troubled by the examination? . . . Is anything worrying you?" Behaviors that seem to present an obstacle to your examination may become the key to understanding your patient's concerns. Adverse reactions may be a sign of prior abuse, and these issues should be explored.

A patient who has never had a pelvic examination is often unsure of what to expect. Try to shape the experience so that she learns about her body and the steps of the pelvic examination, and becomes more comfortable with them. Before she undresses, explain the relevant anatomy with the help of three-dimensional models. Show her the speculum and other equipment and encourage her to handle them during the examination so that she can better understand your explanations and procedures. It is especially important to avoid hurting the patient during her first encounter.

TIPS FOR THE SUCCESSFUL PELVIC EXAMINATION

The Patient	*The Examiner*
■ Avoids intercourse, douching, or use of vaginal suppositories for 24 to 48 hours before examination ■ Empties bladder before examination ■ Lies supine, with head and shoulders elevated, arms at sides or folded across chest to enhance eye contact and reduce tightening of abdominal muscles	■ Explains each step of the examination in advance ■ Drapes patient from midabdomen to knees; depresses drape between knees to provide eye contact with patient ■ Avoids unexpected or sudden movements ■ Warms speculum with tap water ■ Monitors comfort of the examination by watching the patient's face ■ Uses excellent but gentle technique, especially when inserting the speculum (see below)

Indications for a pelvic examination during adolescence include menstrual abnormalities such as amenorrhea, excessive bleeding, or dysmenorrhea, unexplained abdominal pain; vaginal discharge; the prescription of contraceptives; bacteriologic and cytologic studies in a sexually active girl; and the patient's own desire for assessment. (See Chap. 18, Assessing Children: Infancy Through Adolescence, pp. 766–769).

Regardless of age, *rape* merits special evaluation, usually requiring gynecologic consultation and documentation. Often there is a special rape kit, provided in many emergency departments, that must be used to ensure a chain of custody for evidence. Specimens must be labeled carefully with name, date, and time. Additional information may be needed for further legal investigation.

Be sure always to wear gloves, both during the examination and when handling equipment and specimens. Plan ahead, so that any needed equipment and culture media are readily at hand.

Helping the patient to relax is essential for an adequate examination. Adopting the tips above will help ensure the patient's comfort.

Note that male examiners should be accompanied by female assistants. Female examiners should also be assisted if the patient is physically or emotionally disturbed.

Choosing Equipment. You should have within reach a good light, a vaginal speculum of appropriate size, water-soluble lubricant, and equipment for taking Papanicolaou smears, bacteriologic cultures, or other diagnostic tests. Review the supplies and procedures of your own facility before taking cultures and other samples.

Specula are made of metal or plastic and come in two basic shapes, named for Pedersen and Graves. Both are available in small, medium, and large sizes. The medium Pedersen speculum is usually most comfortable for sexually active women. The narrow-bladed Pedersen speculum is best for the patient with a relatively small introitus, such as a virgin or an elderly woman. The Graves specula are best suited for parous women with vaginal prolapse.

Before using a speculum, become thoroughly familiar with how to open and close its blades, lock the blades in an open position, and release them again. Although the instructions in this chapter refer to a metal speculum, you can easily adapt them to a plastic one by handling the speculum before using it.

Plastic specula typically make a loud click or may pinch when locked or released. Forewarning the patient helps to avoid unnecessary surprise.

Positioning the Patient. Drape the patient appropriately and then assist her into the lithotomy position. Help her to place first one heel and then the other into the stirrups. She may be more comfortable with shoes on than with bare feet. Then ask her to slide all the way down the examining

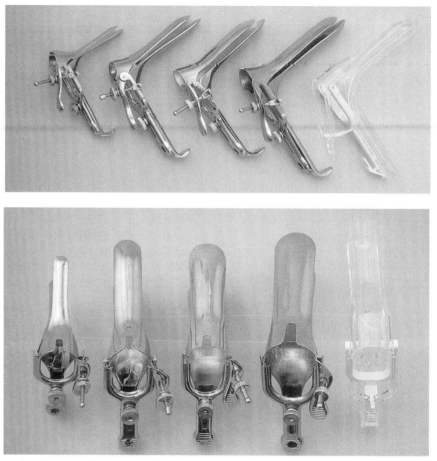

Speculae, from left to right: small metal Pedersen, medium metal Pedersen, medium metal Graves, large metal Graves, and large plastic Pedersen

table until her buttocks extend slightly beyond the edge. Her thighs should be flexed, abducted, and externally rotated at the hips. A pillow should support her head.

EXTERNAL EXAMINATION

Assess the Sexual Maturity of an Adolescent Patient. You can assess pubic hair during either the abdominal or the pelvic examination. Note its character and distribution, and rate it according to Tanner's stages described on p. 783.

Delayed puberty is often familial or related to chronic illness. It may also be from abnormalities in the hypothalamus, anterior pituitary gland, or ovaries.

Examine the External Genitalia. Seat yourself comfortably and warn the patient that you will be touching her genital area. Inspect the mons pubis, labia, and perineum. Separate the labia and inspect:

Excoriations or itchy, small, red maculopapules suggest *pediculosis pubis* (lice or "crabs"). Look for nits or lice at the bases of the pubic hairs.

■ The labia minora

■ The clitoris

Enlarged clitoris in masculinizing conditions

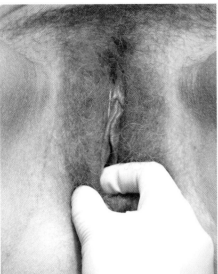

PALPATING BARTHOLIN'S GLAND

- The urethral meatus

- The vaginal opening, or introitus

Note any inflammation, ulceration, discharge, swelling, or nodules. If there are any lesions, palpate them.

If there is a history or an appearance of labial swelling, check Bartholin's glands. Insert your index finger into the vagina near the posterior end of the introitus. Place your thumb outside the posterior part of the labium majus. On each side in turn, palpate between your finger and thumb for swelling or tenderness. Note any discharge exuding from the duct opening of the gland. If any is present, culture it.

Urethral caruncle, prolapse of the urethral mucosa (p. 451)

Herpes simplex, Behcet's disease, syphilitic chancre, epidermoid cyst. See Table 12-1, Lesions of the Vulva (p. 450).

A *Bartholin's gland* may become acutely or chronically infected and then produce a swelling. See Table 12-2, Bulges and Swelling of Vulva, Vagina, and Urethra (p. 451).

■ INTERNAL EXAMINATION

Assess the Support of the Vaginal Walls. With the labia separated by your middle and index fingers, ask the patient to bear down. Note any bulging of the vaginal walls.

Insert the Speculum. Select a speculum of appropriate size and shape, and lubricate it with warm, but not hot, water. (Other lubricants may interfere with cytologic studies and bacterial or viral cultures.) You can enlarge the vaginal introitus by lubricating one finger with water and applying downward pressure at its lower margin. Check the location of the cervix to help angle the

Bulging from a *cystocele* or *rectocele.* See Table 12-2, Bulges and Swelling of Vulva, Vagina, and Urethra (p. 451).

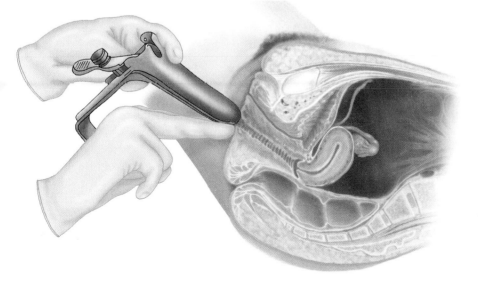

speculum more accurately. Enlarging the introitus greatly eases insertion of the speculum and the patient's comfort. With your other hand (usually the left), introduce the closed speculum past your fingers at a somewhat downward slope. Be careful not to pull on the pubic hair or pinch the labia with the speculum. Separating the labia majora with your other hand can help to avoid this.

THE SMALL INTROITUS

Many virginal vaginal orifices admit a single examining finger. Modify your technique so as to use your index finger only. A small Pedersen speculum may make inspection possible. When the vaginal orifice is even smaller, a fairly good bimanual examination can be performed by placing one finger in the rectum rather than in the vagina, but warn the patient first!

Similar techniques may be indicated in elderly women if the introitus has become atrophied and tight.

Two methods help you to avoid placing pressure on the sensitive urethra. (1) When inserting the speculum, hold it at an angle (shown below on the left), and then (2) slide the speculum inward along the posterior wall of the vagina, applying downward pressure to keep the vaginal introitus relaxed.

An *imperforate hymen* occasionally delays menarche. Be sure to check for this possibility when menarche seems unduly late in relation to the development of a girl's breasts and pubic hair.

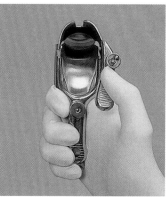

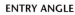

| ENTRY ANGLE | ANGLE AT FULL INSERTION |

After the speculum has entered the vagina, remove your fingers from the introitus. You may wish to switch the speculum to the right hand to enhance maneuverability of the speculum and subsequent collection of specimens. Rotate the speculum into a horizontal position, maintaining the pressure posteriorly, and insert it to its full length. Be careful not to open the blades of the speculum prematurely.

Inspect the Cervix.   Open the speculum carefully. Rotate and adjust the speculum until it cups the cervix and brings it into full view. Position the light until you can visualize the cervix well. When the uterus is retroverted, the cervix points more anteriorly than illustrated. If you have difficulty finding the cervix, withdraw the speculum slightly and reposition it on a different slope. If discharge obscures your view, wipe it away gently with a large cotton swab.

See retroversion of the uterus, p. 455.

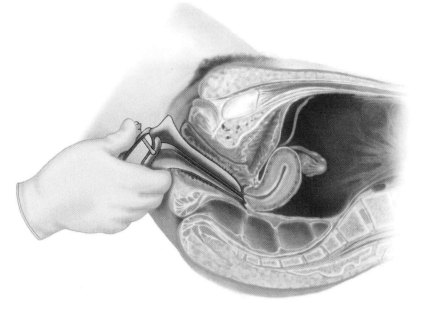

Note the color of the cervix, its position, the characteristics of its surface, and any ulcerations, nodules, masses, bleeding, or discharge. Inspect the cervical os for discharge.

See Table 12-3, Variations in the Cervical Surface (p. 452), Table 12-4, Shapes of the Cervical Os (p. 453), and Table 12-5, Abnormalities of the Cervix (p. 453).

Maintain the open position of the speculum by tightening the thumb screw.

A yellowish discharge on the endocervical swab suggests a mucopurulent cervicitis, commonly caused by *Chlamydia trachomatis, Neisseria gonorrhoeae,* or herpes simplex (p. 454). Raised, friable, or lobed wartlike lesions in *condylomata* or *cervical cancer.*

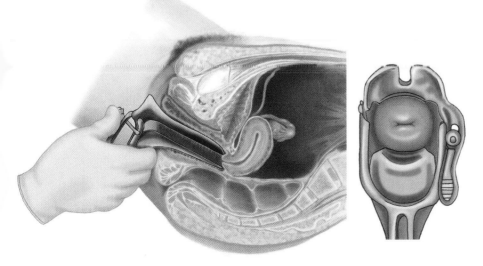

Obtain Specimens for Cervical Cytology (Papanicolaou Smears).
Obtain one specimen from the endocervix and another from the ectocervix, or a combination specimen using the cervical brush ("broom"). For
best results the patient should not be menstruating. She should avoid intercourse and use of douches, tampons, contraceptive foams or creams, or
vaginal suppositories for 48 hours before the examination. In addition to
obtaining the Pap smear, for sexually active women age 25 or younger,

Chlamydial infection is linked to
urethritis, cervicitis, pelvic inflammatory disease, ectopic pregnancy,
infertility, and chronic pelvic pain.
Risk factors include age younger
than 25, multiple partners, and
prior history of STDs.

OBTAINING THE PAP SMEAR: OPTIONS FOR SPECIMEN COLLECTION

Cervical Scrape and Endocervical Brush

Cervical Scrape. Place the longer end of
the scraper in the cervical os. Press,
turn, and scrape in a full circle, making
sure to include the *transformation zone*
and the *squamocolumnar junction.*
Smear the specimen on a glass slide.
Set the slide in a safe spot that is easy to
reach. Note that doing the cervical
scrape first reduces obscuring cells with
blood, which sometimes appears with
use of the endocervical brush.

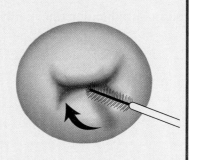

Endocervical Brush. Take the endocervical
brush and place it in the cervical os. Roll it
between your thumb and index finger,
clockwise and counterclockwise. Remove
the brush and pick up the slide you have
set aside. Smear the slide with the brush,
using a gentle painting motion to avoid de-
stroying any cells. Place the slide into an
ether–alcohol solution at once, or spray it
promptly with a special fixative.

Note that for pregnant women, a cotton-tip applicator, moistened with
saline, is advised in place of the endocervical brush.

Cervical Broom

Many clinicians now use a plastic brush
tipped with a broomlike fringe for collection of a single specimen containing both
squamous and columnar epithelial cells.
Rotate the tip of the brush in the cervical
os, in a full clockwise direction, then stroke
each side of the brush on the glass slide.
Promptly place the slide in solution or
spray with a fixative as described above.

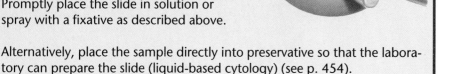

Alternatively, place the sample directly into preservative so that the laboratory can prepare the slide (liquid-based cytology) (see p. 454).

---

and for other asymptomatic women at increased risk for infection, plan to culture the cervix routinely for *Chlamydia trachomatis.*[12]

Inspect the Vagina. Withdraw the speculum slowly while observing the vagina. As the speculum clears the cervix, release the thumb screw and maintain the open position of the speculum with your thumb. Close the speculum as it emerges from the introitus, avoiding both excessive stretching and pinching of the mucosa. During withdrawal, inspect the vaginal mucosa, noting its color and any inflammation, discharge, ulcers, or masses.

See Table 12-6, Vaginal Discharge (p. 454).

Cancer of the vagina

Perform a Bimanual Examination. Lubricate the index and middle fingers of one of your gloved hands, and *from a standing position,* insert them into the vagina, again exerting pressure primarily posteriorly. Your thumb should be abducted, your ring and little fingers flexed into your palm. Pressing inward on the perineum with your flexed fingers causes little if any discomfort and allows you to position your palpating fingers correctly. Note any nodularity or tenderness in the vaginal wall, including the region of the urethra and the bladder anteriorly.

Stool in the rectum may simulate a rectovaginal mass, but, unlike a tumor mass, can usually be dented by digital pressure. Rectovaginal examination confirms the distinction.

Palpate the cervix, noting its position, shape, consistency, regularity, mobility, and tenderness. Normally the cervix can be moved somewhat without pain. Feel the fornices around the cervix.

Pain on movement of the cervix, together with adnexal tenderness, suggests *pelvic inflammatory disease.*

Palpate the uterus. Place your other hand on the abdomen about midway between the umbilicus and the symphysis pubis. While you elevate the cervix and uterus with your pelvic hand, press your abdominal hand in and down, trying to grasp the uterus between your two hands. Note its size, shape, consistency, and mobility, and identify any tenderness or masses.

See Table 12-7, Positions of the Uterus (p. 455) and Table 12-8, Abnormalities of the Uterus (p. 456).

Uterine enlargement suggests pregnancy or benign or malignant tumors.

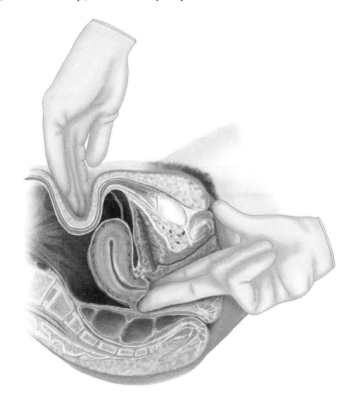

Now slide the fingers of your pelvic hand into the anterior fornix and palpate the body of the uterus between your hands. In this position your pelvic fingers can feel the anterior surface of the uterus, and your abdominal hand can feel part of the posterior surface.

If you cannot feel the uterus with either of these maneuvers, it may be tipped posteriorly (retrodisplaced). Slide your pelvic fingers into the posterior fornix and feel for the uterus butting against your fingertips. An obese or poorly relaxed abdominal wall may also prevent you from feeling the uterus even when it is located anteriorly.

Palpate each ovary. Place your abdominal hand on the right lower quadrant, your pelvic hand in the right lateral fornix. Press your abdominal hand in and down, trying to push the adnexal structures toward your pelvic hand. Try to identify the right ovary or any adjacent adnexal masses. By moving your hands slightly, slide the adnexal structures between your fingers, if possible, and note their size, shape, consistency, mobility, and tenderness. Repeat the procedure on the left side.

Normal ovaries are somewhat tender. They are usually palpable in slender, relaxed women but are difficult or impossible to feel in others who are obese or poorly relaxed.

Nodules on the uterine surfaces suggest *myomas* (see p. 456).

See *retroversion* and *retroflexion of the uterus* (p. 455).

Three to 5 years after menopause, the ovaries have usually atrophied and are no longer palpable. If you can feel an ovary in a post-menopausal woman, consider an abnormality such as a cyst or a tumor.

Adnexal masses include ovarian cysts, tumors, and abscesses, also the swollen fallopian tube(s) of pelvic inflammatory disease, and a tubal pregnancy. A uterine myoma may simulate an adnexal mass. See Table 12-9, Adnexal Masses (p. 457).

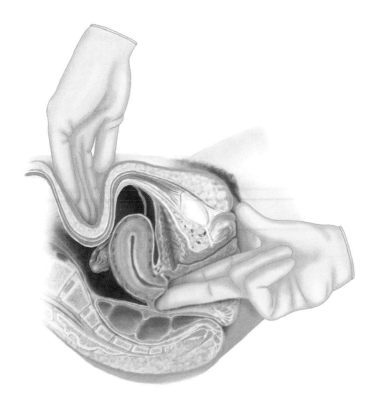

Assess the Strength of the Pelvic Muscles.   Withdraw your two fingers slightly, just clear of the cervix, and spread them to touch the sides of the vaginal walls. Ask the patient to squeeze her muscles around them as hard and long as she can. A squeeze that compresses your fingers snugly, moves them upward and inward, and lasts 3 seconds or more is full strength.

Impaired strength may be because of age, vaginal deliveries, or neurologic deficits. Weakness may be associated with urinary stress incontinence.

Do a Rectovaginal Examination.   Withdraw your fingers. Lubricate and change your gloves again if necessary. (See note on using lubricant below.) Then slowly reintroduce your index finger into the vagina, your middle finger into the rectum. Ask the patient to strain down as you do this so that her anal sphincter will relax. Tell her that this examination may make her feel as if she has to move her bowels but that she will not do so. Repeat the maneuvers of the bimanual examination, giving special attention to the region behind the cervix that may be accessible only to the rectal finger.

Rectovaginal palpation is especially valuable in assessing a retrodisplaced uterus, as illustrated. It also allows palpation of the uterosacral ligaments, the cul-de-sac, and the adnexa.

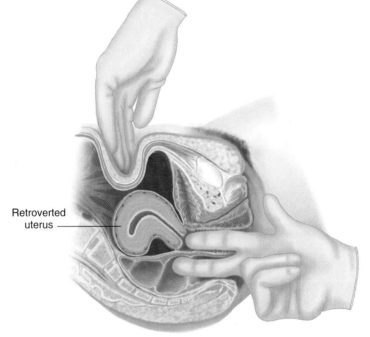

Retroverted uterus

Proceed to the rectal examination (see Chap. 13). If a hemoccult test is planned, you should change gloves to avoid contaminating fecal material with any blood provoked by the Pap smear. After the examination, wipe off the external genitalia and rectum, or offer the patient some tissue so she can do it herself.

USING LUBRICANTS

If you use a tube of lubricant during a pelvic or rectal examination, you may inadvertently contaminate it by touching the tube with your gloved fingers after touching the patient. To avoid this problem, let the lubricant drop onto your gloved fingers without allowing contact between the tube and the gloves. If you or your assistant should inadvertently contaminate the tube, discard it. Small disposable tubes for use with one patient circumvent this problem.

◼ HERNIAS

Hernias of the groin occur in women as well as in men, but they are much less common. The examination techniques (see pp. 419–420) are basically the same as for men. A woman too should stand up to be examined. To feel an indirect inguinal hernia, however, palpate in the labia majora and upward to just lateral to the pubic tubercles.

An indirect inguinal hernia is the most common hernia that occurs in the female groin. A femoral hernia ranks next in frequency.

◼ SPECIAL TECHNIQUES

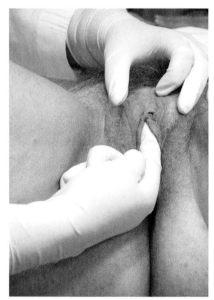

MILKING THE URETHRA

If you suspect urethritis or inflammation of the paraurethral glands, insert your index finger into the vagina and milk the urethra gently from inside outward. Note any discharge from or about the urethral meatus. If present, culture it.

Urethritis may arise from infection with *Chlamydia trachomatis* or *Neisseria gonorrhoeae*.

RECORDING YOUR FINDINGS

Note that initially you may use sentences to describe your findings; later you will use phrases. The style below contains phrases appropriate for most write-ups.

Recording the Pelvic Examination—Female Genitalia

"No inguinal adenopathy. External genitalia without erythema or lesions; no lesions or masses. Vaginal mucosa pink. Cervix parous, pink, and without discharge. Uterus anterior, midline, smooth, and not enlarged. No adnexal tenderness. Pap smear obtained. Rectovaginal wall intact."

OR

"Bilateral spotty inguinal adenopathy. External genitalia without erythema or lesions. Vaginal mucosa and cervix coated with thin white homogeneous discharge with mild fishy odor. After swabbing cervix, no discharge visible in cervical os. Uterus midline; no adnexal masses. Rectal vault without masses. Stool brown and hemoccult negative."

Suggests bacterial vaginosis

BIBLIOGRAPHY

Bibliography

CITATIONS

1. van Noord PA, Dubas JA, Dorland M, et al. Age at natural menopause in a population-based screening cohort: the role of menarche, fecundity, and lifestyle factors. Fertil Steril 68(1): 95–102, 1997.
2. U.S. Preventive Services Task Force. Screening for cervical cancer: recommendations and rationale. January 2003. Available at: www.ahrq.gov. Accessed December 23, 2004.
3. American College of Obstetricians and Gynecologists (ACOG): Clinical practice guidelines for obstetrician-gynecologists: cervical cytology screening. ACOG Practice Bulletin No. 45. Obstet Gynecol 102:417–427, 2003.
4. American College of Obstetricians and Gynecologists. Cervical cancer screening: testing can start later and occur less often under new ACOG recommendations. ACOG News Release, July 31, 2003. Available at: www.acog.org. Accessed December 19, 2004.
5. American Cancer Society (ACS): ACS cancer detection guidelines—cervical cancer. Available at: www.cancer.org/docroot/ PED/content/PED_2_3X_ACS_Cancer_Detection_ Guidelines_36.asp?sitearea=PED. Accessed November 18, 2004.
6. Marshall Austin R: The detection of precancerous cervical lesions can be significantly increased. Arch Pathol Lab Med 127: 143–145, 2003.
7. Solomon D, Davey D, Kurman R, et al, for the Bethesda 2001 Workshop, National Cancer Institute. The 2001 Bethesda System: terminology for reporting results of cervical cytology. JAMA 287(16):2114–2119, 2002. Available at: http:// bethesda2001.cancer.gov. Accessed December 27, 2004.
8. Wright TC, Cox JT, Stewart M, et al, for the 2001 ASCCP-Sponsored Consensus Conference. 2001 Consensus guidelines for the management of women with cervical cytological abnormalities. JAMA 287(16):2120–2129, 2002. Available at: http://www.cancer.org, Can cervical cancer be prevented? Accessed December 27, 2004.
9. U.S. Preventive Services Task Force. Counseling to Prevent Unwanted Pregnancy. Chapter 15. Guide to Clinical Preventive Services, 2nd ed, pp. 739–740. Baltimore, Williams & Wilkins, 1996.
10. North American Menopause Society: Recommendations for estrogen and progestogen use in peri- and postmenopausal women: October 2004 position statement of the North American Menopause Society. Nebioayse 11(6):589–596, 2004.
11. American College of Obstetricians and Gynecologists (ACOG). Clinical management guidelines for obstetric gynecologists—use of botanicals for management of menopausal symptoms. ACOG Practice Bulletin No. 28, June 2001. Available at: http://www. acog.org/from_home/publications/misc/pb028.htm. Accessed December 17, 2004.
12. U.S. Preventive Services Task Force. Screening for chlamydial infection: recommendations and rationale. 2001. Available at: www.ahrq.gov. Accessed December 27, 2004.

ADDITIONAL REFERENCES

Anderson MR, Klink K, Cohrsson A. Evaluation of vaginal complaints. JAMA 291(11):368–379, 2004.

Bachmann GA, Nevadunsky NS. Diagnosis and treatment of atrophic vaginitis. Am Fam Phys 61(10):3090–3096, 2000.

Bent S, Nallamothu BK, Simel DL, et al. Does this woman have an acute uncomplicated urinary tract infection? JAMA 287(20):2701–2710, 2002.

Bickley LS. Acute vaginitis (Chapter 22). In Black ER, Panzer RJ, Bordley DR, et al (eds). Diagnostic Strategies in Common Medical Problems. Philadelphia, American College of Physicians, 2006.

Brink CA, Wells TJ, Sampselle CM, et al. A digital test for pelvic muscle strength in women with urinary incontinence. Nurs Res 43(6):352–356, 1994.

Fox J, Remington P, Layde P et al. The effect of hysterectomy on the risk of an abnormal screening Papanicolaou test result. Am J Obstet Gynecol 180(5):1104–1109, 1999.

Goff BA, Mandel LS, Melancon CH. Frequency of symptoms of ovarian cancer in women presenting to primary care clinics. JAMA 291(22):2705–2712, 2004.

Holroyd-Leduc JM, Straus SE. Management of urinary incontinence in women. JAMA 291(8):996–999, 2004.

Kimberlin DW, Rouse DJ. Genital herpes. N Engl J Med 350(19):1970–1977, 2004.

Novak E, Berek JS (eds). Novak's Gynecology, 13th ed. Philadelphia, Lippincott Williams & Wilkins, 2002.

Levine AM. Evaluation and management of HIV-infected women. Ann Intern Med 136(3):228–242, 2002.

Mandelblatt JS, Lawrence WF, Womack SM, et al. Benefits and costs of using HPV testing to screen for cervical cancer. JAMA 287(18):2372–2381, 2002.

Peipert JF. Genital chlamydial infections. N Engl J Med 349(25):2424–2430, 2003.

Peipert JF, Ness RB, Blume J, et al. Clinical predictors of endometritis in women with symptoms and signs of pelvic inflammatory disease. Am J Obstet Gynecol 184(5):856–864, 2001.

Sawaya GF, Brown AD, Washington AE, et al. Current approaches to cervical cancer screening. N Engl J Med 344(21):1603–1607, 2001.

Scott JR, Di Saia PJ, Hammond CB, et al (eds). Danforth's Obstetrics and Gynecology, 9th ed. Philadelphia, Lippincott Williams & Wilkins, 2003.

Sirovich BE, Welch HG. Cervical cancer screening among women without a cervix. JAMA 291(24):2990–2993, 2004.

Stenchever MA, Droegemueller W, Herbst A, et al. Comprehensive Gynecology, 4th ed. St. Louis, Mosby, 2001.

Wright TC, Cox JT, Massad LS, et al. 2001 Consensus guidelines for the management of women with cervical cytological abnormalities. JAMA 287(16):2120–2129, 2002.

Wooster R, Weber BL. Breast and ovarian cancer. N Engl J Med 348(23):2339–2347, 2003.

TABLE 12-1   **Lesions of the Vulva**

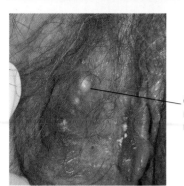

Cystic nodule in skin

Epidermoid Cyst

A small, firm, round cystic nodule in the labia suggests an epidermoid cyst. These are yellowish in color. Look for the dark punctum marking the blocked opening of the gland.

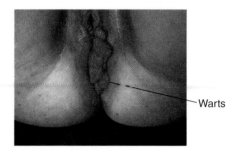

Warts

Venereal Wart
(Condyloma Acuminatum)

Warty lesions on the labia and within the vestibule suggest condyloma acuminatum. They result from infection with human papillomavirus.

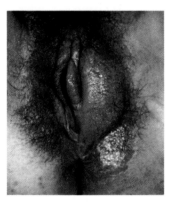

Syphilitic Chancre

A firm, painless ulcer suggests the chancre of primary syphilis. Because most chancres in women develop internally, they often go undetected.

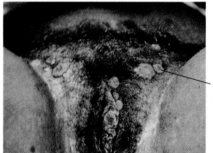

Flat, gray papules

Secondary Syphilis
(Condyloma Latum)

Slightly raised, round or oval, flat-topped papules covered by a gray exudate suggest condylomata lata. These constitute one manifestation of secondary syphilis and are contagious.

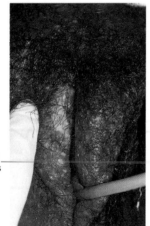

Shallow ulcers on red bases

Genital Herpes

Shallow, small, painful ulcers on red bases suggest a herpes infection. Initial infection may be extensive, as shown. Recurrent infections usually are confined to a small local patch.

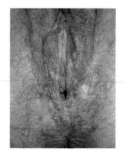

Carcinoma of the Vulva

An ulcerated or raised red vulvar lesion in an elderly woman may indicate vulvar carcinoma.

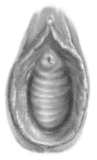

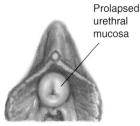

Cystocele

A cystocele is a bulge of the upper two thirds of the anterior vaginal wall, together with the bladder above it. It results from weakened supporting tissues.

Cystourethrocele

When the entire anterior vaginal wall, together with the bladder and urethra, is involved in the bulge, a cystourethrocele is present. A groove sometimes defines the border between urethrocele and cystocele, but is not always present.

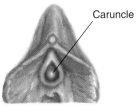

Urethral Caruncle

A urethral caruncle is a small, red, benign tumor visible at the posterior part of the urethral meatus. It occurs chiefly in post-menopausal women and usually causes no symptoms. Occasionally, a carcinoma of the urethra is mistaken for a caruncle. To check, palpate the urethra through the vagina for thickening, nodularity, or tenderness, and feel for inguinal lymphadenopathy.

Prolapse of the Urethral Mucosa

Prolapsed urethral mucosa forms a swollen red ring around the urethral meatus. It usually occurs before menarche or after menopause. Identify the urethral meatus at the center of the swelling to make this diagnosis.

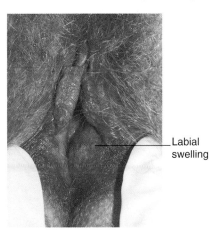

Bartholin's Gland Infection

Causes of a Bartholin's gland infection include trauma, gonococci anaerobes like bacteroides and peptostreptococci, and *Chlamydia trachomatis*. Acutely, it appears as a tense, hot, very tender abscess. Look for pus coming out of the duct or erythema around the duct opening. Chronically, a nontender cyst is felt. It may be large or small.

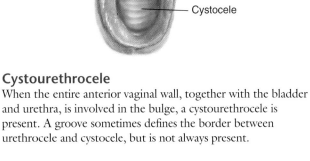

Rectocele

A rectocele is a herniation of the rectum into the posterior wall of the vagina, resulting from a weakness or defect in the endopelvic fascia.

TABLE 12-3   **Variations in the Cervical Surface**

Two kinds of epithelia may cover the cervix: (1) shiny pink *squamous epithelium*, which resembles the vaginal epithelium, and (2) deep red, plushy *columnar epithelium*, which is continuous with the endocervical lining. These two meet at the *squamocolumnar junction*. When this junction is at or inside the cervical os, only squamous epithelium is seen. A ring of columnar epithelium is often visible to a varying extent around the os—the result of a normal process that accompanies fetal development, menarche, and the first pregnancy.*

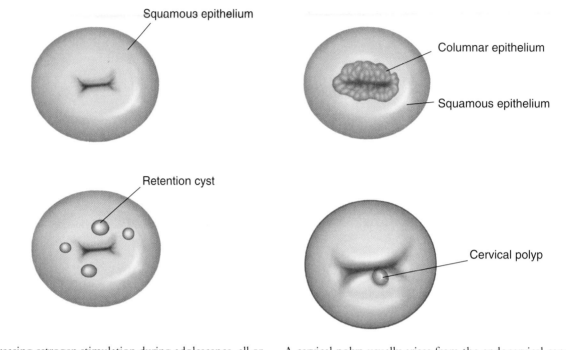

With increasing estrogen stimulation during adolescence, all or part of this columnar epithelium is transformed into squamous epithelium by a process termed *metaplasia*. This change may block the secretions of columnar epithelium and cause *retention cysts* (sometimes called *nabothian cysts*). These appear as one or more translucent nodules on the cervical surface and have no pathologic significance.

A cervical polyp usually arises from the endocervical canal, becoming visible when it protrudes through the cervical os. It is bright red, soft, and rather fragile. When only the tip is seen, it cannot be differentiated clinically from a polyp originating in the endometrium. Polyps are benign but may bleed.

---

* Terminology is in flux. Other terms for the columnar epithelium that is visible on the ectocervix are *ectropion*, *ectopy*, and *eversion*.

TABLE 12-4	Shapes of the Cervical Os

Normal

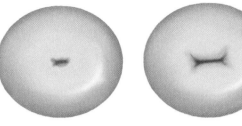

Oval · Slit-like

Types of Lacerations from Delivery

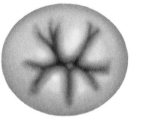

Unilateral transverse · Bilateral transverse · Stellate

TABLE 12-5	Abnormalities of the Cervix

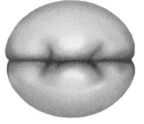

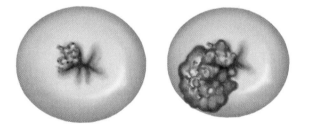

Mucopurulent Cervicitis

Mucopurulent cervicitis produces purulent yellow drainage from the cervical os, usually as a result of infection from *Chlamydia trachomatis, Neisseria gonorrhoeae,* or herpes. These infections are sexually transmitted and may occur without symptoms or signs.

Carcinoma of the Cervix

Carcinoma of the cervix begins in an area of metaplasia. In its earliest stages, it cannot be distinguished from a normal cervix. In a late stage, an extensive, irregular, cauliflower-like growth may develop. Early frequent intercourse, multiple partners, smoking, and infection with human papillomavirus increase the risk for cervical cancer.

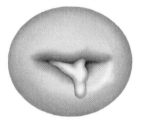

— Vaginal adenosis

— Columnar epithelium

— Collar

Fetal Exposure to Diethylstilbestrol (DES)

Daughters of women who took DES during pregnancy are at greatly increased risk for several abnormalities, including (1) columnar epithelium that covers most or all of the cervix, (2) vaginal adenosis, i.e., extension of this epithelium to the vaginal wall, and (3) a circular collar or ridge of tissue, of varying shapes, between the cervix and vagina. Much less common is an otherwise rare carcinoma of the upper vagina.

TABLE 12-6   Vaginal Discharge

The vaginal discharge that often accompanies vaginitis must be distinguished from a physiologic discharge. The latter is clear or white and may contain white clumps of epithelial cells; it is not malodorous. It is also important to distinguish vaginal from cervical discharges. Use a large cotton swab to wipe off the cervix. If no cervical discharge is present in the os, suspect a vaginal origin and consider the causes below. Remember that diagnosis of cervicitis or vaginitis hinges on careful collection and analysis of the appropriate laboratory specimens.

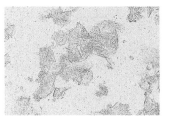

	Trichomonal Vaginitis	Candidal Vaginitis	Bacterial Vaginosis
Cause	*Trichomonas vaginalis*, a protozoa; often but not always acquired sexually	*Candida albicans*, a yeast (normal overgrowth of vaginal flora); many factors predispose, including antibiotic therapy.	Bacterial overgrowth probably from anaerobic bacteria; may be transmitted sexually
Discharge	Yellowish green or gray, possibly frothy; often profuse and pooled in the vaginal fornix; may be malodorous	White and curdy; may be thin but typically thick; not as profuse as in trichomonal infection; not malodorous	Gray or white, thin, homogeneous, malodorous; coats the vaginal walls; usually not profuse, may be minimal
Other Symptoms	Pruritus (though not usually as severe as with *Candida* infection); pain on urination (from skin inflammation or possibly urethritis); dyspareunia	Pruritus; vaginal soreness; pain on urination (from skin inflammation); dyspareunia	Unpleasant fishy or musty genital odor
Vulva and Vaginal Mucosa	Vestibule and labia minora may be reddened. Vaginal mucosa may be diffusely reddened, with small red granular spots or petechiae in the posterior fornix. In mild cases, the mucosa looks normal.	The vulva and even the surrounding skin are often inflamed and sometimes swollen to a variable extent. Vaginal mucosa often reddened, with white, often tenacious patches of discharge. The mucosa may bleed when these patches are scraped off. In mild cases, the mucosa looks normal.	Vulva usually normal. Vaginal mucosa usually normal
Laboratory Evaluation	Scan saline wet mount for trichomonads	Scan potassium hydroxide (KOH) preparation for branching hyphae of *Candida*.	Scan saline wet mount for *clue cells* (epithelial cells with stippled borders); sniff for fishy odor after applying KOH ("whiff test"); vaginal secretions with pH >4.5

TABLE 12-7 ■ Positions of the Uterus

Both retroversion and retroflexion are usually normal variants.

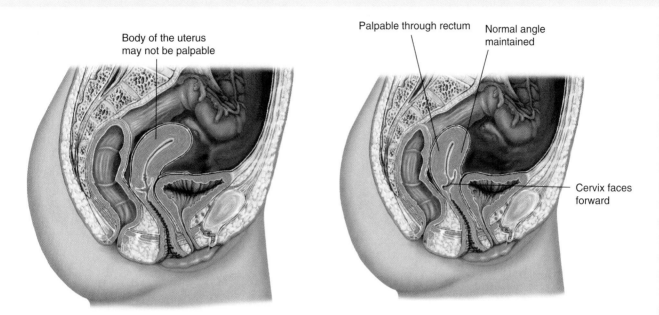

Retroversion of the Uterus

Retroversion of the uterus refers to a tilting backward of the entire uterus, including both body and cervix. It is a common variant occurring in approximately 20% of women. Early clues on pelvic examination are a cervix that faces forward and a uterine body that cannot be felt by the abdominal hand. In *moderate retroversion*, the body may not be palpable with either hand. In *marked retroversion*, the body can be felt posteriorly, either through the posterior fornix or through the rectum. A retroverted uterus is usually both mobile and asymptomatic. Occasionally, such a uterus is fixed and immobile, held in place by conditions such as endometriosis or pelvic inflammatory disease.

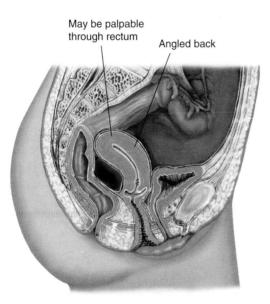

Retroflexion of the Uterus

Retroflexion of the uterus refers to a backward angulation of the body of the uterus in relation to the cervix. The cervix maintains its usual position. The body of the uterus is often palpable through the posterior fornix or through the rectum.

TABLE 12-8   **Abnormalities of the Uterus**

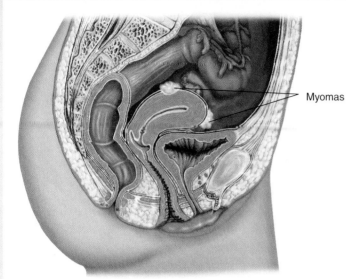

Myomas of the Uterus (Fibroids)

Myomas are very common benign uterine tumors. They may be single or multiple and vary greatly in size, occasionally reaching massive proportions. They feel like firm, irregular nodules in continuity with the uterine surface. Occasionally, a myoma projecting laterally can be confused with an ovarian mass; a nodule projecting posteriorly can be mistaken for a retroflexed uterus. Submucous myomas project toward the endometrial cavity and are not themselves palpable, although they may be suspected because of an enlarged uterus.

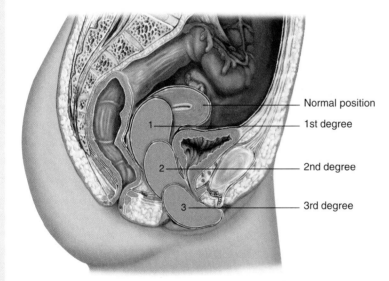

Prolapse of the Uterus

Prolapse of the uterus results from weakness of the supporting structures of the pelvic floor and is often associated with a cystocele and rectocele. In progressive stages, the uterus becomes retroverted and descends down the vaginal canal to the outside:

- In first-degree prolapse, the cervix is still well within the vagina.
- In second-degree prolapse, it is at the introitus.
- In third-degree prolapse (procidentia), the cervix and vagina are outside the introitus.

TABLE 12-9   **Adnexal Masses**

Adnexal masses most commonly result from disorders of the fallopian tubes or ovaries. Three examples—often hard to differentiate—are described. In addition, inflammatory disease of the bowel (such as diverticulitis), carcinoma of the colon, and a pedunculated myoma of the uterus may simulate an adnexal mass.

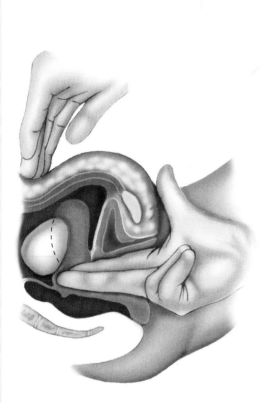

Ovarian Cysts and Tumors

Ovarian cysts and tumors may be detected as adnexal masses on one or both sides. Later, they may extend out of the pelvis. Cysts tend to be smooth and compressible, tumors more solid and often nodular. Uncomplicated cysts and tumors are not usually tender.

Small (≤6 cm in diameter), mobile, cystic masses in a young woman are usually benign and often disappear after the next menstrual period.

Ruptured Tubal Pregnancy

A ruptured tubal pregnancy spills blood into the peritoneal cavity, causing severe abdominal pain and tenderness. Guarding and rebound tenderness are sometimes associated. A unilateral adnexal mass may be palpable, but tenderness often prevents its detection. Faintness, syncope, nausea, vomiting, tachycardia, and shock may be present, reflecting the hemorrhage. There may be a prior history of amenorrhea or other symptoms of a pregnancy.

Pelvic Inflammatory Disease

Pelvic inflammatory disease (PID) is most often a result of sexually transmitted infection of the fallopian tubes (salpingitis) or of the tubes and ovaries (salpingo-oophoritis). It is caused by *Neisseria gonorrhoeae, Chlamydia trachomatis,* and other organisms. *Acute* disease is associated with very tender, bilateral adnexal masses, although pain and muscle spasm usually make it impossible to delineate them. Movement of the cervix produces pain. If not treated, a *tubo-ovarian abscess* or infertility may ensue.

Infection of the fallopian tubes and ovaries may also follow delivery of a baby or gynecologic surgery.

13

The Anus, Rectum, and Prostate

ANATOMY AND PHYSIOLOGY

The gastrointestinal tract terminates in a short segment, the *anal canal.* Its external margin is poorly demarcated, but the skin of the anal canal can usually be distinguished from the surrounding perianal skin by its moist, hairless appearance. The anal canal is normally held in a closed position by the muscle action of the voluntary *external anal sphincter* and involuntary *internal anal sphincter*, the latter an extension of the muscular coat of the rectal wall.

Note carefully the direction of the anal canal on a line roughly between the anus and umbilicus. Unlike the rectum above it, the canal is liberally sup-

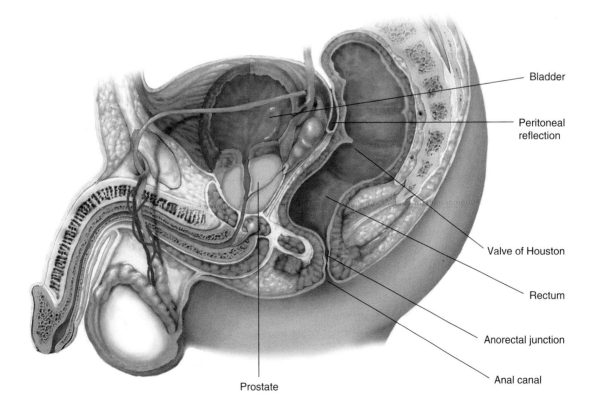

Bladder

Peritoneal reflection

Valve of Houston

Rectum

Anorectal junction

Anal canal

Prostate

plied by somatic sensory nerves, and a poorly directed finger or instrument will produce pain.

The anal canal is demarcated from the rectum superiorly by a serrated line marking the change from skin to mucous membrane. This anorectal junction, often called the *pectinate* or *dentate line*, also denotes the boundary between somatic and visceral nerve supplies. It is readily visible on proctoscopic examination, but it is not palpable.

Above the anorectal junction, the rectum balloons out and turns posteriorly into the hollow of the coccyx and the sacrum. In the male, the three lobes of the *prostate gland* surround the urethra. The prostate gland is small during childhood, but between puberty and the age of about 20 years, it increases roughly five-fold in size. Prostate volume further expands as the gland becomes hyperplastic (see p. 471). The two lateral lobes lie against the anterior rectal wall, where they are palpable as a rounded, heart-shaped structure about 2.5 cm long. They are separated by a shallow median sulcus or groove, also palpable. The third, or median, lobe is anterior to the urethra and cannot be examined. The *seminal vesicles,* shaped like rabbit ears above the prostate, are also not normally palpable.

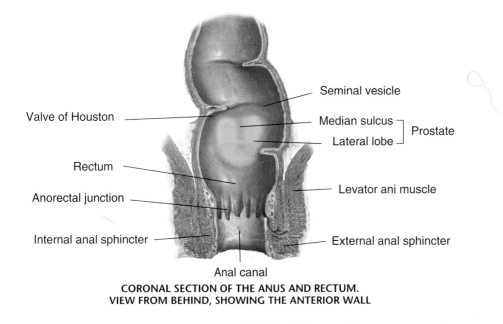

CORONAL SECTION OF THE ANUS AND RECTUM.
VIEW FROM BEHIND, SHOWING THE ANTERIOR WALL

In the female, the uterine *cervix* can usually be felt through the anterior wall of the rectum.

The rectal wall contains three inward foldings, called *valves of Houston*. The lowest of these can sometimes be felt, usually on the patient's left. Most of the rectum that is accessible to digital examination does not have a peritoneal surface. The anterior rectum usually does, however, and you may reach it with the tip of your examining finger. You may thus be able to identify the tenderness of peritoneal inflammation or the nodularity of peritoneal metastases.

THE HEALTH HISTORY

Common or Concerning Symptoms

- Change in bowel habits
- Blood in the stool
- Pain with defecation; rectal bleeding or tenderness
- Anal warts or fissures
- Weak stream of urine
- Burning with urination

Many questions concerning symptoms related to the anorectal area and the prostate have been addressed in other chapters. For example, you will need to ask if there has been any change in the pattern of bowel function or the size or caliber of the stools. What about diarrhea or constipation? You will need to ask about the color of the stools. Turn to pp. 366–367 and review the health history regarding these symptoms, as well as queries about *blood in the stool,* ranging from black stools, suggesting *melena,* to the red blood of *hematochezia,* to *bright-red blood per rectum.* Also, is any mucus present?

See Table 10-3, Constipation, p. 397, and Table 10-5, Black and Bloody Stools, p. 400.

Change in bowel pattern, especially stools of thin pencil-like caliber, may warn of cancer. Blood in the stool may be from polyps or cancer, also from gastrointestinal bleeding or local hemorrhoids; mucus may appear in villous adenoma.

Is there any pain on defecation? Any itching? Any extreme tenderness in the anus or rectum? Is there any mucopurulent discharge or bleeding? Any ulcerations? Does the patient have anal intercourse?

Proctitis with anorectal pain, pruritus, tenesmus, discharge or bleeding in anorectal infection from gonorrhea, *Chlamydia,* lymphogranuloma venereum, receptive anal intercourse, ulcerations in *herpes simplex,* chancre in *primary syphilis.* Itching in younger patients from pinworms.

Is there any history of anal warts, or anal fissures?

Genital warts from *human papillomavirus, condylomata lata* in secondary syphilis. Anal fissures in *proctitis, Crohn's disease*

In men, review the pattern of urination (see pp. 368–370). Does the patient have any difficulty starting the urine stream or holding back urine? Is the flow weak? What about frequent urination, especially at night? Or pain or burning as urine is passed? Any blood in the urine or semen or pain with ejaculation? Is there frequent pain or stiffness in the lower back, hips, or upper thighs?

These symptoms suggest urethral obstruction as in *benign prostatic hyperplasia* or *prostate cancer,* especially in men older than age 70.

Also in men, is there any feeling of discomfort or heaviness in the prostate area at the base of the penis? Any associated malaise, fever, or chills?

Suggests possible *prostatitis*

HEALTH PROMOTION AND COUNSELING

Important Topics for Health Promotion and Counseling

- Screening for prostate cancer
- Screening for polyps and colorectal cancer

Clinicians should discuss screening issues related to prostate cancer to promote health for men and provide screening recommendations to both men and women for detection of colorectal cancer and adenomatous colonic polyps.

Prostate cancer is the leading cancer diagnosed in men in the United States, and the second leading cause of death in men following lung cancer.[1] Age, ethnicity, and family history strongly influence risk. Although rare in men younger than age 45, risk increases sharply with each advancing decade—about 70% of cases occur in men older than age 65.[2] Median age at diagnosis is 72. African American men have the highest incidence of prostate cancer and present most commonly with advanced disease.[3] Incidence rates are lowest in Asian and Native American men. For men with a first-degree relative with prostate cancer, namely a brother or father, risk for prostate cancer is about doubled, and risk may increase 5- to 10-fold in men with two or three affected first-degree relatives.[4] Investigations of diet, intake of nutrients such as selenium and vitamin E, nonsteroidal anti-inflammatory drugs, vasectomy, and testosterone supplements as possible risk factors have been inconclusive.

Several issues complicate decisions to pursue screening. To educate and advise *asymptomatic* patients, clinicians must be knowledgeable about several controversies. Autopsy studies show that many men older than age 50, and even some who are younger, have nests of cancerous prostate cells that never cause disease. Because many of these tumors are quiescent, early detection may increase unnecessary testing and treatment with no benefit to survival. Interventions like prostate surgery, for example, carry up to a 20% risk for erectile dysfunction and a 5% risk for urinary incontinence. Further, neither of the two principal screening tests, the digital rectal examination (DRE) and the serum prostate specific antigen (PSA) test, is highly sensitive or specific.

It is important to review the limitations of DRE and PSA testing with your patients. DRE alone has not been shown to reduce morbidity and mortality and has a high rate of false-positive results, leading to further testing. The DRE reaches only the lateral and posterior surfaces of the prostate, missing 25% to 35% of tumors that are nonpalpable or in other areas.[5] Sensitivity of the DRE for prostate cancer is low, ranging from 20% to 68%, and specificity is approximately 94%.[6] Nonetheless, findings of induration, marked asymmetry, or nodularity should be pursued, especially when accompanying risk factors or an elevated PSA.

The PSA test is also problematic. PSA is a glycoprotein produced by prostate epithelial cells. It can be elevated in benign conditions like hyperplasia and prostatitis and transiently elevated by ejaculation, prostate biopsy, and urinary retention. On the other hand, there is evidence that PSA production can be low in aggressive prostate cancers.

Fewer than one in three men with an elevated PSA will have confirmed prostate cancer.[7] Numerous modifications of the test have been investigated, but none has improved performance of this test. Using the cutoff of 4 nanograms/milliliter (ng/ml), sensitivity is approximately 70% to 80%, with specificity at approximately 60% to 70%.[8] Elevations between 4 and 10 ng/ml and higher than 10 ng/ml increase the likelihood of finding extracapsular tumors, but still have suboptimal sensitivity and specificity for detecting malignancies.

Several groups recommend annual combined screening with DRE and PSA for men older than age 50 and for African Americans and men with a positive family history at age 40, after ensuring that the patient is well informed about risks and benefits and has at least a 10-year life expectancy.[9] The PSA is minimally affected by the DRE, so both can be measured during the same clinician visit. Despite studies showing that DRE and PSA screening can detect prostate cancer in its early stages, evidence that screening improves health outcomes remains inconclusive.[10]

For men *with symptoms* of prostate disorders, the clinician's role is more straightforward. As men approach 50, risk for prostate cancer begins to increase. Review the symptoms of prostate disorders—incomplete emptying of the bladder, urinary frequency or urgency, weak or intermittent stream or straining to initiate flow, hematuria, nocturia, or even bony pains in the pelvis. Men may be reluctant to report such symptoms but should be encouraged to seek evaluation and treatment early.

To increase detection of *colorectal cancer,* clinicians are turning increasingly to colonoscopy, despite its expense and risk for morbidity. Colorectal cancer is the second leading cause of death in the United States and the third most common malignancy. Screening options include DRE, the fecal occult blood test (FOBT), sigmoidoscopy, and colonoscopy. The DRE reaches only 7 to 8 cm of the rectum (usually about 11 cm in length)—only about 10% of colorectal cancers arise in this zone. The FOBT (see discussion on p. 373) detects only 2% to 11% of colorectal cancers and 20% to 30% of adenomas in people older than age 50, and it generates a high rate of false-positive results.[11] Sigmoidoscopy permits good surveillance of the distal third of the colon but misses approximately 35% of more proximal lesions. It may miss up to half of patients with advanced proximal neoplasia. Further, studies have shown that adherence to screening by FOBT and sigmoidoscopy is less than 50%.[12] Colonoscopy offers the potential for detection and excision of most polyps and malignant lesions, especially those larger than 10 mm. Clinicians should explore several options with patients and begin screening for average-risk patients at age 50, and at ages 35 to 40 for those with inflammatory bowel disease or a family history of adenomatous polyps or colorectal cancer (see discussion on pp. 372–373).

TECHNIQUES OF EXAMINATION

For many patients, the rectal examination is the least popular segment of the physical examination. It may cause discomfort and even embarrassment for the patient, but if the examination is skillfully done, it should not be truly painful. You may choose to omit the rectal examination in adolescents who have no relevant complaints; however, in middle-aged or older adults, omission risks missing an asymptomatic carcinoma. A successful examination requires a calm demeanor, an explanation to the patient of what he or she may feel, gentleness, and slow movement of your finger.

MALE

Choose one of several suitable patient positions for conducting the examination. Often, the clinician asks the patient to stand and lean forward with his upper body resting across the examining table and hips flexed. For most purposes, the side-lying position, depicted below, is satisfactory and allows good visualization of the perianal and sacrococcygeal areas.

No matter how you position the patient, your examining finger cannot reach the full length of the rectum. If a rectosigmoid cancer is suspected or screening is warranted, turn to sigmoidoscopy, or colonoscopy.

Ask the patient to lie on his left side with his buttocks close to the edge of the examining table near you. Flexing the patient's hips and knees, especially in the top leg, stabilizes his position and improves visibility. Drape the patient appropriately and adjust the light for the best view. Glove your hands and spread the buttocks apart.

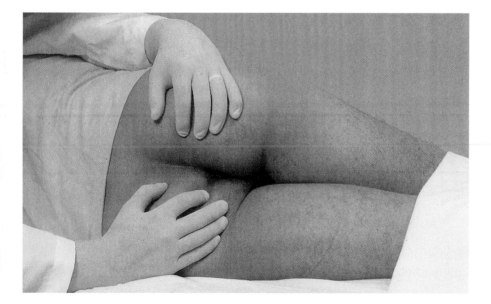

■ *Inspect the sacrococcygeal and perianal areas* for lumps, ulcers, inflammation, rashes, or excoriations. Adult perianal skin is normally more pigmented and somewhat coarser than the skin over the buttocks. Palpate any abnormal areas, noting lumps or tenderness.

■ *Examine the anus and rectum.* Lubricate your gloved index finger, explain to the patient what you are going to do, and tell him that the examination may make him feel as if he were moving his bowels but that he will not do so. Ask him to strain down. Inspect the anus, noting any lesions.

As the patient strains, place the pad of your gloved and lubricated index finger over the anus.

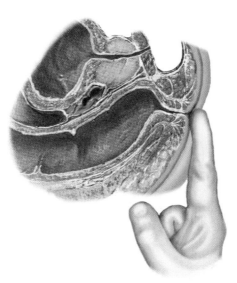

As the sphincter relaxes, gently insert your fingertip into the anal canal in the direction pointing toward the umbilicus. If you feel the sphincter tighten, pause and reassure the patient. When in a moment the sphincter relaxes, proceed.

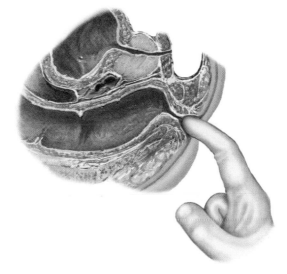

Anal and perianal lesions include hemorrhoids, venereal warts, herpes, syphilitic chancre, and carcinoma. A *perianal abscess* produces a painful, tender, indurated, and reddened mass. Pruritus ani causes swollen, thickened, fissured skin with excoriations.

Soft, pliable tags of redundant skin at the anal margin are common. Though sometimes caused by past anal surgery or previously thrombosed hemorrhoids, they are often unexplained.

See Table 13-1, Abnormalities of the Anus, Surrounding Skin, and Rectum (pp. 469–470).

Occasionally, severe tenderness prevents entry and internal examination. Do not try to force it. Instead, place your fingers on both sides of the anus, gently spread the orifice, and ask the patient to strain down. Look for a lesion, such as an anal fissure, that might explain the tenderness.

If you can proceed without undue discomfort, note:

- The sphincter tone of the anus. Normally, the muscles of the anal sphincter close snugly around your finger.

- Tenderness, if any

- Induration

- Irregularities or nodules

Insert your finger into the rectum as far as possible. Rotate your hand clockwise to palpate as much of the rectal surface as possible on the patient's right side, then counterclockwise to palpate the surface posteriorly and on the patient's left side.

Note any nodules, irregularities, or induration. To bring a possible lesion into reach, take your finger off the rectal surface, ask the patient to strain down, and palpate again.

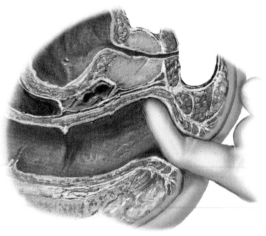

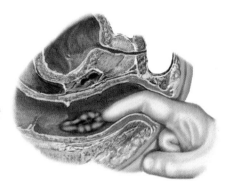

Then rotate your hand further counterclockwise so that your finger can examine the *posterior surface of the prostate gland*. By turning your body somewhat away from the patient, you can feel this area more easily. Tell the patient that you are going to feel his prostate gland, and that this may prompt an urge to urinate.

Sphincter tightness in anxiety, inflammation, or scarring; laxity in some neurologic diseases

Induration may be caused by inflammation, scarring, or malignancy.

The irregular border of a rectal cancer is shown below.

Sweep your finger carefully over the prostate gland, identifying its lateral lobes and the median sulcus between them. Note the size, shape, and consistency of the prostate, and identify any nodules or tenderness. The normal prostate is rubbery and nontender.

See Table 13-2, Abnormalities of the Prostate (p. 471).

If possible, *extend your finger above the prostate* to the region of the seminal vesicles and the peritoneal cavity. Note any nodules or tenderness.

Gently withdraw your finger, and wipe the anus or give the patient tissues. Note the color of any fecal matter on your glove, and test it for occult blood.

A rectal "shelf" of peritoneal metastases (see p. 470) or the tenderness of peritoneal inflammation

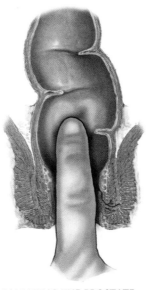

**PALPATING THE PROSTATE—
VIEW FROM BELOW**

FEMALE

The rectum is usually examined after the female genitalia, while the woman is in the lithotomy position. This position allows you to conduct the bimanual examination and delineate a possible adnexal or pelvic mass. It is suitable for testing the integrity of the rectovaginal wall and may also help you to palpate a cancer high in the rectum.

If you only need to examine the rectum, the lateral position is satisfactory and affords a much better view to the perianal and sacrococcygeal areas. Use the same techniques for examination that you use for men. Note that the cervix is readily palpated through the anterior wall. Sometimes a retroverted uterus is also palpable. Do not mistake either of these, or a vaginal tampon, for a tumor.

RECORDING YOUR FINDINGS

Note that initially you may use sentences to describe your findings; later you will use phrases. The style below contains phrases appropriate for most write-ups.

Recording the Physical Examination— The Anus, Rectum, and Prostate

"No perirectal lesions or fissures. External sphincter tone intact. Rectal vault without masses. Prostate smooth and nontender with palpable median sulcus. (Or in a female, uterine cervix nontender.) Stool brown and hemoccult negative."

OR

"Perirectal area inflamed; no ulcerations, warts, or discharge. Unable to examine external sphincter, rectal vault, or prostate because of spasm of external sphincter and marked inflammation and tenderness of anal canal."

Raises concern of proctitis from infectious cause

OR

"No perirectal lesions or fissures. External sphincter tone intact. Rectal vault without masses. Left lateral prostate lobe with 1 × 1 cm firm hard nodule; right lateral lobe smooth; median sulcus obscured. Stool brown and hemoccult negative."

Raises concern of prostate cancer

Bibliography

CITATIONS

1. Jemal A, Tiwari RC, Murray T, et al. Cancer statistics 2004. CA Cancer J Clin 54:8–29, 2004.
2. Ries LA, Eisner MP, Kosary CL, et al (eds). SEER Cancer Statistics Review 1973–1999. Bethesda, MD, National Cancer Institute. Available at: http://www3.cancer.gov/prevention/plco/facts.html. Accessed November 18, 2004.
3. Hoffman RM, Gilliland FD, Eley JW, et al. Racial and ethnic differences in advanced-stage prostate cancer: the Prostate Cancer Outcomes Study. J Natl Cancer Inst 93:388–395, 2001.
4. Brawley O. Risk factors for prostate cancer. Available at: www.utdol.com. Accessed November 18, 2004.
5. U.S. Preventive Services Task Force. Screening for Prostate Cancer, Chapter 10. In Guide to Clinical Preventive Services, 2nd ed. Baltimore, Williams & Wilkins: 119–134, 1996.
6. Hoogendam A, Buntinx F, de Vet HC. The diagnostic value of digital rectal examination in primary care screening for prostate cancer: a meta-analysis. Fam Pract 16:621–626, 1999.
7. Hoffman RM. Screening for prostate cancer. Available at: www.utdol.com. Accessed November 18, 2004.
8. Brawer MK. Prostate-specific antigen: current status. CA Cancer J Clin 11:264–281, 1999.
9. American Cancer Society. ACS cancer detection guidelines. Available at: www.cancer.org. Accessed November 18, 2004.
10. U.S. Preventive Services Task Force. Screening for prostate cancer: recommendation and rationale. Ann Intern Med 137:915–916, 2002.
11. National Cancer Institute. Colorectal cancer: screening (Health Professional version). Available at www.cancer.gov/cancertopics. Accessed November 18, 2004.
12. Vernon SW. Participation in colorectal cancer screening: a review. J Natl Cancer Inst 89(19):1406–1422, 1997

ADDITIONAL REFERENCES

Schrock TR. Examination and diseases of the anorectum. In Feldmen M, Friedman M, Sleisinger MH (eds): Sleisinger's and Fortran's Gastrointestinal and Liver Disease: Pathophysiology/Diagnosis/Management, 7th ed. Philadelphia, Elsevier Saunders, 2000.

Pilonidal Cyst and Sinus

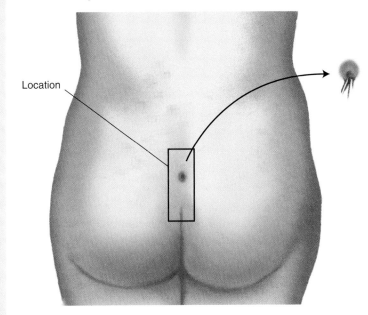

Location

A pilonidal cyst is a fairly common, probably congenital, abnormality located in the midline superficial to the coccyx or the lower sacrum. Look for the opening of a sinus tract. This opening may exhibit a small tuft of hair and be surrounded by a halo of erythema. Although pilonidal cysts are generally asymptomatic, except perhaps for slight drainage, abscess formation and secondary sinus tracts may complicate the picture.

External Hemorrhoids *(Thrombosed)*

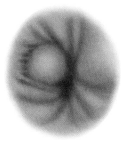

External hemorrhoids are dilated hemorrhoidal veins that originate below the pectinate line and are covered with skin. They seldom produce symptoms unless thrombosis occurs. This causes acute local pain that increases with defecation and sitting. A tender, swollen, bluish, ovoid mass is visible at the anal margin.

Internal Hemorrhoids *(Prolapsed)*

Anterior

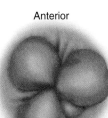

Posterior

Internal hemorrhoids are enlargements of the normal vascular cushions located above the pectinate line. Here, they are not usually palpable. Sometimes, especially during defecation, internal hemorrhoids may cause bright-red bleeding. They may also prolapse through the anal canal and appear as reddish, moist, protruding masses, typically located in one or more of the positions illustrated.

Prolapse of the Rectum

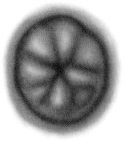

On straining for a bowel movement, the rectal mucosa, with or without its muscular wall, may prolapse through the anus, appearing as a doughnut or rosette of red tissue. A prolapse involving only mucosa is relatively small and shows radiating folds, as illustrated. When the entire bowel wall is involved, the prolapse is larger and covered by concentrically circular folds.

(table continues next page)

Anal Fissure

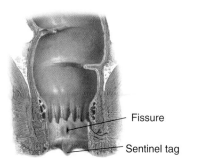

Fissure

Sentinel tag

An anal fissure is a very painful oval ulceration of the anal canal, found most commonly in the midline posteriorly, less commonly in the midline anteriorly. Its long axis lies longitudinally. There may be a swollen "sentinel" skin tag just below it, and gentle separation of the anal margins may reveal the lower edge of the fissure. The sphincter is spastic; the examination is painful. Local anesthesia may be required.

Anorectal Fistula

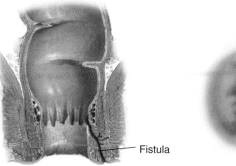

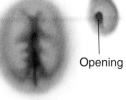

Opening

Fistula

An anorectal fistula is an inflammatory tract or tube that opens at one end into the anus or rectum and at the other end onto the skin surface (as shown here) or into another viscus. An abscess usually antedates such a fistula. Look for the fistulous opening or openings anywhere in the skin around the anus.

Polyps of the Rectum

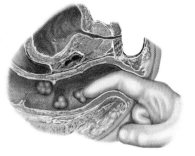

Polyps of the rectum are fairly common. Variable in size and number, they can develop on a stalk (*pedunculated*) or lie on the mucosal surface (*sessile*). They are soft and may be difficult or impossible to feel even when in reach of the examining finger. Proctoscopy and biopsy are needed for differentiation of benign from malignant lesions.

Rectal Shelf

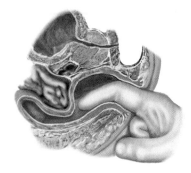

Cancer of the Rectum

Asymptomatic carcinoma of the rectum makes routine rectal examination important for adults. Illustrated here is the firm, nodular, rolled edge of an ulcerated cancer.

Widespread peritoneal metastases from any source may develop in the area of the peritoneal reflection anterior to the rectum. A firm to hard nodular rectal "shelf" may be just palpable with the tip of the examining finger. In a woman, this shelf of metastatic tissue develops in the rectouterine pouch, behind the cervix and the uterus.

TABLE 13-2   **Abnormalities of the Prostate**

Normal Prostate Gland

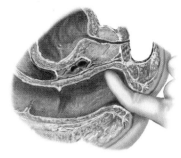

As palpated through the anterior rectal wall, the normal prostate is a rounded, heart-shaped structure about 2.5 cm long. The median sulcus can be felt between the two lateral lobes. Only the posterior surface of the prostate is palpable. Anterior lesions, including those that may obstruct the urethra, are not detectable by physical examination.

Prostatitis

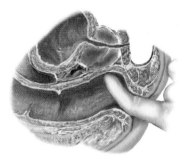

Acute prostatitis (illustrated here) is an acute, febrile condition caused by bacterial infection. The gland is very tender, swollen, firm, and warm. Examine it gently.

Chronic prostatitis does not produce consistent physical findings and must be evaluated by other methods.

Benign Prostatic Hyperplasia

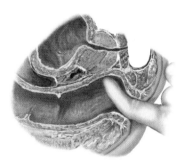

Starting in the 3rd decade of life, benign prostatic hyperplasia (BPH) becomes increasingly prevalent. The affected gland usually feels symmetrically enlarged, smooth, and firm though slightly elastic. It seems to protrude more into the rectal lumen. The median sulcus may be obliterated. Finding a normal-sized gland by palpation, however, does not rule out BPH. Prostatic hyperplasia may obstruct urinary flow, causing symptoms, yet not be palpable.

Cancer of the Prostate

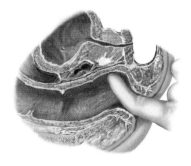

Cancer of the prostate is suggested by an area of hardness in the gland. A distinct hard nodule that alters the contour of the gland may or may not be palpable. As the cancer enlarges, it feels irregular and may extend beyond the confines of the gland. The median sulcus may be obscured. Hard areas in the prostate are not always malignant. They may also result from prostatic stones, chronic inflammation, and other conditions.

14

The Peripheral Vascular System

ANATOMY AND PHYSIOLOGY

This chapter focuses on circulation to the arms and legs. It includes the arteries, the veins, the capillary bed that connects them, and the lymphatic system with its lymph nodes.

ARTERIES

Arterial pulses are palpable when an artery lies close to the body surface. In the arms, there are two or sometimes three such locations. Pulsations of the *brachial artery* can be felt in and above the bend of the elbow, just medial to the biceps tendon and muscle. The brachial artery divides into the radial and ulnar arteries. *Radial artery* pulsations can be felt on the flexor surface of the wrist laterally. Medially, pulsations of the *ulnar artery* may be palpable, but overlying tissues frequently obscure them.

The radial and ulnar arteries are interconnected by two vascular arches within the hand. Circulation to the hand and fingers is thereby doubly protected against possible arterial occlusion.

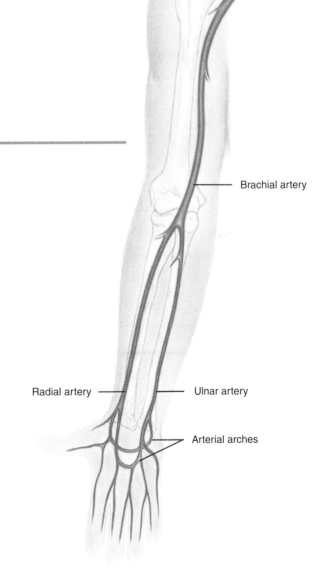

Brachial artery

Radial artery — Ulnar artery

Arterial arches

In the legs, arterial pulsations can usually be felt in four places. Those of the *femoral artery* are palpable below the inguinal ligament, midway between the anterior superior iliac spine and the symphysis pubis. The femoral artery travels downward deep within the thigh, passes medially behind the femur, and becomes the *popliteal artery*. Popliteal pulsations can be felt in the tissues behind the knee. Below the knee, the popliteal artery divides into two branches which both continue to the foot. There the anterior branch becomes the *dorsalis pedis artery*. Its pulsations are palpable on the dorsum of the foot just lateral to the extensor tendon of the big toe. The posterior branch, the *posterior tibial artery,* can be felt as it passes behind the medial malleolus of the ankle.

Like the hand, the foot is protected by an interconnecting arch between its two chief arterial branches.

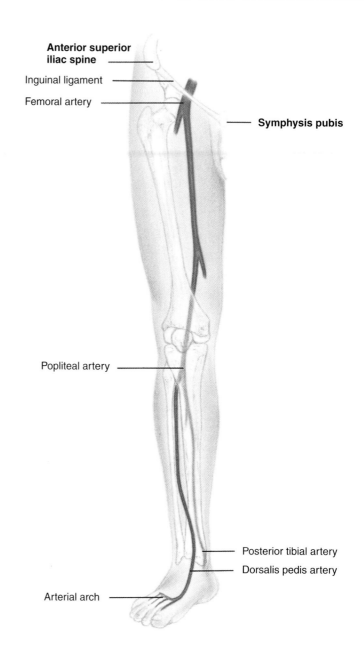

Anterior superior iliac spine

Inguinal ligament

Femoral artery

Symphysis pubis

Popliteal artery

Posterior tibial artery

Dorsalis pedis artery

Arterial arch

VEINS

The veins from the arms, together with those from the upper trunk and the head and neck, drain into the superior vena cava and on into the right atrium. Veins from the legs and the lower trunk drain upward into the inferior vena cava. Because the leg veins are especially susceptible to dysfunction, they warrant special attention.

The *deep veins* of the legs carry approximately 90% of the venous return from the lower extremities. They are well supported by surrounding tissues.

In contrast, the *superficial veins* are located subcutaneously and are supported relatively poorly. The superficial veins include (1) the *great saphenous vein,* which originates on the dorsum of the foot, passes just in front of the medial malleolus, and then continues up the medial aspect of the leg to join the femoral vein of the deep venous system, below the inguinal ligament; and (2) the *small saphenous vein,* which begins at the side of the foot and passes upward along the back of the leg to join the deep system in the popliteal space. Anastomotic veins connect the two saphenous veins superficially and, when dilated, are readily visible. In addition, *communicating,* or *perforating, veins* connect the saphenous system with the deep venous system.

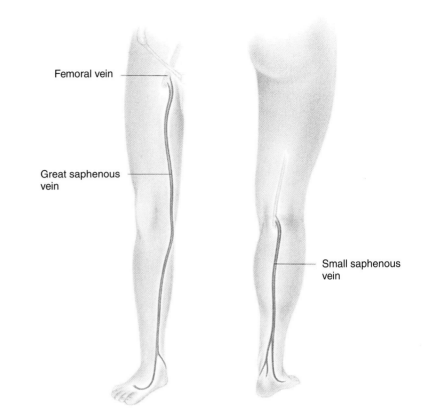

Deep, superficial, and communicating veins all have one-way valves. These allow venous blood to flow from the superficial to the deep system and toward the heart, but not in the opposite directions. Muscular activity contributes importantly to venous blood flow. As calf muscles contract in walking, for example, blood is squeezed upward against gravity, and competent valves keep it from pooling and falling back.

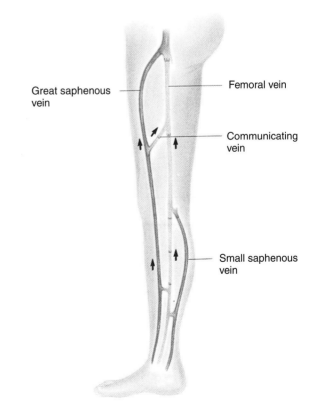

THE LYMPHATIC SYSTEM AND LYMPH NODES

The lymphatic system comprises an extensive vascular network that drains lymph fluid from bodily tissues and returns it to the venous circulation. The system starts peripherally as blind lymphatic capillaries, and continues centrally as thin vascular channels and then collecting ducts that finally empty into major veins at the root of the neck. The lymph transported in these channels is filtered through lymph nodes that are interposed along the way.

Lymph nodes are round, oval, or bean-shaped structures that vary in size according to their location. Some lymph nodes, such as the preauriculars, if palpable at all, are typically very small. The inguinal nodes, in contrast, are relatively larger—often 1 cm in diameter and occasionally even 2 cm in an adult.

In addition to its vascular functions, the lymphatic system plays an important role in the body's immune system. Cells within the lymph nodes engulf cellular debris and bacteria and produce antibodies.

Only the superficial lymph nodes are accessible to physical examination. These include the cervical nodes (p. 170), the axillary nodes (p. 339), and nodes in the arms and legs.

Recall that the axillary lymph nodes drain most of the arm. Lymphatics from the ulnar surface of the forearm and hand, the little and ring fingers, and the adjacent surface of the middle finger, however, drain first into the *epitrochlear nodes*. These are located on the medial surface of the arm approximately 3 cm above the elbow. Lymphatics from the rest of the arm drain mostly into the axillary nodes. A few may go directly to the infraclaviculars.

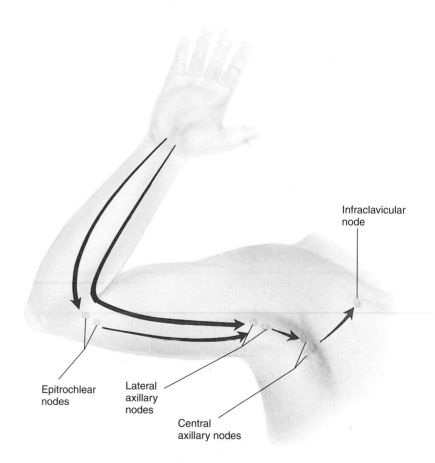

Infraclavicular node

Epitrochlear nodes

Lateral axillary nodes

Central axillary nodes

The lymphatics of the lower limb, following the venous supply, consist of both deep and superficial systems. Only the superficial nodes are palpable. The *superficial inguinal nodes* include two groups. The *horizontal group* lies in a chain high in the anterior thigh below the inguinal ligament. It drains the superficial portions of the lower abdomen and buttock, the external genitalia (but not the testes), the anal canal and perianal area, and the lower vagina.

The *vertical group* clusters near the upper part of the saphenous vein and drains a corresponding region of the leg. In contrast, lymphatics from the portion of leg drained by the small saphenous vein (the heel and outer aspect of the foot) join the deep system at the level of the popliteal space. Lesions in this area, therefore, are not usually associated with palpable inguinal lymph nodes.

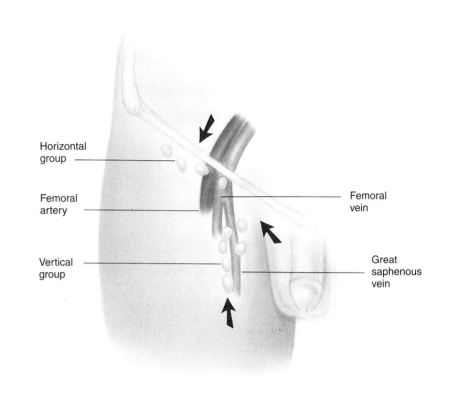

Horizontal group

Femoral artery

Vertical group

Femoral vein

Great saphenous vein

FLUID EXCHANGE AND THE CAPILLARY BED

Blood circulates from arteries to veins through the capillary bed. Here fluids diffuse across the capillary membrane, maintaining a dynamic equilibrium between the vascular and interstitial spaces. Blood pressure (*hydrostatic pressure*) within the capillary bed, especially near the arteriolar end, forces fluid out into the tissue spaces. In effecting this movement, it is aided by the relatively weak osmotic attraction of proteins within the tissues (*interstitial colloid oncotic pressure*) and is opposed by the hydrostatic pressure of the tissues.

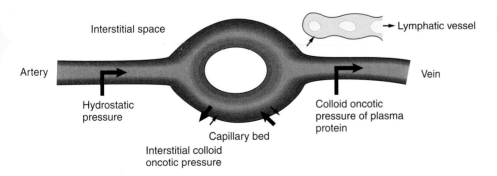

Interstitial space

Lymphatic vessel

Artery

Vein

Hydrostatic pressure

Colloid oncotic pressure of plasma protein

Capillary bed

Interstitial colloid oncotic pressure

As blood continues through the capillary bed toward the venous end, its hydrostatic pressure falls, and another force gains dominance. This is the *colloid oncotic pressure of plasma proteins*, which pulls fluid back into the vascular tree. Net flow of fluid, which was directed outward on the arteriolar side of the capillary bed, reverses itself and turns inward on the venous side. Lymphatic capillaries, which also play an important role in this equilibrium, remove excessive fluid, including protein, from the interstitial space.

Lymphatic dysfunction or disturbances in hydrostatic or osmotic forces can all disrupt this equilibrium. The most common clinical result is the increased interstitial fluid known as edema (see Table 14-4, Some Peripheral Causes of Edema, p. 496).

THE HEALTH HISTORY

Common or Concerning Symptoms

- Pain in the arms or legs
- Intermittent claudication
- Cold, numbness, pallor in the legs; hair loss
- Color change in fingertips or toes in cold weather
- Swelling in calves, legs, or feet
- Swelling with redness or tenderness

To assess possible peripheral vascular disease, begin by asking patients about any *pain in the arms or legs.* Be aware that pain in the extremities may arise from the skin, the peripheral vascular system, the musculoskeletal system, or the nervous system. In addition, visceral pain may be referred to the extremities, like the pain of myocardial infarction that radiates to the left arm or cervical arthritis that radiates to the shoulder.

To elicit symptoms of *arterial peripheral vascular disease* in the legs, inquire about *intermittent claudication,* which is exercise-induced pain that is absent at rest, makes the patient stop exertion, and remits within about 10 minutes. Ask "Have you ever had any pain or cramping in your legs when you walk or exercise?" and "How far can you walk without stopping to rest?" Also, "Does the pain get better with rest?" These questions clarify what makes the patient stop and how quickly the pain is relieved. Ask also about *coldness, numbness,* or *pallor* in the legs or feet or *loss of hair* over the anterior tibial surfaces.

Many patients with arterial peripheral vascular disease have few symptoms, so it is important to identify background risk factors. Assess the patient's his-

See Table 14-1, Painful Peripheral Vascular Disorders and Their Mimics, pp. 492–493.

Atherosclerosis can cause symptomatic limb ischemia with exertion; distinguish this from *spinal stenosis,* which produces leg pain with exertion that may be reduced by leaning forward (stretching the spinal cord in the narrowed vertebral canal) and less readily relieved by rest.

Hair loss over the anterior tibiae occurs with decreased arterial perfusion. "Dry" or brown-black ulcers from gangrene may ensue.

Only about 10% of affected patients have the classic symptoms

tory of tobacco abuse. Ask if the patient has had hypertension, diabetes, or hyperlipidemia. Further, is there any history of myocardial infarction or stroke? Such patients warrant further evaluation, even if without symptoms in the extremities (see p. 480).

To elicit symptoms of arterial spasm in the fingers or toes, ask "Do your fingertips ever change color in cold weather or when you handle cold objects?" . . . "What color changes do you notice?" . . . "What about your toes?"

There may be symptoms of *venous peripheral vascular disease,* such as *swelling of the feet and legs.* Ask about any ulcers on the lower legs, often near the ankles.

The redness, swelling, and tenderness of local inflammation are seen in some vascular disorders and in other conditions that mimic them. In contrast, relatively brief leg cramps that commonly occur at night in otherwise healthy people do not indicate a circulatory problem, and cold hands and feet are so common in healthy people that they have relatively little predictive value.

of exertional calf pain relieved by rest.

Digital ischemic changes of blanching, followed by cyanosis, then rubor with cold exposure and rewarming occur in *Raynaud's phenomenon* or *disease.*

Hyperpigmentation, edema, and possible cyanosis, especially when legs are dependent, occur with *venous stasis ulcers.*

Inflammation may be from *cellulitis, superficial thrombophlebitis,* and *erythema nodosum.*

Etiology of common leg cramps and "restless legs" is not well understood. Leg cramps sometimes arise from diuretic use with hypokalemia.

HEALTH PROMOTION AND COUNSELING

Important Topics for Health Promotion and Counseling

- Detection of peripheral arterial disease (PAD)
- Risk factors for PAD
- Screening for PAD: the ankle–brachial index (ABI)

Peripheral arterial disease (PAD) generally refers to atherosclerotic occlusion of arteries in the lower extremities. The femoral and popliteal arteries are involved most commonly, followed by the tibial and peroneal arteries. PAD affects from 12% to 25% of community populations; however, recent studies have shown that despite significant associations with cardiovascular and cerebrovascular disease, PAD often is underdiagnosed in office practices.[1,2] Most patients with PAD have either no symptoms or a range of nonspecific leg symptoms, such as aching, cramping, numbness, or fatigue. The classic triad for vascular claudication, exercise-induced calf pain that causes stopping of exercise, with relief of pain in 10 minutes or less, may be present in only about

10% of affected patients.[1] The low symptom rate may reflect functional declines in walking even though PAD is present or progressing.[3]

Patients with current or past tobacco use, diabetes, hypertension, hyperlipidemia, or cardiovascular or cerebrovascular disease are at increased risk for atherosclerotic PAD. Such patients should be screened for subclinical PAD and targeted for aggressive risk factor intervention. For screening, clinicians should consider use of the ankle–brachial index (ABI), a highly accurate test for detecting 50% or greater stenoses of 50% or more in major vessels of the legs. The ABI is readily performed by clinicians or office staff, and consists of measuring the systolic blood pressure with Doppler ultrasonography in each arm and in the dorsalis pedis and posterior tibial pulses. The ABI is calculated on both the right and left by dividing the higher right ankle pressure by the higher right arm pressure, and the higher left ankle pressure by the higher left arm pressure. ABI values are as follows: 0.90–1.30 is considered normal; 0.41–0.90, mild to moderate peripheral arterial disease, usually with symptoms of claudication; and 0.00–0.40, severe peripheral vascular disease with critical leg ischemia.

The severity of peripheral vascular disease closely parallels the risk for myocardial infarction, ischemic stroke, and death from vascular causes. Patients with ABIs in the lowest category have a 20% to 25% annual risk for death.[1] A wide range of interventions is available to reduce both onset and progression of subclinical PAD, including meticulous foot care and well-fitting shoes, tobacco cessation, treatment of hyperlipidemia, optimal control and treatment of diabetes and hypertension, use of antiplatelet agents, and, if needed, surgical revascularization.

(Students should consult specialty texts for less common forms of vascular occlusion from arterial or venous thrombosis or endarteritis from infection, inflammation, or autoimmune disease.)

TECHNIQUES OF EXAMINATION

Important Areas of Examination

The Arms

- Size, symmetry, skin color
- Radial pulse, brachial pulse
- Epitrochlear lymph nodes

The Legs

- Size, symmetry, skin color
- Femoral pulse and inguinal lymph nodes
- Popliteal, dorsalis pedis, and posterior tibial pulses
- Peripheral edema

Assessment of the peripheral vascular system relies primarily on inspection of the arms and legs, palpation of the pulses, and a search for edema. See Chapter 4 for a method of integrating these techniques into your examination of the limbs. Additional techniques may be useful when you suspect an abnormality.

ARMS

Inspect both arms from the fingertips to the shoulders. Note:

- Their size, symmetry, and any swelling

Lymphedema of the arm and hand may follow axillary node dissection and radiation therapy.

- The venous pattern

Prominent veins in an edematous arm suggest venous obstruction.

- The color of the skin and nail beds and the texture of the skin

Palpate the radial pulse with the pads of your fingers on the flexor surface of the wrist laterally. Partially flexing the patient's wrist may help you feel this pulse. Compare the pulses in both arms.

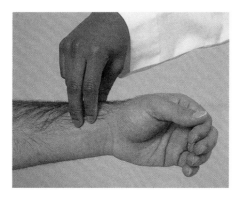

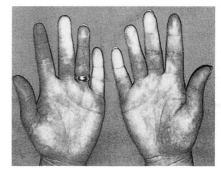

(Source of photo above: Marks R: Skin Disease in Old Age. Philadelphia, JB Lippincott, 1987)

In *Raynaud's disease,* wrist pulses are typically normal, but spasm of more distal arteries causes episodes of sharply demarcated pallor of the fingers (see Table 14-1, Painful Peripheral Vascular Disorders and Their Mimics, pp. 492–493).

There are several systems for grading the amplitude of the arterial pulses. One system is to use a scale of 0 to 4, as below; however, you should check to see what scale is used in your institution.

Note that if an artery is widely dilated, it is *aneurysmal.*

4+	Bounding
3+	Increased
2+	Brisk, expected
1+	Diminished, weaker than expected
0	Absent, unable to palpate

Bounding carotid, radial, and femoral pulses in *aortic insufficiency*; asymmetric diminished pulses in *arterial occlusion* from atherosclerosis or embolism

If you suspect arterial insufficiency, feel for the *brachial pulse.* Flex the patient's elbow slightly, and with the thumb of your opposite hand palpate the artery just medial to the biceps tendon at the antecubital crease. The brachial artery can also be felt higher in the arm in the groove between the biceps and triceps muscles.

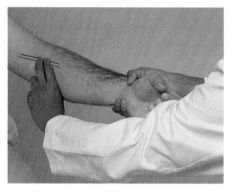

Feel for one or more *epitrochlear nodes.* With the patient's elbow flexed to about 90° and the forearm supported by your hand, reach around behind the arm and feel in the groove between the biceps and triceps muscles, about 3 cm above the medial epicondyle. If a node is present, note its size, consistency, and tenderness.

Medial aspect of left arm

An enlarged epitrochlear node may be secondary to a lesion in its drainage area or may be associated with generalized lymphadenopathy.

Epitrochlear nodes are difficult or impossible to identify in most normal people.

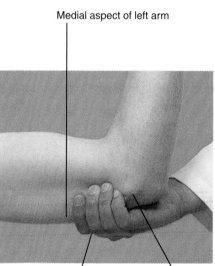

Right hand of examiner
Medial epicondyle of humerus

 LEGS

The patient should be lying down and draped so that the external genitalia are covered and the legs fully exposed. A good examination is impossible through stockings or socks!

Inspect both legs from the groin and buttocks to the feet. Note:

- Their size, symmetry, and any swelling

- The venous pattern and any venous enlargement

- Any pigmentation, rashes, scars, or ulcers

- The color and texture of the skin, the color of the nail beds, and the distribution of hair on the lower legs, feet, and toes.

See Table 14-2, Chronic Insufficiency of Arteries and Veins (p. 494).

See Table 14-3, Common Ulcers of the Feet and Ankles (p. 495).

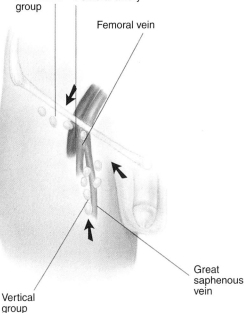

Palpate the *superficial inguinal nodes,* including both the horizontal and the vertical groups. Note their size, consistency, and discreteness, and note any tenderness. Nontender, discrete inguinal nodes up to 1 cm or even 2 cm in diameter are frequently palpable in normal people.

Lymphadenopathy refers to enlargement of the nodes, with or without tenderness. Try to distinguish between local and generalized lymphadenopathy, respectively, by finding either (1) a causative lesion in the drainage area, or (2) enlarged nodes in at least two other noncontiguous lymph node regions.

Palpate the pulses in order to assess the arterial circulation.

- *The femoral pulse.* Press deeply, below the inguinal ligament and about midway between the anterior superior iliac spine and the symphysis pubis. As in deep abdominal palpation, the use of two hands, one on top of the other, may facilitate this examination, especially in obese patients.

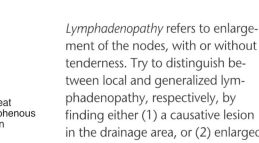

A diminished or absent pulse indicates partial or complete occlusion proximally; for example, at the aortic or iliac level, all pulses distal to the occlusion are typically affected. Chronic arterial occlusion, usually from atherosclerosis, causes *intermittent claudication,* (p. 492, postural color changes (p. 489), and trophic changes in the skin (p. 489)

An exaggerated, widened femoral pulse suggests a femoral aneurysm, a pathologic dilatation of the artery.

■ *The popliteal pulse.* The patient's knee should be somewhat flexed, the leg relaxed. Place the fingertips of both hands so that they just meet in the midline behind the knee and press them deeply into the popliteal fossa. The popliteal pulse is often more difficult to find than other pulses. It is deeper and feels more diffuse.

An exaggerated, widened popliteal pulse suggests an aneurysm of the popliteal artery. Neither popliteal nor femoral aneurysms are common. They are usually due to atherosclerosis, and occur primarily in men older than age 50.

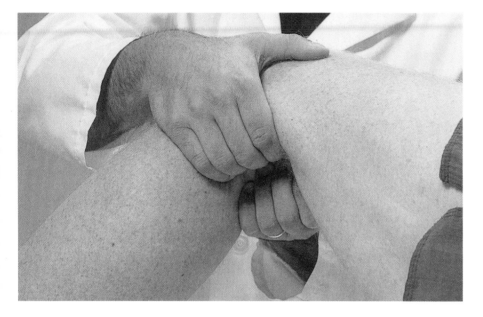

If you cannot feel the popliteal pulse with this approach, try with the patient prone. Flex the patient's knee to about 90°, let the lower leg relax against your shoulder or upper arm, and press your two thumbs deeply into the popliteal fossa.

Atherosclerosis (arteriosclerosis obliterans) most commonly obstructs arterial circulation in the thigh. The femoral pulse is then normal, the popliteal decreased or absent.

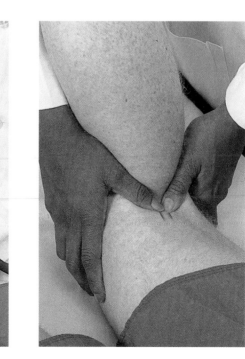

■ *The dorsalis pedis pulse.* Feel the dorsum of the foot (not the ankle) just lateral to the extensor tendon of the great toe. If you cannot feel a pulse, explore the dorsum of the foot more laterally.

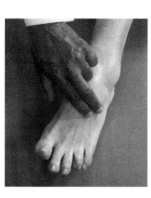

The dorsalis pedis artery may be congenitally absent or may branch higher in the ankle. Search for a pulse more laterally.

Decreased or absent pedal pulses (assuming a warm environment) with normal femoral and popliteal pulses suggest occlusive disease in the lower popliteal artery or its branches— a pattern often associated with diabetes mellitus.

■ *The posterior tibial pulse.* Curve your fingers behind and slightly below the medial malleolus of the ankle. (This pulse may be hard to feel in a fat or edematous ankle.)

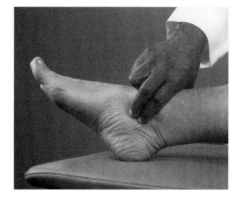

Sudden arterial occlusion, as from embolism or thrombosis, causes pain and numbness or tingling. The limb distal to the occlusion becomes cold, pale, and pulseless. Emergency treatment is required. If collateral circulation is good, only numbness and coolness may result.

Tips on feeling difficult pulses: (1) Position your own body and examining hand comfortably; awkward positions decrease your tactile sensitivity. (2) Place your hand properly and linger there, varying the pressure of your fingers to pick up a weak pulsation. If unsuccessful, then explore the area deliberately. (3) Do not confuse the patient's pulse with your own pulsating fingertips. If you are unsure, count your own heart rate and compare it with the patient's. The rates are usually different. Your carotid pulse is convenient for this comparison.

Note the temperature of the feet and legs with the backs of your fingers. Compare one side with the other. Bilateral coldness is most often due to a cold environment or anxiety.

Coldness, especially when unilateral or associated with other signs, suggests arterial insufficiency from inadequate arterial circulation.

Look for edema. Compare one foot and leg with the other, noting their relative size and the prominence of veins, tendons, and bones.

Edema causes swelling that may obscure the veins, tendons, and bony prominences.

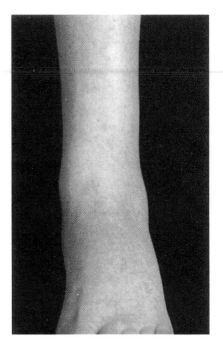

Check for pitting edema. Press firmly but gently with your thumb for at least 5 seconds (1) over the dorsum of each foot, (2) behind each medial malleolus, and (3) over the shins. Look for *pitting*—a depression caused by pressure from your thumb. Normally there is none. The severity of edema is graded on a four-point scale, from slight to very marked.

See Table 14-4, Some Peripheral Causes of Edema (p. 496).

Shown below is 3+ pitting edema.

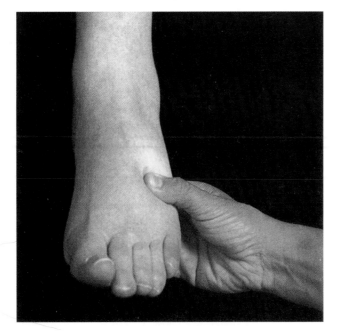

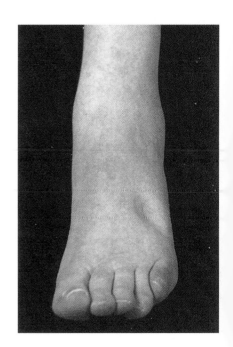

If you suspect edema, *measurement of the legs* may help you to identify it and to follow its course. With a flexible tape, measure (1) the forefoot, (2) the smallest possible circumference above the ankle, (3) the largest circumference at the calf, and (4) the midthigh, a measured distance above the patella with the knee extended. Compare one side with the other. A difference of more than 1 cm just above the ankle or 2 cm at the calf is unusual in normal people and suggests edema.

Conditions such as muscular atrophy can also cause different circumferences in the legs.

If edema is present, look for possible causes in the peripheral vascular system. These include (1) recent deep venous thrombosis, (2) chronic venous insufficiency due to previous deep venous thrombosis or to incompetence of the venous valves, and (3) lymphedema. Note the extent of the swelling. How far up the leg does it go?

In *deep venous thrombosis,* the extent of edema suggests the location of the occlusion: the calf when the lower leg or the ankle is swollen, the iliofemoral veins when the entire leg is swollen.

Is the swelling unilateral or bilateral? Are the veins unusually prominent?

Venous distention suggests a venous cause of edema.

Try to identify any venous tenderness that may accompany deep venous thrombosis. Palpate the groin just medial to the femoral pulse for tenderness of the femoral vein. Next, with the patient's leg flexed at the knee and relaxed, palpate the calf. With your fingerpads, gently compress the calf muscles against the tibia, and search for any tenderness or cords. Deep venous thrombosis, however, may have no demonstrable signs, and diagnosis often depends on high clinical suspicion and other testing.

A painful, pale swollen leg, together with tenderness in the groin over the femoral vein, suggests deep *iliofemoral thrombosis.* Only half of patients with *deep venous thrombosis* in the calf have tenderness and cords deep in the calf. Calf tenderness is nonspecific, however, and may be present without thrombosis.

Note the *color of the skin.*

- Is there a local area of redness? If so, note its temperature, and gently try to feel the firm cord of a thrombosed vein in the area. The calf is most often involved.

Local swelling, redness, warmth, and a subcutaneous cord suggest *superficial thrombophlebitis.*

- Are there brownish areas near the ankles?

A brownish color or ulcers just above the ankle suggest *chronic venous insufficiency.*

- Note any ulcers in the skin. Where are they?

- Feel the thickness of the skin.

Thickened brawny skin occurs in lymphedema and advanced venous insufficiency.

Ask the patient to stand, and *inspect the saphenous system for varicosities.* The standing posture allows any varicosities to fill with blood and makes them visible. You can easily miss them when the patient is in a supine position. Feel for any varicosities, noting any signs of thrombophlebitis.

Varicose veins are dilated and tortuous. Their walls may feel somewhat thickened. Many varicose veins can be seen in the leg on p. 490.

SPECIAL TECHNIQUES

Evaluating the Arterial Supply to the Hand. If you suspect arterial insufficiency in the arm or hand, try to feel the *ulnar pulse* as well as the radial and brachial pulses. Feel for it deeply on the flexor surface of the wrist medially. Partially flexing the patient's wrist may help you. The pulse of a normal ulnar artery, however, may not be palpable.

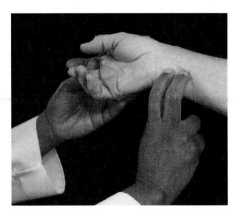

Arterial occlusive disease is much less common in the arms than in the legs. Absent or diminished pulses at the wrist in acute embolic occlusion and in *Buerger's disease,* or thromboangiitis obliterans.

The *Allen test* gives further information. This test is also useful to ensure the patency of the ulnar artery before puncturing the radial artery for blood samples. The patient should rest with hands in lap, palms up.

Ask the patient to make a tight fist with one hand; then compress both radial and ulnar arteries firmly between your thumbs and fingers.

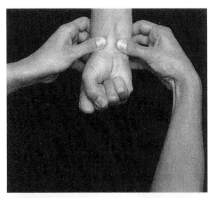

Next, ask the patient to open the hand into a relaxed slightly flexed position. The palm is pale.

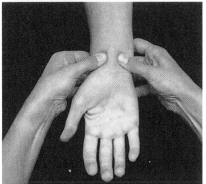

Extending the hand fully may cause pallor and a falsely positive test.

Release your pressure over the ulnar artery. If the ulnar artery is patent, the palm flushes within about 3 to 5 seconds.

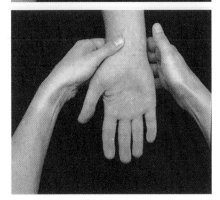

Persisting pallor indicates occlusion of the ulnar artery or its distal branches.

Patency of the radial artery may be tested by releasing the radial artery while still compressing the ulnar.

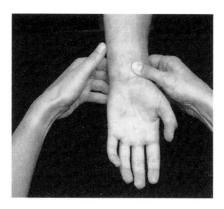

Postural Color Changes of Chronic Arterial Insufficiency. If pain or diminished pulses suggest arterial insufficiency, look for postural color changes. Raise both legs, as shown at the right, to about 60° until maximal pallor of the feet develops—usually within a minute. In light-skinned persons, either maintenance of normal color, as seen in this right foot, or slight pallor is normal.

Marked pallor on elevation suggests *arterial insufficiency.*

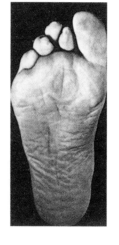
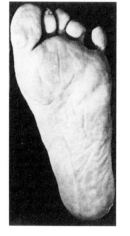

Then ask the patient to sit up with legs dangling down. Compare both feet, noting the time required for:

The foot below is still pale, and the veins are just starting to fill—signs of arterial insufficiency.

- Return of pinkness to the skin, normally about 10 seconds or less

- Filling of the veins of the feet and ankles, normally about 15 seconds

This right foot has normal color and the veins on the foot have filled. These normal responses suggest an adequate circulation.

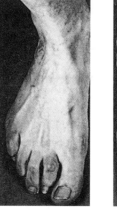
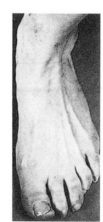

(Source of foot photos: Kappert A, Winsor T: Diagnosis of Peripheral Vascular Disease. Philadelphia, FA Davis, 1972).

Look for any unusual *rubor* (dusky redness) to replace the pallor of the dependent foot. Rubor may take a minute or more to appear.

Normal responses accompanied by diminished arterial pulses suggest that a good collateral circulation has developed around an arterial occlusion.

Color changes may be difficult to see in darker-skinned persons. Inspect the soles of the feet for these changes, and use tangential lighting to see the veins.

Persisting rubor on dependency suggests arterial insufficiency (see p. 495). When veins are incompetent, dependent rubor and the timing of color return and venous filling are not reliable tests of arterial insufficiency.

Mapping Varicose Veins. You can map out the course and connections of varicose veins by transmitting pressure waves along the blood-filled veins. With the patient standing, place your palpating fingers gently on a vein and, with your other hand below it, compress the vein sharply. Feel for a pressure wave transmitted to the fingers of your upper hand. A palpable pressure wave indicates that the two parts of the vein are connected.

A wave may also be transmitted downward, but not as easily.

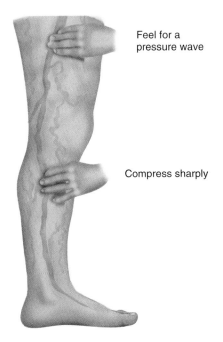

Feel for a pressure wave

Compress sharply

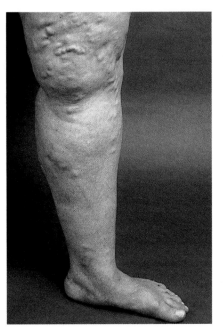

Evaluating the Competency of Venous Valves. By the *retrograde filling (Trendelenburg) test,* you can assess the valvular competency in both the communicating veins and the saphenous system. Start with the patient supine. Elevate one leg to about 90° to empty it of venous blood.

Next, occlude the great saphenous vein in the upper thigh by manual compression, using enough pressure to occlude this vein but not the deeper vessels. Ask the patient to stand. While you keep the vein occluded, watch for venous filling in the leg. Normally the saphenous vein fills from below, taking about 35 seconds as blood flows through the capillary bed into the venous system.

Rapid filling of the superficial veins while the saphenous vein is occluded indicates incompetent valves in the communicating veins. Blood flows quickly in a retrograde direction from the deep to the saphenous system.

After the patient stands for 20 seconds, release the compression and look for sudden additional venous filling. Normally there is none; competent valves in the saphenous vein block retrograde flow. Slow venous filling continues.

Sudden additional filling of superficial veins after release of compression indicates incompetent valves in the saphenous vein.

When both steps of this test are normal, the response is termed negative–negative. Negative–positive and positive–negative responses may also occur.

When both steps are abnormal, the test is positive–positive.

RECORDING YOUR FINDINGS

Note that initially you may use sentences to describe your findings; later you will use phrases. The style below contains phrases appropriate for most write-ups. Recall that the written description of lymph nodes appears after the Head and Neck section (see p. 203). Likewise, assessment of the carotid pulse is recorded in the Cardiovascular section (see p. 305–306).

Recording the Physical Examination— The Peripheral Vascular System

"Extremities are warm and without edema. No varicosities or stasis changes. Calves are supple and nontender. No femoral or abdominal bruits. Brachial, radial, femoral, popliteal, dorsalis pedis (DP), and posterior tibial (PT) pulses are 2+ and symmetric."

OR

"Extremities are pale below the midcalf, with notable hair loss. Rubor noted when legs dependent but no edema or ulceration. Bilateral femoral bruits; no abdominal bruits heard. Brachial and radial pulses 2+; femoral, popliteal, DP and PT pulses 1+." (Alternatively, pulses can be recorded as below.)

Suggests atherosclerotic peripheral arterial disease

	Radial	Brachial	Femoral	Popliteal	Dorsalis Pedis	Posterior Tibial
RT	2+	2+	1+	1+	1+	1+
LT	2+	2+	1+	1+	1+	1+

Bibliography

CITATIONS

1. Hirsh AT, Criqui MH, Treat-Jacobson D, et al: Peripheral arterial disease: detection, awareness, and treatment in primary care. JAMA 286(11):1317–1324, 2001.
2. Hiatt WR: Medical treatment of peripheral arterial disease and claudication. N Engl J Med 344(21):1608–1620, 2001.
3. McDermott MM, Liu K, Greenland, et al: Functional decline in peripheral arterial disease—associations with the ankle brachial index and leg symptoms. JAMA 292(4):453–461, 2004.

ADDITIONAL REFERENCES

Anand SS, Wells PS, Hunt D, et al. Does this patient have a deep vein thrombosis? JAMA 279(14):1094–1099, 1998.

Bates SM, Gionsberg JS. Treatment of deep-vein thrombosis. N Engl J Med 351(3):268–276, 2004.

Colman RW, Marder VJ, Clowes AW, et al (eds). Hemostasis and Thrombosis: Basic Principles and Clinical Practice, 4th ed. Philadelphia, Lippincott Williams & Wilkins, 2005.

Creager MA, Loscalzo J, Dzau VJ (eds). Vascular Medicine: A Companion to Braunwald's Heart Disease. Philadelphia, WB Saunders, 2006.

De Araujo T, Valencia I, Federman DG, et al. Managing the patient with venous ulcers. Ann Intern Med 138(4):326–334, 2003.

Falagas ME, Vergidis PI. Narrative review: diseases that masquerade as infectious cellulitis. Ann Intern Med 142(1):47–55, 2005.

Olson KWP, Treat-Jacobson D. Symptoms of peripheral arterial disease: a critical review. J Vasc Nurs 22(3):72–77, 2004.

Rauch U, Osende JI, Fuster V, et al. Thrombus formation on atherosclerotic plaques: pathogenesis and clinical consequences. Ann Intern Med 134(10):224–238, 2001.

Sumpio BE. Foot ulcers. N Engl J Med 343(11):787–793, 2000.

Wigley FM. Raynaud's phenomenon. N Engl J Med 347(13): 1001–1008, 2002.

| TABLE 14-1 | Painful Peripheral Vascular Disorders and Their Mimics |

Problem	Process	Location of Pain
Arterial Disorders		
Atherosclerosis (arteriosclerosis obliterans)		
■ Intermittent claudication	Episodic muscular ischemia induced by exercise, due to obstruction of large or medium-sized arteries by atherosclerosis	Usually the calf, but also may be in the buttock, hip, thigh, or foot, depending on the level of obstruction
■ Rest pain	Ischemia even at rest	Distal pain, in the toes or forefoot
Acute Arterial Occlusion	Embolism or thrombosis, possibly superimposed on arteriosclerosis obliterans	Distal pain, usually involving the foot and leg
Raynaud's Disease and Phenomenon	*Raynaud's disease:* Episodic spasm of the small arteries and arterioles; no vascular occlusion *Raynaud's phenomenon:* Syndrome is secondary to other conditions such as collagen vascular disease, arterial occlusion, trauma, drugs	Distal portions of one or more fingers. Pain is usually not prominent unless fingertip ulcers develop. Numbness and tingling are common.
Venous Disorders		
Superficial Thrombophlebitis	Clot formation and acute inflammation in a superficial vein	Pain in a local area along the course of a superficial vein, most often in the saphenous system
Deep Venous Thrombosis	Clot formation in a deep vein	Pain, if present, is usually in the calf, but the process more often is painless.
Chronic Venous Insufficiency (deep)	Chronic venous engorgement secondary to venous occlusion or incompetency of venous valves	Diffuse aching of the leg(s)
Thromboangiitis Obliterans (*Buerger's disease*)	Inflammatory and thrombotic occlusions of small arteries and also of veins, occurring in smokers	■ Intermittent claudication, particularly in the arch of the foot ■ Rest pain in the fingers or toes
Acute Lymphangitis	Acute bacterial infection (usually streptococcal) spreading up the lymphatic channels from a portal of entry such as an injured area or an ulcer	An arm or a leg
Mimics*		
Acute Cellulitis	Acute bacterial infection of the skin and subcutaneous tissues	Arms, legs, or elsewhere
Erythema Nodosum	Subcutaneous inflammatory lesions associated with a variety of systemic conditions such as pregnancy, sarcoidosis, tuberculosis, and streptococcal infections	Anterior surfaces of both lower legs

* Mistaken primarily for acute superficial thrombophlebitis.

Timing	Factors That Aggravate	Factors That Relieve	Associated Manifestations
Fairly brief; pain usually forces the patient to rest.	Exercise such as walking	Rest usually stops the pain in 1–3 min.	Local fatigue, numbness, diminished pulses, often signs of arterial insufficiency (see p. 495)
Persistent, often worse at night	Elevation of the feet, as in bed	Sitting with legs dependent	Numbness, tingling, trophic signs and color changes of arterial insufficiency (see p. 495)
Sudden onset; associated symptoms may occur without pain.			Coldness, numbness, weakness, absent distal pulses
Relatively brief (minutes) but recurrent	Exposure to cold, emotional upset	Warm environment	Color changes in the distal fingers: severe pallor (essential for the diagnosis) followed by cyanosis and then redness
An acute episode lasting days or longer			Local redness, swelling, tenderness, a palpable cord, possibly fever
Often hard to determine because of lack of symptoms			Possibly swelling of the foot and calf and local calf tenderness; often nothing
Chronic, increasing as the day wears on	Prolonged standing	Elevation of the leg(s)	Chronic edema, pigmentation, possibly ulceration (see p. 495)
■ Fairly brief but recurrent ■ Chronic, persistent, may be worse at night	■ Exercise	■ Rest ■ Permanent cessation of smoking helps both kinds of pain (but patients seldom stop)	Distal coldness, sweating, numbness, and cyanosis; ulceration and gangrene at the tips of fingers or toes; migratory thrombophlebitis
An acute episode lasting days or longer			Red streak(s) on the skin, with tenderness, enlarged, tender lymph nodes, and fever
An acute episode lasting days or longer			A local area of diffuse swelling, redness, and tenderness with enlarged, tender lymph nodes and fever; no palpable cord
Pain associated with a series of lesions over several weeks			Raised, red, tender swellings recurring in crops; often malaise, joint pains, and fever

TABLE 14-2 — Chronic Insufficiency of Arteries and Veins

Chronic Arterial Insufficiency (Advanced)

Chronic Venous Insufficiency (Advanced)

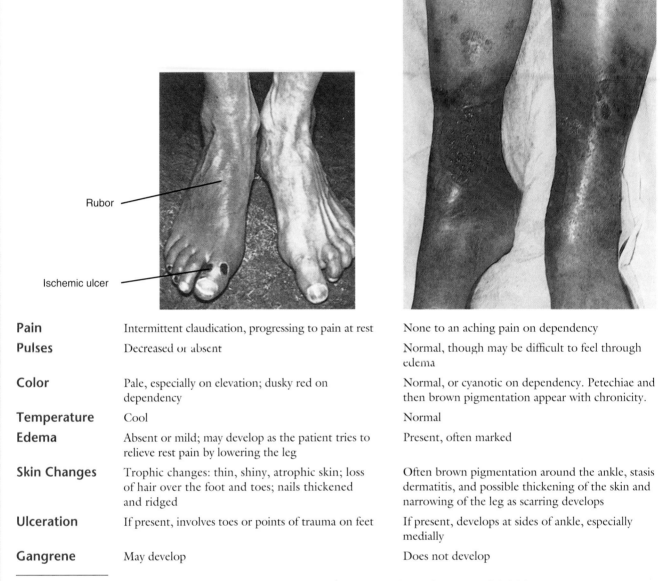

Rubor

Ischemic ulcer

	Chronic Arterial Insufficiency (Advanced)	Chronic Venous Insufficiency (Advanced)
Pain	Intermittent claudication, progressing to pain at rest	None to an aching pain on dependency
Pulses	Decreased or absent	Normal, though may be difficult to feel through edema
Color	Pale, especially on elevation; dusky red on dependency	Normal, or cyanotic on dependency. Petechiae and then brown pigmentation appear with chronicity.
Temperature	Cool	Normal
Edema	Absent or mild; may develop as the patient tries to relieve rest pain by lowering the leg	Present, often marked
Skin Changes	Trophic changes: thin, shiny, atrophic skin; loss of hair over the foot and toes; nails thickened and ridged	Often brown pigmentation around the ankle, stasis dermatitis, and possible thickening of the skin and narrowing of the leg as scarring develops
Ulceration	If present, involves toes or points of trauma on feet	If present, develops at sides of ankle, especially medially
Gangrene	May develop	Does not develop

(Sources of photos: *Arterial Insufficiency*—Kappert A, Winsor T. Diagnosis of Peripheral Vascular Disease. Philadelphia, FA Davis, 1972; *Venous Insufficiency*—Marks R. Skin Disease in Old Age. Philadelphia, JB Lippincott, 1987)

TABLE 14-3   **Common Ulcers of the Feet and Ankles**

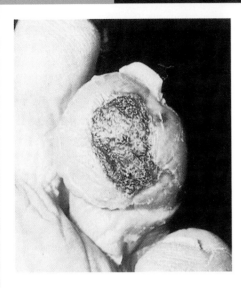

Arterial Insufficiency

This condition occurs in the toes, feet, or possibly in areas of trauma (e.g., the shins). Surrounding skin shows no callus or excess pigment, although it may be atrophic. Pain often is severe unless neuropathy masks it. Gangrene may be associated, along with decreased pulses, trophic changes, foot pallor on elevation, and dusky rubor on dependency.

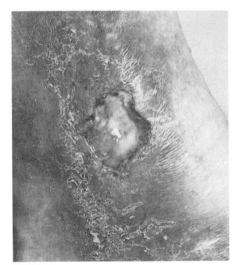

Chronic Venous Insufficiency

This condition appears on the inner or sometimes outer ankle. Surrounding skin is pigmented and sometimes fibrotic. Pain is not severe, with no gangrene. Associated signs include edema, pigmentation, stasis dermatitis, and possibly cyanosis of the foot on dependency.

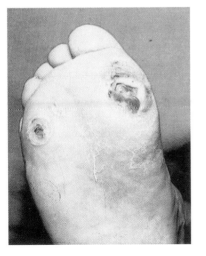

Neuropathic Ulcer

This condition develops in pressure points of areas with diminished sensation (e.g., with diabetic polyneuropathy). Surrounding skin is calloused. There is no pain, which sometimes results in the ulcer going unnoticed. In uncomplicated cases, there is no gangrene. Associated signs include decreased sensation and absent ankle jerks.

(Source of photos: Marks R: Skin Disease in Old Age. Philadelphia, JB Lippincott, 1987)

TABLE 14-4   **Some Peripheral Causes of Edema**

Approximately one third of total body water is extracellular, or outside the body's cells. Approximately 25% of extracellular fluid is plasma; the remainder is interstitial fluid. At the arteriolar end of the capillaries, *hydrostatic pressure* in the blood vessels and *colloid oncotic pressure* in the interstitium cause fluid to move into the tissues; at the venous end of the capillaries and in the lymphatics, hydrostatic pressure in the interstitium and the colloid oncotic pressure of plasma proteins cause fluid to return to the vascular compartment. Several clinical conditions disrupt this balance, resulting in *edema*, or a clinically evident accumulation of interstitial fluid. Not depicted below is capillary leak syndrome, in which protein leaks into the interstitial space, seen in burns, angioedema, snake bites, and allergic reactions.

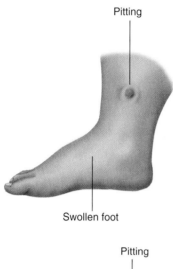

Pitting

Swollen foot

Pitting Edema

Edema is soft, bilateral, with pitting on pressure, and including the feet. There is no skin thickening, ulceration, or pigmentation. Pitting edema results when legs are dependent in cases of prolonged standing or sitting, which leads to increased hydrostatic pressure in the veins and capillaries; congestive heart failure leading to decreased cardiac output; increased hydrostatic pressure in the veins or capillaries; nephrotic syndrome, cirrhosis, or malnutrition leading to low albumin and decreased intravascular colloid oncotic pressure; and drug use.

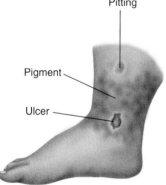

Pitting

Pigment

Ulcer

Advanced

Chronic Venous Insufficiency

Edema is soft, with pitting on pressure; it may progress to brawny (hard). Skin may be thickened, especially near the ankle. Ulceration, pigmentation, and edema in the feet are common, occasionally in a bilateral presentation. Examples include chronic obstruction or valvular incompetence of the deep veins.

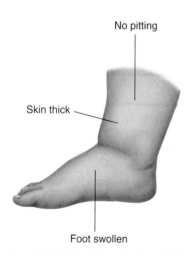

No pitting

Skin thick

Foot swollen

Lymphedema

Edema is soft in the early stages, then becomes indurated, hard, and nonpitting. Skin is markedly thickened; ulceration is rare. There is no pigmentation. Edema is found in the feet and toes, often bilaterally. Lymphedema develops in cases of lymph channels obstructed by tumor, fibrosis, or inflammation, as well as in cases of axillary node dissection and radiation.

The Musculoskeletal System

ASSESSING THE MUSCULOSKELETAL SYSTEM

GUIDE TO NEW ORGANIZATION OF THIS CHAPTER

Musculoskeletal complaints and disorders are leading causes of health care visits in clinical practice. Low back pain alone ranks fifth among reasons for clinical visits and is the second most common symptom of patients seeking care.[1] This chapter has been redesigned to help strengthen your approach and examination skills as you master assessment of common conditions of the joints.

This chapter presents the structure and function of the major joints and their connecting bony structures, muscles, and soft tissues. Because of the specialized nature of joint assessment, the organization of the chapter is a unique departure from other regional examination chapters in this book. Physical assessment of joint complaints requires both visualization and thorough knowledge of surface landmarks and underlying anatomy. To help students pair their knowledge of each joint's structure and function with its related methods of examination, the Anatomy and Physiology and Techniques of Examination for each joint *are combined*. The format of the chapter is as follows:

FORMAT OF THIS CHAPTER

- Structure and Function of Joints
- The Health History
- Health Promotion and Counseling
- Examination of Specific Joints: Anatomy and Physiology and Related Techniques of Examination. To promote a systematic approach to the examination of the musculoskeletal system, the sections on p. 498 follow a "head-to-toe" sequence, beginning with the jaw and joints of the upper extremities, then proceeding to the spine and hip and the joints of the lower extremities:

(continued)

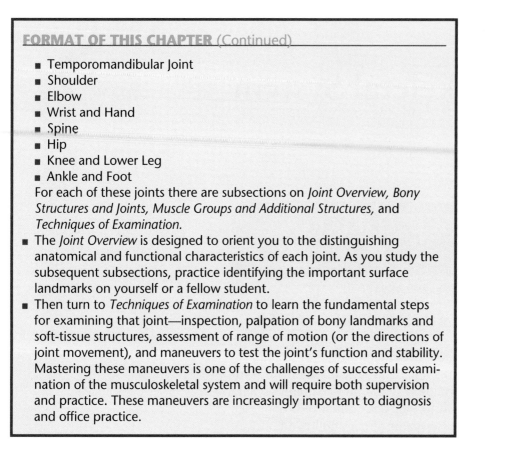

FORMAT OF THIS CHAPTER (Continued)

- Temporomandibular Joint
- Shoulder
- Elbow
- Wrist and Hand
- Spine
- Hip
- Knee and Lower Leg
- Ankle and Foot

For each of these joints there are subsections on *Joint Overview, Bony Structures and Joints, Muscle Groups and Additional Structures,* and *Techniques of Examination.*

- The *Joint Overview* is designed to orient you to the distinguishing anatomical and functional characteristics of each joint. As you study the subsequent subsections, practice identifying the important surface landmarks on yourself or a fellow student.

- Then turn to *Techniques of Examination* to learn the fundamental steps for examining that joint—inspection, palpation of bony landmarks and soft-tissue structures, assessment of range of motion (or the directions of joint movement), and maneuvers to test the joint's function and stability. Mastering these maneuvers is one of the challenges of successful examination of the musculoskeletal system and will require both supervision and practice. These maneuvers are increasingly important to diagnosis and office practice.

STRUCTURE AND FUNCTION OF JOINTS

It is helpful to begin by reviewing some anatomical terminology.

- *Articular structures* include the joint capsule and articular cartilage, the synovium and synovial fluid, intra-articular ligaments, and juxta-articular bone.

- *Nonarticular structures* include periarticular ligaments, tendons, bursae, muscle, fascia, bone, nerve, and overlying skin.

- *Ligaments* are ropelike bundles of collagen fibrils that connect bone to bone.

- *Tendons* are collagen fibers connecting muscle to bone. Another type of collagen matrix forms the *cartilage* that overlies bony surfaces.

- *Bursae* are pouches of synovial fluid that cushion the movement of tendons and muscles over bone or other joint structures.

To understand joint function, study the various types of joints and how they articulate, or interconnect, and the role of bursae in easing joint movement.

■ TYPES OF JOINTS

There are three primary types of joint articulation—synovial, cartilaginous, and fibrous—allowing varying degrees of joint movement.

■ Joints

Type of Joint	Extent of Movement	Example
Synovial	Freely movable	Knee, shoulder
Cartilaginous	Slightly movable	Vertebral bodies of the spine
Fibrous	Immovable	Skull sutures

Synovial Joints.   The bones do not touch each other, and the joint articulations are *freely moveable.* The bones are covered by *articular cartilage* and separated by a *synovial cavity* that cushions joint movement, as shown. A *synovial membrane* lines the synovial cavity and secretes a small amount of viscous lubricating fluid—the *synovial fluid.* The membrane is attached at the margins of the articular cartilage and pouched or folded to accommodate joint movement. Surrounding the synovial membrane is a fibrous *joint capsule,* which is strengthened by ligaments extending from bone to bone.

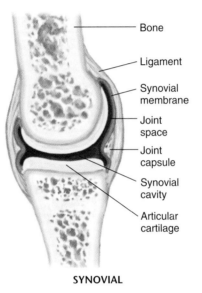

SYNOVIAL

Cartilaginous Joints.   These joints, such as those between vertebrae and the symphysis pubis, are *slightly moveable.* Fibrocartilaginous discs separate the bony surfaces. At the center of each disc is the *nucleus pulposus,* fibrocartilaginous material that serves as a cushion or shock absorber between bony surfaces.

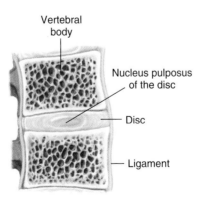

CARTILAGINOUS

Fibrous Joints.   In these joints, such as the sutures of the skull, intervening layers of fibrous tissue or cartilage hold the bones together. The bones are almost in direct contact, which allows *no appreciable movement.*

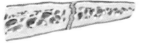

FIBROUS

◼ STRUCTURE OF SYNOVIAL JOINTS

As you learn about the examination of the musculoskeletal system, think about how the anatomy of the joint relates to its movement.

◼ Synovial Joints

Type of Joint	Articular Shape	Movement	Example
Spheroidal (ball and socket)	Convex surface in concave cavity	Wide-ranging flexion, extension, abduction, adduction, rotation, circumduction	Shoulder, hip
Hinge	Flat, planar	Motion in one plane; flexion, extension	Interphalangeal joints of hand and foot; elbow
Condylar	Convex or concave	Movement of two articulating surfaces not dissociable	Knee; temporomandibular joint

Many of the joints we examine are *synovial,* or movable, *joints.* The shape of the articulating surfaces of synovial joints determines the direction and extent of joint motion.

- *Spheroidal joints* have a ball-and-socket configuration—a rounded, convex surface articulating with a cuplike cavity, allowing a wide range of rotatory movement, as in the shoulder and hip.

- *Hinge joints* are flat, planar, or slightly curved, allowing only a gliding motion in a single plane, as in flexion and extension of the digits.

- In *condylar joints,* such as the knee, the articulating surfaces are convex or concave, termed condyles.

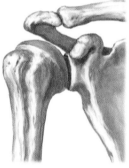

SPHEROIDAL JOINT (BALL AND SOCKET)

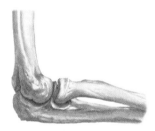

HINGE JOINT

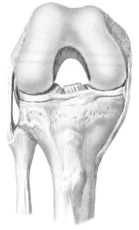

CONDYLAR JOINT

Bursae.   Easing joint action are *bursae,* roughly disc-shaped synovial sacs that allow adjacent muscles or muscles and tendons to glide over each other during movement. They lie between the skin and the convex surface of a bone or joint (as in the prepatellar bursa of the knee, p. 546) or in areas where tendons or muscles rub against bone, ligaments, or other tendons or muscles (as in the subacromial bursa of the shoulder, p. 514).

Knowledge of the underlying joint anatomy and movement will help you assess joints subjected to trauma. Your knowledge of the soft-tissue structures, ligaments, tendons, and bursae will help you evaluate the changes of aging, as well as arthritis.

THE HEALTH HISTORY

Common or Concerning Symptoms

- Low back pain
- Neck pain
- Monoarticular or polyarticular joint pain
- Inflammatory or infectious joint pain
- Joint pain with systemic features such as fever, chills, rash, anorexia, weight loss, weakness
- Joint pain with symptoms from other organ systems

Joint pain is one of the leading complaints of patients seeking health care. In addition to obtaining the seven features of any joint pain, three tips help guide your subsequent examination and diagnosis:

- Ask the patient to *"point to the pain."* This may save considerable time because the patient's verbal description may be imprecise.

- Clarify and record the *mechanism of injury,* particularly if there is a history of trauma.

- Determine whether the pain is *localized or diffuse, acute or chronic, inflammatory or noninflammatory.*

Low Back Pain.   You may wish to begin with "Any pains in your back?" because *backache* is the most common and widespread disorder of the musculoskeletal system. Using your usual interviewing style, get a clear picture of the problem, especially its location. Establish whether the pain

See Table 15-1, Low Back Pain, p. 560.

is on the midline, in the area of the vertebrae, or off the midline. If the pain radiates into the legs, ask about any associated numbness, tingling, or weakness.

Causes of *midline back pain* include musculoskeletal strain, vertebral collapse, disc herniation, or spinal cord metastases. *Pain off the midline* may arise from sacroiliitis, trochanteric bursitis, sciatica, or arthritis in the hips.

Neck Pain. Neck pain is also common, especially after trauma. Approach it in the same manner. For both neck and back pain, be especially alert for symptoms such as weakness, loss of sensation, or loss of bladder or bowel function.

See Table 15-2, Pains in the Neck, p. 561.

Motor or sensory deficits, loss of bladder or bowel function in spinal cord compression at S2–S4

Joint Pain. To pursue other musculoskeletal disorders, ask "Do you have any pains in your joints?"

Joint pain may be *localized, diffuse, or systemic.* Ask the patient to *point to the pain.* If the joint pain is localized and involves only one joint, it is *monoarticular.* Pain originating in the small joints of the hands and feet is more sharply localized than that from the larger joints. Pain from the hip joint is especially deceptive. Although it is typically felt in the groin or buttock, it is sometimes felt in the anterior thigh or partly or solely in the knee.

Pain in one joint suggests trauma, monoarticular arthritis, possible tendinitis, or bursitis. Hip pain near the greater trochanter suggests *trochanteric bursitis.*

More diffuse joint pain may be *polyarticular,* involving several joints. Ask whether the pain involves one joint or several joints. If polyarticular, what is the pattern of involvement . . . migrating from joint to joint or steadily spreading from one joint to multiple joint involvement? Is the involvement symmetric, affecting similar joints on both sides of the body?

Migratory pattern of spread in *rheumatic fever* or *gonococcal arthritis;* progressive additive pattern with symmetric involvement typically in *rheumatoid arthritis*

Note that joint pain may also be *nonarticular,* involving bones, muscles, and tissues around the joint such as the tendons, bursae, or even overlying skin. Generalized "aches and pains" are called *myalgias* if in muscles and *arthralgias* if there is pain but no evidence of arthritis.

Problems in tissues around joints include inflammation of bursae (*bursitis*), tendons (*tendinitis*), or tendon sheaths (*tenosynovitis*); also *sprains* from stretching or tearing of ligaments

Assess the chronicity, quality, and severity of the joint symptoms. *Timing* is especially important. Did the pain or discomfort develop rapidly over the course of a few hours or insidiously over weeks or even months? Has the pain progressed slowly or fluctuated, with periods of improvement and worsening? How long has the pain lasted? What is it like over the course of a day? . . . In the morning? . . . As the day wears on?

Severe pain of rapid onset in a swollen joint in the absence of trauma seen in *acute septic arthritis* or *gout.* In children consider *osteomyelitis* in bone contiguous to a joint.

If more rapid in onset, how did the pain arise? Was there an acute injury or overuse from repetitive motion of the same part of the body? If the pain comes from trauma, what was the *mechanism of injury* or the series of events that caused the joint pain? Further, what aggravates or relieves the pain? What are the effects of exercise, rest, and treatment?

See Table 15-3, Patterns of Pain In and Around the Joints, pp. 562–563.

Try to determine whether the problem is *inflammatory* or *noninflammatory*. Is there *tenderness, warmth,* or *redness*? These features are best assessed on examination, but patients can sometimes guide you to points of tenderness. Ask about systemic symptoms such as fever or chills.

Fever, chills, warmth, redness in *septic arthritis;* also consider *gout* or possible *rheumatic fever*

Additional symptoms can help you decide if the pain is *articular* in origin, such as *swelling, stiffness,* or *decreased range of motion.* Localize any *swelling* as accurately as possible. If *stiffness* is present, it may be difficult to assess because people use the term differently. In the context of musculoskeletal problems, stiffness refers to a perceived tightness or resistance to movement, the opposite of feeling limber. It is often associated with discomfort or pain. If the patient does not report stiffness spontaneously, ask about it and try to calculate its duration. Find out when the patient gets up in the morning and when the joints feel the most limber. Healthy people experience stiffness and muscular soreness after unusually strenuous muscular exertion; such symptoms tend to peak around the second day after exertion.

Pain, swelling, loss of active and passive motion, "locking," deformity in *articular joint pain;* loss of active but not passive motion, tenderness outside the joint, absence of deformity often in *nonarticular pain*

Stiffness and limited motion after inactivity, sometimes called *gelling,* in degenerative joint disease but usually lasts only a few minutes; stiffness lasting ≥ 30 minutes in rheumatoid arthritis and other inflammatory arthritides. Stiffness also with *fibromyalgia* and *polymyalgia rheumatica (PMR)*

To assess *limitations of motion,* ask about changes in level of activity because of problems with the involved joint. When relevant, inquire specifically about the patient's ability to walk, stand, lean over, sit, sit up, rise from a sitting position, climb, pinch, grasp, turn a page, open a door handle or jar, and care for bodily needs such as combing hair, brushing teeth, eating, dressing, and bathing.

Finally, some joint problems have *systemic* features such as fever, chills, rash, anorexia, weight loss, and weakness.

Generalized symptoms are common in *rheumatoid arthritis, systemic lupus erythematosus (SLE), PMR,* and other inflammatory arthritides. High fever and chills suggest an infectious cause.

Other joint disorders may be linked to *organ systems outside the musculoskeletal system.* Symptoms elsewhere in the body can give important clues to these conditions. Be alert to such symptoms as:

■ *Skin conditions*

A butterfly rash on the cheeks

Systemic lupus erythematosus

The scaly rash and pitted nails of psoriasis

Psoriatic arthritis

A few papules, pustules, or vesicles on reddened bases, located on the distal extremities

Gonococcal arthritis

An expanding erythematous patch early in an illness

Lyme disease

Hives

Serum sickness, drug reaction

Erosions or scale on the penis and crusted scaling papules on the soles and palms

Reiter's syndrome, which also includes arthritis, urethritis, and uveitis

The maculopapular rash of rubella

Arthritis of *rubella*

Clubbing of the fingernails (see p. 150)

Hypertrophic osteoarthropathy

- Red, burning, and itchy eyes (*conjunctivitis*)

Reiter's syndrome, Behçet's syndrome[2]

- Preceding *sore throat*

Acute rheumatic fever or *gonococcal arthritis*

- *Diarrhea, abdominal pain, cramping*

Arthritis with *ulcerative colitis, regional enteritis, scleroderma*

- Symptoms of *urethritis*

Reiter's syndrome or possibly *gonococcal arthritis*

- Mental status change, facial or other weakness, stiff neck

Lyme disease with central nervous system involvement

HEALTH PROMOTION AND COUNSELING

Important Topics for Health Promotion and Counseling

- Balanced nutrition, exercise, appropriate weight
- Lifting and the biomechanics of the back
- Risk factor screening and prevention of falls
- Prevention and treatment of osteoporosis

Maintaining the integrity of the musculoskeletal system brings many features of daily life into play—balanced nutrition, regular exercise, appropriate weight. As shown in this chapter, each joint has its specific vulnerabilities to trauma and wear. Care with lifting, avoidance of falls, household safety measures, and exercise help to protect and preserve well-functioning muscles and joints.

The habits of a healthy lifestyle convey direct benefit to the skeleton. Good nutrition supplies calcium needed for bone mineralization and bone density. Exercise appears to maintain and possibly increase bone mass, in addition to improving outlook and management of stress. Weight appropriate to height and body frame reduces excess mechanical wear on weight-bearing joints such as hips and knees. Regular physical activity has been shown to help prevent osteoporosis, obesity, cardiovascular disease, hypertension, and type 2 diabetes, and may reduce all-cause morbidity and lengthen life span.[3] Even modest activity, such as walking or bicycling 30 minutes each day, benefits health. Twenty to 30% of adult Americans report sedentary lifestyles and may benefit from routine counseling (although evidence linking counseling to behavior change is still preliminary).

One of the most vulnerable parts of the skeleton is the low back, especially L5–S1, where the sacral vertebrae make a sharp posterior angle. From 60% to 80% of the population experiences *low back pain* at least once in a lifetime.[4] Usually symptoms are short lived, but 30% to 60% of people experience recurrences when onset is work related. Exercises to strengthen the low back, especially in flexion and extension, and risk factor modification are often recommended (although studies have not demonstrated a consistent benefit for these interventions).[5] Alternatively, fitness exercises appear equally effective. Education on lifting strategies, posture, and the biomechanics of injury is prudent for patients doing repetitive lifting such as nurses, heavy-machinery operators, and construction workers. For occupational back pain, increasing graded physical activity and behavioral counseling show promise in improving functional status and return to work.[6] Such programs focus on improvements in function and do not make pain relief as a condition for resuming work.

Among elderly persons in the United States, *falls* exact a heavy toll in morbidity and mortality. They are the leading cause of nonfatal injuries and account for a dramatic rise in death rates after age 65, increasing from ~5/100,000 in the general population to ~10/100,000 between the ages of 65 and 74 to ~147/100,000 after age 85.[7] Approximately 5% of falls result in fractures, usually of the wrist, hip, pelvis, or femur. Risk factors are both cognitive and physiologic, including unstable gait, imbalanced posture, reduced strength, cognitive loss as in dementia, deficits in vision and proprioception, and osteoporosis. Poor lighting, stairs, chairs at awkward heights, slippery or irregular surfaces, and ill-fitting shoes are environmental dangers that can often be corrected. Clinicians should work with patients and families to help modify such risks whenever possible. Home health assessments have proven useful in reducing environmental hazards, as have exercise programs to improve patient balance and strength. (See also Chapter 20, The Older Adult, pp. 839–873.)

Finally, it is important to counsel selected postmenopausal women and some men about *osteoporosis,* a major threat to public health for 44 million Americans, of whom 68% are women.[8] One of every two women and one in four men older than 50 will have a fracture related to osteoporosis. The National Institutes of Health define osteoporosis as a "skeletal disorder characterized by compromised bone strength predisposing a person to an increased risk of fracture."[9] Bone strength reflects both *bone density* and *bone quality. Bone density* reflects the interaction between bone mass (highest in the second decade), new bone formation, and bone resorption. The World Health Organization uses bone density to define osteoporosis, namely bone density 2.5 standard deviations below the mean for young white adult women. A 10% drop in bone density, equivalent to one standard deviation, is associated with a 20% increase in risk for fracture. Bone *quality* refers to bone structure, including "architecture, turnover, damage accumulation (e.g., microfractures) and mineralization"—in osteoporosis the microarchitecture of the bone also deteriorates.[9]

The U.S. Preventive Services Task Force recommends routine bone density screening for women 65 years or older.[10] Additional risk factors for osteoporosis and guidelines for screening include low body weight, estrogen deficiency, white race (although risks for African Americans are also substantial), family history of osteoporosis, smoking, and prior vertebral fractures. Low body weight is the single best predictor of low bone density, and bone density at the femoral neck is the best predictor of subsequent hip fracture.[11,12] Fracture risk is also consistently linked to the risk factors for falls detailed above.

Several agents inhibit bone resorption—calcium, vitamin D, calcitonin, bisphosphonates, and estrogen—but consensus on several clinical management decisions has yet to emerge. Criteria are unclear for identifying those women at menopause at greatest risk for bone loss and fractures one to two decades later. In addition, guidelines for tailoring dosage of medication to level of bone density have yet to be determined. Estrogen therapy helps reduce occurrence of hip fracture, although there are no trials of estrogen therapy with hip fracture as a primary outcome.[9] Despite the benefits of estrogen on bone density, three recent trials have shown increased risk for stroke in women taking hormone replacement therapy and absence of added protection against coronary heart disease; the two trials of estrogen-progestin therapy also found increased risk for breast cancer.[13–15] The U.S. Preventive Services Task Force now recommends against the routine use of estrogen and progestin for the prevention of chronic conditions in postmenopausal women.[16] Learn the therapeutic uses of the bisphosphonates, calcitonin, and the newer selective estrogen-receptor modulators (SERMs).[17] At present, despite public interest, the natural estrogens, including the plant-derived phytoestrogens, have not been shown to reduce risk for fracture in humans.[9]

EXAMINATION OF SPECIFIC JOINTS: ANATOMY AND PHYSIOLOGY AND TECHNIQUES OF EXAMINATION

Important Areas of Examination for Each of the Major Joints

- Inspection for joint symmetry, alignment, bony deformities
- Inspection and palpation of surrounding tissues for skin changes, nodules, muscle atrophy, crepitus
- Range of motion and maneuvers to test joint function and stability, integrity of ligaments, tendons, bursae, especially if pain or trauma
- Assessment of inflammation or arthritis, especially swelling, warmth, tenderness, redness

---

During the interview you have evaluated the patient's ability to carry out normal activities of daily living. Keep these abilities in mind during your physical examination.

In your initial survey of the patient you have assessed general appearance, body proportions, and ease of movement. Now, as you apply techniques of examination to the musculoskeletal system, visualize the underlying anatomy and recall the key elements of the history—for example, the mechanism of injury if there is trauma, or the time course of symptoms and limitations in function in arthritis.

Your examination should be systematic. It should include inspection, palpation of bony landmarks as well as related joint and soft-tissue structures, assessment of range of motion, and *special maneuvers* to test specific movements. Recall that the anatomical shape of each joint determines its range of motion.[18]

TIPS FOR SUCCESSFUL EXAMINATION OF THE MUSCULOSKELETAL SYSTEM

- During inspection, look for *symmetry* of involvement. Is there a symmetric change in joints on both sides of the body, or is the change only in one or two joints?

Acute involvement of only one joint suggests trauma, septic arthritis, gout. *Rheumatoid arthritis* typically involves several joints, symmetrically distributed.[19–21]

Also note any *joint deformities* or *malalignment of bones*.

Dupuytren's contracture (p. 568), bowlegs or knock-knees

(continued)

TIPS FOR SUCCESSFUL EXAMINATION OF THE MUSCULOSKELETAL SYSTEM (Continued)

- Use inspection and palpation to assess the *surrounding tissues,* noting skin changes, subcutaneous nodules, and muscle atrophy. Note any *crepitus,* an audible or palpable crunching during movement of tendons or ligaments over bone. This may occur in normal joints but is more significant when associated with symptoms or signs.

- Testing range of motion and maneuvers (described for each joint) may demonstrate *limitations in range of motion* or increased mobility and joint instability from excess mobility of joint ligaments, called *ligamentous laxity.*

- Finally, testing *muscle strength* may aid in the assessment of joint function (for these techniques, see Chap. 17).

Be especially alert to *signs of inflammation and arthritis.*

- *Swelling.* Palpable swelling may involve: (1) the synovial membrane, which can feel boggy or doughy; (2) effusion from excess synovial fluid within the joint space; or (3) soft-tissue structures such as bursae, tendons, and tendon sheaths.

- *Warmth.* Use the backs of your fingers to compare the involved joint with its unaffected contralateral joint, or with nearby tissues if both joints are involved.

- *Tenderness.* Try to identify the specific anatomical structure that is tender. Trauma may also cause tenderness.

- *Redness.* Redness of the overlying skin is the *least* common sign of inflammation near the joints.

Subcutaneous nodules in rheumatoid arthritis or rheumatic fever; effusions in trauma; crepitus over inflamed joints, in osteoarthritis, or inflamed tendon sheaths

Decreased range of motion in arthritis, inflammation of tissues around a joint, fibrosis in or around a joint, or bony fixation (*ankylosis*). Ligamentous laxity of the ACL in knee trauma

Muscle atrophy or weakness in *rheumatoid arthritis*

Palpable bogginess or doughiness of the synovial membrane indicates *synovitis,* which is often accompanied by effusion. Palpable joint fluid in effusion, tenderness over the tendon sheaths in *tendinitis*

Arthritis, tendinitis, bursitis, osteomyelitis

Tenderness and warmth over a thickened synovium may suggest arthritis or infection.

Redness over a tender joint suggests septic or gouty arthritis, or possibly *rheumatoid arthritis.*

If the person has painful joints, move the person gently. Patients may move more comfortably by themselves. Let them show you how they manage. If joint trauma is present, consider an x-ray before attempting movement.

The detail needed for examining the musculoskeletal system may vary widely. This section presents examination techniques for both comprehensive and targeted assessment of joint function. Patients with extensive or severe musculoskeletal problems will require more time. A briefer survey for those without musculoskeletal symptoms is outlined in Chapter 4 (see p. 105).

■ TEMPOROMANDIBULAR JOINT

OVERVIEW, BONY STRUCTURES, AND JOINTS

The temporomandibular joint is the most active joint in the body, opening and closing up to 2000 times a day. It is formed by the fossa and articular tubercle of the temporal bone and the condyle of the mandible. It lies midway between the external acoustic meatus and the zygomatic arch.

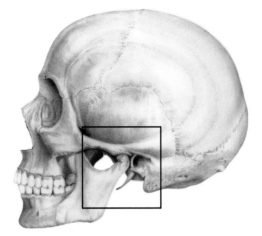

A fibrocartilaginous disc cushions the action of the condyle of the mandible against the synovial membrane and capsule of the articulating surfaces of the temporal bone. Hence, it is a condylar synovial joint.

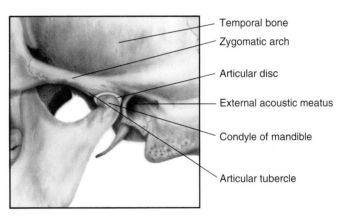

Temporal bone

Zygomatic arch

Articular disc

External acoustic meatus

Condyle of mandible

Articular tubercle

MUSCLE GROUPS AND ADDITIONAL STRUCTURES

The principal muscles opening the mouth are the *external pterygoids.* Closing the mouth are the muscles innervated by Cranial Nerve V, the trigeminal nerve (see p. 613)—the *masseter,* the *temporalis,* and the *internal pterygoids.*

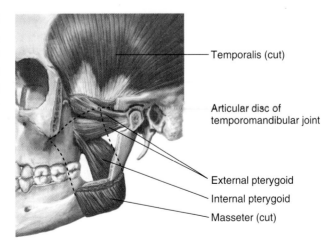

Temporalis (cut)

Articular disc of temporomandibular joint

External pterygoid

Internal pterygoid

Masseter (cut)

TECHNIQUES OF EXAMINATION

INSPECTION AND PALPATION

Inspect the face for symmetry. Inspect the TMJ for swelling or redness. Swelling may appear as a rounded bulge approximately ½ cm anterior to the external auditory meatus.

Facial asymmetry associated with *TMJ syndrome,* or unilateral chronic pain with chewing, jaw clenching, or teeth grinding, often associated with stress (may also present as headache)

Swelling, tenderness, and decreased range of motion in inflammation or arthritis

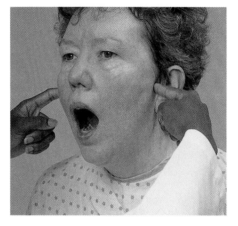

To locate and palpate the joint, place the tips of your index fingers just in front of the tragus of each ear and ask the patient to open his or her mouth. The fingertips should drop into the joint spaces as the mouth opens. Check for smooth range of motion; note any swelling or tenderness. Snapping or clicking may be felt or heard in normal people.

Dislocation of the TMJ may be seen in trauma.

Palpable crepitus or clicking in poor occlusion, meniscus injury, or synovial swelling from trauma.

Also palpate the muscles of mastication:

■ The *masseters* externally at the angle of the mandible

■ The *temporal muscles,* externally during clenching and relaxation of the jaw

■ The *pterygoid muscles,* internally between the tonsillar pillars at the mandible

Pain and tenderness on palpation in *TMJ syndrome.*

RANGE OF MOTION AND MANEUVERS

The temporomandibular joint has glide and hinge motions in its upper and lower portions, respectively. Grinding or chewing consists primarily of gliding movements in the upper compartments.

Range of motion is three-fold: ask the patient to demonstrate opening and closing, protrusion and retraction (by jutting the jaw forward), and lateral, or side-to-side, motion. Normally as the mouth is opened wide, three fingers can be inserted between incisors. During normal protrusion of the jaw, the bottom teeth can be placed in front of the upper teeth.

THE SHOULDER

OVERVIEW

The shoulder is distinguished by wide-ranging movement in all directions. The humerus virtually dangles from the scapula, suspended from the shallow glenoid fossa by the joint capsule, the intra-articular capsular ligaments, the glenoid labrum, and a meshwork of muscles and tendons. The shoulder derives its mobility from a complex interconnected structure of four joints, three large bones, and three principal muscle groups, often referred to as the *shoulder girdle*. The clavicle and acromion stabilize the shoulder girdle, allowing the humerus to swing out and away from the body, giving the shoulder its remarkable range of motion.

BONY STRUCTURES

The bony structures of the shoulder include the humerus, the clavicle, and the scapula. The scapula is anchored to the axial skeleton only by the sternoclavicular joint and inserting muscles, often called the *scapulothoracic articulation* because it is not a true joint.

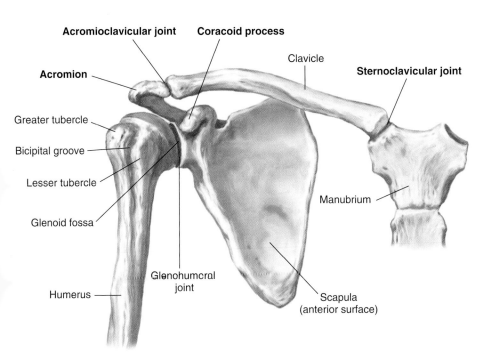

Identify the manubrium, the sternoclavicular joint, and the clavicle. With your fingers, trace the clavicle laterally. Now, from behind, follow the bony spine of the scapula laterally and upward until it becomes the *acromion*, the summit of the shoulder. Its upper surface is rough and slightly convex.

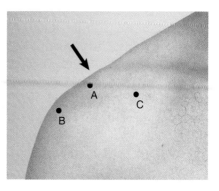

■ Identify the anterior tip of the acromion (**A**) and mark it with ink. With your index finger on top of the acromion, just behind its tip, press medially to find the slightly elevated ridge that marks the distal end of the clavicle at the *acromioclavicular joint* (shown by the arrow).

■ Move your finger laterally and down a short step to the next bony prominence, the *greater tubercle of the humerus* (**B**). Mark this with ink.

■ Now sweep your finger medially until you feel a large bony prominence, the *coracoid process* of the scapula (**C**). Mark this also.

These three points—the tip of the acromion, the greater tubercle of the humerus, and the coracoid process—orient you to the anatomy of the shoulder.

JOINTS

Three different joints articulate at the shoulder:

■ The *glenohumeral joint.* In this joint, the head of the humerus articulates with the shallow glenoid fossa of the scapula. This joint is deeply situated and not normally palpable. It is a ball-and-socket joint, allowing the arm its wide arc of movement—flexion, extension, abduction (movement away from the trunk), adduction (movement toward the trunk), rotation, and circumduction.

■ The *sternoclavicular joint.* The convex medial end of the clavicle articulates with the concave hollow in the upper sternum.

■ The *acromioclavicular joint.* The lateral end of the clavicle articulates with the acromion process of the scapula.

MUSCLE GROUPS

Three groups of muscles attach at the shoulder:

The Scapulohumeral Group. This group extends from the scapula to the humerus and includes the muscles inserting directly on the humerus, known as *"SITS muscles"* of the *rotator cuff*:

- *Supraspinatus*—runs above the glenohumeral joint; inserts on the greater tubercle

- *Infraspinatus* and *teres minor*—cross the glenohumeral joint posteriorly; insert on the greater tubercle

- *Subscapularis* (not illustrated)—originates on the anterior surface of the scapula and crosses the joint anteriorly; inserts on the lesser tubercle.

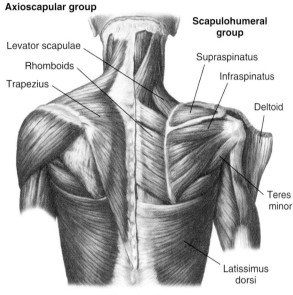

Axioscapular group

Scapulohumeral group

Levator scapulae
Rhomboids
Trapezius
Supraspinatus
Infraspinatus
Deltoid
Teres minor
Latissimus dorsi

Posterior view

Axioscapular group (pulls shoulder backward)
Scapulohumeral group (rotates shoulder laterally; includes rotator cuff)

The scapulohumeral group rotates the shoulder laterally (the *rotator cuff*) and depresses and rotates the head of the humerus. (See pp. 564–565 for discussion of rotator cuff injuries.)

The Axioscapular Group. This group attaches the trunk to the scapula and includes the trapezius, rhomboids, serratus anterior, and levator scapulae. These muscles rotate the scapula.

The Axiohumeral Group. This group attaches the trunk to the humerus and includes the pectoralis major and minor and the latissimus dorsi. These muscles produce internal rotation of the shoulder.

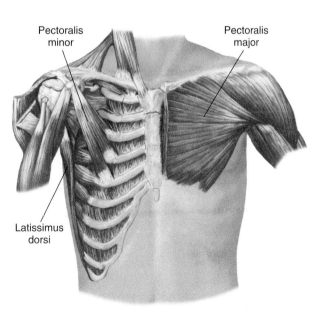

Pectoralis minor
Pectoralis major
Latissimus dorsi

Anterior view

Axiohumeral group (rotates shoulder internally)

The biceps and triceps, which connect the scapula to the bones of the forearm, are also involved in shoulder movement, particularly abduction.

ADDITIONAL STRUCTURES

Also important to shoulder movement are the *articular capsule and bursae*. Surrounding the glenohumeral joint is a fibrous articular capsule formed by the tendon insertions of the rotator cuff and other capsular muscles. The loose fit of the capsule allows the shoulder bones to separate, and contributes to the shoulder's wide range of movement. The capsule is lined by a synovial membrane with two outpouchings—the *subscapular bursa* and the *synovial sheath of the tendon of the long head of the biceps*.

To locate the biceps tendon, rotate your arm externally and find the tendinous cord that runs just medial to the greater tubercle. Roll it under your fingers. This is the tendon of the long head of the biceps. It runs in the bicipital groove between the greater and lesser tubercles.

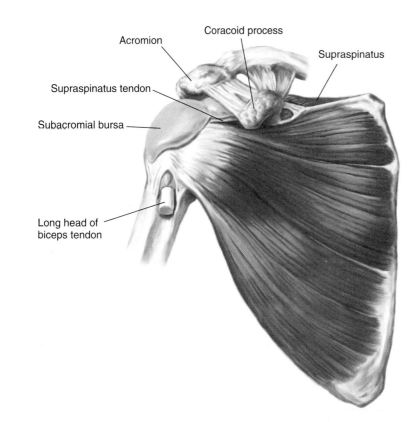

The principal bursa of the shoulder is the *subacromial bursa,* positioned between the acromion and the head of the humerus and overlying the supraspinatus tendon. Abduction of the shoulder compresses this bursa. Normally, the supraspinatus tendon and the subacromial bursa are not palpable. However, if the bursal surfaces are inflamed (subacromial bursitis), there may be tenderness just below the tip of the acromion, pain with abduction and rotation, and loss of smooth movement.

TECHNIQUES OF EXAMINATION

INSPECTION

Observe the shoulder and shoulder girdle anteriorly, and inspect the scapulae and related muscles posteriorly. Note any swelling, deformity, muscle atrophy or fasciculations (fine tremors of the muscles), or abnormal positioning.

Scoliosis may cause elevation of one shoulder. With *anterior dislocation of the shoulder*, the rounded lateral aspect of the shoulder appears flattened.[22,23]

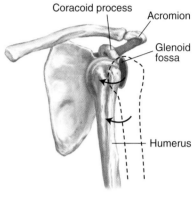

**ANTERIOR DISLOCATION
OF HUMERUS**

With posterior dislocation of the shoulder (relatively rare), the anterior aspect of the shoulder is flattened, and the humeral head appears more prominent.

Look for swelling of the joint capsule anteriorly or a bulge in the subacromial bursa under the deltoid muscle. Survey the entire upper extremity for color change, skin alteration, or unusual bony contours.

A significant amount of synovial fluid is needed before the joint capsule appears distended.

PALPATION

If there is a history of shoulder pain, ask the patient to point to the painful area. The location of the pain provides clues to its origin:

See Table 15-4, Painful Shoulders (pp. 564–565).

■ Top of the shoulder, radiating toward the neck—acromioclavicular joint

■ Lateral aspect of the shoulder, radiating toward the deltoid insertion—rotator cuff

■ Anterior shoulder—bicipital tendon

Now identify the bony landmarks of the shoulder and then palpate the area of pain. Locate the *acromion process* and press medially to locate the distal tip of the clavicle at the *acromioclavicular joint*. Palpate laterally and down a short step to the greater tubercle of the humerus, and then press medially to locate the *coracoid process* of the scapula. Next palpate the painful area and identify the structures involved.

RANGE OF MOTION AND MANEUVERS

The six motions of the shoulder girdle are flexion, extension, abduction, adduction, and internal and external rotation.

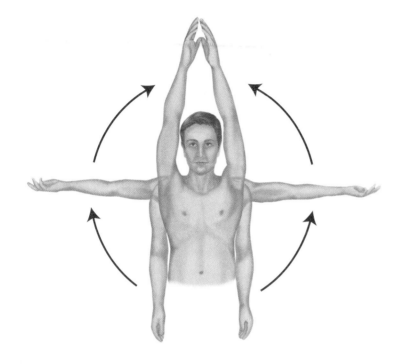

Watch for smooth, fluid movement as you stand in front of the patient and ask the patient to:

(1) raise (*abduct*) the arms to shoulder level (90°) with palms facing down (tests pure glenohumeral motion)

(2) raise the arms to a vertical position above the head with the palms facing each other (tests scapulothoracic motion for 60°, and combined glenohumeral and scapulothoracic motion during adduction for the final 30°

(3) place both hands behind the neck, with elbows out to the side (tests *external rotation* and *abduction*) and

(4) place both hands behind the small of the back (tests *internal rotation* and *adduction*). (Placing your hand on the shoulder during these movements allows you to detect any crepitus.)

Crepitus during movement suggests osteoarthritis.

The examination of the shoulder often requires selective evaluation of the acromioclavicular joint, the subacromial and subdeltoid bursae, the rotator cuff, the bicipital groove and tendon, and the articular capsule and synovial membrane of the glenohumeral joint.[24] Techniques for examining these structures are described on following pages.

■ Techniques for Examining the Shoulder[25]

Structure	Technique	
Acromioclavicular Joint	Palpate and compare both joints for swelling or tenderness. Adduct the patient's arm across the chest, sometimes called the *"crossover test."*	
Subacromial and Subdeltoid Bursae	Passively extend the shoulder by lifting the elbow posteriorly. This exposes the bursa anterior to the acromion. Palpate carefully over the sub-acromial and subdeltoid bursae.	

Localized tenderness or pain with adduction suggests inflammation or arthritis of the acromioclavicular joint. See Table 15-4, Painful Shoulders (pp. 564–565).

Localized tenderness arises from *subacromial* or *subdeltoid bursitis,* degenerative changes or calcific deposits in the rotator cuff.

Swelling suggests a *bursal tear* with communication into the articular cavity.

Overall Shoulder Rotation

Ask the patient to touch the opposite scapula using the two motions shown below (the Apley scratch test).

Difficulty with these motions suggests rotator cuff disorder.

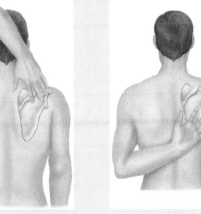

Tests abduction and external rotation.

Tests adduction and internal rotation.

(continued)

■ *Techniques for Examining the Shoulder*[25] *(Continued)*

Structure	Technique
Rotator Cuff	With the patient's arm hanging at the side, palpate the three "SITS" muscles that insert on the greater tuberosity of the humerus. (The fourth muscle, the subscapularis, inserts anteriorly and is not palpable.) ■ **S**upraspinatus—directly under the acromion ■ **I**nfraspinatus—posterior to supraspinatus ■ **T**eres minor—posterior and inferior to the supraspinatus Passively extend the shoulder by lifting the elbow posteriorly. This maneuver also moves the rotator cuff out from under the acromion. Palpate the rounded SITS muscle insertions near the greater tuberosity of the humerus. Subacromial bursa Rotator cuff

Tenderness over the "SITS" muscle insertions and inability to lift the arm above shoulder level are seen in sprains, tears, and tendon rupture of the rotator cuff, most commonly the *supraspinatus*. See Table 15-4, Painful Shoulders (pp. 564–565).

	Check the *"drop-arm" sign*. Ask the patient to fully abduct the arm to shoulder level (or up to 90°) and lower it slowly. (Note that abduction above shoulder level, from 90° to 120°, reflects action of the deltoid muscle.)
Bicipital Groove and Tendon	Rotate the arm and forearm externally and locate the biceps muscle distally near the elbow. Track the muscle and its tendon proximally into the bicipital groove along the anterior aspect of the humerus. As you check for tendon tenderness, rolling the tendon under the fingertips may be helpful. **PALPATION OF THE BICIPITAL GROOVE AND TENDON**

If the patient is unable to hold the arm fully abducted at shoulder level, the "drop arm" test is positive, indicating a tear in the rotator cuff.

See also Bicipital Tendinitis in Table 15-4 Painful Shoulders (pp. 564–565).

Finally, hold the patient's elbow against the body with the forearm flexed at a right angle. Ask the patient to supinate the forearm against resistance.

(continued)

Tenderness or pain against resistance occurs with tenosynovitis of the bicipital tendon sheath, tendinitis, or biceps tendon rupture.

■ *Techniques for Examining the Shoulder[25] (Continued)*

Structure	Technique
Articular Capsule, Synovial Membrane, and Glenohumeral Joint	The fibrous articular capsule and the broad flat tendons of the rotator cuff are so closely associated that they must be examined simultaneously. Swelling in the capsule and synovial membrane is often best detected by looking down on the shoulder from above. Palpate the capsule and synovial membrane beneath the anterior and posterior acromion.

Tenderness and effusion suggest synovitis of the glenohumeral joint. If the margins of the capsule and synovial membrane are palpable, a moderate to large effusion is present. Minimal degrees of synovitis at the glenohumeral joint cannot be detected on palpation.

The following maneuvers test individual muscles of the shoulder girdle and help localize pain. Note that medial rotation against resistance also tests the pectoralis major, teres major, and latissimus dorsi. Additional evaluation of muscle strength, sensation over the neck, shoulder, and arm, and upper extremity reflexes is often warranted to complete your assessment (see pp. 618–621).

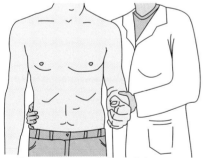

Supraspinatus: Patient abducts against resistance.

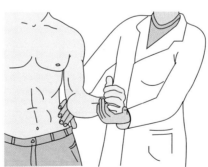

Subscapularis: Patient rotates forearm medially against resistance

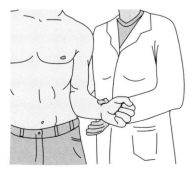

Infraspinatus, teres minor: Patient rotates forearm laterally against resistance.

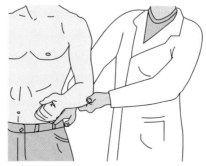

Thoracohumeral group: Patient adducts forearm against resistance.

THE ELBOW

OVERVIEW, BONY STRUCTURES, AND JOINTS

The elbow helps position the hand in space and stabilizes the lever action of the forearm. The elbow joint is formed by the humerus and the two bones of the forearm, the radius, and the ulna. Identify the medial and lateral epi condyles of the humerus and the olecranon process of the ulna.

These bones have three articulations: the *humeroulnar joint*, the *radiohumeral joint*, and the *radioulnar joint*. All three share a large common articular cavity and an extensive synovial lining.

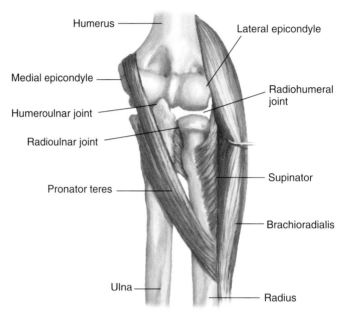

MUSCLE GROUPS AND ADDITIONAL STRUCTURES

Muscles traversing the elbow include the *biceps* and *brachioradialis* (flexion), the *triceps* (extension), the *pronator teres* (pronation), and the *supinator* (supination).

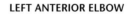

LEFT ANTERIOR ELBOW

Note the location of the *olecranon bursa* between the olecranon process and the skin. The bursa is not normally palpable but swells and becomes tender when inflamed. The *ulnar nerve* runs posteriorly in the ulnar groove between the medial epicondyle and the olecranon process. On the ventral forearm, the *median nerve* is just medial to the brachial artery.

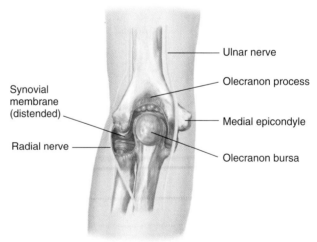

LEFT POSTERIOR ELBOW

TECHNIQUES OF EXAMINATION

INSPECTION AND PALPATION

Support the patient's forearm with your opposite hand so the elbow is flexed to about 70°. Identify the medial and lateral epicondyles and the olecranon process of the ulna. Inspect the contours of the elbow, including the extensor surface of the ulna and the olecranon process. Note any nodules or swelling.

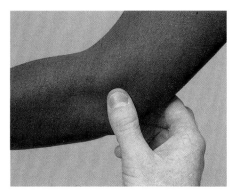

See Table 15-5, Swollen or Tender Elbows (p. 566).

Swelling over the olecranon process in olecranon bursitis; inflammation or synovial fluid in arthritis.

Palpate the olecranon process and press on the epicondyles for tenderness. Note any displacement of the olecranon.

Tenderness in *lateral epicondylitis* (tennis elbow) and less commonly in *medial epicondylitis* (pitcher's or golfer's elbow)

The olecranon is displaced posteriorly in *posterior dislocation of the elbow* and *supracondylar fracture.*

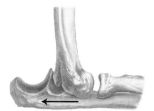

**POSTERIOR DISLOCATION
OF THE ELBOW**

**SUPRACONDYLAR FRACTURE
OF THE ELBOW**

Palpate the grooves between the epicondyles and the olecranon, noting any tenderness, swelling, or thickening. The synovium is most accessible to examination between the olecranon and the epicondyles. (Normally neither synovium nor bursa is palpable.) The sensitive ulnar nerve can be felt posteriorly between the olecranon process and the medial epicondyle.

RANGE OF MOTION AND MANEUVERS

Range of motion includes *flexion* and *extension* at the elbow and *pronation* and *supination* of the forearm. To test flexion and extension, ask the patient to bend and straighten the elbow. Elbow extension reduces intra-articular volume.

Full elbow extension makes intra-articular process, effusion, or hemarthrosis unlikely.

With the patient's arms at the sides and elbows flexed to minimize shoulder movement, ask the patient to *supinate*, or turn up the palms, and to *pronate*, or turn the palms down.

THE WRIST AND HANDS

OVERVIEW

The wrist and hands form a complex unit of small, highly active joints used almost continuously during waking hours. There is little protection from overlying soft tissue, increasing vulnerability to trauma and disability.

BONY STRUCTURES

The wrist includes the distal radius and ulna and eight small carpal bones. At the wrist, identify the bony tips of the radius and the ulna.

The carpal bones lie distal to the wrist joint within each hand. Identify the carpal bones, each of the five meta-carpals, and the proximal, middle, and distal phalanges. Note that the thumb lacks a middle phalanx.

JOINTS

The numerous joints of the wrist and hand lend unusual dexterity to the hands.

■ *Wrist joints.* The wrist joints include the *radiocarpal* or *wrist joint*, the *distal radioulnar joint*, and the *intercarpal joints.* The joint capsule, articular disc, and syno-vial membrane of the wrist join the radius to the ulna and to the proximal carpal bones. On the dor-sum of the wrist, locate the groove of the *radiocarpal joint*, which provides most of the flexion and extension at the wrist because the ulna does not articulate directly with the carpal bones.

■ *Hand joints.* The joints of the hand include the *metacarpopha-langeal joints* (MCPs), the *proxi-mal interphalangeal joints* (PIPs), and the *distal interphalangeal joints* (DIPs). Flex the hand and find the groove marking the MCP joint of each finger. It is distal to the knuckle and is best felt on either side of the extensor tendon.

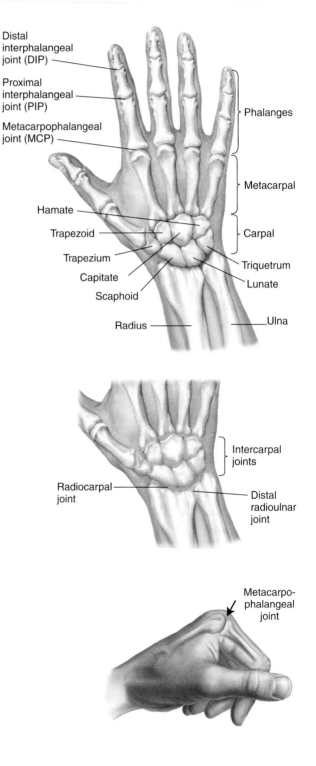

522

MUSCLE GROUPS

Wrist flexion arises from the two carpal muscles, located on the radial and ulnar surfaces. Two radial and one ulnar muscle provide wrist extension. Supination and pronation result from muscle contraction in the forearm.

The thumb is powered by three muscles that form the thenar eminence and provide flexion, abduction, and opposition. The muscles of extension are at the base of the thumb along the radial margin. Movement in the digits depends on action of the flexor and extensor tendons of muscles in the forearm and wrist.

The intrinsic muscles of the hand attaching to the metacarpal bones are involved in flexion (*lumbricals*), abduction (*dorsal interossei*), and adduction (*palmar interossei*) of the fingers.

ADDITIONAL STRUCTURES

Soft-tissue structures, especially tendons and tendon sheaths, are extremely important in the wrist and hand. Six extensor tendons and two flexor tendons pass across the wrist and hand to insert on the fingers. Through much of their course these tendons travel in tunnel-like sheaths, generally palpable only when swollen or inflamed.

Be familiar with the structures in the *carpal tunnel,* a channel beneath the palmar surface of the wrist and proximal hand. The canal contains the sheath and flexor tendons of the forearm muscles and the *median nerve.*

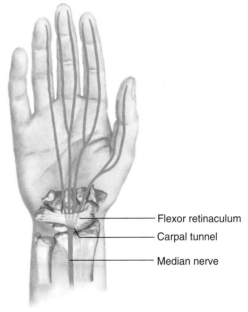

Holding the tendons and tendon sheath in place is a transverse ligament, the *flexor retinaculum.* The median nerve lies between the flexor retinaculum and the tendon sheath. It provides sensation to the palm and the palmar surface of most of the thumb, the second and third digits, and half of the fourth digit. It also innervates the thumb muscles of flexion, abduction, and opposition.

— Flexor retinaculum
— Carpal tunnel
— Median nerve

TECHNIQUES OF EXAMINATION

INSPECTION

Observe the position of the hands in motion to see if movements are smooth and natural. At rest, the fingers should be slightly flexed and aligned almost in parallel.

Guarded movement suggests injury. Poor finger alignment is seen in flexor tendon damage.

Inspect the palmar and dorsal surfaces of the wrist and hand carefully for swelling over the joints.

Diffuse swelling in arthritis or infection; local swelling from cystic ganglion. See Table 15 6, Arthritis in the Hands (p. 567) and Table 15-7, Swellings and Deformities of the Hands (p. 568).

Note any deformities of the wrist, hand, or finger bones, as well as any angulation from radial or ulnar deviation.

In *osteoarthritis,* Heberden's nodes at the DIP joints, Bouchard's nodes at the PIP joints. In *rheumatoid arthritis,* symmetric deformity in the PIP, MCP, and wrist joints, with ulnar deviation

Observe the contours of the palm, namely the thenar and hypothenar eminences.

Thenar atrophy in median nerve compression from *carpal tunnel syndrome*; hypothenar atrophy in *ulnar nerve compression.*

Note any thickening of the flexor tendons or flexion contractures in the fingers.

Flexion contractures in the ring, 5th, and 3rd fingers, or *Dupuytren's contractures,* arise from thickening of the palmar fascia (see p. 568).

PALPATION

At the wrist, palpate the distal radius and ulna on the lateral and medial surfaces. Palpate the groove of each wrist joint with your thumbs on the dorsum of the wrist, your fingers beneath it. Note any swelling, bogginess, or tenderness.

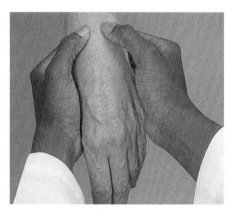

Tenderness over the distal radius in *Colles' fracture.* Any tenderness or bony step-offs are suspicious for fracture.

Swelling and/or tenderness suggests *rheumatoid arthritis* if bilateral and of several weeks' duration.

Palpate the radial styloid bone and the *anatomical snuffbox,* a hollowed depression just distal to the radial styloid process formed by the abductor and extensor muscles of the thumb. The "snuffbox" becomes more visible with lateral extension of the thumb away from the hand.

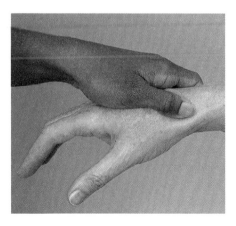

Tenderness over the extensor and abductor tendons of the thumb at the radial styloid in *de Quervain's tenosynovitis* and *gonococcal tenosynovitis.* See Table 15-8, Tendon Sheath and Palmar Space Infections; Felons (p. 569).

Tenderness over the "snuffbox" in *scaphoid fracture,* the most common injury of the carpal bones. Poor blood supply puts the scaphoid bone at risk for *avascular necrosis.*

Palpate the eight carpal bones lying distal to the wrist joint, and then each of the five metacarpals and the proximal, middle, and distal phalanges.

Palpate any other area where you suspect an abnormality.

Compress the MCP joints by squeezing the hand from each side between the thumb and fingers. Alternatively, use your thumb to palpate each MCP joint just distal to and on each side of the knuckle as your index finger feels the head of the metacarpal in the palm. Note any swelling, bogginess, or tenderness.

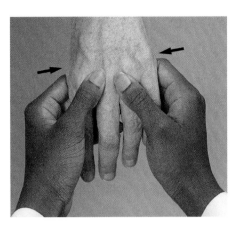

Synovitis in the MCPs is painful with this pressure—a point to remember when shaking hands.

The MCPs are often boggy or tender in *rheumatoid arthritis* (but rarely involved in osteoarthritis). Pain with compression also in *posttraumatic arthritis*.

Now examine the fingers and thumb. Palpate the medial and lateral aspects of each PIP joint between your thumb and index finger, again checking for swelling, bogginess, bony enlargement, or tenderness.

PIP changes seen in *rheumatoid arthritis*, Bouchard's nodes in *osteoarthritis*. Pain at the base of the thumb in first *carpometacarpal arthritis*.

Hard dorsolateral nodules on the DIP joints, or *Heberden's nodes*, common in osteoarthritis; DIP joint involvement in *psoriatic arthritis*

Using the same techniques, examine the DIP joints.

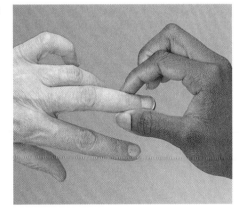

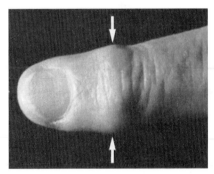

In any area of swelling or inflammation, palpate along the tendons inserting on the thumb and fingers.

Tenderness and swelling in *tenosynovitis,* or inflammation of the tendon sheaths. *De Quervain's tenosynovitis* over the extensor and abductor tendons of the thumb as they cross the radial styloid. See Table 15-8, Tendon Sheath and Palmar Space Infections; Felons (p. 569).

RANGE OF MOTION AND MANEUVERS

Now assess range of motion for the wrists, fingers, and thumbs.

Wrists.   At the *wrist*, test flexion, extension, and ulnar and radial deviation.

- *Flexion.* With the patient's forearm stabilized, place the wrist in extension and place your fingertips in the patient's palm. Ask the patient to flex the wrist against gravity, then against graded resistance.

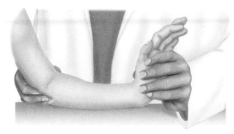

FLEXION

- *Extension.* With the patient's forearm stabilized, place the wrist in flexion and put your hand on the patient's dorsal metacarpals. Ask the patient to extend the wrist against gravity, then against graded resistance.

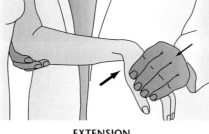

EXTENSION

- *Ulnar and radial deviation.* With palms down, ask the patient to move the wrists laterally and medially.

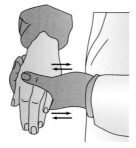

**ULNAR AND RADIAL
DEVIATION**

Make an approximate test of *grip strength* by asking the patient to grasp your second and third finger. This maneuver tests function of the intrinsic muscles and joints of the hand, the joints of the wrist, and the flexor tendons and muscles of the forearm. (Use a dynometer for more accurate measurements.)

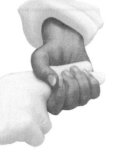

GRIP STRENGTH

Conditions that impair range of motion include *arthritis, tenosynovitis, Dupuytren's contracture.* See Table 15-7, Swelling and Deformities of the Hands (p. 568).

Wrist pain and grip weakness in *de Quervain's tenosynovitis.* Decreased grip strength in *arthritis, carpal tunnel syndrome,* epicondylitis, and *cervical radiculopathy.*[26]

Fingers. Test flexion, extension, abduction, and adduction of the *fingers:*

■ *Flexion and extension.* Ask the patient to make a tight fist with each hand, thumb across the knuckles, and then extend and spread the fingers. The fingers should close and open smoothly and easily. At the MCPs, the fingers may extend beyond the neutral position. This maneuver also tests overall thumb function. Also test flexion and extension at the PIP and DIP joints.

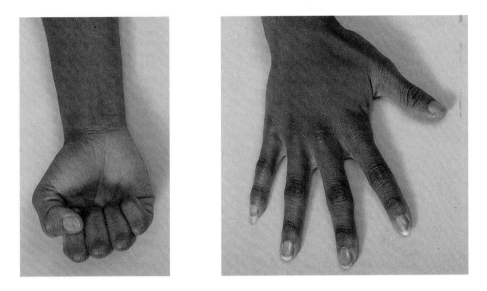

Impaired hand movement in arthritis, trigger finger, Dupuytren's contracture

■ *Abduction and adduction.* Ask the patient to spread the fingers apart (abduction) and back together (adduction). Check for smooth, coordinated movement.

Thumbs. At the *thumb,* assess *flexion, extension, abduction, adduction,* and *opposition.* Ask the patient to move the thumb across the palm and touch the base of the 5th finger to test *flexion,* and then to move the thumb back across the palm and away from the fingers to test *extension.*

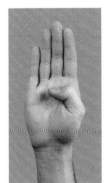
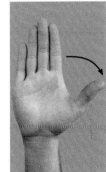

FLEXION   **EXTENSION**

Next, ask the patient to place the fingers and thumb in the neutral position with the palm up, then have the patient move the thumb anteriorly away from the palm to assess abduction and back down for adduction. To test opposition, or movements of the thumb across the palm, ask the patient to touch the thumb to each of the other fingertips.

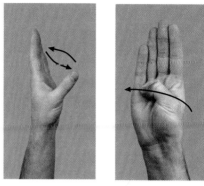

ABDUCTION AND ADDUCTION

OPPOSITION

Test sensation in the fingers only along the lateral and medial surfaces to isolate any alterations in the digital nerves. Test median, ulnar, and radial nerve function by checking sensation as follows:

- Pulp of the index finger—median nerve

- Pulp of the 5th finger—ulnar nerve

Decreased sensation in the median nerve distribution in carpal tunnel syndrome.

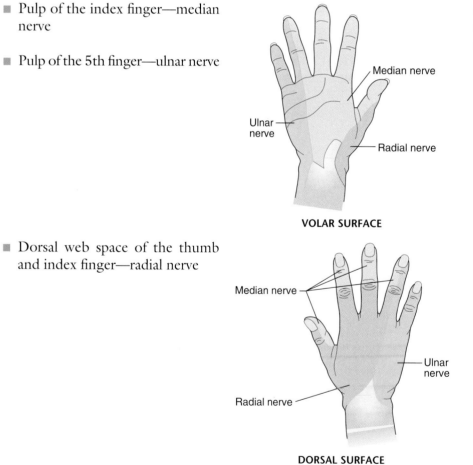

Median nerve

Ulnar nerve

Radial nerve

VOLAR SURFACE

- Dorsal web space of the thumb and index finger—radial nerve

Median nerve

Ulnar nerve

Radial nerve

DORSAL SURFACE

THE SPINE

OVERVIEW

The vertebral column, or spine, is the central supporting structure of the trunk and back. Note the *concave curves* of the cervical and lumbar spine and the *convex curves* of the thoracic and sacrococcygeal spine. These curves help distribute upper body weight to the pelvis and lower extremities and cushion the concussive impact of walking or running.

The complex mechanics of the back reflect the coordinated action of:

■ The vertebrae and intervertebral discs

■ An interconnecting system of ligaments between anterior vertebrae and posterior vertebrae, ligaments between the spinous processes, and ligaments between the lamina of two adjacent vertebrae

■ Large superficial muscles, deeper intrinsic muscles, and muscles of the abdominal wall.

Viewing the patient from behind, identify the following landmarks:

1. Spinous processes, usually more prominent at C7 and T1 and more evident on forward flexion

2. Paravertebral muscles on either side of the midline

3. Scapulae

4. Iliac crests

5. Posterior superior iliac spines, usually marked by skin dimples.

A line drawn above the posterior iliac crests crosses the spinous process of L4.

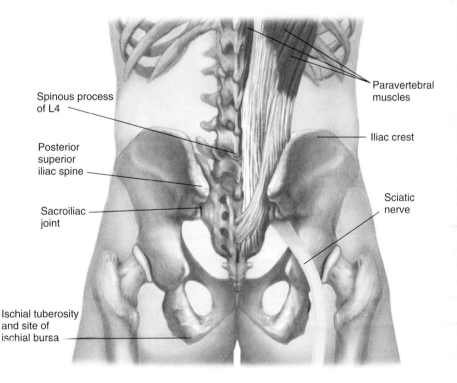

Spinous process of L4

Posterior superior iliac spine

Sacroiliac joint

Ischial tuberosity and site of ischial bursa

Paravertebral muscles

Iliac crest

Sciatic nerve

BONY STRUCTURES

The vertebral column contains 24 vertebrae stacked on the sacrum and coccyx. A typical vertebra contains sites for joint articulations, weight bearing, and muscle attachments, as well as foramina for the spinal nerve roots and peripheral nerves. Anteriorly, the *vertebral body* supports weight bearing. The posterior *vertebral arch* encloses the spinal cord. Review the location of the vertebral processes and foramina, with particular attention to:

- The *spinous process* projecting posteriorly in the midline and the two transverse processes at the junction of the *pedicle* and the *lamina*. Muscles attach at these processes.

- The *articular processes*—two on each side of the vertebra, one facing up and one facing down, at the junction of the pedicles and laminae, often called *articular facets*

- The *vertebral foramen*, which encloses the spinal cord, the *intervertebral foramen*, formed by the inferior and superior articulating process of adjacent vertebrae, creating a channel for the spinal nerve roots; and in the cervical vertebrae, the *transverse foramen* for the vertebral artery.

The proximity of the spinal cord and spinal nerve roots to their bony vertebral casing and the intervertebral discs makes them especially vulnerable to disc herniation, impingement from degenerative changes in the vertebrae, and trauma.

JOINTS

The spine has slightly movable cartilaginous joints between the vertebral bodies and between the articular facets. Between the vertebral bodies are the *intervertebral discs*, each

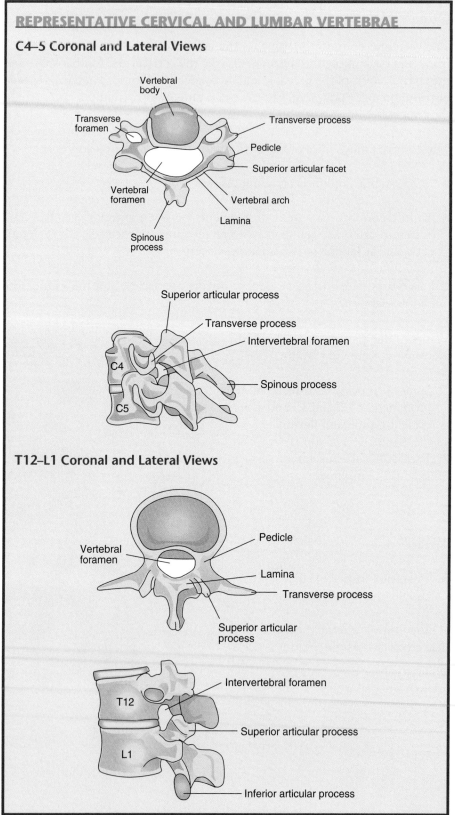

REPRESENTATIVE CERVICAL AND LUMBAR VERTEBRAE

C4–5 Coronal and Lateral Views

Vertebral body

Transverse foramen

Transverse process

Pedicle

Superior articular facet

Vertebral foramen

Vertebral arch

Lamina

Spinous process

Superior articular process

Transverse process

Intervertebral foramen

C4

Spinous process

C5

T12–L1 Coronal and Lateral Views

Pedicle

Vertebral foramen

Lamina

Transverse process

Superior articular process

Intervertebral foramen

T12

Superior articular process

L1

Inferior articular process

consisting of a soft mucoid central core, the *nucleus pulposus*, rimmed by the tough fibrous tissue of the *annulus fibrosis*. The intervertebral discs cushion movement between vertebrae and allow the vertebral column to curve, flex, and bend. The flexibility of the spine is largely determined by the angle of the articular facet joints relative to the plane of the vertebral body, and varies at different levels of the spine. Note that the vertebral column angles sharply posterior at the *lumbosacral junction* and becomes immovable. The mechanical stress at this angulation contributes to the risk for disc herniation and subluxation, or slippage, of L5 on S1.

MUSCLE GROUPS

The *trapezius* and *latissimus dorsi* form the large outer layer of muscles attaching to each side of the spine. They overlie two deeper muscle layers—a layer attaching to the head, neck, and spinous processes (*splenius capitis, splenius cervicis,* and *sacrospinalis*) and a layer of smaller intrinsic muscles between vertebrae. Muscles attaching to the anterior surface of the vertebrae, including the *psoas* muscle and muscles of the abdominal wall, assist with flexion.

Muscles moving the neck and lower vertebral column are summarized below.

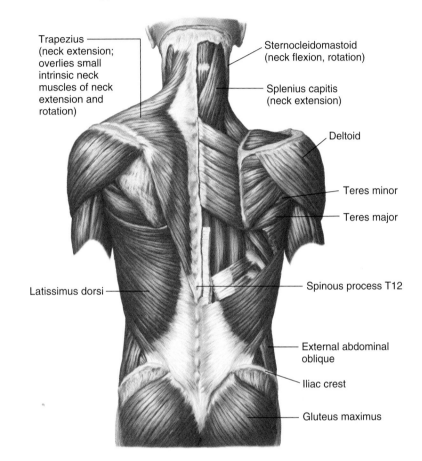

Trapezius (neck extension; overlies small intrinsic neck muscles of neck extension and rotation)

Sternocleidomastoid (neck flexion, rotation)

Splenius capitis (neck extension)

Deltoid

Teres minor

Teres major

Latissimus dorsi

Spinous process T12

External abdominal oblique

Iliac crest

Gluteus maximus

■ Muscles of the Neck and Lower Vertebrae	
Movement	**Principal Muscle Group**
Cervical Spine (neck)	
Flexion	Sternocleidomastoid, scalene, and prevertebral muscles
Extension	Splenius, trapezius, small intrinsic neck muscles
Rotation	Sternocleidomastoid, small intrinsic neck muscles
Lateral bending	Scalene and small intrinsic neck muscles
Lumbar Spine	
Flexion	Psoas major, psoas minor, quadratus lumborum; abdominal muscles such as the internal and external obliques and rectus abdominis, attaching to the anterior vertebrae
Extension	Intrinsic muscles of the back, sacrospinalis
Rotation	Abdominal muscles, intrinsic muscles of the back
Lateral bending	Abdominal muscles, intrinsic muscles of the back

TECHNIQUES OF EXAMINATION

INSPECTION

Begin by observing the patient's posture, including the position of both the neck and trunk, when entering the room.

Assess the patient for erect position of the head, smooth, coordinated neck movement, and ease of gait.

> Neck stiffness signals arthritis, muscle strain, or other underlying pathology that should be pursued.

Drape or gown the patient to expose the entire back for complete inspection. If possible, the patient should be upright in the natural standing position—with feet together and arms hanging at the sides. The head should be midline in the same plane as the sacrum, and the shoulders and pelvis should be level.

> Lateral deviation and rotation of the head suggests *torticollis*, from contraction of the sternocleidomastoid muscle.

Inspect the patient from the side. Evaluate the spinal curvatures.

PALPATION

From a sitting or standing position, palpate the *spinous processes* of each vertebra with your thumb.

> Tenderness suggests fracture or dislocation if preceded by trauma, underlying infection, or arthritis.

In the neck, also palpate the *facet joints* that lie between the cervical vertebrae about 1 inch lateral to the spinous processes of C2–C7. These joints lie deep to the trapezius muscle and may not be palpable unless the neck muscles are relaxed.

> Tenderness in arthritis, especially at the facet joints between C5 and C6

In the lower lumbar area, check carefully for any vertebral "step-offs" to determine whether one spinous process seems unusually prominent (or recessed) in relation to the one above it. Identify any tenderness.

> Step-offs in *spondylolisthesis,* or forward slippage of one vertebra, which may compress the spinal cord. Vertebral tenderness is suspicious for fracture or infection.

Palpate over the sacroiliac joint, often identified by the dimple overlying the posterior superior iliac spine.

> Tenderness over the sacroiliac joint in sacroiliitis. *Ankylosing spondylitis* may produce sacroiliac tenderness.

You may wish to percuss the spine for tenderness by thumping, but not too roughly, with the ulnar surface of your fist.

> Pain on percussion may arise from *osteoporosis, infection,* or *malignancy.*

Inspect and palpate the paravertebral muscles for tenderness and spasm. Muscles in spasm feel firm and knotted and may be visible.

> Spasm occurs in degenerative and inflammatory processes of muscles, prolonged contraction from abnormal posture, or anxiety.

With the hip flexed and the patient lying on the opposite side, palpate the sciatic nerve, the largest nerve in the body, consisting of nerve roots from L4, L5, S1, S2, and S3. The nerve lies midway between the greater trochanter and the ischial tuberosity as it leaves the pelvis through the sciatic notch.

> *Sciatic nerve tenderness* suggests a herniated disc or mass lesion impinging on the contributing nerve roots.

■ *Inspection of the Spine*

View of Patient	Focus of Inspection	
From the side	Cervical, thoracic, and lumbar curves.	

Cervical concavity

Thoracic convexity

Lumbar concavity

Increased *thoracic kyphosis* occurs with aging. In children a correctable structural deformity should be pursued.

From behind	Upright spinal column (an imaginary line should fall from C7 through the gluteal cleft)	
	Alignment of the shoulders, the iliac crests, and the skin creases below the buttocks (gluteal folds)	
	Skin markings, tags, or masses	

In *scoliosis,* there is lateral and rotatory curvature of the spine to bring the head back to midline. Scoliosis often becomes evident during adolescence, before symptoms appear.

Unequal shoulder heights seen in: scoliosis; Sprengel's deformity of the scapula (from the attachment of an extra bone or band between the upper scapula and C7); in "winging" of the scapula (from loss of innervation of the serratus anterior muscle by the long thoracic nerve); and in contralateral weakness of the trapezius.

Unequal heights of the iliac crests, or *pelvic tilt,* suggest unequal lengths of the legs and disappear when a block is placed under the short leg and foot. Scoliosis and hip abduction or adduction may also cause a pelvic tilt. "Listing" of the trunk to one side is seen with a herniated lumbar disc.

Birthmarks, port-wine stains, hairy patches, and lipomas often overlie bony defects such as *spina bifida*.

Café-au-lait spots (discolored patches of skin), skin tags, and fibrous tumors in *neurofibromatosis*

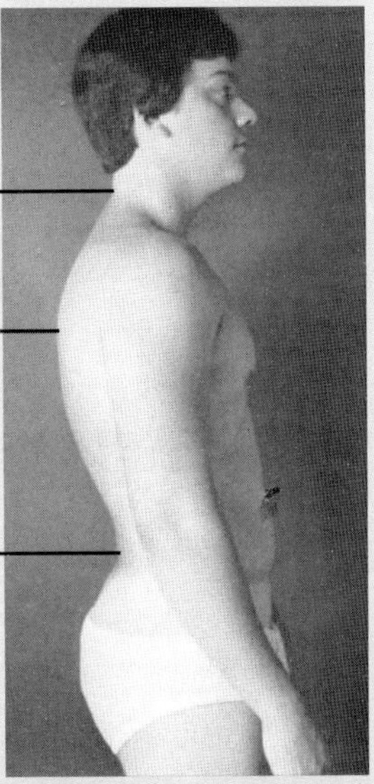

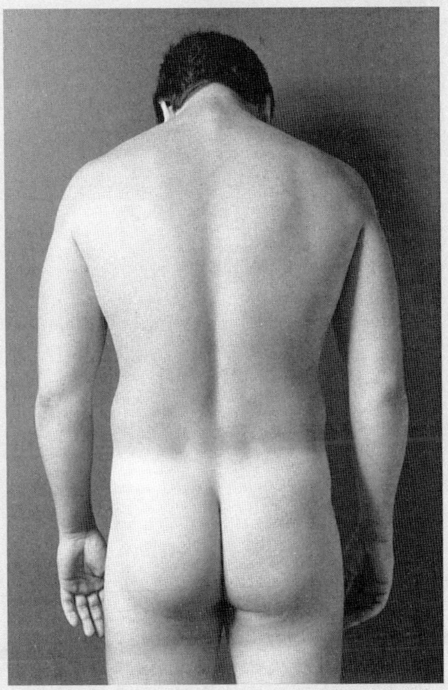

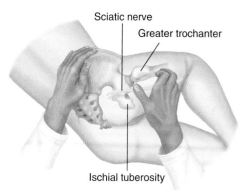

Sciatic nerve

Greater trochanter

Ischial tuberosity

Palpate for tenderness in any other areas that are suggested by the patient's symptoms. Recall that low back pain warrants careful assessment for cord compression, the most serious cause of pain, because of risk for paralysis of the affected limb.

Herniated intervertebral discs, most common between L5 and S1 or between L4 and L5, may produce tenderness of the spinous processes, the intervertebral joints, the paravertebral muscles, the sacrosciatic notch, and the sciatic nerve.

Rheumatoid arthritis may also cause tenderness of the intervertebral joints.

Remember that tenderness in the costovertebral angles may signify kidney infection rather than a musculoskeletal problem.

See Table 15-1, Low Back Pain (p. 560).

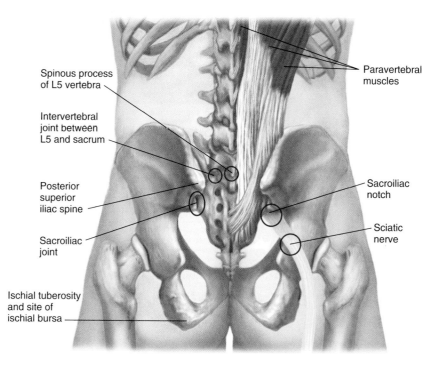

Spinous process of L5 vertebra

Intervertebral joint between L5 and sacrum

Posterior superior iliac spine

Sacroiliac joint

Ischial tuberosity and site of ischial bursa

Paravertebral muscles

Sacroiliac notch

Sciatic nerve

RANGE OF MOTION AND MANEUVERS

The neck is the most mobile portion of the spine, remarkable for its seven fragile vertebrae supporting the 10- to 15-pound head. Flexion and extension occur primarily between the skull and C1 (the atlas), rotation at C1–C2 (the axis), and lateral bending at C2–C7.

Ask the patient to perform the following maneuvers, and check for smooth, coordinated motion:

■ *Flexion.* Touch the chin to the chest.

■ *Extension.* Look up at the ceiling.

Limitations in range of motion can arise from stiffness from arthritis, pain from trauma, or muscle spasm such as *torticollis.*

It is important to assess any complaints or findings of neck, shoulder, or arm pain or numbness for possible cervical cord or nerve root compression. See Table 15-2, Pains in the Neck (p. 561).

- *Rotation.* Turn the head to each side, looking directly over the shoulder.

- *Lateral bending.* Tilt the head, touching each ear to the corresponding shoulder.

Tenderness, loss of sensation, or impaired movement warrants careful neurologic testing of the neck and upper extremities.

Now assess range of motion in the spinal column.

- *Flexion.* Ask the patient to bend forward to touch the toes (flexion). Note the smoothness and symmetry of movement, the range of motion, and the curve in the lumbar area. As flexion proceeds, the lumbar concavity should flatten out.

Tenderness at C1–C2 in *rheumatoid arthritis* suggests possible risk for subluxation and high cervical cord compression.

Deformity of the thorax on forward bending in *scoliosis.*

Persistence of lumbar lordosis suggests muscle spasm or *ankylosing spondylitis.*

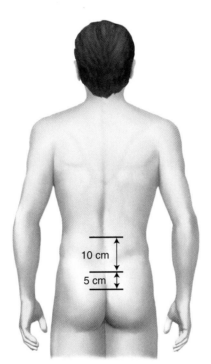

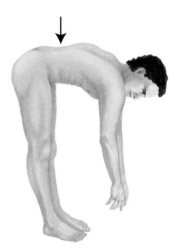

You may wish to measure the degree of flexion of the spine with the patient standing and bending forward. Mark the spine at the lumbosacral junction, then 10 cm above and 5 cm below this point. A 4-cm increase between the two upper marks is normally seen. The distance between the lower two marks should be unchanged.

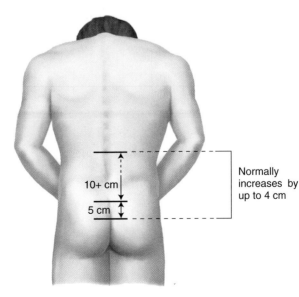

Normally increases by up to 4 cm

- *Extension.* Place your hand on the posterior superior iliac spine, with your fingers pointing toward the midline, and ask the patient to bend backward as far as possible.

- *Rotation.* Stabilize the pelvis by placing one hand on the patient's hip and the other on the opposite shoulder. Then rotate the trunk by pulling the shoulder and then the hip posteriorly. Repeat these maneuvers for the opposite side.

- *Lateral bending.* Again stabilize the pelvis by placing your hand on the patient's hip. Ask the patient to lean to both sides as far as possible.

Decreased spinal mobility in *osteo-arthritis* and *ankylosing spondylitis,* among other conditions[27]

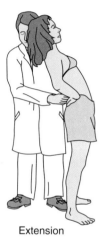

Extension

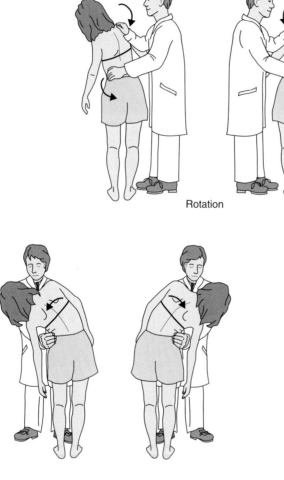

Rotation

Lateral bending

As with the neck, pain or tenderness with these maneuvers, particularly with radiation into the leg, warrants careful neurologic testing of the lower extremities.

Underlying cord or nerve root compression should be considered. Note that arthritis or infection in the hip, rectum, or pelvis may cause symptoms in the lumbar spine. See Table 15-1, Low Back Pain (p. 560).

THE HIP

OVERVIEW

The hip joint is deeply embedded in the pelvis, and is notable for its strength, stability, and wide range of motion. The stability of the hip joint, so essential for weight bearing, arises from the deep fit of the head of the femur into the *acetabulum*, its strong fibrous articular capsule, and the powerful muscles crossing the joint and inserting below the femoral head, providing leverage for movement of the femur.

BONY STRUCTURES AND JOINTS

The hip joint lies below the middle third of the inguinal ligament but in a deeper plane. It is a ball-and-socket joint—note how the rounded head of the femur articulates with the cuplike cavity of the acetabulum. Because of its overlying muscles and depth, it is not readily palpable. Review the bones of the pelvis—the *acetabulum*, the *ilium*, and the *ischium*—and the connection inferiorly at the *symphysis pubis* and posteriorly with the sacroiliac bone.

On the *anterior aspect* of the hip, identify the *iliac crest* at the upper margin of the pelvis at the level of L4. Follow the downward anterior curve and locate the *iliac tubercle*, marking the widest point of the crest, and continue tracking downward to the *anterior superior iliac spine*. Place your thumbs on the anterior superior spines and move your fingers downward from the iliac tubercles to the *greater trochanter* of the femur. Then move your thumbs medially and obliquely to the *pubic symphysis*, which lies at the same level as the greater trochanter.

On the *posterior aspect* of the hip, locate the *posterior superior iliac spine* directly underneath the visible dimples just above the buttocks. Placing your left thumb and index finger over the posterior superior iliac spine, next locate the *greater trochanter* laterally with your fingers at the level of the gluteal fold and place your thumb medially on the *ischial tuberosity*. The *sacroiliac joint* is not always

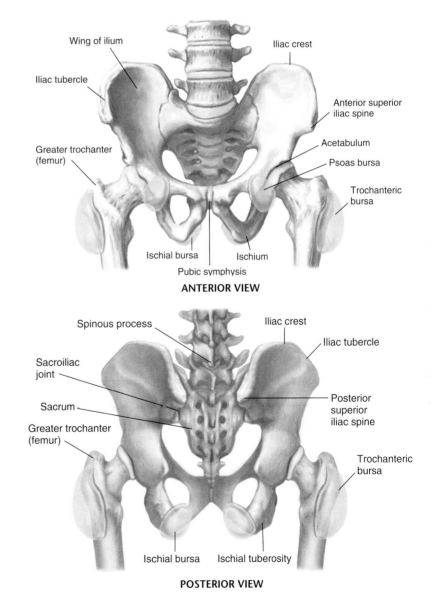

Wing of ilium

Iliac crest

Iliac tubercle

Anterior superior iliac spine

Greater trochanter (femur)

Acetabulum

Psoas bursa

Trochanteric bursa

Ischial bursa

Ischium

Pubic symphysis

ANTERIOR VIEW

Spinous process

Iliac crest

Iliac tubercle

Sacroiliac joint

Sacrum

Greater trochanter (femur)

Posterior superior iliac spine

Trochanteric bursa

Ischial bursa

Ischial tuberosity

POSTERIOR VIEW

palpable. Note that an imaginary line between the posterior superior iliac spines crosses the joint at S2.

MUSCLE GROUPS

Four powerful muscle groups move the hip. Picture these groups as you examine patients, and remember that to move the femur or any bone in a given direction, the proximal and distal muscle insertions must **extend across the joint line.**

The *flexor group* lies anteriorly and flexes the thigh. The primary hip flexor is the *iliopsoas*, extending from above the iliac crest to the lesser trochanter. The *extensor group* lies posteriorly and extends the thigh. The *gluteus maximus* is the primary extensor of the hip. It forms a band crossing from its origin along the medial pelvis to its insertion below the trochanter.

The *adductor group* is medial and swings the thigh toward the body. The muscles in this group arise from the rami of the pubis and ischium and insert on the posteromedial aspect of the femur. The *abductor group* is lateral, extending from the iliac crest to the head of the femur, and moves the thigh away from the body. This group includes the *gluteus medius* and *minimus*. These muscles help stabilize the pelvis during the stance phase of gait.

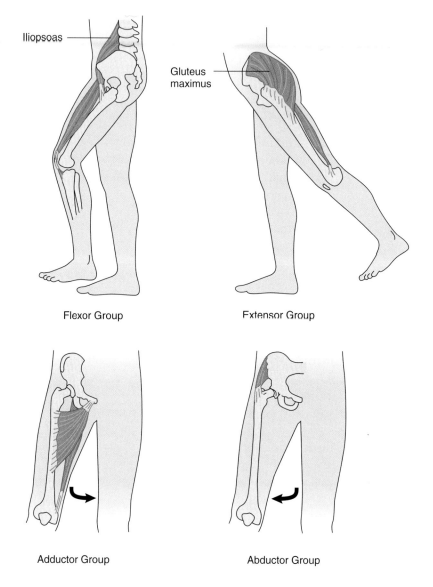

Iliopsoas

Gluteus maximus

Flexor Group

Extensor Group

Adductor Group

Abductor Group

ADDITIONAL STRUCTURES

A strong dense articular capsule, extending from the acetabulum to the femoral neck, encases and strengthens the hip joint, reinforced by three overlying ligaments and lined with synovial membrane. There are three principal bursae at the hip. Anterior to the joint is the psoas (also termed *iliopectineal* or *iliopsoas*) *bursa*, overlying the articular capsule and the psoas muscle. Find the bony prominence lateral to the hip joint—the *greater trochanter* of the femur. The large multilocular *trochanteric bursa* lies on its posterior surface. The *ischial* (or *ischiogluteal*) *bursa*—not always present—lies under the *ischeal tuberosity*, on which a person sits. Note its proximity to the sciatic nerve, as shown on p. 529.

TECHNIQUES OF EXAMINATION

INSPECTION

Inspection of the hip begins with careful observation of the patient's gait on entering the room. Observe the two phases of gait:

■ *Stance*—when the foot is on the ground and bears weight (60% of the walking cycle)

Most problems appear during the weight-bearing stance phase.

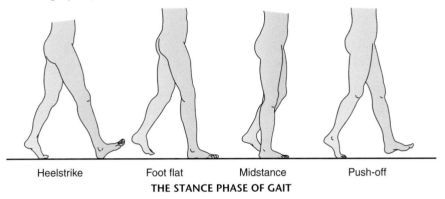

| Heelstrike | Foot flat | Midstance | Push-off |

THE STANCE PHASE OF GAIT

■ *Swing*—when the foot moves forward and does not bear weight (40% of the cycle)

Observe the gait for the width of the base, the shift of the pelvis, and flexion of the knee. The width of the base should be 2 to 4 inches from heel to heel. Normal gait has a smooth, continuous rhythm, achieved in part by contraction of the abductors of the weight-bearing limb. Abductor contraction stabilizes the pelvis and helps maintain balance, raising the opposite hip. The knee should be flexed throughout the stance phase, except when the heel strikes the ground to counteract motion at the ankle.

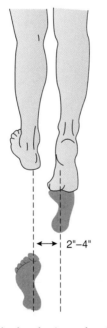

2"–4"

A wide base suggests cerebellar disease or foot problems.

Hip dislocation, arthritis, or abductor weakness can cause the pelvis to drop on the opposite side, producing a waddling gait.

Lack of knee flexion interrupts the smooth pattern of gait.

Observe the lumbar portion of the spine for slight lordosis and, with the patient supine, assess the length of the legs for symmetry. (To measure leg length, see Special Techniques, p. 557).

Loss of lordosis may reflect *paravertebral spasm*; excess lordosis suggests a *flexion deformity* of the hip.

Changes in leg length are seen in abduction or adduction deformities and scoliosis. Leg shortening and external rotation suggest *hip fracture.*

Inspect the anterior and posterior surfaces of the hip for any areas of muscle atrophy or bruising.

PALPATION

Review the surface landmarks of the hip. On the *anterior surface* locate the *iliac crest*, the *iliac tubercle*, and the *anterior superior iliac spine*. On the *posterior surface* identify the *posterior superior iliac spine*, the *greater trochanter*, the *ischial tuberosity*, and the *sciatic nerve*.

With the patient supine, ask the patient to place the heel of the leg being examined on the opposite knee. Then palpate along the *inguinal ligament,* which extends from the anterior superior iliac spine to the pubic tubercle. The femoral nerve, artery, and vein bisect the overlying inguinal ligament; lymph nodes lie medially. The mnemonic **NAVEL** may help you remember the lateral-to-medial sequence of Nerve—Artery—Vein—Empty space—Lymph node.

If the hip is painful, palpate the *(psoas) bursa,* below the inguinal ligament but on a deeper plane.

With the patient resting on one side and the hip flexed and internally rotated, palpate the *trochanteric bursa* lying over the greater trochanter. Normally, the *ischiogluteal bursa,* over the ischial tuberosity, is not palpable unless inflamed.

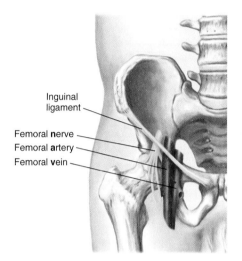

Inguinal ligament

Femoral nerve
Femoral artery
Femoral vein

Bulges along the ligament may suggest an *inguinal hernia* or, on occasion, an *aneurysm.*

Enlarged lymph nodes suggest infection in the lower extremity or pelvis.

Tenderness in the groin area may be due to *synovitis* of the hip joint, *bursitis*, or possibly *psoas abscess.*

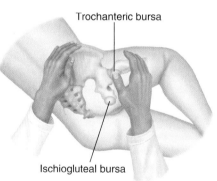

Trochanteric bursa

Ischiogluteal bursa

TROCHANTERIC BURSA

Focal tenderness over the trochanter in *trochanteric bursitis.* Tenderness over the posterolateral surface of the greater trochanter in localized tendinitis or muscle spasm from referred hip pain

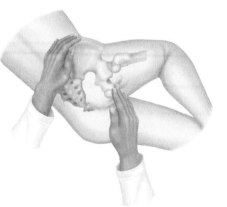

ISCHIOGLUTEAL BURSA

Tenderness in *ischiogluteal bursitis* or "weaver's bottom"—because of the adjacent sciatic nerve, this may mimic sciatica.

RANGE OF MOTION AND MANEUVERS

Motions at the hip include *flexion, extension, abduction, adduction,* and *rotation.* Note that the hip can flex farther when the knee is also flexed. The direction of rotation at the hip while the knee is flexed may be confusing at first: when the lower leg swings laterally, the femur rotates internally. It is the motion of the femur at the hip joint that identifies these movements.

■ *Flexion.* With the patient supine, place your hand under the patient's lumbar spine. Ask the patient to bend each knee in turn up to the chest and pull it firmly against the abdomen. Note when the back touches your hand, indicating normal flattening of the lumbar lordosis—further flexion must arise from the hip joint itself.

In *flexion deformity of the hip,* as the opposite hip is flexed (with the thigh against the chest), the affected hip does not allow full leg extension, and the affected thigh appears flexed.

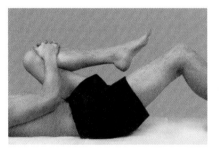

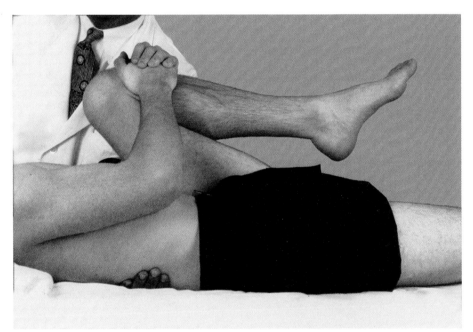

HIP FLEXION AND FLATTENING OF LUMBAR LORDOSIS

As the thigh is held against the abdomen, observe the degree of flexion at the hip and knee. Normally the anterior portion of the thigh can almost touch the chest wall. Note whether the opposite thigh remains fully extended, resting on the table.

Flexion deformity may be masked by an increase, rather than flattening, in lumbar lordosis and an anterior pelvic tilt.

■ *Extension.* With the patient lying face down, extend the thigh toward you in a posterior direction. Alternatively, carefully position the supine patient near the edge of the table and extend the leg posteriorly.

■ *Abduction.* Stabilize the pelvis by pressing down on the opposite anterior superior iliac spine with one hand. With the other hand, grasp the ankle and abduct the extended leg until you feel the iliac spine move. This movement marks the limit of hip abduction.

Restricted abduction is common in hip *osteoarthritis.*

Alternatively, stand at the foot of the table, grasp both ankles, and spread them maximally, abducting both extended legs at the hips. This method

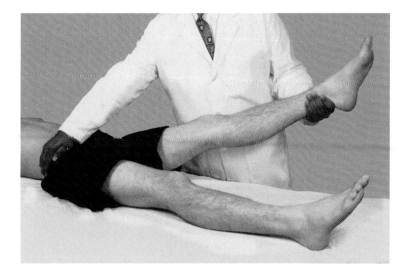

provides easy comparison of two sides when movements are restricted, but it is impractical when range of motion is full.

- *Adduction.* With the patient supine, stabilize the pelvis, hold one ankle, and move the leg medially across the body and over the opposite extremity.

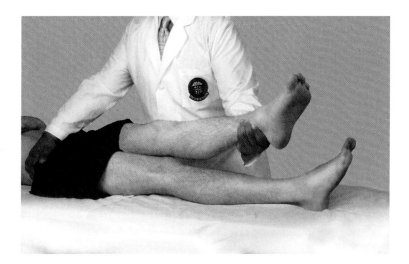

- *External and internal rotation.* Flex the leg to 90° at hip and knee, stabilize the thigh with one hand, grasp the ankle with the other, and swing the lower leg—medially for external rotation at the hip and laterally for internal rotation.

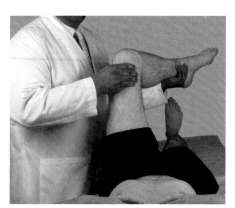

Restriction of internal rotation is an especially sensitive indicator of hip disease such as arthritis. External rotation is also often restricted.

◢ THE KNEE

OVERVIEW

The knee joint is the largest joint in the body. It is a hinge joint involving three bones: the femur, the tibia, and the patella (or knee cap), with three articular surfaces, two between the femur and the tibia and one between the femur and the patella. Note how the two rounded condyles of the femur rest on the relatively flat tibial plateau. There is no inherent stability in the knee joint itself, making it dependent on ligaments to hold its articulating bones in place. This feature, in addition to the lever action of the femur on the tibia and lack of padding from fat or muscle, makes the knee highly vulnerable to injury.

BONY STRUCTURES

Landmarks in and around the knee will orient you to this complicated joint. Bring your fingertips firmly down the medial surface of the thigh along a line analogous to the inner seam of a pant leg. Your fingers will run up against an abrupt bony prominence, the *adductor tubercle*. Just below this is the *medial epicondyle*. The *lateral epicondyle* is comparably situated on the other side.

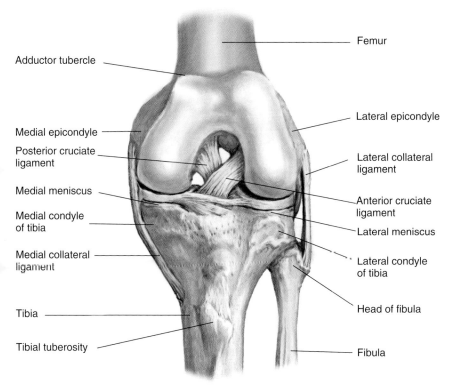

ANTERIOR ASPECT OF THE KNEE

Identify the flat medial surface of the tibia—the shin. Follow its anterior border upward to the *tibial tuberosity* (**A**). Mark this point with a dot of ink. Now follow the medial border of the tibia upward until it merges into a bony prominence—the *medial condyle* of the tibia (**B**). This is somewhat higher than the tibial tuberosity. In a comparable location on the other side of the knee, find a similar prominence—the *lateral condyle* (**C**). Mark both condyles with ink. On the lateral surface of the knee, somewhat below the level of the lateral tibial condyle, find the head of the fibula.

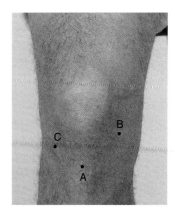

The *patella* rests on the anterior articulating surface of the femur, midway between the epicondyles, embedded in the tendon of the quadriceps muscle. This tendon continues below the knee joint as the *patellar tendon* and inserts on the tibial tuberosity.

JOINTS

Two condylar *tibiofemoral joints* are formed by the convex curves of the medial and lateral condyles of the femur as they articulate with the concave condyles of the tibia. The third articular surface is the *patello-femoral joint*. The patella slides in a groove on the anterior aspect of the distal femur, called the *trochlear groove*, during flexion and extension of the knee.

With the knee flexed about 90°, you can press your thumbs—one on each side of the patellar tendon—into the groove of the tibiofemoral joint. Note that the patella lies just above this joint line. As you press your thumbs downward, you can feel the edge of the tibial plateau, the upper surface of the tibia. Follow it medially, then laterally until you are stopped by the converging femur and tibia. By moving your thumbs upward toward the midline to the top of the patella, you can follow the articulating surface of the femur and identify the margins of the joint.

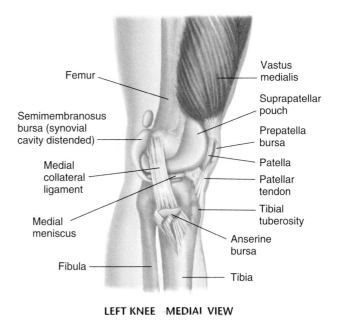

LEFT KNEE   MEDIAL VIEW

MUSCLE GROUPS

Powerful muscles move and support the knee. The *quadriceps femoris* extends the leg, covering the anterior, medial, and lateral aspects of the thigh. The *hamstring muscles* lie on the posterior aspect of the thigh and flex the knee.

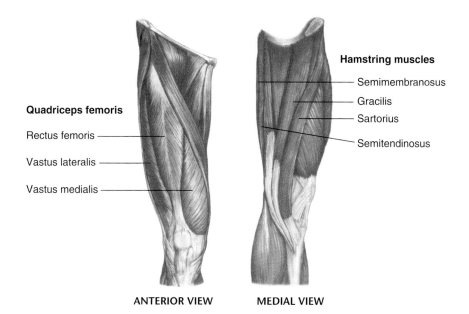

Quadriceps femoris

Rectus femoris

Vastus lateralis

Vastus medialis

Hamstring muscles

Semimembranosus

Gracilis

Sartorius

Semitendinosus

ANTERIOR VIEW   MEDIAL VIEW

ADDITIONAL STRUCTURES

Two important pairs of ligaments, the collateral ligaments and the cruciate ligaments, and the menisci provide stability to the knee (see pp. 550 and 551).

■ The *medial collateral ligament* (MCL), not easily palpable, is a broad flat ligament connecting the medial condyles of the femur and the tibia. To locate the anatomical region of the MCL, move your fingers medially and posteriorly along the joint line, then palpate along the ligament from its origin to insertion.

■ The *lateral collateral ligament* (LCL) connects the lateral femoral condyle and the head of the fibula. To feel the LCL, cross one leg so the ankle rests on the opposite knee and find the firm cord that runs from the lateral epicondyle of the femur to the head of the fibula. The MCL and LCL provide medial and lateral stability to the knee.

■ The *anterior cruciate ligament* (ACL) crosses obliquely from the lateral femoral condyle to the medial tibia, preventing the tibia from sliding forward on the femur.

■ The *posterior cruciate ligament* (PCL) crosses from the lateral tibia and lateral meniscus to the medial femoral condyle, preventing the tibia from slipping backward on the femur. Because these ligaments lie within the knee joint, they are not palpable. They are nonetheless crucial to the anteroposterior stability of the knee.

■ The *medial and lateral menisci* cushion the action of the femur on the tibia. These crescent-shaped fibrocartilaginous discs add a cuplike surface to the otherwise flat tibial plateau. Palpate the *medial meniscus* by pressing on the medial soft-tissue depression along the upper edge of the tibial plateau. Place the knee in slight flexion and palpate the *lateral meniscus* along the lateral joint line.

Observe the concavities that are usually evident at each side of the patella and also above it. Occupying these areas is the synovial cavity of the knee, the largest joint cavity in the body. This cavity includes an extension 6 centimeters above the upper border of the patella, lying upward and deep to the quadriceps muscle—the *suprapatellar pouch*. The joint cavity covers the anterior, medial, and lateral surfaces of the knee, as well as the condyles of the femur and tibia posteriorly. Although the synovium is not normally detectable, these areas may become swollen and tender when the joint is inflamed.

Several bursae lie near the knee. The *prepatellar bursa* lies between the patella and the overlying skin. The *anserine bursa* lies 1 to 2 inches below the knee joint on the medial surface, proximal and medial to the attachments of the medial hamstring muscles on the proximal tibia. It cannot be palpated due to these overlying tendons. Now identify the large *semimembranosus bursa* that communicates with the joint cavity, also on the posterior and medial surfaces of the knee.

TECHNIQUES OF EXAMINATION

INSPECTION

Observe the gait for a smooth, rhythmic flow as the patient enters the room. The knee should be extended at heel strike and flexed at all other phases of swing and stance.

Stumbling or pushing the knee into extension with the hand during heel strike suggests *quadriceps weakness*.

Check the alignment and contours of the knees. Observe any atrophy of the quadriceps muscles.

Bowlegs (*genu varum*) and knock-knees (*genu valgum*) are common; flexion contracture (inability to extend fully) in limb paralysis

Look for loss of the normal hollows around the patella, a sign of swelling in the knee joint and suprapatellar pouch; note any other swelling in or around the knee.

Swelling over the patella suggests *prepatellar bursitis*. Swelling over the tibial tubercle suggests *infrapatellar* or, if more medial, *anserine bursitis*.

PALPATION

Ask the patient to sit on the edge of the examining table with the knees in flexion. In this position, bony landmarks are more visible, and the muscles, tendons, and ligaments are more relaxed, making them easier to palpate.

First review the important bony landmarks of the knee. Facing the knee, place your thumbs in the soft-tissue depressions on either side of the *patellar tendon*. On the medial aspect, move your thumb upward and then downward and identify the *medial femoral condyle* and the upper margin of the *medial tibial plateau*. Trace the patellar tendon distally to the *tibial tubercle*. The *adductor tubercle* is posterior to the *medial femoral condyle*.

Lateral to the patellar tendon, identify the *lateral femoral condyle* and the *lateral tibial plateau*. The medial and lateral femoral *epicondyles* are lateral to the condyles with the knee in flexion. Locate the *patella*.

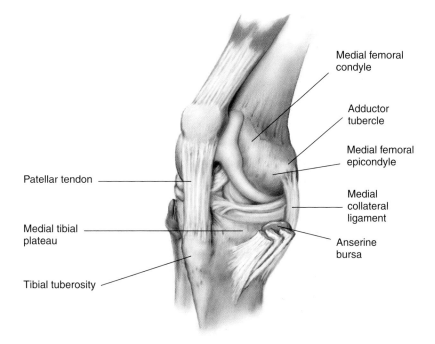

Medial femoral condyle

Adductor tubercle

Medial femoral epicondyle

Medial collateral ligament

Anserine bursa

Patellar tendon

Medial tibial plateau

Tibial tuberosity

Palpate the ligaments, the borders of the menisci, and the bursae of the knee, paying special attention to any areas of tenderness. Pain is a common complaint in knee problems, and localizing the structure causing pain is important for accurate evaluation.

In the *patellofemoral compartment*, palpate the patellar tendon and ask the patient to extend the leg to make sure the tendon is intact.

Tenderness over the tendon or inability to extend the leg suggests a partial or complete tear of the patellar tendon.

With the patient supine and the knee extended, compress the patella against the underlying femur. Ask the patient to tighten the quadriceps as the patella moves distally in the trochlear groove. Check for a smooth sliding motion (the *patellofemoral grinding test*).

Pain and crepitus suggest roughening of the patellar undersurface that articulates with the femur. Similar pain may occur with climbing stairs or getting up from a chair.

Pain with compression and with patellar movement during quadriceps contraction suggests *chondromalacia,* or degenerative patella (the patellofemoral syndrome).

Now assess the *medial and lateral compartments* of the *tibiofemoral joint*. Flex the patient's knee to about 90°. The patient's foot should rest on the examining table. Palpate the *medial collateral ligament* (MCL) between the medial

MCL tenderness after injury is suspicious for an MCL tear. (The LCL is less subject to injury.)

femoral epicondyle and the femur; then palpate the cordlike *lateral collateral ligament* (LCL) between the lateral femoral epicondyle and the fibular head.

Palpate the *medial and lateral menisci* along the medial and lateral joint lines. It is easier to palpate the medial meniscus if the tibia is internally rotated. Note any swelling or tenderness.

Tenderness from tears following injury are more common in the medial meniscus.

Note any irregular bony ridges along the joint margins.

Tender bony ridges along the joint margins may be felt in osteoarthritis.[28,29]

Try to feel any thickening or swelling in the suprapatellar pouch and along the sides of the patella. Start 10 centimeters above the superior border of the patella (well above the pouch) and feel the soft tissues between your thumb and fingers. Move your hand distally in progressive steps, trying to identify the pouch. Continue your palpation along the sides of the patella. Note any tenderness or warmth greater than in the surrounding tissues.

Swelling above and adjacent to the patella suggests synovial thickening or effusion in the knee joint.

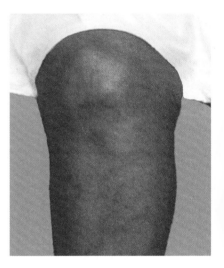

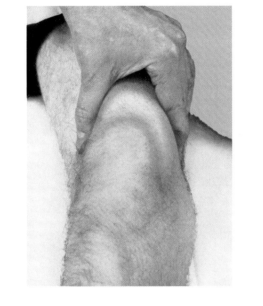

Thickening, bogginess, or warmth in these areas indicates synovitis or nontender effusions from osteoarthritis.

Check three other bursae for bogginess or swelling. Palpate the *prepatellar bursa*, and over the *anserine bursa* on the posteromedial side of the knee between the medial collateral ligament and the tendons inserting on the medial tibial and plateau. On the posterior surface, with the leg extended, check the medial aspect of the popliteal fossa.

Prepatellar bursitis ("housemaid's knee") from excessive kneeling. *Anserine bursitis* from running, valgus knee deformity, fibromyalgias, osteoarthritis. A *popliteal or "baker's" cyst* from distention of the gastrocnemius semimembranosus bursa

Three further tests will help you detect fluid in the knee joint.

■ The *Bulge Sign* (*for minor effusions*). With the knee extended, place the left hand above the knee and apply pressure on the suprapatellar pouch, displacing or "milking" fluid downward. Stroke downward on the medial aspect of the knee and apply pressure to force fluid into the lateral area. Tap the knee just behind the lateral margin of the patella with the right hand.

A fluid wave or bulge on the medial side between the patella and the femur is considered a positive bulge sign consistent with an effusion.

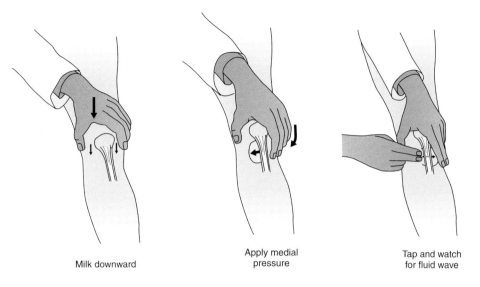

Milk downward

Apply medial pressure

Tap and watch for fluid wave

- The *Balloon Sign (for major effusions)*. Place the thumb and index finger of your right hand on each side of the patella; with the left hand, compress the suprapatellar pouch against the femur. Feel for fluid entering (or ballooning into) the spaces next to the patella under your right thumb and index finger.

When the knee joint contains a large effusion, suprapatellar compression ejects fluid into the spaces adjacent to the patella. A palpable fluid wave signifies a positive "balloon sign." A returning fluid wave into the suprapatellar pouch confirms an effusion.

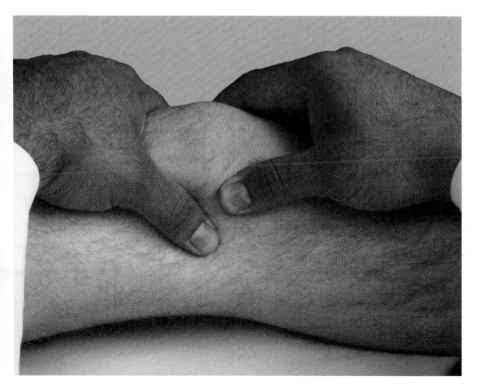

■ *Ballotting the patella*. To assess large effusions, you can also compress the suprapatellar pouch and "ballotte" or push the patella sharply against the femur. Watch for fluid returning to the suprapatellar pouch.

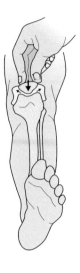

Palpable fluid returning into the pouch further confirms the presence of a large effusion.

A palpable patellar click with compression may also occur, but yields more false positives.

RANGE OF MOTION AND MANEUVERS

The principal movements of the knee are flexion, extension, and internal and external rotation. Ask the patient to flex and extend the knee while sitting. To check internal and external rotation, instruct the patient to rotate the foot medially and laterally. Knee flexion and extension can also be assessed by asking the patient to squat and stand up—provide support if needed to maintain balance.

Crepitus uteri flexion and extension in osteoarthritis (Altman; Cibere).

You will often need to test ligamentous stability and integrity of the menisci, particularly when there is a history of trauma or palpable tenderness.[30,31] Always examine both knees and compare findings.

■ *Techniques for Examining the Knee*

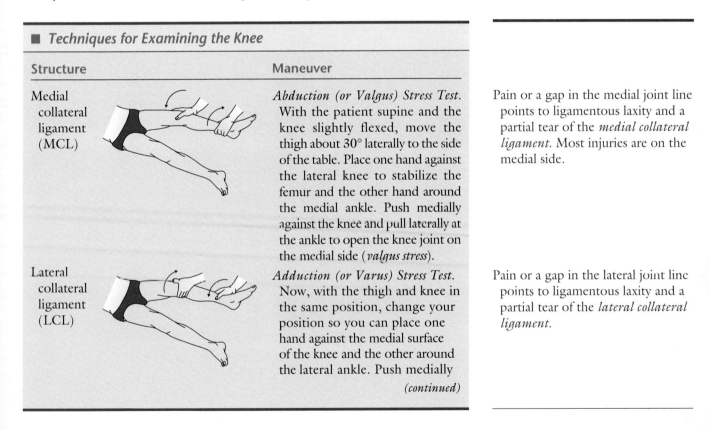

Structure		Maneuver
Medial collateral ligament (MCL)		*Abduction (or Valgus) Stress Test.* With the patient supine and the knee slightly flexed, move the thigh about 30° laterally to the side of the table. Place one hand against the lateral knee to stabilize the femur and the other hand around the medial ankle. Push medially against the knee and pull laterally at the ankle to open the knee joint on the medial side (*valgus stress*).
Lateral collateral ligament (LCL)		*Adduction (or Varus) Stress Test.* Now, with the thigh and knee in the same position, change your position so you can place one hand against the medial surface of the knee and the other around the lateral ankle. Push medially *(continued)*

Pain or a gap in the medial joint line points to ligamentous laxity and a partial tear of the *medial collateral ligament.* Most injuries are on the medial side.

Pain or a gap in the lateral joint line points to ligamentous laxity and a partial tear of the *lateral collateral ligament.*

■ *Techniques for Examining the Knee (Continued)*

Structure	Maneuver	
	against the knee and pull laterally at the ankle to open the knee joint on the lateral side (*varus stress*).	
Anterior cruciate ligament (ACL)	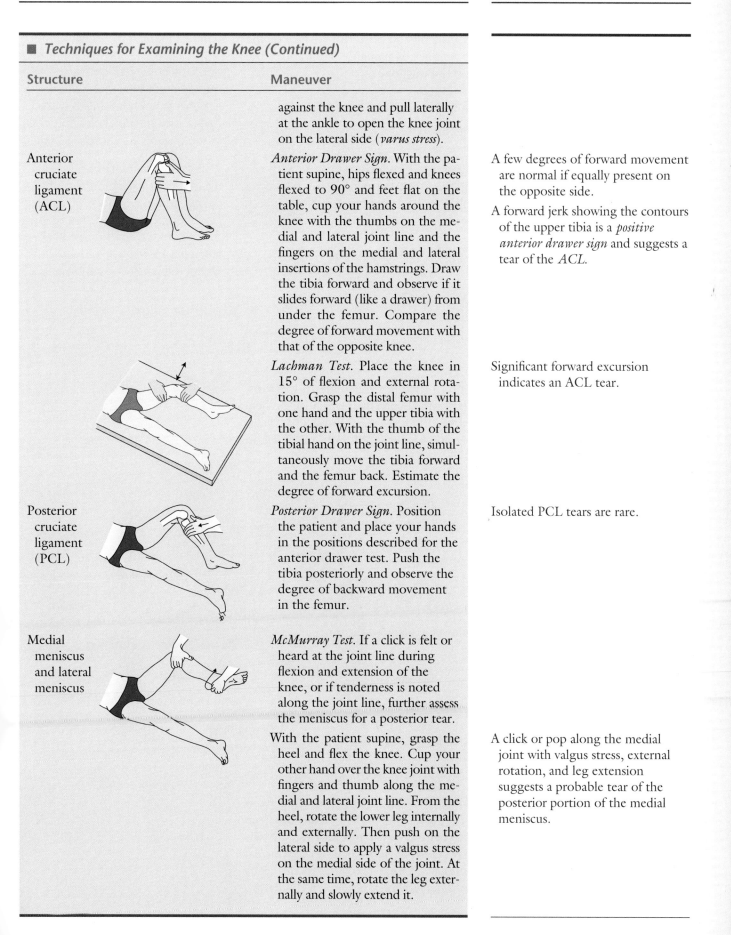 *Anterior Drawer Sign.* With the patient supine, hips flexed and knees flexed to 90° and feet flat on the table, cup your hands around the knee with the thumbs on the medial and lateral joint line and the fingers on the medial and lateral insertions of the hamstrings. Draw the tibia forward and observe if it slides forward (like a drawer) from under the femur. Compare the degree of forward movement with that of the opposite knee.	A few degrees of forward movement are normal if equally present on the opposite side. A forward jerk showing the contours of the upper tibia is a *positive anterior drawer sign* and suggests a tear of the *ACL*.
	Lachman Test. Place the knee in 15° of flexion and external rotation. Grasp the distal femur with one hand and the upper tibia with the other. With the thumb of the tibial hand on the joint line, simultaneously move the tibia forward and the femur back. Estimate the degree of forward excursion.	Significant forward excursion indicates an ACL tear.
Posterior cruciate ligament (PCL)	*Posterior Drawer Sign.* Position the patient and place your hands in the positions described for the anterior drawer test. Push the tibia posteriorly and observe the degree of backward movement in the femur.	Isolated PCL tears are rare.
Medial meniscus and lateral meniscus	*McMurray Test.* If a click is felt or heard at the joint line during flexion and extension of the knee, or if tenderness is noted along the joint line, further assess the meniscus for a posterior tear. With the patient supine, grasp the heel and flex the knee. Cup your other hand over the knee joint with fingers and thumb along the medial and lateral joint line. From the heel, rotate the lower leg internally and externally. Then push on the lateral side to apply a valgus stress on the medial side of the joint. At the same time, rotate the leg externally and slowly extend it.	A click or pop along the medial joint with valgus stress, external rotation, and leg extension suggests a probable tear of the posterior portion of the medial meniscus.

Palpate the *gastrocnemius* and *soleus muscles* on the posterior surface of the lower leg. Their common tendon, the Achilles, is palpable from about the lower third of the calf to its insertion on the calcaneus.

A defect in the muscles with tenderness and swelling in a *ruptured Achilles tendon;* tenderness and thickening of the tendon above the calcaneus, sometimes with a protuberant posterolateral bony process of the calcaneus in *Achilles tendinitis*

To test the integrity of the *Achilles tendon,* place the patient prone with the knee and ankle flexed at 90°, or alternatively, ask the patient to kneel on a chair. Squeeze the calf and watch for plantar flexion at the ankle.

Absence of plantar flexion is a positive test indicating rupture of the Achilles tendon. Sudden severe pain "like a gunshot wound," an ecchymosis from the calf into the heel, and a flat-footed gait with absence of "toe-off" may also be present.

◥ THE ANKLE AND FOOT

OVERVIEW

The total weight of the body is transmitted through the ankle to the foot. The ankle and foot must balance the body and absorb the impact of the heel strike and gait. Despite thick padding along the toes, sole, and heel and stabilizing ligaments at the ankles, the ankle and foot are frequent sites of sprain and bony injury.

BONY STRUCTURES AND JOINTS

The ankle is a hinge joint formed by the *tibia,* the *fibula,* and the *talus.* The tibia and fibula act as a mortise, stabilizing the joint while bracing the talus like an inverted cup.

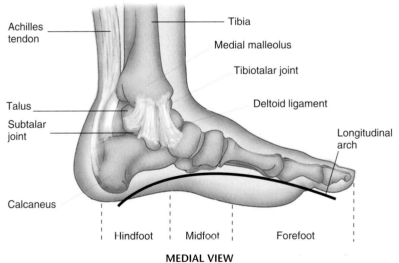

MEDIAL VIEW

The principal joints of the ankle are the *tibiotalar joint,* between the tibia and the talus, and the *subtalar (talocalcaneal) joint.*

Note the principal landmarks of the ankle: the *medial malleolus,* the bony prominence at the distal end of the tibia, and the *lateral malleolus,* at the distal end of the fibula. Lodged under the talus and jutting posteriorly is the *calcaneus,* or heel.

An imaginary line, the *longitudinal arch,* spans the foot, extending from the calcaneus of the hind foot along the tarsal bones of the midfoot (see cuneiforms, navicular, and cuboid bones below) to the forefoot metatarsals and toes. The *heads of the metatarsals* are palpable in the ball of the foot. In the forefoot, identify the *metatarsophalangeal joints,* proximal to the webs of the toes, and the *proximal and distal interphalangeal joints* of the toes.

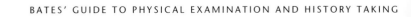

MUSCLE GROUPS AND ADDITIONAL STRUCTURES

Movement at the ankle joint is limited to dorsiflexion and plantar flexion. *Plantar flexion* is powered by the gastrocnemius, the posterior tibial muscle, and the toe flexors. Their tendons run behind the malleoli. The *dorsiflexors* include the anterior tibial muscle and the toe extensors. They lie prominently on the anterior surface, or dorsum, of the ankle, anterior to the malleoli.

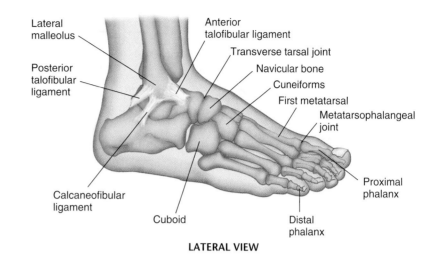

LATERAL VIEW

Ligaments extend from each malleolus onto the foot. Medially, the triangle-shaped *deltoid ligament* fans out from the inferior surface of the medial malleolus to the talus and proximal tarsal bones, protecting against stress from eversion (ankle bows inward). The three ligaments on the lateral side are less substantial, with higher risk for injury: the *anterior talofibular ligament*—most at risk in injury from inversion (ankle bows outward) injuries; the *calcaneofibular ligament*; and the *posterior talofibular ligament*. The strong Achilles tendon inserts on the heel posteriorly. The plantar fascia inserts on the medial tubercle of the calcaneus.

TECHNIQUES OF EXAMINATION

INSPECTION

Observe all surfaces of the ankles and feet, noting any deformities, nodules, or swellings, and any calluses or corns.

See Table 15-9, Abnormalities of the Feet and Toes (p. 570) and Table 15-10, Abnormalities of the Toes and Soles (p. 571).

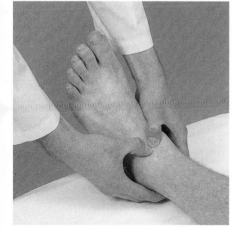

PALPATION

With your thumbs, palpate the anterior aspect of each *ankle joint*, noting any bogginess, swelling, or tenderness.

Localized tenderness in arthritis, ligamentous injury, or infection of the ankle

Feel along the *Achilles tendon* for nodules and tenderness.

Rheumatoid nodules; tenderness in Achilles tendinitis, bursitis, or partial tear from trauma

Palpate the heel, especially the posterior and inferior calcaneus, and the plantar fascia for tenderness.

Bone spurs may be present on the calcaneus. Focal heel pain on palpation of the plantar fascia suggests *plantar fasciitis;* seen in prolonged standing or heel-strike exercise, also in rheumatoid arthritis, gout.[32,33]

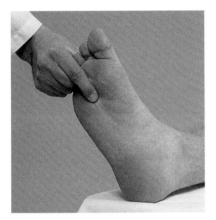

Palpate the *metatarsophalangeal joints* for tenderness. Compress the forefoot between the thumb and fingers. Exert pressure just proximal to the heads of the 1st and 5th metatarsals.

Tenderness on compression is an early sign of *rheumatoid arthritis.* Acute inflammation of the first metatarsophalangeal joint is associated with gout.

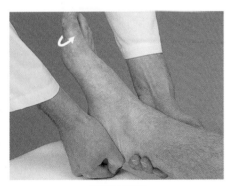

Palpate the heads of the five metatarsals and the grooves between them with your thumb and index finger. Place your thumb on the dorsum of the foot and your index finger on the plantar surface.

Pain and tenderness, called *metatarsalgia,* seen in trauma, arthritis, vascular compromise

Tenderness over the 3rd and 4th metatarsal heads on the plantar surface in Morton's neuroma (see p. 570).

RANGE OF MOTION AND MANEUVERS

Range of motion at the ankle includes *flexion* and *extension at the ankle (tibiotalar) joint* and, *in the foot, inversion* and *eversion* at the subtalar and transverse tarsal joints.

- *The Ankle (Tibiotalar) Joint.* Dorsiflex and plantar flex the foot at the ankle.

Pain during movements of the ankle and the foot helps to localize possible arthritis.

- *The Subtalar (Talocalcaneal) Joint.* Stabilize the ankle with one hand, grasp the heel with the other, and invert and evert the foot.

An arthritic joint is frequently painful when moved in any direction, whereas a ligamentous sprain produces maximal pain when the ligament is stretched. For example, in a common form of sprained ankle, inversion and plantar flexion of the foot cause pain, whereas eversion and plantar flexion are relatively pain free.

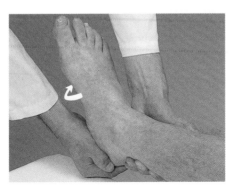

INVERSION   **EVERSION**

- *The Transverse Tarsal Joint.* Stabilize the heel and invert and evert the forefoot.

- *The Metatarsophalangeal Joints.* Flex the toes in relation to the feet.

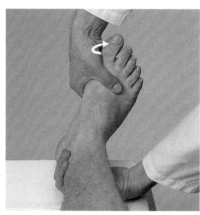

INVERSION

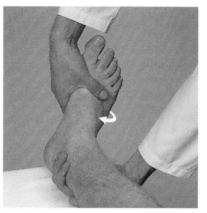

EVERSION

■ SPECIAL TECHNIQUES

For Carpal Tunnel Syndrome. Pain and numbness on the ventral surface of the first three digits of the hand (but not in the palm), especially at night, suggest median nerve compression in the carpal tunnel, which lies between the carpal bones dorsally and a ventral band of more superficial fascia, the *flexor retinaculum.*

Appropriate symptoms and objective loss of sensation on the ventral surface of the hand in the distribution of the median nerve (see p. 528), and *weak abduction of the thumb* on muscle strength testing are the most helpful for making the diagnosis.[34] Two additional clinical tests are also used—when positive, Tinel's test appears more likely to be confirmed by further diagnostic testing.[35]

Onset often related to repetitive motion with wrists flexed (e.g., keyboard use, mail-sorting), pregnancy, rheumatoid arthritis, diabetes, hypothyroidism

Thenar atrophy may also be present.

Thumb Abduction. Ask the patient to raise the thumb perpendicular to the palm as you apply downward pressure on the distal phalanx. (This maneuver reliably tests the strength of the abductor pollicis brevis, which is innervated only by the median nerve.)

Tinel's Sign. With your finger, percuss lightly over the course of the median nerve in the carpal tunnel at the spot indicated by the arrow.

Tingling or electric sensations in the distribution of the median nerve constitute a positive test, suggesting *carpal tunnel syndrome.*

Phalen's Test. Hold the patient's wrists in acute flexion for 60 seconds. Alternatively, ask the patient to press the backs of both hands together to form right angles. These maneuvers compress the median nerve.

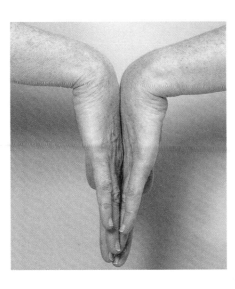

If numbness and tingling develop over the distribution of the median nerve (e.g., the palmar surface of the thumb, and the index, middle, and part of the ring fingers), the sign is positive, suggesting *carpal tunnel syndrome.*

For Low Back Pain With Radiation Into the Leg. If the patient has noted low back pain that radiates down the leg, check straight leg raising on each side in turn. The patient should be supine. Raise the patient's relaxed and straightened leg until pain occurs. Then dorsiflex the foot.

Record the degree of elevation at which pain occurs, the quality and distribution of the pain, and the effects of dorsiflexion. Tightness and mild discomfort in the hamstrings with these maneuvers are common and do not indicate radicular pain.

Sharp pain radiating from the back down the leg in an L5 or S1 distribution (*radicular pain*) highly suggestive of compression of the nerve root(s), typically due to a herniated lumbar disc.[1] Dorsiflexion of the foot increases the pain. Increased pain in the affected leg when the opposite leg is raised strongly confirms radicular pain and constitutes a positive *crossed straight leg-raising sign.*

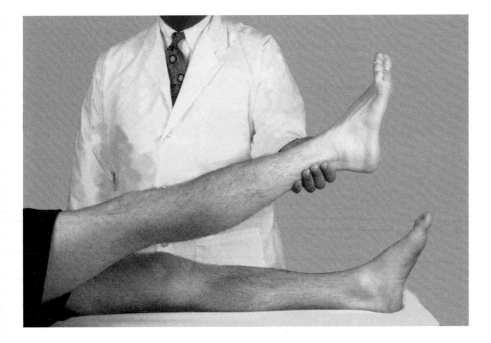

Examine the patient neurologically, focusing on the motor and sensory function and the reflexes at the lumbosacral levels. These are outlined in the next chapter.

See Table 15-1, Low Back Pain (p. 560).

Measuring the Length of Legs.   If you suspect that the patient's legs are unequal in length, measure them. Get the patient relaxed in the supine position and symmetrically aligned with legs extended. With a tape, measure the distance between the anterior superior iliac spine and the medial malleolus. The tape should cross the knee on its medial side.

Unequal leg length may explain a scoliosis.

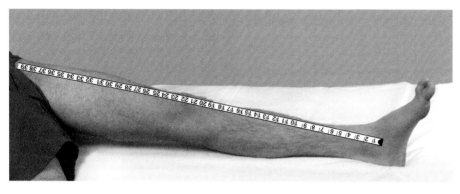

Describing Limited Motion of a Joint.   Although measurement of motion is seldom necessary, limitations can be described in degrees. Pocket goniometers are available for this purpose. In the two examples shown below, the red lines indicate the range of the patient's movement, and the black lines suggest the normal range.

Observations may be described in several ways. The numbers in parentheses are suitably abbreviated recordings.

A. The elbow flexes from 45° to 90° (45° → 90°),

          -or-

    The elbow has a flexion deformity of 45° and can be flexed farther to 90° (45° → 90°).

B. Supination at elbow = 30° (0° → 30°)
Pronation at elbow = 45° (0° → 45°)

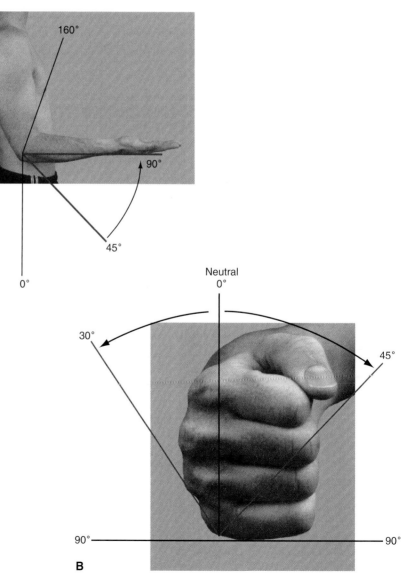

RECORDING YOUR FINDINGS

The examples below contain phrases appropriate for most write-ups. Note that use of the anatomical terms specific to the structure and function of individual joint problems makes your write-up of musculoskeletal findings more meaningful and informative.

Recording the Examination—The Musculoskeletal System

"Good range of motion in all joints. No evidence of swelling or deformity."

OR

"Good range of motion in all joints. Hand with degenerative changes of Heberden's nodes at the distal interphalangeal joints, Bouchard's nodes at proximal interphalangeal joints. Mild pain with flexion, extension, and rotation of both hips. Good range of motion in the knees, with moderate crepitus; no effusion but boggy synovium and osteophytes along the tibiofemoral joint line bilaterally. Both feet with hallux valgus at the first metatarsophalangeal joints."

OR

"Right knee with moderate effusion and tenderness over medial meniscus along the joint line. Moderate laxity of anterior cruciate ligament (ACL) on anterior drawer test; posterior cruciate ligament (PCL) and medial and lateral collateral ligaments (MCL, LCL) intact—no posterior drawer sign or tenderness with varus or valgus stress. Patellar tendon intact—patient able to extend lower extremity. All other joints with good range of motion, no other deformity or swelling."

Suggests osteoarthritis

Suggests partial tear of medial meniscus and ACL, possibly from sports injury or trauma

---

Bibliography

CITATIONS

1. Atlas SJ, Deyo RA. Evaluating and managing acute low back pain in the primary care setting. J Gen Intern Med 16(2): 120–131, 2001.
2. Sakane T, Takleno M, Suzuki N, et al. Behcet's disease. N Engl J Med 341(17):1284–1291, 1999.
3. U.S. Preventive Services Task Force. Behavioral Counseling in Primary Care to Promote Physical Activity: Recommendations and Rationale. Rockville, MD, Agency for Healthcare Research and Quality, July 2002. Available at: http://www.ahrq.gov/clinic/3rduspstf/physactivity/physactrr.htm. Accessed January 15, 2005.
4. U.S. Preventive Services Task Force. Counseling to Prevent Low Back Pain, Chapter 60, Guide to Clinical Preventive Services, 2nd ed., Baltimore, Williams & Wilkins. 699–709, 1996.
5. U.S. Preventive Services Task Force. Primary Care Interventions to Prevent Low Back Pain in Adults: Recommendation Statement. Rockville, MD, Agency for Healthcare Research

and Quality, February 2004. Available at: http://www.ahrq.gov/clinic/3rduspstf/lowback/lowbackrs.htm. Accessed January 15, 2005.
6. Staal JB, Hlobil H, Twoisk JWR, et al. Graded activity for low back pain in occupational health care. Ann Intern Med 140(2): 77–84, 2004.
7. U.S. Preventive Services Task Force. Counseling to prevent household and recreational injuries. In Guide to Clinical Preventive Services, 2nd ed. Baltimore, Williams & Wilkins. 659–686, 1996.
8. National Institutes of Health Osteoporosis and Related Bone Disease National Resource Center. Osteoporosis Overview–Facts and Figures. Revised January 2003. Available at: http://www.osteo.org. Accessed January 15, 2005.
9. NIH Consensus Development Panel on Osteoporosis Prevention, Diagnosis, and Therapy—Consensus Conference. Osteoporosis prevention, diagnosis, and therapy. JAMA 285(6): 785–795, 2001.
10. Nelson HD, Helfand M, Woolf SH, et al. Screening for postmenopausal osteoporosis: summary of the evidence. [Originally in Ann Intern Med 2002;137:529–541.] Rockville, MD,

BIBLIOGRAPHY

Agency for Healthcare Research and Quality. Available at: http://www.ahrq.gov/clinic/3rduspstf/osteoporosis/osteosumm1.htm. Accessed January 15, 2005.

11. U.S. Preventive Services Task Force. Screening for Osteoporosis in Postmenopausal Women: Recommendations and Rationale. Rockville, MD, Agency for Healthcare Research and Quality, September 2002. Available at: http://www.ahrq.gov/clinic/3rduspstf/osteoporosis/osteorr.htm. Accessed January 15, 2005.

12. Margolis KL, Ensrud KE, Schreiner PJ, et al. Body size and risk for clinical fractures in older women. Ann Intern Med 133(2):123–127, 2000.

13. Hulley S, Grady D, Bush T, et al. Randomized trial of estrogen plus progestin for secondary prevention of coronary heart disease in postmenopausal women. Heart and Estrogen/Progestin Replacement Study (HERS) Research Group. JAMA 280(7):605–613, 1998.

14. Writing Group for the Women's Health Initiative Investigators. Risks and benefits of estrogen plus progestin in healthy postmenopausal women: principal results from the Women's Health Initiative randomized controlled trial. JAMA 288:321–333, 2002.

15. Women's Health Initiative Steering Committee. Effects of conjugated equine estrogen in postmenopausal women with hysterectomy: the Women's Health Initiative randomized controlled trial. JAMA 291:1701–1712, 2004.

16. U.S. Preventive Services Task Force. Hormone Replacement Therapy for Primary Prevention of Chronic Conditions: Recommendations and Rationale. Rockville, MD, Agency for Healthcare Research and Quality, October 2002. Available at: http://www.ahrq.gov/clinic/3rduspstf/hrt/hrtrr.htm. Accessed January 15, 2005.

17. Greenspan SL, Emkey RD, Bone HG, et al. Significant differential effects of alendronate, estrogen, or combination therapy on the rate of bone loss after discontinuation of treatment of postmenopausal osteoporosis. Ann Intern Med 137(11):875–883, 2002.

18. American College of Rheumatology Ad Hoc Committee on Clinical Guidelines. Guidelines for the initial evaluation of the adult patient with acute musculoskeletal symptoms. Arthritis Rheum 39(1):1–8, 1996.

19. Arnett FC, Edworthy SM, Bloch DA, et al. The American Rheumatism Association 1987 revised criteria for the classification of rheumatoid arthritis. Arthritis Rheum 31:315–324, 1988.

20. Goldring SR. A 55-year-old woman with rheumatoid arthritis. JAMA 283(4):524–529, 2000.

21. Lee DM, Weinblatt ME. Rheumatoid arthritis. Lancet 358:903–911, 2001.

22. Woodward TW, Best TM. The painful shoulder. Part II. Acute and chronic disorders. Am Fam Physician 61(11):3291–3300, 2000.

23. Liume JJ, Verhagen AP, Meidema HS, et al. Does this patient have an instability of the shoulder or a labrum lesion? The rational clinical examination. JAMA 292:1989–1999, 2004.

24. Burkhardt SS. A 26-year-old woman with shoulder pain. JAMA 284(12):1559–1567, 2000.

25. Woodward TW, Best TM. The painful shoulder. Part I. Clinical evaluation. Am Fam Physician 61(10):3079–3088, 2000.

26. Anderson BC. Office Orthopedics for Primary Care: Diagnosis and Treatment, 2nd ed. Philadelphia, WB Saunders, 1999.

27. Haywood KL, Garratt AM, Jordan K, et al. Spinal mobility in ankylosing spondylitis: reliability, validity and responsiveness. Rheumatology 43:750–757, 2004.

28. Altman R, Asch E, Bloch D, et al. Development of criteria for the classification and reporting of osteoarthritis. Classification of osteoarthritis of the knee. Arthritis Rheum 29(8):1039–1049, 1986.

29. Cibere J, Bellamy N, Thorne A, et al. Reliability of the knee examination in osteoarthritis. Arthritis Rheum 50(2):458–468, 2004.

30. Solomon DH, Simel DL, Bates DW, et al. Does this patient have a torn meniscus or ligament of the knee? Value of the physical examination. The rational physical examination. JAMA 286:1610–1620, 2001.

31. Jackson JL, O'Malley PG, Kroenke K. Evaluation of acute knee pain in primary care. Ann Intern Med 139(7):575–588, 2003.

32. Young CC, Rutherford DS, Niedfeldt MW. Treatment of plantar fasciitis. Am Fam Physician 63:467–474, 477–478, 2001.

33. Buchbinder R. Plantar Fasciitis. N Engl J Med 350(21):2159–2166, 2004.

34. D'Arcy CA, McGee S. Does this patient have carpal tunnel syndrome? The rational clinical examination. JAMA 283(23):3110–3117, 2000.

35. Katz JN, Simmons BP. Carpal tunnel syndrome. N Engl J Med 346(23):1807–1811, 2002.

36. Goldenberg DL, Burckhardt C, Crofford L. Management of fibromyalgia syndrome. JAMA 292(19):2388–2395, 2004.

37. Levanthal LJ. Management of fibromyalgia. Ann Intern Med 131(11):850–858, 1999.

38. Wolfe F, Smythe HA, Yunus MB, et al. The American College of Rheumatology 1990 Criteria for the Classification of Fibromyalgia. Report of the Multicenter Criteria Committee. Arthritis Rheum 33(2):160–172, 1990.

ADDITIONAL REFERENCES

Deyo RA, Rainville J, Kent DL. What can the history and physical examination tell us about low back pain? JAMA 268(6):760–765, 1992.

Gerritsen AAM, de Vet HCW, Scholten RJPM et al. Splinting vs surgery in the treatment of carpal tunnel syndrome. A randomized controlled trial. JAMA 288(10):1245–1251, 2002.

Greene WB, American Academy of Orthopaedic Surgeons, American Academy of Pediatrics Essentials of Musculoskeletal Care, 2nd ed. Rosemont, IL, American Academy of Orthopaedic Surgeons, 2001.

Harris ED, Kelley WN. Kelley's Textbook of Rheumatology, 7th ed. Philadelphia, Elsevier Saunders, 2005.

Hoppenfeld S, Hutton R. Physical Examination of the Spine and Extremities. New York, Appleton-Century-Crofts, 1976.

Koopman WJ, Moreland LW. Arthritis and Allied Conditions: A Textbook of Rheumatology, 15th ed. Philadelphia, Lippincott Williams & Wilkins, 2005.

Lew DP, Waldvogel FA. Osteomyelitis. N Engl J Med 336(14):999–1007, 1997.

Murrell GAC, Walton JR. Diagnosis of rotator cuff tears. Lancet 357(9258):769–770, 2001.

TABLE 15-1   **Low Back Pain**

Patterns	Possible Causes	Possible Physical Signs
Mechanical Low Back Pain Acute, often recurrent, or possibly chronic aching pain in the lumbosacral area, possibly radiating into the posterior thighs but not below the knees. Often precipitated or aggravated by moving, lifting, or twisting motions and relieved by rest. Spinal movement typically limited by pain. Common from the teenage years through the 40s.	Causes cannot usually be proven; include intervertebral disc disease, congenital disorders of the spine, such as spondylolisthesis, in older women or people on long-term corticosteroid therapy, osteoporosis complicated by a collapsed vertebra.	Local tenderness, muscle spasm, pain on movement of the back, and loss of the normal lumbar lordosis, but no motor or sensory loss or reflex abnormalities. In osteoporosis there may be a thoracic kyphosis, percussion tenderness over a spinous process, or fractures elsewhere such as in the thoracic spine or in a hip.
Radicular Low Back Pain A radicular nerve root pain, usually superimposed on low back pain. The sciatic pain is shooting and radiates down one or both legs, usually to below the knee(s) in a dermatomal distribution, often with associated numbness and tingling and possibly local weakness. The pain is usually worsened by spinal movement such as bending and by sneezing, coughing, or straining.[1]	A *herniated intervertebral disc* with compression or traction of nerve root(s) is the most common cause in persons ≤ age 50. Nerve roots of L5 or S1 are most often affected. Spinal cord tumors or abscesses are much less common and tend to affect more nerve roots, producing more neurologic deficits.	Pain on straight leg raising (see p. 556), tenderness of the sciatic nerve, loss of sensation in a dermatomal distribution, local muscular weakness and atrophy, and decreased to absent reflex(es), especially affecting the ankle jerks. Dermatomal signs and reflex changes may be absent when only a single root is affected.
Back and Leg Pain From Lumbar Spinal Stenosis Pseudoclaudication is a pain in the back or legs that worsens with walking and improves with flexing of the spine, as by sitting or bending forward.	*Lumbar stenosis,* or a combination of degenerative disc disease and osteoarthritis that narrows the spinal canal and impinges on the spinal nerves, often after age 60.	Posture may become flexed forward, with motor weakness and hyporeflexia in the lower extremities.
Chronic Persistent Low Back Stiffness	*Ankylosing spondylitis,* a chronic inflammatory polyarthritis, most common in young men	Loss of the normal lumbar lordosis, muscle spasm, and limitation of anterior and lateral flexion
	Diffuse idiopathic skeletal hyperostosis (DISH), which affects middle-aged and older men	Flexion and immobility of the spine
Aching Nocturnal Back Pain, Unrelieved by Rest	Consider *metastatic malignancy* in the spine from cancer of the prostate, breast, lung, thyroid, and kidney, and multiple myeloma.	Variable with the source. Local bone tenderness may be present
Back Pain Referred From the Abdomen or Pelvis Usually a deep, aching pain; the level varies with the source	Peptic ulcer, pancreatitis, pancreatic cancer, chronic prostatitis, endometriosis, dissecting aortic aneurysm, retroperitoneal tumor, and other causes	Spinal movements are not painful and range of motion is not affected. Look for signs of the primary disorder.

TABLE 15-2	Pains in the Neck	

Patterns	Possible Causes	Possible Physical Signs
"Simple Stiff Neck" Acute, episodic, localized pain in the neck, often appearing on awakening and lasting 1–4 days. No dermatomal radiation	Mechanisms are not understood.	Local muscular tenderness and pain from certain movements
Aching Neck A persistent dull aching in the back of the neck, often spreading to the occiput. Common from postural strain, as in prolonged typing or studying; may also accompany tension and depression.	Poorly understood; may be related to sustained muscle contraction	Local muscular tenderness. When areas of pain and tenderness are also present elsewhere in the body, consider the fibromyalgia syndrome (see Table 15-3, Patterns of Pain In and Around the Joints).
"Cervical Sprain" Acute and often recurrent neck pains that are often more severe and last longer than simple stiff neck. There may be a precipitating factor such as a whiplash injury, heavy lifting, or a sudden movement, but there is no dermatomal radiation.	Poorly understood	Local tenderness and pain on movement
Neck Pain With Dermatomal Radiation Neck pain as in cervical sprain, but with radiation of the pain to the shoulder, back, or arm in a dermatomal distribution. This radicular pain is typically sharp, burning, or tingling in quality.	Compression of one or more nerve roots caused by either a herniated cervical disc or degenerative disease of the intervertebral discs with bony spurring*	Muscle tenderness and spasm, limited range of neck motion, increase in pain on coughing or straining, and possible sensory loss, weakness, muscular atrophy, and decreased reflexes in the areas involved
Neck Pain From Possible Compression of the Cervical Spinal Cord Associated here is weakness or paralysis of the legs, often with a decrease in or loss of sensation. These symptoms may occur in addition to the radicular symptoms or by themselves. Neck pain may be mild or even absent.	Compression of the spinal cord in the neck caused by either a herniated cervical disc or degenerative disease of the intervertebral discs with bony spurring. Trauma may also be the cause.*	Limited range of motion in the neck, weakness or paralysis in the legs of the central nervous system type, Babinski responses, loss of position and vibration sense in the legs, and, less commonly, loss of pain and temperature sensation. Radicular signs in the arms may also be present.

* Tumors or abscesses of the cervical spinal cord, though less common, should also be considered.

TABLE 15-3   Patterns of Pain In and Around the Joints

Problem	Process	Common Locations	Pattern of Spread	Onset	Progression and Duration
Rheumatoid Arthritis	Chronic inflammation of *synovial membranes* with secondary erosion of adjacent cartilage and bone, and damage to ligaments and tendons	Hands (proximal interphalangeal and metacarpophalangeal joints), feet (metatarsophalangeal joints), wrists, knees, elbows, ankles	Symmetrically additive: progresses to other joints while persisting in the initial ones	Usually insidious	Often chronic, with remissions and exacerbations
Osteoarthritis (*degenerative joint disease*)	Degeneration and progressive loss of *cartilage* within the joints, damage to underlying bone, and formation of new bone at the margins of the cartilage	Knees, hips, hands (distal, sometimes proximal interphalangeal joints), cervical and lumbar spine, and wrists (first carpometacarpal joint); also joints previously injured or diseased	Additive; however, only one joint may be involved.	Usually insidious	Slowly progressive, with temporary exacerbations after periods of overuse
Gouty Arthritis *Acute Gout*	An inflammatory reaction to microcrystals of sodium urate	Base of the big toe (the first metatarsophalangeal joint), the instep or dorsum of feet, the ankles, knees, and elbows	Early attacks are usually confined to one joint.	Sudden, often at night, often after injury, surgery, fasting, or excessive food or alcohol intake	Occasional isolated attacks lasting days up to 2 weeks; they may get more frequent and severe, with persisting symptoms.
Chronic Tophaceous Gout	Multiple local accumulations of sodium urate in the joints and other tissues (tophi), with or without inflammation	Feet, ankles, wrists, fingers, and elbows	Additive, not so symmetric as rheumatoid arthritis	Gradual development of chronicity with repeated attacks	Chronic symptoms with acute exacerbations
Polymyalgia Rheumatica	A disease of unclear nature in people older than 50, especially women; may be associated with giant cell arteritis	Muscles of the hip girdle and shoulder girdle; symmetric		Insidious or abrupt, even appearing overnight	Chronic but ultimately self-limiting
Fibromyalgia Syndrome[36-38]	Widespread musculoskeletal pain and tender points. May accompany other diseases. Mechanisms unclear	"All over," but especially in the neck, shoulders, hands, low back, and knees	Shifts unpredictably or worsens in response to immobility, excessive use, or chilling	Variable	Chronic, with "ups and downs"

The vagueness of these characteristics is in itself a clue to the fibromyalgia syndrome.

Associated Symptoms

Swelling	Redness, Warmth, and Tenderness	Stiffness	Limitation of Motion	Generalized Symptoms
Frequent swelling of synovial tissue in joints or tendon sheaths; also subcutaneous nodules	Tender, often warm, but seldom red	Prominent, often for an hour or more in the mornings, also after inactivity	Often develops	Weakness, fatigue, weight loss, and low fever are common.
Small effusions in the joints may be present, especially in the knees; also bony enlargement.	Possibly tender, seldom warm, and rarely red	Frequent but brief (usually 5–10 min), in the morning and after inactivity	Often develops	Usually absent
Present, within and around the involved joint	Exquisitely tender, hot, and red	Not evident	Motion is limited primarily by pain.	Fever may be present.
Present, as tophi, in joints, bursae, and subcutaneous tissues	Tenderness, warmth, and redness may be present during exacerbations.	Present	Present	Possibly fever; patient may also develop symptoms of renal failure and renal stones.
None	Muscles often tender, but not warm or red	Prominent, especially in the morning	Usually none	Malaise, a sense of depression, possibly anorexia, weight loss, and fever, but no true weakness
None	Multiple specific and symmetric tender "trigger points," often not recognized until the examination	Present, especially in the morning	Absent, though stiffness is greater at the extremes of movement	A disturbance of sleep, usually associated with morning fatigue

TABLE 15-4   Painful Shoulders[22,25]

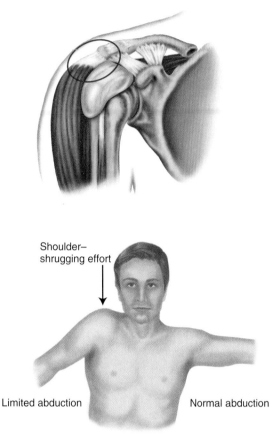

Rotator Cuff Tendinitis

Repeated shoulder motion, as in throwing or swimming, can cause edema and hemorrhage followed by inflammation, most commonly involving the supraspinatus tendon. Acute, recurrent, or chronic pain may result, often aggravated by activity. Patients may report sharp catches of pain, grating, and weakness when lifting the arm overhead. When the supraspinatus tendon is involved, tenderness is maximal just below the tip of the acromion. Patients are typically athletically active.

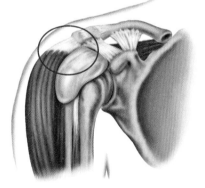

Shoulder–shrugging effort

Limited abduction   Normal abduction

Rotator Cuff Tears

When the arm is raised in forward flexion, the rotator cuff may impinge against the undersurface of the acromion and the coracoacromial ligament. Injury from a fall or repeated impingement may weaken the rotator cuff, causing a partial or complete tear, usually after age 40. Weakness, atrophy of the supraspinatus and infraspinatus muscles, pain, and tenderness may ensue. In a complete tear of the supraspinatus tendon (illustrated), active abduction and forward flexion at the glenohumeral joint is severely impaired, producing a characteristic shrugging of the shoulder and a positive "drop arm" test (see p. 518).

Calcific Tendinitis

Calcific tendinitis refers to a degenerative process in the tendon associated with the deposition of calcium salts. Usually involves the supraspinatus tendon. Acute, disabling attacks of shoulder pain may occur, usually in patients older than 30 years and more often in women. The arm is held close to the side, and all motions are severely limited by pain. Tenderness is maximal below the tip of the acromion. The subacromial bursa, which overlies the supraspinatus tendon, may be inflamed. Chronic, less severe pain may also occur.

(table continues next page)

TABLE 15-4   Painful Shoulders[22,25] *(Continued)*

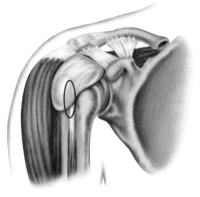

Bicipital Tendinitis

Inflammation of the long head of the biceps tendon and its sheath causes anterior shoulder pain that may resemble rotator cuff tendinitis and may coexist with it. Often this is a sign of shoulder instability. This tendon, like the cuff, may suffer impingement injury. Tenderness is maximal in the bicipital groove. By externally rotating and abducting the arm, you can more easily separate this area from the subacromial tenderness of supraspinatus tendinitis. With the patient's arm at the side, elbow flexed to 90°, ask the patient to supinate the forearm against your resistance. Increased pain in the bicipital groove confirms this condition.

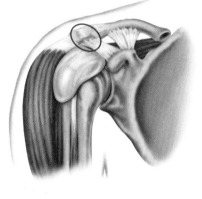

Acromioclavicular Arthritis

Acromioclavicular arthritis is not a common cause of shoulder pain. When present, it usually is the result of direct injury to the shoulder girdle with resulting degenerative changes. Tenderness is localized over the acromioclavicular joint. Although motion in the glenohumeral joint is not painful in acromioclavicular arthritis, as it is in many other painful conditions of the shoulder, movements of the scapula, such as shoulder shrugging, are.

Adhesive Capsulitis (Frozen Shoulder)

Adhesive capsulitis refers to a mysterious fibrosis of the glenohumeral joint capsule, manifested by diffuse, dull, aching pain in the shoulder and progressive restriction of active and passive range of motion, but usually no localized tenderness. The condition is usually unilateral and occurs in people aged 50 to 70. There is often an antecedent painful disorder of the shoulder or possibly another condition (such as myocardial infarction) that has decreased shoulder movements. The course is chronic, lasting months to years, but the disorder often resolves spontaneously, at least partially.

| TABLE 15-5 | Swollen or Tender Elbows |

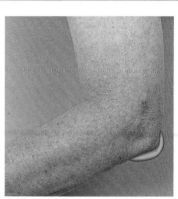

Olecranon bursitis

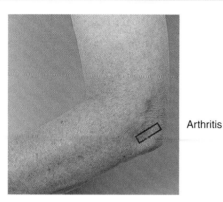

Arthritis

Olecranon Bursitis

Swelling and inflammation of the olecranon bursa may result from trauma or may be associated with rheumatoid or gouty arthritis. The swelling is superficial to the olecranon process.

Arthritis of the Elbow

Synovial inflammation or fluid is felt best in the grooves between the olecranon process and the epicondyles on either side. Palpate for a boggy, soft, or fluctuant swelling and for tenderness.

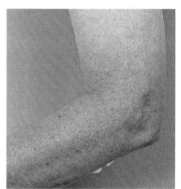

Rheumatoid nodules

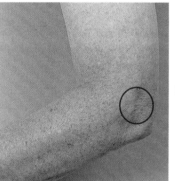

Epicondylitis

Rheumatoid Nodules

Subcutaneous nodules may develop at pressure points along the extensor surface of the ulna in patients with rheumatoid arthritis or acute rheumatic fever. They are firm and nontender, and are not attached to the overlying skin. They may or may not be attached to the underlying periosteum. Although they may develop in the area of the olecranon bursa, they often occur more distally.

Epicondylitis

Lateral epicondylitis (tennis elbow) follows repetitive extension of the wrist or pronation–supination of the forearm. Pain and tenderness develop at the lateral epicondyle and possibly in the extensor muscles close to it. When the patient tries to extend the wrist against resistance, pain increases.

Medial epicondylitis (pitcher's, golfer's, or Little League elbow) follows repetitive wrist flexion, as in throwing. Tenderness is maximal at the medial epicondyle. Wrist flexion against resistance increases the pain.

TABLE 15-6   Arthritis in the Hands

Acute Rheumatoid Arthritis

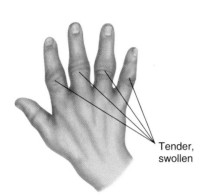

Tender, swollen

Tender, painful, stiff joints in *rheumatoid arthritis*, usually with *symmetric* involvement on both sides of the body. The proximal interphalangeal, metacarpophalangeal, and wrist joints are the most frequently affected. Note the fusiform or spindle-shaped swelling of the proximal interphalangeal joints in acute disease.

Chronic Rheumatoid Arthritis

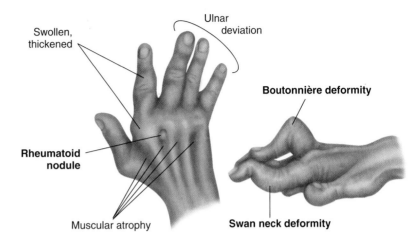

Swollen, thickened

Ulnar deviation

Boutonnière deformity

Rheumatoid nodule

Muscular atrophy

Swan neck deformity

In chronic disease, note the swelling and thickening of the metacarpophalangeal and proximal interphalangeal joints. Range of motion becomes limited, and fingers may deviate toward the ulnar side. The interosseous muscles atrophy. The fingers may show *"swan neck" deformities* (hyperextension of the proximal interphalangeal joints with fixed flexion of the distal interphalangeal joints). Less common is a *boutonnière deformity* (persistent flexion of the proximal interphalangeal joint with hyperextension of the distal interphalangeal joint). Rheumatoid nodules seen in acute or the chronic stage.

Osteoarthritis (*Degenerative Joint Disease*)

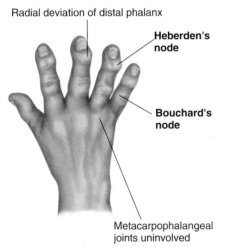

Radial deviation of distal phalanx

Heberden's node

Bouchard's node

Metacarpophalangeal joints uninvolved

Heberden's nodes on the dorsolateral aspects of the distal interphalangeal joints from bony overgrowth of osteoarthritis. Usually hard and painless, they affect the middle-aged or elderly; often associated with arthritic changes in other joints. Flexion and deviation deformities may develop. *Bouchard's nodes* on the proximal interphalangeal joints are less common. The metacarpophalangeal joints are spared.

Chronic Tophaceous Gout

Swollen

Draining tophus

Knobby swelling

The deformities of long-standing chronic tophaceous gout can mimic rheumatoid arthritis and osteoarthritis. Joint involvement is usually not as symmetric as in rheumatoid arthritis. Acute inflammation may be present. Knobby swellings around the joints ulcerate and discharge white chalklike urates.

TABLE 15-7	Swellings and Deformities of the Hands

Dupuytren's Contracture

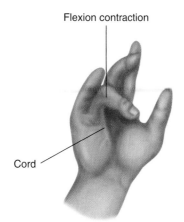

The first sign of a *Dupuytren's contracture* is a thickened plaque overlying the flexor tendon of the ring finger and possibly the little finger at the level of the distal palmar crease. Subsequently, the skin in this area puckers, and a thickened fibrotic cord develops between palm and finger. Flexion contracture of the fingers may gradually ensue.

Trigger Finger

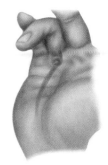

Caused by a painless nodule in a flexor tendon in the palm, near the head of the metacarpal. The nodule is too big to enter easily into the tendon sheath during extension of the fingers from a flexed position. With extra effort or assistance, the finger extends and flexes with a palpable and audible snap as the nodule pops into the tendon sheath. Watch and listen as the patient flexes and extends the fingers, and feel for both the nodule and the snap.

Thenar Atrophy

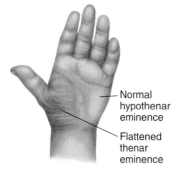

Thenar atrophy suggests a disorder of the median nerve or its components. Pressure on the nerve at the wrist is a common cause (*carpal tunnel syndrome*). Hypothenar atrophy suggests an *ulnar nerve disorder*.

Ganglion

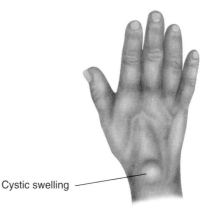

Ganglia are cystic, round, usually nontender swellings located along tendon sheaths or joint capsules, frequently at the dorsum of the wrist. Flexion of the wrist makes ganglia more prominent; extension tends to obscure them. Ganglia may also develop elsewhere on the hands, wrists, ankles, and feet.

TABLE 15-8   **Tendon Sheath and Palmar Space Infections; Felons**

Acute Tenosynovitis

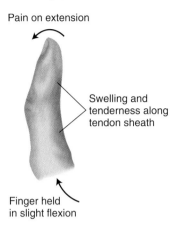

Pain on extension

Swelling and tenderness along tendon sheath

Finger held in slight flexion

Infection of the flexor tendon sheaths (acute tenosynovitis) may follow local injury, even when trivial in nature. Unlike arthritis, tenderness and swelling develop not in the joint but along the course of the tendon sheath, from the distal phalanx to the level of the metacarpophalangeal joint. The finger is held in slight flexion; finger extension is very painful.

Acute Tenosynovitis and Thenar Space Involvement

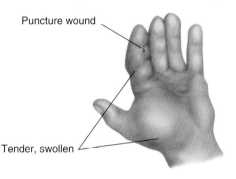

Puncture wound

Tender, swollen

If the infection progresses, it may extend from the tendon sheath into the adjacent fascial spaces within the palm. Infections of the index finger and thenar space are illustrated. Early diagnosis and treatment are important.

Felon

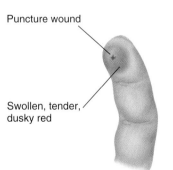

Puncture wound

Swollen, tender, dusky red

Injury to the fingertip may result in infection in the enclosed fascial spaces of the finger pad. Severe pain, localized tenderness, swelling, and dusky redness are characteristic. Early diagnosis and treatment are important.

TABLE 15-9   **Abnormalities of the Feet**

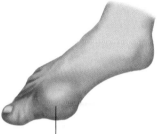

Acute Gouty Arthritis

The metatarsophalangeal joint of the great toe may be the first joint involved in *acute gouty arthritis*. It is characterized by a very painful and tender, hot, dusky red swelling that extends beyond the margin of the joint. It is easily mistaken for a cellulitis. Acute gout may also involve the dorsum of the foot.

Hot, red, tender, swollen

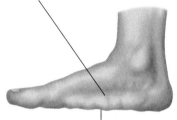

Medial border becomes convex

Sole touches floor

Flat Feet

Signs of *flat feet* may be apparent only when the patient stands, or they may become permanent. The longitudinal arch flattens so that the sole approaches or touches the floor. The normal concavity on the medial side of the foot becomes convex. Tenderness may be present from the medial malleolus down along the medial-plantar surface of the foot. Swelling may develop anterior to the malleoli. Inspect the shoes for excess wear on the inner side of the soles and heels.

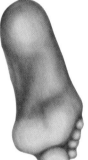

Hallux Valgus

In *hallux valgus,* the great toe is abnormally abducted in relationship to the first metatarsal, which itself is deviated medially. The head of the first metatarsal may enlarge on its medial side, and a bursa may form at the pressure point. This bursa may become inflamed.

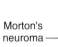

Morton's neuroma

Morton's Neuroma

Tenderness over the plantar surface, third and fourth metatarsal heads, from probable entrapment of the medial and lateral plantar nerves. Symptoms include hyperesthesia, numbness, aching, and burning from the metatarsal heads into the third and fourth toes.

TABLE 15-10 **Abnormalities of the Toes and Soles**

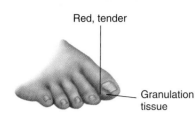

Red, tender

Granulation tissue

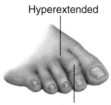

Hyperextended

Flexed

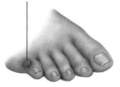

Red, thickened

Ingrown Toenail

The sharp edge of a toenail may dig into and injure the lateral nail fold, resulting in inflammation and infection. A tender, reddened, overhanging nail fold, sometimes with granulation tissue and purulent discharge, results. The great toe is most often affected.

Hammer Toe

Most commonly involving the second toe, a hammer toe is characterized by hyperextension at the metatarso-phalangeal joint with flexion at the proximal interphalangeal joint. A corn frequently develops at the pressure point over the proximal interphalangeal joint.

Corn

A corn is a painful conical thickening of skin that results from recurrent pressure on normally thin skin. The apex of the cone points inward and causes pain. Corns characteristically occur over bony prominences (e.g., the 5th toe). When located in moist areas (e.g., at pressure points between the 4th and 5th toes), they are called soft corns.

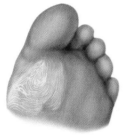

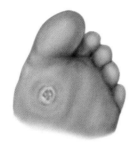

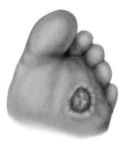

Callus

Like a corn, a callus is an area of greatly thickened skin that develops in a region of recurrent pressure. Unlike a corn, however, a callus involves skin that is normally thick, such as the sole, and is usually painless. If a callus is painful, suspect an underlying plantar wart.

Plantar Wart

A plantar wart is a common wart (verruca vulgaris) located in the thickened skin of the sole. It may look somewhat like a callus or even be covered by one. Look for the characteristic small dark spots that give a stippled appearance to a wart. Normal skin lines stop at the wart's edge.

Neuropathic Ulcer

When pain sensation is diminished or absent (as in diabetic neuropathy, for example), neuropathic ulcers may develop at pressure points on the feet. Although often deep, infected, and indolent, they are painless. Callus formation about the ulcer is diagnostically helpful. Like the ulcer itself, it results from chronic pressure.

16

The Nervous System: Mental Status and Behavior

Examining the nervous system calls on many skills. You will learn to assess the mood, speech, behaviors, and cognition that constitute the patient's mental status, the initial segment of the examination. Then you will come to master the techniques for physical examination of the nervous system. Be careful and systematic, and you will learn to accurately gauge the patient's motor strength, bulk, and tone, as well as sensation and reflexes. Learning these techniques requires practice and often humility—be open to asking your teachers to check your techniques and your findings until you are confident that you are truly examining the nervous system accurately and reliably.

To facilitate our learning of this complex area of patient assessment, the Nervous System is divided into two chapters:

- **Chapter 16, Mental Status and Behavior** includes related sections on overview, health history, health promotion and counseling, techniques of examination, and tables of abnormalities.

- **Chapter 17, Cranial Nerves, Motor System, Sensory System, and Reflexes,** also has related sections on overview, health history, health promotion and counseling, techniques of examination, the written record, and tables of abnormalities. Note that because the mental status and remaining examination are so intertwined during assessment of the actual patient, the examples of the write-up are combined and can be found in Chapter 17 on pp. 646–647.

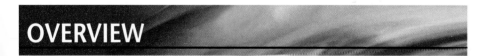

OVERVIEW

As with the General Survey, your assessment of mental status begins with the first words of the interview. As you gather the health history, you will quickly discern the patient's level of *alertness* and *orientation, mood, attention,* and *memory.* As the history unfolds, you will learn about the patient's *insight* and *judgment,* as well as any *recurring or unusual thoughts or perceptions.* For some, you will need to supplement your interview with specific questions and a more formal evaluation of mental status. Just as symptoms, blood pressure, and valvular murmurs help you to distinguish, for example, health from disease in the cardiovascular system, specific components of mental function illuminate the workings of the mind. Although these components do not encompass all the aspects of human thought and feeling, they serve as useful and continually important clinical tools.

Many of the terms used to describe the mental status examination are familiar to you from social conversation. Take the time to learn their precise meanings in the context of the formal evaluation of mental status.

TERMINOLOGY: THE MENTAL STATUS EXAMINATION

Level of consciousness	Alertness or state of awareness of the environment
Attention	The ability to focus or concentrate over time on one task or activity—an inattentive or distractible person with impaired consciousness has difficulty giving a history or responding to questions.
Memory	The process of registering or recording information, tested by asking for immediate repetition of material, followed by storage or retention of information. *Recent or short-term memory* covers minutes, hours, or days; *remote or long-term memory* refers to intervals of years.
Orientation	Awareness of personal identity, place, and time; requires both memory and attention
Perceptions	Sensory awareness of objects in the environment and their interrelationships (external stimuli); also refers to internal stimuli such as dreams or hallucinations
Thought processes	The logic, coherence, and relevance of the patient's thought as it leads to selected goals, or *how* people think
Thought content	*What* the patient thinks about, including level of insight and judgment
Insight	Awareness that symptoms or disturbed behaviors are normal or abnormal; for example, distinguishing between daydreams and hallucinations that seem real
Judgment	Process of comparing and evaluating alternatives when deciding on a course of action; reflects values that may or may not be based on reality and social conventions or norms
Affect	An observable, usually episodic, feeling or tone expressed through voice, facial expression, and demeanor
Mood	A more sustained emotion that may color a person's view of the world (mood is to affect as climate is to weather)
Language	A complex symbolic system for expressing, receiving, and comprehending words; as with consciousness, attention, and memory, language is essential for assessing other mental functions
Higher cognitive functions	Assessed by vocabulary, fund of information, abstract thinking, calculations, construction of objects that have two or three dimensions

Distinguishing the interplay of body and mind in relation to these attributes is very important but not always easy. Mental disorders such as anxiety or depression may take the form of somatic complaints. Likewise, physical illness can cause mental and emotional responses and in older patients, can impair mental function without causing typical symptoms or signs such as fever or pain. Always look carefully for physical or pharmacologic causes as you try to understand the context and emotional meaning of changes in mental status. Some mental status evaluations are complicated by personality factors, psychodynamics, or the patient's personal experiences, areas that can be explored during the interview (but not covered in this chapter). By integrating and correlating all the relevant data, the clinician tries to understand the person as a whole.

As a student, you may feel reluctant to perform mental status examinations, wondering if they will upset patients, invade their privacy, or result in labeling their thoughts or behavior as pathologic. Such concerns are understandable and appropriate. An insensitive examination of mental status may alarm a patient, and even a skillful examination may bring to conscious awareness an embarrassing or upsetting deficit that the patient is trying to ignore. You may wish to discuss some of these concerns with your instructor or other experienced clinicians. As with other realms of interviewing and assessment, your skills and confidence will improve with practice, and rewards will follow. Remember that patients appreciate an understanding listener, and some will owe their health, their safety, or even their lives to your attention.

THE HEALTH HISTORY

Common or Concerning Symptoms

- Changes in attention, mood, or speech
- Changes in insight, judgment, orientation, or memory
- Anxiety, panic, ritualistic behavior, and phobias
- Delirium or dementia

Much of the information about the patient's *mental status* becomes evident during the interview. As you talk with the patient and listen to the patient's story, assess *level of consciousness*; general *appearance*; *mood*, including depression or mania;[1] and *ability to pay attention, remember, understand*, and *speak*. By placing the patient's vocabulary and general fund of information in the context of his or her cultural and educational background, you can often make a rough estimate of intelligence. Likewise, the patient's responses to illness and life circumstances often tell you about his or her degree of *insight and judgment*. If you suspect a problem in orientation and memory, you can ask, "Let's see, your last clinic appointment was when . . . ?" "And the date today?" The more you can integrate your exploration of mental status into a sensitive patient history, the less it will seem like an interrogation.

See Table 16-1, Disorders of Mood, p. 590, and Table 16-2, Disorders of Speech, p. 591.

If the patient has unusual thoughts, preoccupations, beliefs, or perceptions, you should explore them as they arise during the interview. For example, worries persisting over a 6-month period suggest a possible *generalized anxiety disorder*, the most prevalent psychiatric condition in the United States following substance abuse, with a lifetime prevalence of approximately 5%.[2] Over time, you will come to recognize some of its mimics: *panic disorder*, with its recurrent panic attacks followed by a period of anxiety about further attacks; *obsessive-compulsive disorder*, with its intrusive thoughts and ritualistic behaviors; *posttraumatic stress disorder*, characterized by "avoidance, numbing, and hyperarousal;[2] and *social phobia*, with its marked anticipatory anxiety in social situations. For such patients, you will need to supplement your interview with questions in specific areas. You may determine the need to go further and pursue a formal mental status examination. The components of the mental status examination are described in the section on Techniques of Examination, pp. 578–588.

See Table 16-3, Anxiety Disorders, p. 592, and Table 16-4, Psychotic Disorders, p. 593.

All patients with documented or suspected brain lesions, psychiatric symptoms, or reports from family members of vague or changed behavioral symptoms need further systematic assessment. Patients may have subtle behavioral changes, difficulty taking medications properly, problems attending to household chores or paying bills, or loss of interest in their usual activities. See Table 20-1, Delirium and Dementia, p. 873. Other patients may behave strangely after surgery or during an acute illness. Each problem should be identified as expeditiously as possible. Mental function influences the ability to hold a job and is often important in evaluating disability.

Possible signs of depression or dementia

HEALTH PROMOTION AND COUNSELING

Important Topics for Health Promotion and Counseling

- Screening for depression and suicidality
- Screening for dementia

A high proportion of primary care visits, with estimates ranging from 10% to 50%, involve mental health concerns, particularly depression, but also anxiety, somatic complaints, and less frequent but equally serious disorders of mood and mental function.[3,4] The burden of suffering imposed by these disorders is great, yet they are often underdiagnosed and not adequately treated. For the general population, focus health promotion and counseling on depression, suicidality, and dementia, three important conditions often overlooked. You should also screen routinely for addiction to alcohol or drugs (see pp. 50–51).

Major depression is a common medical illness and frequently coexists with other mental disorders. The lifetime prevalence of major depression meeting formal diagnostic criteria in the U.S. population is high, approximately 16%, with an annual prevalence of approximately 6%.[4] The lifetime risk for women (20% to 25%) is approximately double that of men. Clinicians should search also for depressive symptoms, which may be two to three times more in the community and the office.[5] Primary care providers fail to diagnose major depression in up to 50% of affected patients, often missing early clues such as low self-esteem, anhedonia, or the failure to find pleasure in daily life activities, sleep disorders, and difficulty concentrating or making decisions. Watch carefully for depressive symptoms, especially in patients who are young, female, single, divorced, separated, seriously or chronically ill, or bereaved. Patients with a prior history of depression or positive family history are also at risk.

The U.S. Preventive Services Task Force has found evidence that screening helps identify patients with depression in primary care settings, and that treatment reduces clinical morbidity. The Task Force recommends screening in practices that provide accurate diagnosis, treatment, and follow-up, and cites two questions that may be as effective as use of more formal screening tools, namely: "Over the past 2 weeks, have you felt down, depressed, or hopeless?" and "Over the past 2 weeks, have you felt little interest or pleasure in doing things?"[6, 7] Screening tools suitable for the office are also readily available.[8–10] Positive screening warrants more formal diagnostic evaluation. Failure to diagnose depression can have fatal consequences—suicide rates in patients with major depression are eight times higher than in the general population.[3]

Reducing rates of *suicide* has become a national imperative.[11] Suicide rates in 2001 reached more than 10 per 100,000, and accounted for 1% of U.S. deaths, outnumbering homicides and deaths from AIDS and HIV.[12] Rates are highest in white men older than 85 and are increasing in teenagers and young adults. More than half of deaths are by firearms. Risk factors include suicidal or homicidal ideation, intent, or plan; access to the means for suicide; current symptoms of psychosis or severe anxiety; any history of psychiatric illness, especially if linked to hospital admission; substance abuse or personality disorder; and prior history or family history of suicide.[6, 13] Patients with these risk factors should be immediately referred for psychiatric care and possibly hospitalization.

Dementia is an acquired decline in cognitive function, especially memory, but also language, visual-spatial, or executive function, sufficient to interfere with social or occupational functioning.[14] Dementia affects 3% to 11% of Americans older than 65 and is highly correlated with age, rising to 25% to 47% of those older than 85.[15, 16] Apolipoprotein E, hypertension, and mild cognitive impairment may also increase risk.[17] Most dementias represent Alzheimer's disease (roughly 60% to 70% of cases), or vascular or multi-infarct dementia (approximately 20% to 30% of cases).[18] Individuals with a positive family history have a three times higher risk for dementia than the general population.[19] The U.S. Preventive Services Task Force has deferred recommendations in support of screening because of inconclusive evidence with respect to "accuracy of diagnosis, the feasibility of screening and treatment in routine clinical practice, and the potential harms of screening (e.g., labeling effects)."[18] See also Chapter 20, The Older Adult, pp. 839–873.

TECHNIQUES OF EXAMINATION

Important Areas of Examination

- Appearance and behavior
- Speech and language
- Mood
- Thoughts and perceptions
- Cognition, including memory, attention, information and vocabulary, calculations, abstract thinking, and constructional ability

Your approach to the examination of the nervous system centers on three important questions. Keep all these in mind throughout each segment of your examination, even though you are beginning by focusing on mental status and behavior:

- Is the mental status intact?

- Are right-sided and left-sided findings symmetric?

- If the findings are asymmetric or otherwise abnormal, does the causative lesion lie in the central nervous system or the peripheral nervous system?

The mental status examination consists of the following components:

- Appearance and behavior

- Speech and language

- Mood

- Thoughts and perceptions

- Cognitive function, including memory, attention, information and vocabulary, calculations, and abstract thinking and constructional ability.

The format that follows should help to organize your observations, but it is not intended as a step-by-step guide. When a full examination is indicated, you should be flexible in your approach but thorough in what you cover. In some situations, however, sequence is important. If during your initial interview, the patient's consciousness, attention, comprehension of words, or ability to speak seems impaired, assess this attribute promptly. Such a patient cannot give a reliable history, and you will not be able to test most of the other mental functions.

APPEARANCE AND BEHAVIOR

Use here all the relevant observations made throughout the course of your history and examination. Include these areas:

Level of Consciousness.   Is the patient awake and alert? Does the patient seem to understand your questions and respond appropriately and reasonably quickly, or is there a tendency to lose track of the topic and fall silent or even asleep?

See the table on Level of Consciousness (Arousal), Chapter 17, The Nervous System, p. 643.

If the patient does not respond to your questions, escalate the stimulus in steps:

■ Speak to the patient by name and in a loud voice.

Lethargic patients are drowsy but open their eyes and look at you, respond to questions, and then fall asleep.

■ Shake the patient gently, as if awakening a sleeper.

Obtunded patients open their eyes and look at you, but respond slowly and are somewhat confused.

If there is no response to these stimuli, promptly assess the patient for stupor or coma—severe reductions in the level of consciousness (see p. 643).

Posture and Motor Behavior.   Does the patient lie in bed, or prefer to walk around? Note body posture and the patient's ability to relax. Observe the pace, range, and character of movements. Do they seem to be under voluntary control? Are certain parts immobile? Do posture and motor activity change with topics under discussion or with activities or people around the patient?

Tense posture, restlessness, and fidgeting of anxiety; crying, pacing, and handwringing of agitated depression; hopeless, slumped posture and slowed movements of depression; singing, dancing, and expansive movements of a manic episode.

Dress, Grooming, and Personal Hygiene.   How is the patient dressed? Is clothing clean, pressed, and properly fastened? How does it compare with clothing worn by people of comparable age and social group? Note the patient's hair, nails, teeth, skin, and, if present, beard. How are they groomed? How do the person's grooming and hygiene compare with those of other people of comparable age, lifestyle, and socioeconomic group? Compare one side of the body with the other.

Grooming and personal hygiene may deteriorate in *depression, schizophrenia,* and *dementia.* Excessive fastidiousness may be seen with *obsessive–compulsive disorder.* One-sided neglect may result from a lesion in the opposite parietal cortex, usually the nondominant side.

Facial Expression.   Observe the face, both at rest and when the patient is interacting with others. Watch for variations in expression with topics under discussion. Are they appropriate? Or is the face relatively immobile throughout?

Expressions of anxiety, depression, apathy, anger, elation. Facial immobility of parkinsonism

Manner, Affect, and Relationship to Persons and Things.   Using your observations of facial expressions, voice, and body movements, assess the patient's affect. Does it vary appropriately with topics under discussion, or is the affect labile, blunted, or flat? Does it seem inappropriate or extreme

Anger, hostility, suspiciousness, or evasiveness of patients with *paranoia.* Elation and euphoria of *mania.* Flat affect and remoteness

at certain points? If so, how? Note the patient's openness, approachability, and reactions to others and to the surroundings. Does the patient seem to hear or see things that you do not or seem to be conversing with someone who is not there?

of *schizophrenia*. Apathy (dulled affect with detachment and indifference) of *dementia*. Anxiety, depression

SPEECH AND LANGUAGE

Throughout the interview, note the characteristics of the patient's speech, including the following:

Quantity.   Is the patient talkative or relatively silent? Are comments spontaneous or only responsive to direct questions?

Rate.   Is speech fast or slow?

Slow speech of *depression*; accelerated rapid, loud speech in *mania*

Loudness.   Is speech loud or soft?

Articulation of Words.   Are the words spoken clearly and distinctly? Is there a nasal quality to the speech?

Dysarthria refers to defective articulation. *Aphasia* refers to a disorder of language. See Table 16-2, Disorders of Speech, p. 591.

Fluency.   This involves the rate, flow, and melody of speech and the content and use of words. Be alert for abnormalities of spontaneous speech such as:

- Hesitancies and gaps in the flow and rhythm of words

- Disturbed inflections, such as a monotone

- Circumlocutions, in which phrases or sentences are substituted for a word the person cannot think of, such as "what you write with" for "pen"

- Paraphasias, in which words are malformed ("I write with a den"), wrong ("I write with a bar"), or invented ("I write with a dar").

These abnormalities suggest *aphasia.* The patient may have so much difficulty in talking or in understanding others that you may not be able to obtain a history. You may also falsely suspect a psychotic disorder.

If the patient's speech lacks meaning or fluency, proceed with further testing as outlined in the following table.

■ *Testing for Aphasia*

Word Comprehension	Ask the patient to follow a one-stage command, such as "Point to your nose." Try a two-stage command: "Point to your mouth, then your knee."
Repetition	Ask the patient to repeat a phrase of one-syllable words (the most difficult repetition task): "No ifs, ands, or buts."
Naming	Ask the patient to name the parts of a watch.
Reading Comprehension	Ask the patient to read a paragraph aloud.
Writing	Ask the patient to write a sentence.

These tests help you to decide what kind of aphasia the patient may have. Remember that deficiencies in vision, hearing, intelligence, and education may also affect performance. Two common kinds of aphasia—Wernicke's and Broca's—are compared in Table 16-2, Disorders of Speech, p. 591.

A person who can write a correct sentence does not have aphasia.

MOOD

Assess mood during the interview by exploring the patient's perceptions of his or her mood. Find out about the patient's usual mood level and how it has varied with life events. "How did you feel about that?", for example, or, more generally, "How are your spirits?" The reports of relatives and friends may be of great value.

What has the patient's mood been like? How intense has it been? Has it been labile or fairly unchanging? How long has it lasted? Is it appropriate to the patient's circumstances? In case of depression, have there also been episodes of an elevated mood, suggesting a bipolar disorder?

If you suspect depression, assess its depth and any associated risk of suicide. The following series of questions is useful, proceeding as far as the patient's positive answers warrant:

- Do you get pretty discouraged (or depressed or blue)?

- How low do you feel?

- What do you see for yourself in the future?

- Do you ever feel that life isn't worth living? Or that you would just as soon be dead?

- Have you ever thought of doing away with yourself?

- How did (do) you think you would do it?

- What would happen after you were dead?

Asking about suicidal thoughts does not implant the idea in the patient's mind, and it may be the only way to get the information. Although you may feel uneasy about exploring this topic, most patients can discuss their thoughts and feelings about it freely with you, sometimes with considerable relief. By such discussion, you demonstrate your interest and concern for what may well be a serious and life-threatening problem. By avoiding the issue, you may miss the most important feature of the patient's illness.

Moods include sadness and deep melancholy; contentment, joy, euphoria, and elation; anger and rage; anxiety and worry; and detachment and indifference.

For depressive and bipolar disorders, see Table 16-1, Disorders of Mood, p. 590.

THOUGHT AND PERCEPTIONS

Thought Processes. Assess the logic, relevance, organization, and coherence of the patient's thought processes as they are revealed in words and speech throughout the interview. Does speech progress logically toward a goal? Here you use speech as a window into the patient's mind. Listen for patterns of speech that suggest disorders of thought processes, as outlined in the table below.

■ Variations and Abnormalities in Thought Processes

Circumstantiality	Speech characterized by indirection and delay in reaching the point because of unnecessary detail, although components of the description have a meaningful connection. Many people without mental disorders speak circumstantially.	Observed in people with obsessions
Derailment (Loosening of Associations)	Speech in which a person shifts from one subject to others that are unrelated or related only obliquely without realizing that the subjects are not meaningfully connected. Ideas slip off the track between clauses, not within them.	Observed in *schizophrenia, manic episodes,* and other *psychotic disorders*
Flight of Ideas	An almost continuous flow of accelerated speech in which a person changes abruptly from topic to topic. Changes are usually based on understandable associations, plays on words, or distracting stimuli, but the ideas do not progress to sensible conversation.	Most frequently noted in *manic episodes*
Neologisms	Invented or distorted words, or words with new and highly idiosyncratic meanings	Observed in *schizophrenia,* other *psychotic disorders,* and *aphasia*
Incoherence	Speech that is largely incomprehensible because of illogic, lack of meaningful connections, abrupt changes in topic, or disordered grammar or word use. Shifts in meaning occur within clauses. Flight of ideas, when severe, may produce incoherence.	Observed in severe psychotic disturbances (usually *schizophrenia*)
Blocking	Sudden interruption of speech in midsentence or before completion of an idea. The person attributes this to losing the thought. Blocking occurs in normal people.	Blocking may be striking in *schizophrenia.*
Confabulation	Fabrication of facts or events in response to questions, to fill in the gaps in an impaired memory	Common with *amnesia*
Perseveration	Persistent repetition of words or ideas	Occurs in *schizophrenia* and other *psychotic disorders*
Echolalia	Repetition of the words and phrases of others	Occurs in manic episodes and *schizophrenia*
Clanging	Speech in which a person chooses a word on the basis of sound rather than meaning, as in rhyming and punning speech. For example, "Look at my eyes and nose, wise eyes and rosy nose. Two to one, the ayes have it!"	Occurs in *schizophrenia* and *manic episodes*

Thought Content. You should assess information relevant to thought content during the interview. Follow appropriate leads as they occur rather than using stereotyped lists of specific questions. For example, "You mentioned a few minutes ago that a neighbor was responsible for your entire illness. Can you tell me more about that?" Or, in another situation, "What do you think about at times like these?"

You may need to make more specific inquiries. If so, couch them in tactful and accepting terms. "When people are upset like this, they sometimes can't keep certain thoughts out of their minds," or ". . . things seem unreal. Have you experienced anything like this?"

In these ways, find out about any of the patterns shown in the following table.

■ *Abnormalities of Thought Content*	
Compulsions	Repetitive behaviors or mental acts that a person feels driven to perform in order to produce or prevent some future state of affairs, although expectation of such an effect is unrealistic
Obsessions	Recurrent, uncontrollable thoughts, images, or impulses that a person considers unacceptable and alien
Phobias	Persistent, irrational fears, accompanied by a compelling desire to avoid the stimulus
Anxieties	Apprehensions, fears, tensions, or uneasiness that may be focused (phobia) or free floating (a general sense of ill-defined dread or impending doom)
Feelings of Unreality	A sense that things in the environment are strange, unreal, or remote
Feelings of Depersonalization	A sense that one's self is different, changed, or unreal, or has lost identity or become detached from one's mind or body
Delusions	False, fixed, personal beliefs that are not shared by other members of the person's culture or subculture. Examples include: ■ *Delusions of persecution* ■ *Delusions of grandeur* ■ *Delusional jealousy* ■ *Delusions of reference*, in which a person believes that external events, objects, or people have a particular and unusual personal significance (e.g., that the radio or television might be commenting on or giving instructions to the person) ■ *Delusions of being controlled* by an outside force ■ *Somatic delusions* of having a disease, disorder, or physical defect ■ *Systematized delusions*, a single delusion with many elaborations or a cluster of related delusions around a single theme, all systematized into a complex network

Compulsions, obsessions, phobias, and *anxieties* are often associated with neurotic disorders. See Table 16-3, Anxiety Disorders (p. 592).

Delusions and feelings of unreality or depersonalization are more often associated with *psychotic disorders.* See Table 16-4, Psychotic Disorders (p. 593). Delusions may also occur in delirium, severe mood disorders, and dementia.

Perceptions.   Inquire about false perceptions in a manner similar to that used for thought content. For example, "When you heard the voice speaking to you, what did it say? How did it make you feel?" Or, "After you've been drinking a lot, do you ever see things that aren't really there?" Or, "Sometimes after major surgery like this, people hear peculiar or frightening things. Have you experienced anything like that?" In these ways, find out about the following abnormal perceptions.

■ *Abnormalities of Perception*	
Illusions	Misinterpretations of real external stimuli
Hallucinations	Subjective sensory perceptions in the absence of relevant external stimuli. The person may or may not recognize the experiences as false. Hallucinations may be auditory, visual, olfactory, gustatory, tactile, or somatic. (False perceptions associated with dreaming, falling asleep, and awakening are not classified as hallucinations.)

Illusions may occur in grief reactions, *delirium*, acute and *posttraumatic stress disorders*, and *schizophrenia*.

Hallucinations may occur in *delirium*, *dementia* (less commonly), *posttraumatic stress disorder*, *schizophrenia*, and alcoholism.

Insight and Judgment. These attributes are usually best assessed during the interview.

Insight. Some of your very first questions to the patient often yield important information about insight: "What brings you to the hospital?" "What seems to be the trouble?" "What do you think is wrong?" More specifically, note whether the patient is aware that a particular mood, thought, or perception is abnormal or part of an illness.

Patients with psychotic disorders often lack insight into their illness. Denial of impairment may accompany some neurologic disorders.

Judgment. You can usually assess judgment by noting the patient's responses to family situations, jobs, use of money, and interpersonal conflicts. "How do you plan to get the help you'll need after leaving the hospital?" "How are you going to manage if you lose your job?" "If your husband starts to abuse you again, what will you do?" "Who will attend to your financial affairs while you are in the nursing home?"

Judgment may be poor in delirium, dementia, mental retardation, and psychotic states. Anxiety, mood disorders, intelligence, education, income, and cultural values also influence judgment.

Note whether decisions and actions are based on reality or, for example, on impulse, wish fulfillment, or disordered thought content. What values seem to underlie the patient's decisions and behavior? Allowing for cultural variations, how do these compare with mature adult standards? Because judgment reflects maturity, it may be variable and unpredictable during adolescence.

Disorientation occurs especially when memory or attention is impaired, as in delirium.

COGNITIVE FUNCTIONS

Orientation. By skillful questioning, you can often determine the patient's orientation in the context of the interview. For example, you can ask quite naturally for specific dates and times, the patient's address and telephone number, the names of family members, or the route taken to the hospital. At times—when rechecking the status of a patient with delirium, for example—simple, direct questions may be indicated.

"Can you tell me what time it is now . . . and what day is it?" In either of these ways, determine the patient's orientation for the following:

■ *Time*—the time of day, day of the week, month, season, date and year, duration of hospitalization

■ *Place*—the patient's residence, the names of the hospital, city, and state

■ *Person*—the patient's own name, and the names of relatives and professional personnel

Attention.   These tests of attention are commonly used:

Digit Span.   Explain that you would like to test the patient's ability to concentrate, perhaps adding that this can be difficult when people are in pain, or ill, or feverish. Recite a series of digits, starting with two at a time and speaking each number clearly at a rate of about one per second. Ask the patient to repeat the numbers back to you. If this repetition is accurate, try a series of three numbers, then four, and so on as long as the patient responds correctly. Jot down the numbers as you say them to ensure your own accuracy. If the patient makes a mistake, try once more with another series of the same length. Stop after a second failure in a single series.

Causes of poor performance include *delirium, dementia, mental retardation,* and performance anxiety.

In choosing digits you may use street numbers, zip codes, telephone numbers, and other numerical sequences that are familiar to you, but avoid consecutive numbers, easily recognized dates, and sequences that possibly are familiar to the patient.

Now, starting again with a series of two, ask the patient to repeat the numbers to you backward.

Normally, a person should be able to repeat correctly at least five digits forward and four backward.

Serial 7s.   Instruct the patient, "Starting from a hundred, subtract 7, and keep subtracting 7. . . ." Note the effort required and the speed and accuracy of the responses. Writing down the answers helps you keep up with the arithmetic. Normally, a person can complete serial 7s in 1½ minutes, with fewer than four errors. If the patient cannot do serial 7s, try 3s or counting backward.

Poor performance may be the result of delirium, the late stage of dementia, mental retardation, loss of calculating ability, anxiety, or depression. Also consider the possibility of limited education.

Spelling Backward.   This can substitute for serial 7s. Say a five-letter word, spell it, e.g., W-O-R-L-D, and ask the patient to spell it backward.

Remote Memory.   Inquire about birthdays, anniversaries, social security number, names of schools attended, jobs held, or past historical events such as wars relevant to the patient's past.

Remote memory may be impaired in the late stage of *dementia.*

Recent Memory.   As in the events of the day. Ask questions with answers you can check against other sources so you can see if the patient is confabulating (making up facts to compensate for a defective memory). These might include the day's weather, today's appointment time, and medications or lab-

Recent memory is impaired in *dementia* and *delirium. Amnestic disorders* impair memory or new learning ability significantly and re-

oratory tests taken during the day. (Asking what the patient had for breakfast may be a waste of time unless you can check the accuracy of the answer.)

New Learning Ability.   Give the patient three or four words such as "83 Water Street and blue," or "table, flower, green, and hamburger." Ask the patient to repeat them so that you know that the information has been heard and registered. This step, like digit span, tests registration and immediate recall. Then proceed to other parts of the examination. After about 3 to 5 minutes, ask the patient to repeat the words. Note the accuracy of the response, awareness of whether it is correct, and any tendency to confabulate. Normally, a person should be able to remember the words.

duce a person's social or occupational functioning, but they do not have the global features of delirium or dementia. Anxiety, depression, and mental retardation may also impair recent memory.

 # HIGHER COGNITIVE FUNCTIONS

Information and Vocabulary.   Information and vocabulary, when observed clinically, provide a rough estimate of a person's intelligence. Assess them during the interview. Ask a student, for example, about favorite courses, or inquire about work, hobbies, reading, favorite television programs, or current events. Explore such topics first with simple questions, then with more difficult ones. Note the person's grasp of information, the complexity of the ideas expressed, and the vocabulary used.

More directly, you can ask about specific facts such as:

The name of the president, vice president, or governor

The names of the last four or five presidents

The names of five large cities in the country

If considered in the context of cultural and educational background, information and vocabulary are fairly good indicators of intelligence. They are relatively unaffected by any but the most severe psychiatric disorders, and may be helpful for distinguishing mentally retarded adults (whose information and vocabulary are limited) from those with mild or moderate *dementia* (whose information and vocabulary are fairly well preserved).

Calculating Ability.   Test the patient's ability to do arithmetical calculations, starting at the rote level with simple addition ("What is 4 + 3? . . . 8 + 7?") and multiplication ("What is 5 × 6? . . . 9 × 7?"). The task can be made more difficult by using two-digit numbers ("15 + 12" or "25 × 6") or longer, written examples.

Poor performance may be a useful sign of dementia or may accompany *aphasia*, but it must be assessed in terms of the patient's intelligence and education.

Alternatively, pose practical and functionally important questions, such as "If something costs 78 cents and you give the clerk one dollar, how much should you get back?"

Abstract Thinking.   Test the capacity to think abstractly in two ways.

Proverbs.   Ask the patient what people mean when they use some of the following proverbs:

A stitch in time saves nine.

Don't count your chickens before they're hatched.

The proof of the pudding is in the eating.

Concrete responses are often given by people with mental retardation, *delirium,* or *dementia,* but may also be a function of limited education. Patients with *schizophrenia* may respond concretely or with personal, bizarre interpretations.

A rolling stone gathers no moss.

The squeaking wheel gets the grease.

Note the relevance of the answers and their degree of concreteness or abstractness. For example, "You should sew a rip before it gets bigger" is concrete, whereas "Prompt attention to a problem prevents trouble" is abstract. Average patients should give abstract or semiabstract responses.

Similarities. Ask the patient to tell you how the following are alike:

An orange and an apple   A church and a theater

A cat and a mouse   A piano and a violin

A child and a dwarf   Wood and coal

Note the accuracy and relevance of the answers and their degree of concreteness or abstractness. For example, "A cat and a mouse are both animals" is abstract, "They both have tails" is concrete, and "A cat chases a mouse" is not relevant.

Constructional Ability. The task here is to copy figures of increasing complexity onto a piece of blank unlined paper. Show each figure one at a time and ask the patient to copy it as well as possible.

The three diamonds below are rated poor, fair, and good (but not excellent).[20]

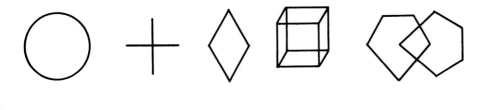

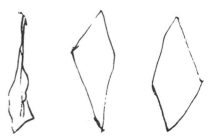

In another approach, ask the patient to draw a clock face complete with numbers and hands. The example below is rated excellent.[20]

These three clocks are poor, fair, and good.[20]

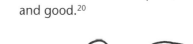

If vision and motor ability are intact, poor constructional ability suggests dementia or parietal lobe damage. Mental retardation may also impair performance.

SPECIAL TECHNIQUES

Mini-Mental State Examination (MMSE). This brief test is useful in screening for cognitive dysfunction or dementia and following their course over time. For more detailed information regarding the MMSE, contact the Publisher, Psychological Assessment Resources, Inc., 16204 North Florida Avenue, Lutz, Florida 33549. Below are some sample questions.

MMSE SAMPLE ITEMS

Orientation to Time
"What is the date?"

Registration
"Listen carefully, I am going to say three words. You say them back after I stop. Ready? Here they are . . .
HOUSE (pause), CAR (pause), LAKE (pause). Now repeat those words back o me." [Repeat up to five times, but score only the first trial.]

Naming
"What is this?" [Point to a pencil or pen.]

Reading
"Please read this and do what it says." [Show examinee the words on the stimulus form.]
CLOSE YOUR EYES

Reproduced by special permission of the Publisher, Psychological Assessment Resources, Inc., 16204 North Florida Avenue, Lutz, Florida 33549, from the Mini Mental State Examination, by Marshal Folstein and Susan Folstein, Copyright 1975, 1998, 2001 by Mini Mental LLC, Inc. Published 2001 by Psychological Assessment Resources, Inc. Further reproduction is prohibited without permission of PAR, Inc. The MMSE can be purchased from PAR, Inc. by calling (800) 331-8378 or (813) 968-3003.

RECORDING YOUR FINDINGS

See Chapter 17, The Nervous System: Cranial Nerves, Motor System, Sensory System, and Reflexes, p. 595–667.

Bibliography

CITATIONS

1. Belmaker RH. Bipolar disorder. N Engl J Med 351(5): 476–486, 2004.

2. Fricchione G. Generalized anxiety disorder. N Engl J Med 351(7):675–682, 2004.

3. U.S. Preventive Services Task Force. Screening for depression. In Guide to Clinical Preventive Services, 2nd ed. pp. 541–546. Baltimore, Williams & Wilkins, 1996. Also available at: Guide to Clinical Preventive Services, 3rd ed., www.ahrq.gov/clinic/uspstix.htm.

4. Kessler RC, Berglund P, Demler O, et al. The epidemiology of major depressive disorder: results from the National Comorbidity Survey Replication (NCS-R). JAMA 289(23):3095–3105, 2003.

5. Katon W, Schulberg H. Epidemiology of depression in primary care. Gen Hosp Psychiatry 14(4):237–247, 1992.

6. U.S. Preventive Services Task Force. Screening for depression: recommendations and rationale. Ann Intern Med 136(10): 760–764, 2002.

7. Whooley MA, Avins AL, Miranda J, et al. Case-finding instruments for depression. Two questions are as good as many. J Gen Intern Med 12:439–445, 1997.

8. Williams JW, Noel PH, Cordes JA, et al. Is this patient clinically depressed? JAMA 287(9):1160–1170, 2002.

9. Beck Depression Inventory (BDI): Available at: http://www.uea.ac.uk/~wp316/depression.pdf.

10. Zung Self-Rating Depression Scale (SDS). Available at: http://www.wellbutrin-sr.com/hcp/depression/zung.html.

11. Goldsmith SK, Pellmar TC, Kleinman AM, et al (Eds). Reducing Suicide: A National Imperative. Washington, DC: Institute of Medicine National Academies Press, 2002.

12. National Institutes of Mental Health. Suicide facts and statistics. Available at: http://www.nimh.nih.gov/suicideprevention/suifact.cfm. Accessed December 4, 2004.

13. Schreiber J, Culpepper L, Fife A. Suicidal ideation and behavior in adults. Available at: www.utdol.com. Accessed December 4, 2004.

14. American Psychiatric Association. Diagnostic and Statistical Manual of Mental Disorders, 4th ed. Washington, DC, APA Press, 1994.

15. Boustani M, Peterson B, Hanson L, et al. Screening for dementia in primary care: a summary of the evidence for the U.S. Preventive Services Task Force. Ann Intern Med 138;927–937, 2003.

16. Hebert LE, Scherr PA, Beckett LA, et al. Age-specific incidence of Alzheimer's disease in a community population. JAMA 273(17):1354–1359, 1995.

17. Kawas CH. Early Alzheimer's disease. N Engl J Med 349(11):1056–1063, 2003.

18. U.S. Preventive Services Task Force. Screening for dementia. Recommendations and rationale. Available at: www.ahrq.gov/clinic/3rduspstf/dementia/dementrr.htm. Accessed December 4, 2004.

19. U.S. Preventive Services Task Force. Screening for dementia. In Guide to Clinical Preventive Services, pp. 531–541. Baltimore, Williams & Wilkins, 1996.

20. Strub RL, Black FW. The Mental Status Examination in Neurology, 2nd ed. Philadelphia, FA Davis, 1985.

ADDITIONAL REFERENCES

American Psychiatric Association. Diagnostic and Statistical Manual of Mental Disorders, 4th ed., text revision. Washington, DC, American Psychiatric Association, 2000.

Antai-Otong D. Managing geriatric psychiatric emergencies: delirium and dementia. Nurs Clin North Am 38(1):123–135, 2003.

Coffey CE, Cummings JL. American Psychiatric Press Textbook of Geriatric Neuropsychiatry, 2nd ed. Washington, DC, American Psychiatric Press, 2000.

Folstein M, Folstein SE, Mchugh PR. "Mini-mental state." A practical method for grading the cognitive state of patients for the clinician. J Psych Res 12(3):189–198, 1975.

Hales RE, Yudofsky SC (eds). Essentials of Clinical Psychiatry, 2nd ed. Washington, DC, American Psychiatric Press, 2004.

Luoma JB, Martin CE, Pearson JL. Contact with mental health and primary care providers before suicide: a review of the evidence. Am J Psychiatry 159(6):909–916, 2002.

Sadock BJ, Sadock VA, Kaplan HI (eds). Kaplan & Sadock's Comprehensive Textbook of Psychiatry, 8th ed. Philadelphia, Lippincott Williams & Wilkins, 2005.

Schiffer RB, Rao SM, Fogel BS (eds.). Neuropsychiatry. Philadelphia, Lippincott Williams & Williams, 2002.

Weisner C, Mertens J, Parthasarathy S, et al. Integrating primary medical care with addition treatment: a randomized controlled trial. JAMA 286(14):1715–1723, 2001.

TABLE 16-1   **Disorders of Mood**

Mood disorders may be either depressive or bipolar. A bipolar disorder can include manic, hypomanic, or depressive features. *Four types of episodes,* described below, are combined in different ways in diagnosis of mood disorders. A major depressive disorder includes only one or more major depressive episodes. A *bipolar I disorder* includes one or more manic or mixed episodes, usually accompanied by major depressive episodes. A *bipolar II disorder* includes one or more major depressive episodes accompanied by at least one hypomanic episode.

Dysthymic and *cyclothymic disorders* are chronic and less severe conditions that do not meet the criteria of the other disorders. Mood disorders due to general medical conditions or substance abuse are classified separately.

Major Depressive Episode

At least five of the symptoms listed below (including one of the first two) must be present during the same 2-week period. They must also represent a change from the person's previous state.

- Depressed mood (may be an irritable mood in children and adolescents) most of the day, nearly every day
- Markedly diminished interest or pleasure in almost all activities most of the day, nearly every day
- Significant weight gain or loss (not dieting) or increased or decreased appetite nearly every day
- Insomnia or hypersomnia nearly every day
- Psychomotor agitation or retardation nearly every day
- Fatigue or loss of energy nearly every day
- Feelings of worthlessness or inappropriate guilt nearly every day
- Inability to think or concentrate or indecisiveness nearly every day
- Recurrent thoughts of death or suicide, or a specific plan for or attempt at suicide

The symptoms cause significant distress or impair social, occupational, or other important functions. In severe cases, hallucinations and delusions may occur.

Mixed Episode

A mixed episode, which must last at least 1 week, meets the criteria for both major and manic depressive episodes.

Dysthymic Disorder

A depressed mood and symptoms for most of the day, for more days than not, over at least 2 years (1 year in children and adolescents). Freedom from symptoms lasts no more than 2 months at a time.

Manic Episode

A distinct period of abnormally and persistently elevated, expansive, or irritable mood must be present for at least a week (any duration if hospitalization is necessary). During this time, at least three of the symptoms listed below have been persistent and significant. (Four of the these symptoms are required if the mood is only irritable).

- Inflated self-esteem or grandiosity
- Decreased need for sleep (feels rested after sleeping 3 hours)
- More talkative than usual or pressure to keep talking
- Flight of ideas or racing thoughts
- Distractibility
- Increased goal-directed activity (either socially at work or school, or sexually) or psychomotor agitation
- Excessive involvement in pleasurable high-risk activities (buying sprees, foolish business ventures, sexual indiscretions)

The disturbance is severe enough to impair social or occupational functions or relationships. It may necessitate hospitalization for the protection of self or others. In severe cases, hallucinations and delusions may occur.

Hypomanic Episode

The mood and symptoms resemble those in a manic episode but are less impairing, do not require hospitalization, do not include hallucinations or delusions, and have a shorter minimum duration—4 days.

Cyclothymic Episode

Numerous periods of hypomanic and depressive symptoms that last for at least 2 years (1 year in children and adolescents). Freedom from symptoms lasts no more than 2 months at a time.

Tables 16-1, 16-3, and 16-4 are based, with permission, on the *Diagnostic and Statistical Manual of Mental Disorders,* 4th ed., text revision (*DSM IV-TR*). Washington, DC, American Psychiatric Association, 2000. For further details and criteria, the reader should consult this manual, its successor, or comprehensive textbooks of psychiatry.

TABLE 16-2   Disorders of Speech

Disorders of speech fall into three groups: those affecting (1) the voice, (2) the articulation of words, and (3) the production and comprehension of language.

Aphonia refers to a loss of voice that accompanies disease affecting the larynx or its nerve supply. *Dysphonia* refers to less severe impairment in the volume, quality, or pitch of the voice. For example, a person may be hoarse or only able to speak in a whisper. Causes include laryngitis, laryngeal tumors, and a unilateral vocal cord paralysis (Cranial Nerve X).

Dysarthria refers to a defect in the muscular control of the speech apparatus (lips, tongue, palate, or pharynx). Words may be nasal, slurred, or indistinct, but the central symbolic aspect of language remains intact. Causes include motor lesions of the central or peripheral nervous system, parkinsonism, and cerebellar disease.

Aphasia refers to a disorder in producing or understanding language. It is often caused by lesions in the dominant cerebral hemisphere, usually the left.

Compared below are two common types of aphasia: (1) Wernicke's, a fluent (receptive) aphasia, and (2) Broca's, a nonfluent (or expressive) aphasia. There are other less common kinds of aphasia, which are distinguished by differing responses on the specific tests listed. Neurologic consultation is usually indicated.

	Wernicke's Aphasia	Broca's Aphasia
Qualities of Spontaneous Speech	Fluent; often rapid, voluble, and effortless. Inflection and articulation are good, but sentences lack meaning and words are malformed (paraphasias) or invented (neologisms). Speech may be totally incomprehensible.	Nonfluent; slow, with few words and laborious effort. Inflection and articulation are impaired but words are meaningful, with nouns, transitive verbs, and important adjectives. Small grammatical words are often dropped.
Word Comprehension	Impaired	Fair to good
Repetition	Impaired	Impaired
Naming	Impaired	Impaired, though the patient recognizes objects
Reading Comprehension	Impaired	Fair to good
Writing	Impaired	Impaired
Location of Lesion	Posterior superior temporal lobe	Posterior inferior frontal lobe

Although it is important to recognize aphasia early in your encounter with a patient, its full diagnostic meaning does not become clear until you integrate this information with your neurologic examination.

TABLE 16-3   **Anxiety Disorders**

Panic Disorder

A *panic disorder* is defined by recurrent, unexpected panic attacks, at least one of which has been followed by a month or more of persistent concern about further attacks, worry over their implications or consequences, or a significant change in behavior in relation to the attacks. A *panic attack* is a discrete period of intense fear or discomfort that develops abruptly and peaks within 10 minutes. It involves at least four of the following symptoms: (1) palpitations, pounding heart, or accelerated heart rate, (2) sweating, (3) trembling or shaking, (4) shortness of breath or a sense of smothering, (5) a feeling of choking, (6) chest pain or discomfort, (7) nausea or abdominal distress, (8) feeling dizzy, unsteady, lightheaded, or faint, (9) feelings of unreality or depersonalization, (10) fear of losing control or going crazy, (11) fear of dying, (12) paresthesias (numbness or tingling), (13) chills or hot flushes. Panic disorder may occur with or without *agoraphobia*.

Agoraphobia

Agoraphobia is an anxiety about being in places or situations where escape may be difficult or embarrassing or help unavailable. Such situations are avoided, require a companion, or cause marked anxiety.

Specific Phobia

A specific phobia is a marked, persistent, and excessive or unreasonable fear that is cued by the presence or anticipation of a specific object or situation, such as dogs, injections, or flying. The person recognizes the fear as excessive or unreasonable, but exposure to the cue provokes immediate anxiety. Avoidance or fear impairs the person's normal routine, occupational or academic functioning, or social activities or relationships.

Social Phobia

A social phobia is a marked, persistent fear of one or more social or performance situations that involve exposure to unfamiliar people or to scrutiny by others. Those afflicted fear that they will act in embarrassing or humiliating ways, as by showing their anxiety. Exposure creates anxiety and possibly a panic attack, and the person avoids precipitating situations. He or she recognizes the fear as excessive or unreasonable. Normal routines, occupational or academic functioning, or social activities or relationships are impaired.

Obsessive-Compulsive Disorder

This disorder involves obsessions or compulsions that cause marked anxiety or distress. Although they are recognized at some point as excessive or unreasonable, they are very time consuming and interfere with the person's normal routine, occupational functioning, or social activities or relationships.

Acute Stress Disorder

The person has been exposed to a traumatic event that involved actual or threatened death or serious injury to self or others and responded with intense fear, helplessness, or horror. During or immediately after this event, the person has at least three of these dissociative symptoms: (1) a subjective sense of numbing, detachment, or absence of emotional responsiveness; (2) a reduced awareness of surroundings, as in a daze; (3) feelings of unreality; (4) feelings of depersonalization; and (5) amnesia for an important part of the event. The event is persistently reexperienced, as in thoughts, images, dreams, illusions, and flashbacks, or distress from reminders of the event. The person is very anxious or shows increased arousal and tries to avoid stimuli that evoke memories of the event. The disturbance causes marked distress or impairs social, occupational, or other important functions. The symptoms occur within 4 weeks of the event and last from 2 days to 4 weeks.

Posttraumatic Stress Disorder

The event, the fearful response, and the persistent reexperiencing of the traumatic event resemble those in acute stress disorder. Hallucinations may occur. The person has increased arousal, tries to avoid stimuli related to the trauma, and has numbing of general responsiveness. The disturbance causes marked distress, impairs social, occupational, or other important functions, and lasts for more than a month.

Generalized Anxiety Disorder

This disorder lacks a specific traumatic event or focus for concern. Excessive anxiety and worry, which the person finds hard to control, are about a number of events or activities. At least three of the following symptoms are associated: (1) feeling restless, keyed up, or on edge; (2) being easily fatigued; (3) difficulty in concentrating or mind going blank; (4) irritability; (5) muscle tension; (6) difficulty in falling or staying asleep, or restless, unsatisfying sleep. The disturbance causes significant distress or impairs social, occupational, or other important functions.

| TABLE 16-4 | Psychotic Disorders |

Psychotic disorders involve grossly impaired reality testing. Specific diagnoses depend on the nature and duration of the symptoms and on a cause when it can be identified. Seven disorders are outlined below.

Schizophrenia	Schizophrenia impairs major functioning, as at work or school or in interpersonal relations or self-care. For this diagnosis, performance of one or more of these functions must have decreased for a significant time to a level markedly below prior achievement. In addition, the person must manifest at least two of the following for a significant part of 1 month: (1) delusions, (2) hallucinations, (3) disorganized speech, (4) grossly disorganized or catatonic behavior,* and (5) negative symptoms such as a flat affect, alogia (lack of content in speech), or avolition (lack of interest, drive, and ability to set and pursue goals). Continuous signs of the disturbance must persist for at least 6 months. Subtypes of this disorder include paranoid, disorganized, and catatonic schizophrenia.
Schizophreniform Disorder	A schizophreniform disorder has symptoms similar to those of schizophrenia, but they last less than 6 months, and the functional impairment seen in schizophrenia need not be present.
Schizoaffective Disorder	A schizoaffective disorder has features of both a major mood disturbance and schizophrenia. The mood disturbance (depressive, manic, or mixed) is present during most of the illness and must, for a time, be concurrent with symptoms of schizophrenia (listed above). During the same period of time, there must also be delusions or hallucinations for at least 2 weeks without prominent mood symptoms.
Delusional Disorder	A delusional disorder is characterized by nonbizarre delusions that involve situations in real life, such as having a disease or being deceived by a lover. The delusion has persisted for at least a month, but the person's functioning is not markedly impaired, and behavior is not obviously odd or bizarre. The symptoms of schizophrenia, except for tactile and olfactory hallucinations related to the delusion, have not been present.
Brief Psychotic Disorder	In this disorder, at least one of the following psychotic symptoms must be present: delusions, hallucinations, disordered speech such as frequent derailment or incoherence, or grossly disorganized or catatonic behavior. The disturbance lasts at least 1 day but less than 1 month, and the person returns to his or her prior functional level.
Psychotic Disorder Due to a General Medical Condition	Prominent hallucinations or delusions may be experienced during a medical illness. For this diagnosis, they should not occur exclusively during the course of delirium. The medical condition should be documented and judged to be causally related to the symptoms.
Substance-Induced Psychotic Disorder	Prominent hallucinations or delusions may be induced by intoxication or withdrawal from a substance such as alcohol, cocaine, or opioids. For this diagnosis, these symptoms should not occur exclusively during the course of delirium. The substance should be judged to be causally related to the symptoms.

*Catatonic behaviors are psychomotor abnormalities that include stupor, mutism, negativistic resistance to instructions or attempts to move the person, rigid or bizarre postures, and excited, apparently purposeless activity.

The Nervous System: Cranial Nerves, Motor System, Sensory System, and Reflexes

ANATOMY AND PHYSIOLOGY

This section deals briefly with structures, functions, and concepts that relate directly to the neurologic examination. After a short description of the brain (anatomy shown below), spinal cord, cranial and peripheral nerves, and reflexes, there are summaries of important motor and sensory pathways. Common or concerning symptoms and health promotion and counseling follow. Next comes *Techniques of Examination* for the nervous system, including the cranial nerves, the motor and sensory systems, and reflexes. Then turn to the write-up combining mental status and the examination of the nervous system.

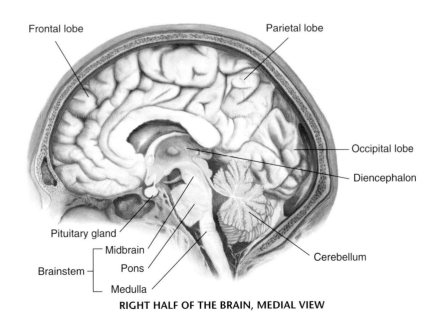

RIGHT HALF OF THE BRAIN, MEDIAL VIEW

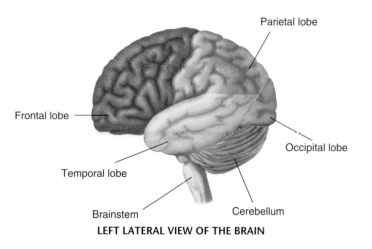

Parietal lobe

Frontal lobe

Occipital lobe

Temporal lobe

Brainstem

Cerebellum

LEFT LATERAL VIEW OF THE BRAIN

As you review this material, note that the *central nervous system* consists of the brain and the spinal cord. The *peripheral nervous system* consists of the 12 pairs of cranial nerves and the spinal and peripheral nerves. Most of the peripheral nerves contain both motor and sensory fibers.

CENTRAL NERVOUS SYSTEM

THE BRAIN

The brain has four regions: the cerebrum, the diencephalon, the brainstem, and the cerebellum. The cerebral hemispheres contain the greatest mass of brain tissue. Each hemisphere is subdivided into frontal, parietal, temporal, and occipital lobes, as shown above.

The brain is a vast network of interconnecting *neurons* (nerve cells). These consist of cell bodies and their *axons*—single long fibers that conduct impulses to other parts of the nervous system.

Brain tissue may be gray or white. *Gray matter* consists of aggregations of neuronal cell bodies. It rims the surfaces of the cerebral hemispheres, forming the cerebral cortex. *White matter* consists of neuronal axons that are coated with myelin. The myelin sheaths, which create the white color, allow nerve impulses to travel more rapidly.

Deep in the brain lie additional clusters of gray matter. These include the *basal ganglia,* which affect movement, and the thalamus and the hypothalamus, structures in the diencephalon. The *thalamus* processes sensory impulses and relays them to the cerebral cortex. The *hypothalamus* maintains homeostasis and regulates temperature, heart rate, and blood pressure. The hypothalamus affects the endocrine system and governs emotional behaviors such as anger and sexual drive. Hormones secreted in the hypothalamus act directly on the pituitary gland.

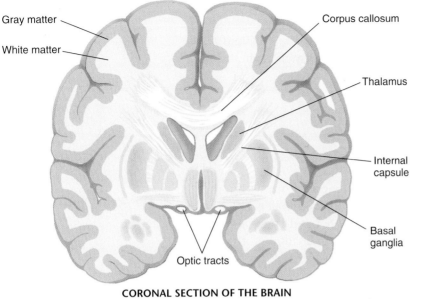

CORONAL SECTION OF THE BRAIN

In contrast, note the *internal capsule,* a white-matter structure where myelinated fibers converge from all parts of the cerebral cortex and descend into the brainstem. The *brainstem,* which connects the upper part of the brain with the spinal cord, has three sections: the midbrain, the pons, and the medulla.

Consciousness depends on the interaction between intact cerebral hemispheres and an important structure in the diencephalon and upper brainstem, the *reticular activating (arousal) system.*

The *cerebellum,* which lies at the base of the brain, coordinates all movement and helps maintain the body upright in space.

THE SPINAL CORD

The *spinal cord* is a cylindrical mass of nerve tissue encased within the bony vertebral column, extending from the medulla to the first or second lumbar vertebra. It contains important motor and sensory nerve pathways that exit and enter the cord through anterior and posterior nerve roots and spinal and peripheral nerves. The spinal cord also mediates reflex activity of the deep tendon reflexes from the spinal nerves.

The spinal cord is divided into five segments: cervical, from C1 to C8; thoracic, from T1 to T12; lumbar, from L1 to L5; sacral, from S1 to S5; and coccygeal.

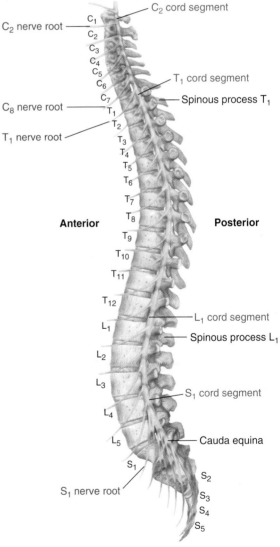

THE SPINAL CORD, LATERAL VIEW

spinal cord is not as long as the vertebral canal. The lumbar
ots travel the longest intraspinal distance and fan out like a
L1 to L2, giving rise to the term *cauda equina*. To avoid injury to the spinal cord, most lumbar punctures are performed at the L2–4
vertebral interspace.

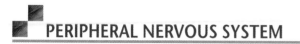

PERIPHERAL NERVOUS SYSTEM

THE CRANIAL NERVES

Twelve pairs of special nerves called *cranial nerves* emerge from within the
skull or *cranium*. Cranial Nerves II through XII arise from the diencephalon
and the brainstem, as illustrated below. Cranial Nerves I and II are actually
fiber tracts emerging from the brain. Some cranial nerves are limited to general motor or sensory functions, whereas others are specialized, producing
smell, vision, or hearing (I, II, VIII).

Functions of the cranial nerves (CN) most relevant to physical examination
are summarized on the next page.

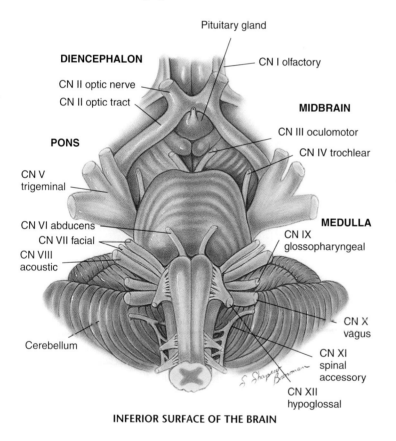

INFERIOR SURFACE OF THE BRAIN

THE PERIPHERAL NERVES

In addition to cranial nerves, the peripheral nervous system also includes spinal
and peripheral nerves that carry impulses to and from the cord. Thirty-one
pairs of nerves attach to the spinal cord: 8 cervical, 12 thoracic, 5 lumbar,

■ *Cranial Nerves*

No.	Name	Function
I	**Olfactory**	Sense of smell
II	**Optic**	Vision
III	**Oculomotor**	Pupillary constriction, opening the eye, and most extraocular movements
IV	**Trochlear**	Downward, inward movement of the eye
VI	**Abducens**	Lateral deviation of the eye
V	**Trigeminal**	*Motor*—temporal and masseter muscles (jaw clenching), also lateral movement of the jaw *Sensory*—facial. The nerve has three divisions: (1) ophthalmic, (2) maxillary, and (3) mandibular.

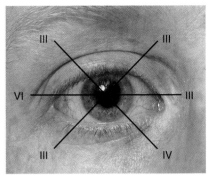

RIGHT EYE (CN III, IV, VI)

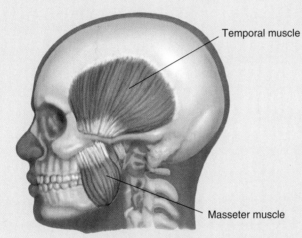

Temporal muscle

Masseter muscle

CN V—MOTOR

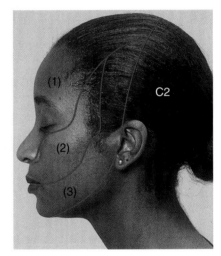

CN V—SENSORY

VII	**Facial**	*Motor*—facial movements, including those of facial expression, closing the eye, and closing the mouth *Sensory*—taste for salty, sweet, sour, and bitter substances on the anterior two thirds of the tongue
VIII	**Acoustic**	Hearing (cochlear division) and balance (vestibular division)
IX	**Glossopharyngeal**	*Motor*—pharynx *Sensory*—posterior portions of the eardrum and ear canal, the pharynx, and the posterior tongue, including taste (salty, sweet, sour, bitter)
X	**Vagus**	*Motor*—palate, pharynx, and larynx *Sensory*—pharynx and larynx
XI	**Spinal accessory**	*Motor*—the sternomastoid and upper portion of the trapezius
XII	**Hypoglossal**	*Motor*—tongue

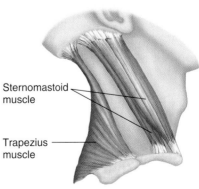

Sternomastoid muscle

Trapezius muscle

CN XI—MOTOR

5 sacral, and 1 coccygeal. Each nerve has an anterior (ventral) root containing motor fibers, and a posterior (dorsal) root containing sensory fibers. The anterior and posterior roots merge to form a short *spinal nerve,* less than 5 mm in length. Spinal nerve fibers commingle with similar fibers from other levels to form *peripheral nerves.* Most peripheral nerves contain both *sensory* (afferent) and *motor* (efferent) fibers.

Like the brain, the spinal cord contains both gray matter and white matter. Nuclei of gray matter, which are aggregations of nerve cell bodies, are surrounded by white tracts of nerve fibers connecting the brain to the peripheral nervous system. Note the butterfly appearance of the gray-matter nuclei, with anterior and posterior horns.

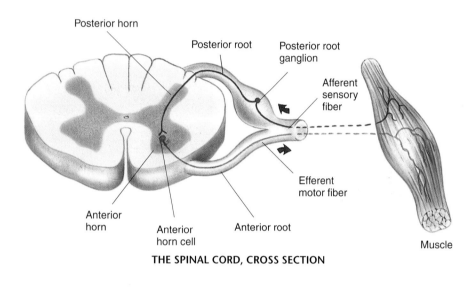

Posterior horn

Posterior root

Posterior root ganglion

Afferent sensory fiber

Efferent motor fiber

Anterior horn

Anterior horn cell

Anterior root

Muscle

THE SPINAL CORD, CROSS SECTION

SPINAL REFLEXES: THE DEEP TENDON RESPONSE

The deep tendon or muscle stretch reflexes are relayed over structures of both the central and peripheral nervous systems. Recall that a *reflex* is an involuntary stereotypical response that may involve as few as two neurons, one afferent (sensory) and one efferent (motor), across a single synapse. The deep tendon reflexes in the arms and legs are such monosynaptic reflexes. They illustrate the simplest unit of sensory and motor function. (Other reflexes are polysynaptic, involving interneurons interposed between sensory and motor neurons.)

To elicit a deep tendon reflex, briskly tap the tendon of a partially stretched muscle. For the reflex to fire, all components of the reflex arc must be intact: sensory nerve fibers, spinal cord synapse, motor nerve fibers, neuromuscular junction, and muscle fibers. Tapping the tendon activates special sensory fibers in the partially stretched muscle, triggering a sensory impulse that travels to the spinal cord via a peripheral nerve. The stimulated sensory fiber synapses directly with the anterior horn cell innervating the same muscle. When the impulse crosses the neuromuscular junction, the muscle suddenly contracts, completing the reflex arc.

Because each deep tendon reflex involves specific spinal segments, together with their sensory and motor fibers, an abnormal reflex can help you to locate a pathologic lesion. Learn the segmental levels of the deep tendon reflexes. You can remember them easily by their numerical sequence in ascending order from ankle to triceps: S1—L2, 3, 4,—C5, 6, 7.

Ankle reflex	Sacral 1 primarily
Knee reflex	Lumbar 2, 3, 4
Supinator (brachioradialis) reflex	Cervical 5, 6
Biceps reflex	Cervical 5, 6
Triceps reflex	Cervical 6, 7

Reflexes may be initiated by stimulating skin as well as muscle. Stroking the skin of the abdomen, for example, produces a localized muscular twitch. These superficial (cutaneous) reflexes and their corresponding spinal segments include:

Abdominal reflexes—upper	Thoracic 8, 9, 10
—lower	Thoracic 10, 11, 12
Plantar responses	Lumbar 5, Sacral 1

MOTOR PATHWAYS

Motor pathways contain upper motor neurons, synapses in the brainstem or spinal cord, and lower motor neurons. Nerve cell bodies or *upper motor neurons* lie in the motor strip of the cerebral cortex and in several brainstem nuclei; their axons synapse with motor nuclei in the brainstem (for cranial nerves) and in the spinal cord (for peripheral nerves). *Lower motor neurons* have cell bodies in the spinal cord, termed anterior horn cells; their axons transmit impulses through the anterior roots and spinal nerves into peripheral nerves, terminating at the neuromuscular junction.

Three kinds of motor pathways impinge on the anterior horn cells: the corticospinal tract, the basal ganglia system, and the cerebellar system. There are additional pathways originating in the brainstem that mediate flexor and extensor tone in limb movement and posture, most notable in coma (see Table 17-11, p. 667).

THE PRINCIPAL MOTOR PATHWAYS

■ The **corticospinal (pyramidal) tract**. The corticospinal tracts mediate voluntary movement and integrate skilled, complicated, or delicate movements by stimulating selected muscular actions and inhibiting others. They also carry impulses that inhibit *muscle tone,* the slight tension maintained by normal muscle even when it is relaxed. The corticospinal tracts originate in the motor cortex of the brain. Motor fibers travel down into the lower medulla, where they form an anatomical structure resembling a pyramid. There, most of these fibers cross to the opposite or *contralateral*

(continued)

> ## THE PRINCIPAL MOTOR PATHWAYS (Continued)
>
> side of the medulla, continue downward, and synapse with anterior horn cells or with intermediate neurons. Tracts synapsing in the brainstem with motor nuclei of the cranial nerves are termed *corticobulbar*.
>
> - The ***basal ganglia system***. This exceedingly complex system includes motor pathways between the cerebral cortex, basal ganglia, brainstem, and spinal cord. It helps to maintain muscle tone and to control body movements, especially gross automatic movements such as walking.
> - The ***cerebellar system***. The cerebellum receives both sensory and motor input and coordinates motor activity, maintains equilibrium, and helps to control posture.

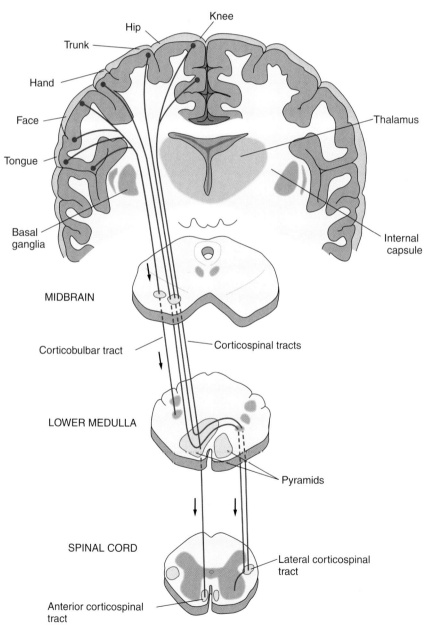

MOTOR PATHWAYS: CORTICOSPINAL AND CORTICOBULBAR TRACTS

All of these higher motor pathways affect movement only through the lower motor neuron systems—sometimes called the "final common pathway." Any movement, whether initiated voluntarily in the cortex, "automatically" in the basal ganglia, or reflexly in the sensory receptors, must ultimately be translated into action via the anterior horn cells. A lesion in any of these areas will affect movement or reflex activity.

When the corticospinal tract is damaged or destroyed, its functions are reduced or lost below the level of injury. *When upper motor neuron systems are damaged above the crossover of its tracts in the medulla, motor impairment develops on the opposite or contralateral side. In damage below the crossover, motor impairment occurs on the same or ipsilateral side of the body.* The affected limb becomes weak or paralyzed, and skilled, complicated, or delicate movements are performed especially poorly when compared with gross movements.

In upper motor neuron lesions, muscle tone is increased and deep tendon reflexes are exaggerated. Damage to the lower motor neuron systems causes ipsilateral weakness and paralysis, but in this case, muscle tone and reflexes are decreased or absent.

Disease of the basal ganglia system or cerebellar system does not cause paralysis but can be disabling. Damage to the basal ganglia system produces changes in muscle tone (most often an increase), disturbances in posture and gait, a slowness or lack of spontaneous and automatic movements termed *bradykinesia*, and a variety of involuntary movements. Cerebellar damage impairs coordination, gait, and equilibrium and decreases muscle tone.

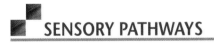

SENSORY PATHWAYS

Sensory impulses not only participate in reflex activity, as previously described, but also give rise to conscious sensation, calibrate body position in space, and help regulate internal autonomic functions like blood pressure, heart rate, and respiration.

A complex system of sensory receptors relays impulses from skin, mucous membranes, muscles, tendons, and viscera. Sensory fibers registering sensations such as pain, temperature, position, and touch pass through the peripheral nerves and posterior roots and enter the spinal cord. Once inside the cord, sensory impulses reach the sensory cortex of the brain via one of the two pathways: the spinothalamic tracts or the posterior columns.

Within one or two spinal segments from their entry into the cord, fibers conducting the sensations of *pain* and *temperature* pass into the posterior horn of the spinal cord and synapse with secondary sensory neurons. Fibers conducting *crude touch*—a sensation perceived as light touch but without accurate localization—also pass into the posterior horn and synapse with secondary neurons. The secondary neurons then cross to the opposite side and pass upward in the *spinothalamic tract* into the thalamus.

Fibers conducting the sensations of *position* and *vibration* pass directly into the *posterior columns* of the cord and travel upward to the medulla, together with fibers transmitting *fine touch*—touch that is accurately localized and finely discriminating. These fibers synapse in the medulla with secondary sensory neurons. Fibers projecting from secondary neurons cross to the opposite side at the medullary level and continue on to the thalamus.

At the *thalamic level,* the general quality of sensation is perceived (e.g., pain, cold, pleasant, and unpleasant), but fine distinctions are not made. For full perception, a third group of sensory neurons sends impulses from the thalamus to the *sensory cortex* of the brain. Here stimuli are localized and higher-order discriminations are made.

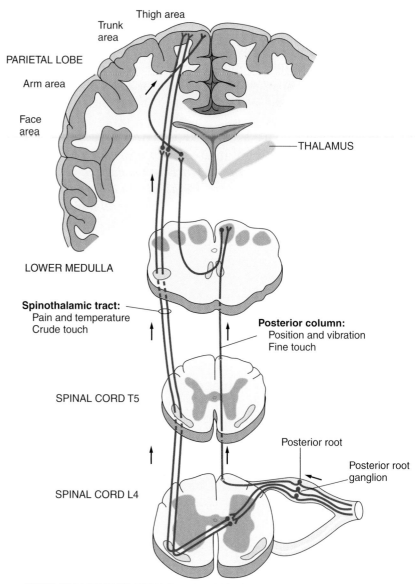

SENSORY PATHWAYS: SPINOTHALAMIC TRACT AND POSTERIOR COLUMNS

Lesions at different points in the sensory pathways produce different kinds of sensory loss. Patterns of sensory loss, together with their associated motor findings, help you to identify where the causative lesions might be. A lesion in the sensory cortex may not impair the perception of pain, touch, and position, for example, but does impair finer discrimination. A person so affected cannot appreciate the size, shape, or texture of an object by feeling it and therefore cannot identify it. Loss of position and vibration sense with preservation of other sensations points to disease of the posterior columns, whereas loss of all sensations from the waist down, together with paralysis and hyperactive reflexes in the legs, indicates transection of the spinal cord (see Table 17-11, p. 667). Crude and light touch are often preserved despite partial damage to the cord because impulses originating on one side of the body travel up both sides of the cord.

Dermatomes. A knowledge of *dermatomes* also aids in localizing neurologic lesions. *A dermatome is the band of skin innervated by the sensory root of a single spinal nerve.* Dermatome patterns are mapped in the next two figures. Their levels are considerably more variable than the diagrams suggest, and dermatomes overlap each other. The sensory nerves from each side of the body overlap slightly across the midline. The distribution of a few key peripheral nerves is shown in the inserts on the left.

Do not try to memorize all the dermatomes. It is useful, however, to remember the locations of some, such as those shaded in green on the right side of the diagrams.

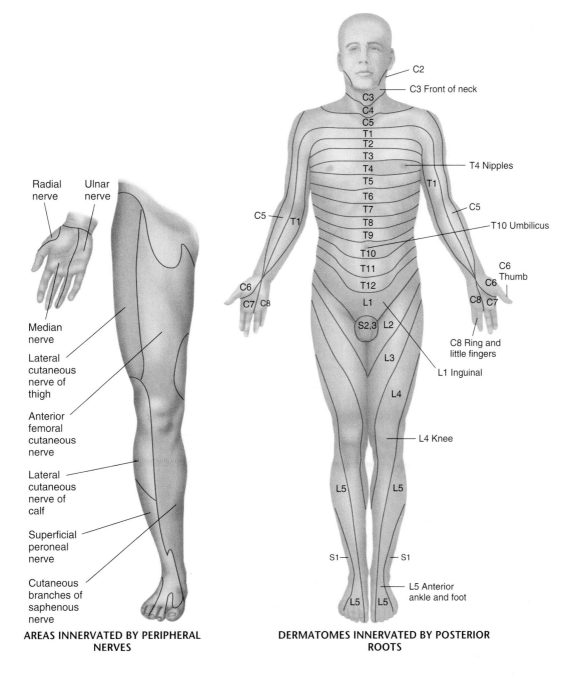

AREAS INNERVATED BY PERIPHERAL NERVES

DERMATOMES INNERVATED BY POSTERIOR ROOTS

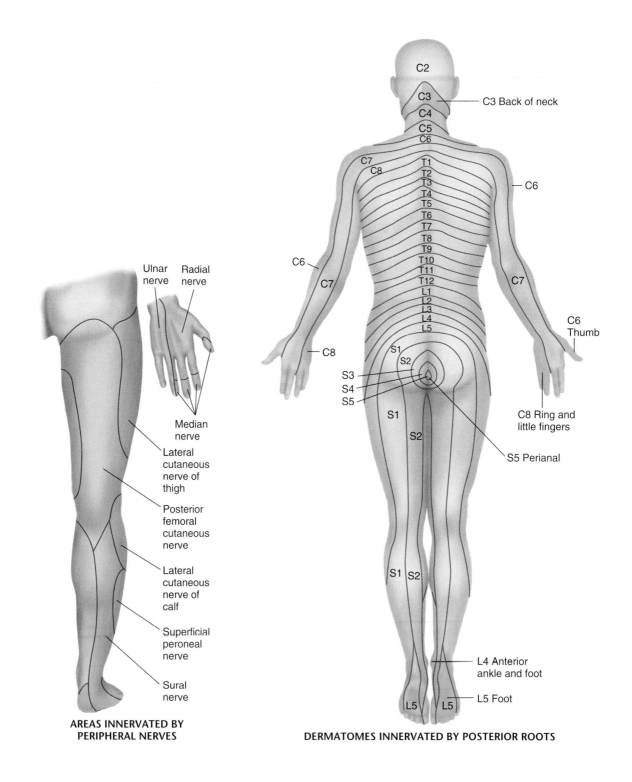

Ulnar nerve

Radial nerve

Median nerve

Lateral cutaneous nerve of thigh

Posterior femoral cutaneous nerve

Lateral cutaneous nerve of calf

Superficial peroneal nerve

Sural nerve

**AREAS INNERVATED BY
PERIPHERAL NERVES**

C2

C3

C3 Back of neck

C4

C5

C6

C7

C8

T1
T2
T3
T4
T5
T6
T7
T8
T9
T10
T11
T12
L1
L2
L3
L4
L5

C6

C6

C7

C7

C6
Thumb

C8

C8

S1

S2

S3

S4

S5

S1

S2

C8 Ring and
little fingers

S5 Perianal

S1 S2

L4 Anterior
ankle and foot

L5 Foot

L5 L5

DERMATOMES INNERVATED BY POSTERIOR ROOTS

THE HEALTH HISTORY

Common or Concerning Symptoms

- Headache
- Dizziness or vertigo
- Generalized, proximal, or distal weakness
- Numbness, abnormal or loss of sensations
- Loss of consciousness, syncope, or near-syncope
- Seizures
- Tremors or involuntary movements

Two of the most common symptoms in neurologic disorders are *headache* and *dizziness*. Turn to p. 171 and p. 173 to review the health history pertinent to these symptoms.

See Table 6-1, Headaches, pp. 206–209.

For *headache,* be sure to ask about location, severity, how long it lasts, and any associated symptoms, such as visual changes, weakness, or loss of sensation. Ask if the headache is affected by coughing, sneezing, or sudden movements of the head.

Subarachnoid hemorrhage may evoke "the worst headache of my life." Dull headache affected by such maneuvers, especially on awakening and recurring in the same location, is seen with mass lesions such as a brain tumor.

The complaint of *dizziness* can have many meanings. You will need to elicit exactly what the patient has experienced. Is the patient light-headed or feeling faint? Or is there *vertigo,* a perception that the room is spinning or rotating?

Light-headedness in palpitations, near syncope from vasovagal stimulation, low blood pressure, febrile illness, and others. Vertigo in middle-ear conditions, brainstem tumor. See Table 6-2, p. 210.

Especially in older patients, are any medications contributing to the dizziness? Are there any associated symptoms such as double vision, or *diplopia,* difficulty forming words, or *dysarthria,* or difficulty with gait or balance, or *ataxia?*

Diplopia, dysarthria, ataxia in posterior circulation *transient ischemic attack* (TIA) or *stroke*

What about any associated *weakness,* either generalized or in the face or a part of the body? Weakness is another common symptom and requires careful attention to detail. Probe for exactly what it means to the patient. Explore whether there is any *paralysis,* or inability to move a part or side of the body. Did the weakness start slowly or suddenly? Has it progressed? How? What areas of the body are involved? Does the weakness affect one or both sides? What movements are affected?

Weakness or paralysis in transient ischemic attack or stroke

Focal weakness may arise from ischemic, vascular, or mass lesions in the central nervous system; also from peripheral nervous system disorders, neuromuscular disorders, or the muscles themselves.

For weakness without light-headedness, try to distinguish between *proximal* and *distal weakness*. For proximal weakness, ask about combing hair, trying to reach something on a high shelf, or difficulty getting up out of a chair or taking a high step up. Does the weakness increase with repeated effort and improve after rest? Are there associated sensory or other symptoms? For distal weakness in the arms, inquire about hand movements such as opening a jar or can, or using hand tools such as scissors, pliers, or a screwdriver. For distal weakness in the legs, ask about frequent tripping.

Find out if the patient has had any *loss of sensation*. Ask if there has been any *numbness*, but clarify its meaning and location. Has there been loss of sensation, difficulty moving a limb, or altered sensations such as tingling or pins and needles? There may be peculiar sensations without an obvious stimulus, called *paresthesias*. These occur commonly when an arm or leg "goes to sleep" following compression of a nerve, and may be described as tingling, prickling, or feelings of warmth, coldness, or pressure. *Dysesthesias* are distorted sensations in response to a stimulus and may last longer than the stimulus itself. For example, a person may perceive a light touch or pinprick as a burning or tingling sensation that is irritating or unpleasant. *Pain* may arise from neurologic causes but is usually reported with symptoms of other body systems, such as the head and neck or the musculoskeletal system.

"Have you ever fainted or passed out?" leads the discussion to any *loss of consciousness*. It is important to begin by exploring what the patient means by loss of consciousness. Did the patient black out completely, or could voices be heard throughout the episode, indicating some consciousness? Be sure to use descriptive terms carefully and precisely. *Syncope* is the sudden but temporary loss of consciousness that occurs with decreased blood flow to the brain, commonly described as *fainting*. Symptoms of feeling faint, light-headed, or weak, but without actual loss of consciousness, are called *near syncope* or *presyncope*.

Get as complete and unbiased a description of the event as you can. What brought on the episode? Were there any warning symptoms? Was the patient standing, sitting, or lying down when the episode began? How long did it last? Could voices be heard while passing out and coming to? How rapidly did the patient recover? In retrospect, were onset and offset slow or fast?

Also ask if anyone observed the episode. If so, what did the patient look like before losing consciousness, during the episode, and afterward? Was there any seizure-like movement of the arms or legs? Any incontinence of the bladder or bowel? Any drowsiness or impaired memory after the episode ended?

Bilateral proximal weakness in myopathy. Bilateral, predominantly distal weakness in polyneuropathy. Weakness made worse with repeated effort and improved with rest suggests myasthenia gravis.

Loss of sensation, paresthesias, and dysesthesias in central lesions in the brain and spinal cord, as well as disorders of peripheral sensory roots and nerves; paresthesias in the hands and around the mouth in hyperventilation. Burning pain in painful sensory neuropathy.

See Table 15-2, Pains in the Neck, p. 561, and Table 15-1, Low Back Pain, p. 560.

See Table 17-1, Syncope and Similar Disorders, pp. 649–650.

Young people with emotional stress and warning symptoms of flushing, warmth, or nausea may have *vasodepressor (or vasovagal) syncope* of slow onset, slow offset. *Cardiac syncope* from arrhythmias, more common in older patients, often with sudden onset, sudden offset.

Tonic–clonic motor activity, bladder or bowel incontinence, and *postictal state* suggest a generalized *seizure*. Unlike syncope, injury such as tongue biting or bruising of limbs may occur.

A *seizure* is a paroxysmal disorder caused by sudden excessive electrical discharge in the cerebral cortex or its underlying structures. Seizures can be of several types. Depending on the type, there may or may not be loss of consciousness. With some types of seizures, there may be abnormal feelings, thought processes, and sensations, including smells, as well as abnormal movements. Asking "Have you ever had any seizures or 'spells'?" . . . "Any fits or convulsions?" can open the discussion. As with syncope, aim for a full and complete description, including precipitating circumstances, warnings, and behavior and feelings both during the attack and afterward. Ask about age at onset, frequency, any change in frequency or symptom pattern, and use of medications. Is there any history of prior head injury or other conditions that may be causally related?

See Table 17-2, Seizure Disorders, pp. 651–652.

Tremors and other *involuntary movements* occur with or without additional neurologic manifestations. Ask about any trembling, shakiness, or body movements that the patient seems unable to control.

See Table 17-3, Tremors and Involuntary Movements, pp. 653–654. Tremor, rigidity and bradykinesia in Parkinson's disease[1]

Distinct from these symptoms is an almost indescribable *restlessness of the legs* that typically develops at rest and is accompanied by an urge to move about. Walking gives relief.

The common but often overlooked restless legs syndrome, usually benign

HEALTH PROMOTION AND COUNSELING

Important Topics for Health Promotion and Counseling

- Prevention of TIAs or stroke

Cerebrovascular disease is the third leading cause of death in the United States and contributes to extensive disability in the workforce and general population. Decreased vascular perfusion results in sudden brain dysfunction from transient ischemic attack (TIA), with temporary loss of blood flow, or permanent cerebral infarction, or stroke. Approximately 85% of strokes are ischemic; approximately 15% are hemorrhagic. Most strokes are caused by thromboembolism. Other causes include local injury in the vascular wall, as in atherosclerosis, inflammation, or dissection; loss of perfusion pressure, as in hypotension from myocardial infarction; changes in blood viscosity, as in polycythemia; and blood vessel rupture into the subarachnoid space or intracerebral tissue.[2,3]

Be alert for transient symptoms of TIAs such as visual loss (especially transient monocular blindness), aphasia, dysarthria, and changes in facial movement or sensation. For TIAs affecting motor or sensory pathways, watch for clumsiness, weakness, paralysis, or tingling or paresthesias of the extremities. The long-standing definition of TIAs that can last up to 24 hours has been revised to symptoms lasting 1 hour or less, without evidence of permanent brain injury.[2-5] Detecting TIAs is especially important—in the first 3 months after a TIA, subsequent stroke is seen in approximately 10% of patients, especially those with diabetes, age older than 60, or changes in speech or motor function.[5]

The clinician's first step in stroke prevention is aggressive management of risk factors and patient education. Risk factors for stroke include hypertension, diet, dyslipidemia, heavy alcohol use, physical inactivity, obesity, and diabetes. Controlling *hypertension* is key because it is a leading contributor to both ischemic and hemorrhagic strokes. Hypertension accelerates atherosclerotic changes in the carotid, vertebral, and cerebral arteries and disturbs autoregulation of cerebral blood pressure. Blood pressure should be less than 140/90 mm Hg and less than 130/80 mm Hg for those with diabetes or nondiabetic renal disease with significant proteinuria[6] (see further discussion in Chap. 8, Cardiovascular System, pp. 295–301). Evidence from trials of lipid-lowering agents in cardiovascular patients suggests benefit in reducing risk for stroke.[7,8] Urge patients with unhealthy diets and *dyslipidemia* to replace saturated and trans-unsaturated fats, found in dairy products, meat, and stick margarine, with polyunsaturated and unhydrogenated monosaturated fats, found in soybean and liquid margarine and fish oils. Or simply recommend increased intake of fruits, vegetables, and fiber. Heavy alcohol users have significantly higher risk for stroke.[9] Counsel patients to maintain regular exercise and body weight. The U.S. Preventive Services Task Force recommends individualized discussion of exercise and optimal body weight. Diabetes should be closely monitored to attain optimal control of blood glucose in the range of 100 mg/dl. The U.S. Preventive Services Task Force recommends discussion of use of aspirin in primary prevention in patients at high risk for coronary heart disease, but notes that aspirin is associated with increased risk for gastrointestinal bleeding and stroke.[10]

TECHNIQUES OF EXAMINATION

Important Areas of Examination

- Cranial Nerves I through XII
- Motor system: muscle bulk, tone, and strength; coordination, gait, and stance
- Sensory system: pain and temperature, position and vibration, light touch, discrimination
- Deep tendon, abdominal, and plantar reflexes

Now return to the three important questions that govern the neurologic examination:

■ Is the mental status intact?

■ Are right-sided and left-sided findings symmetric?

■ If the findings are asymmetric or otherwise abnormal, does the causative lesion lie in the central nervous system or the peripheral nervous system?

In this section, you will learn the techniques for a practical and reasonably comprehensive examination of the nervous system. It is important to master the techniques for a thorough examination. At first these techniques may seem difficult, but with practice, dedication, and supervision, you will come to feel comfortable evaluating neurologic symptoms and disease. You should be active in your learning and ask your instructors or even neurologists to review your skills.

The detail of an appropriate neurologic examination varies widely. As you gain experience, you will find that in healthy people, your examination will come to be relatively brief. When you detect abnormal findings, your examination will become more comprehensive. Be aware that neurologists may use many other techniques in specific situations.

For efficiency, you should integrate certain portions of the neurologic assessment with other parts of your examination. Survey the patient's mental status and speech during the interview, for example, even though you may wish to do further testing during your neurologic evaluation. Assess some of the cranial nerves as you examine the head and neck, and inspect the arms and legs for neurologic abnormalities while you also observe the peripheral vascular and musculoskeletal systems. Chapter 4 provides an outline for this kind of integrated approach. Think about and describe your findings, however, in terms of the nervous system as a unit.

Organize your thinking into five categories: (1) mental status, speech, and language, (2) cranial nerves, (3) the motor system, (4) the sensory system, and (5) reflexes. If your findings are abnormal, begin to group them into patterns of central or peripheral disorders.

THE CRANIAL NERVES

Overview.   The examination of the cranial nerves (abbreviated as CN) can be summarized as follows:

I	Smell
II	Visual acuity, visual fields, and ocular fundi
II, III	Pupillary reactions
III, IV, VI	Extraocular movements

V	Corneal reflexes, facial sensation, and jaw movements
VII	Facial movements
VIII	Hearing
IX, X	Swallowing and rise of the palate, gag reflex
V, VII, X, XII	Voice and speech
XI	Shoulder and neck movements
XII	Tongue symmetry and position

Cranial Nerve I—Olfactory.   Test the *sense of smell* by presenting the patient with familiar and nonirritating odors. First be sure that each nasal passage is open by compressing one side of the nose and asking the patient to sniff through the other. The patient should then close both eyes. Occlude one nostril and test smell in the other with such substances as cloves, coffee, soap, or vanilla. Ask if the patient smells anything and, if so, what. Test the other side. A person should normally perceive odor on each side, and can often identify it.

Loss of smell has many causes, including nasal disease, head trauma, smoking, aging, and the use of cocaine. It may be congenital.

Cranial Nerve II—Optic.   Test *visual acuity* (see pp. 177–178).

Inspect the *optic fundi* with your ophthalmoscope, paying special attention to the optic discs (see pp. 184–188).

Optic atrophy, papilledema

Screen the visual fields by confrontation (see pp. 178–179). Occasionally—in a stroke patient, for example—screening indicates a visual field defect, such as a homonymous hemianopsia, that you cannot confirm by testing one eye at a time. This screening observation, nevertheless, is significant.

These findings suggest visual *extinction,* a subtle impairment detectable only when testing both eyes simultaneously. It suggests a lesion in the parietal cortex.

Cranial Nerves II and III—Optic and Oculomotor.   Inspect the size and shape of the pupils, and compare one side with the other. Test the *pupillary reactions to light*; if these are abnormal, examine the *near response* also (see p. 182).

See Table 6-9, Pupillary Abnormalities (p. 217).

Cranial Nerves III, IV, and VI—Oculomotor, Trochlear, and Abducens.   Test the *extraocular movements* in the six cardinal directions of gaze, and look for loss of conjugate movements in any of the six directions. Check convergence of the eyes. Identify any nystagmus, noting the direction of gaze in which it appears, the plane in which movements occur (horizontal, vertical, rotary, or mixed), and the direction of the quick and slow components (see pp. 655–656).

See Table 6-10, Dysconjugate Gaze (p. 218).

See Table 17-4, Nystagmus (pp. 655–656).

Look for *ptosis* (drooping of the upper eyelids). A slight difference in the width of the palpebral fissures may be noted in about one third of all normal people.

Ptosis in 3rd nerve palsy, Horner's syndrome (ptosis, meiosis, anhidrosis), myasthenia gravis

Cranial Nerve V—Trigeminal

Motor. While palpating the temporal and masseter muscles in turn, ask the patient to clench his or her teeth. Note the strength of muscle contraction.

Weak or absent contraction of the temporal and masseter muscles on one side suggests a lesion of CN V. Bilateral weakness may result from peripheral or central involvement. When the patient has no teeth, this test may be difficult to interpret.

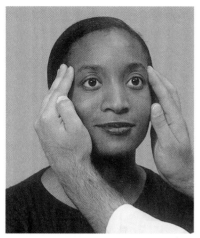

PALPATING TEMPORAL MUSCLES

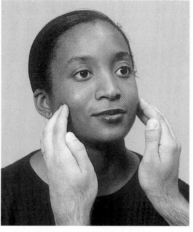

PALPATING MASSETER MUSCLES

Sensory. After explaining what you plan to do, test the forehead, cheeks, and jaw on each side for *pain sensation.* Suggested areas are indicated by the circles. The patient's eyes should be closed. Use a safety pin or other suitable sharp object,* occasionally substituting the blunt end for the point as a stimulus. Ask the patient to report whether it is "sharp" or "dull" and to compare sides.

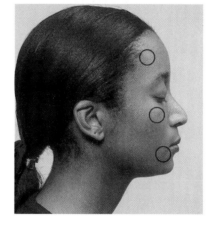

Unilateral decrease in or loss of facial sensation suggests a lesion of CN V or of interconnecting higher sensory pathways. Such a sensory loss may also be associated with a conversion reaction.

If you find an abnormality, confirm it by testing *temperature sensation.* Two test tubes, filled with hot and ice-cold water, are the traditional stimuli. A tuning fork may also be used. It usually feels cool. If you are near running water, the fork is easily made colder or warm. Dry it before use. Touch the skin and ask the patient to identify "hot" or "cold."

Then test for *light touch,* using a fine wisp of cotton. Ask the patient to respond whenever you touch the skin.

Test *the corneal reflex.* Ask the patient to look up and away from you. Approaching from the other side, out of the patient's line of vision, and avoiding the eyelashes, touch the cornea (not just the conjunctiva) lightly with a fine wisp of cotton. If the patient is apprehensive, however, first touching the conjunctiva may allay fear.

---

*To avoid transmitting infection, use a new object with each patient. You can create a sharp wood splinter by breaking or twisting a cotton swab. The cotton end of the swab can also be used as a dull stimulus.

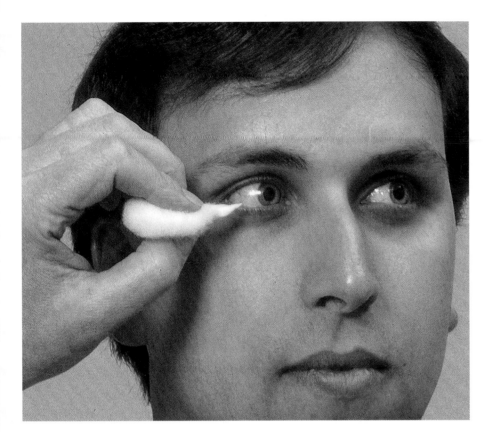

Look for blinking of the eyes, the normal reaction to this stimulus. (The sensory limb of this reflex is carried in CN V, the motor response in CN VII.) Use of contact lenses frequently diminishes or abolishes this reflex.

Absence of blinking suggests a lesion of CN V. A lesion of CN VII (innervates the muscles that close the eyes) may also impair this reflex.

Cranial Nerve VII—Facial. Inspect the face, both at rest and during conversation with the patient. Note any asymmetry (e.g., of the nasolabial folds), and observe any tics or other abnormal movements.

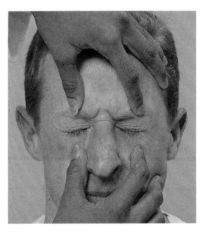

Ask the patient to:

1. Raise both eyebrows.

2. Frown.

3. Close both eyes tightly so that you cannot open them. Test muscular strength by trying to open them, as illustrated.

4. Show both upper and lower teeth.

Flattening of the nasolabial fold and drooping of the lower eyelid suggest facial weakness.

A peripheral injury to CN VII, as in Bell's palsy, affects both the upper and the lower face; a central lesion affects mainly the lower face. See Table 17-5, Types of Facial Paralysis (pp. 657–658).

In unilateral facial paralysis, the mouth droops on the paralyzed side when the patient smiles or grimaces.

5. Smile.

6. Puff out both cheeks.

Note any weakness or asymmetry.

Cranial Nerve VIII—Acoustic.   Assess *hearing*. If hearing loss is present, (1) test for *lateralization*, and (2) compare *air and bone conduction* (see p. 191).

See Table 6-19, Patterns of Hearing Loss (p. 229).

Specific tests of *vestibular function* are seldom included in the usual neurologic examination. Consult textbooks of neurology or otolaryngology as the need arises.

Nystagmus may indicate vestibular dysfunction. See Table 17-4, Nystagmus (pp. 655–656).

Cranial Nerves IX and X—Glossopharyngeal and Vagus.   Listen to the patient's *voice*. Is it hoarse, or does it have a nasal quality?

Hoarseness in vocal cord paralysis; a nasal voice in paralysis of the palate

Is there difficulty in swallowing?

Pharyngeal or palatal weakness

Ask the patient to say "ah" or to yawn as you watch the *movements of the soft palate and the pharynx*. The soft palate normally rises symmetrically, the uvula remains in the midline, and each side of the posterior pharynx moves medially, like a curtain. The slightly curved uvula seen occasionally in a normal person should not be mistaken for a uvula deviated by a lesion of CN X.

The palate fails to rise with a bilateral lesion of the vagus nerve. In unilateral paralysis, one side of the palate fails to rise and, together with the uvula, is pulled toward the normal side (see p. 194).

Warn the patient that you are going to test the *gag reflex*. Stimulate the back of the throat lightly on each side in turn and note the gag reflex. It may be symmetrically diminished or absent in some normal people.

Unilateral absence of this reflex suggests a lesion of CN IX, perhaps CN X.

Cranial Nerve XI—Spinal Accessory.   From behind, look for atrophy or fasciculations in the trapezius muscles, and compare one side with the

Weakness with atrophy and fasciculations indicates a peripheral nerve disorder. When the trapezius is paralyzed, the shoulder droops, and the scapula is displaced downward and laterally.

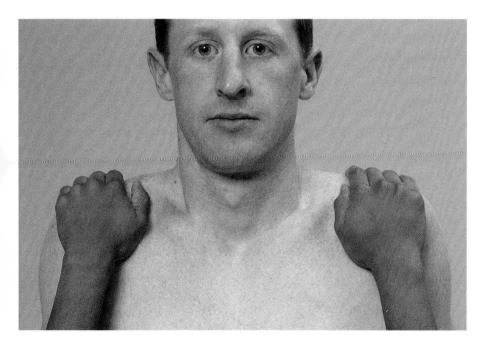

other. Ask the patient to shrug both shoulders upward against your hands. Note the strength and contraction of the trapezii.

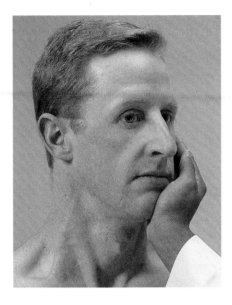

Ask the patient to turn his or her head to each side against your hand. Observe the contraction of the opposite sternomastoid and note the force of the movement against your hand.

A supine patient with bilateral weakness of the sternomastoids has difficulty raising the head off the pillow.

Cranial Nerve XII—Hypoglossal. Listen to the articulation of the patient's words. This depends on Cranial Nerves V, VII, and X as well as XII. Inspect the patient's tongue as it lies on the floor of the mouth. Look for any atrophy or *fasciculations* (fine, flickering, irregular movements in small groups of muscle fibers). Some coarser restless movements are often seen in a normal tongue. Then, with the patient's tongue protruded, look for asymmetry, atrophy, or deviation from the midline. Ask the patient to move the tongue from side to side, and note the symmetry of the movement. In ambiguous cases, ask the patient to push the tongue against the inside of each cheek in turn as you palpate externally for strength.

For poor articulation, or *dysarthria*, see Table 16-2, Disorders of Speech (p. 591). Atrophy and fasciculations in *amyotrophic lateral sclerosis, polio*

In a unilateral cortical lesion, the protruded tongue deviates transiently in a direction away from the side of the cortical lesion.

THE MOTOR SYSTEM

As you assess the motor system, focus on body position, involuntary movements, characteristics of the muscles (bulk, tone, and strength), and coordination. These components are described below in sequence. You may either use this sequence or check each component in the arms, legs, and trunk in turn. If you see an abnormality, identify the muscle(s) involved. Think about whether the abnormality is central or peripheral in origin, and begin to learn which nerves innervate the affected muscles.

Body Position. Observe the patient's body position during movement and at rest.

Abnormal positions alert you to neurologic deficits such as paralysis.

Involuntary Movements. Watch for involuntary movements such as tremors, tics, or fasciculations. Note their location, quality, rate, rhythm, and amplitude, and their relation to posture, activity, fatigue, emotion, and other factors.

See Table 17-3, Tremors and Involuntary Movements (pp. 653–654).

Muscle Bulk. Compare the size and contours of muscles. Do the muscles look flat or concave, suggesting atrophy? If so, is the process unilateral or bilateral? Is it proximal or distal?

When looking for atrophy, pay particular attention to the hands, shoulders, and thighs. The thenar and hypothenar eminences should be full and convex, and the spaces between the metacarpals, where the dorsal interosseous muscles lie, should be full or only slightly depressed. Atrophy of hand muscles may occur with normal aging, however, as shown on the right below.

Muscular *atrophy* refers to a loss of muscle bulk (wasting). It results from diseases of the peripheral nervous system such as diabetic neuropathy, as well as diseases of the muscles themselves. *Hypertrophy* refers to an increase in bulk with proportionate strength, whereas increased bulk with diminished strength is called *pseudohypertrophy* (seen in the *Duchenne form of muscular dystrophy*).

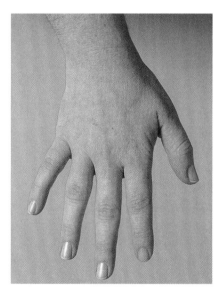
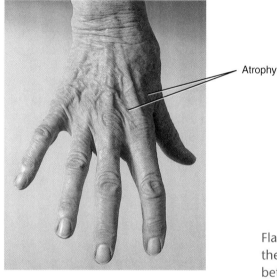

Atrophy

Hand of a 44-year-old woman   Hand of an 84-year-old woman

Flattening of the thenar and hypothenar eminences and furrowing between the metacarpals suggest atrophy. Localized atrophy of the thenar and hypothenar eminences suggests damage to the median and ulnar nerves, respectively.

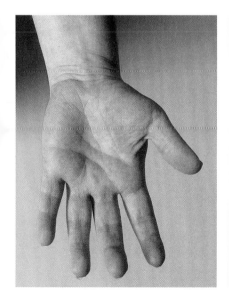
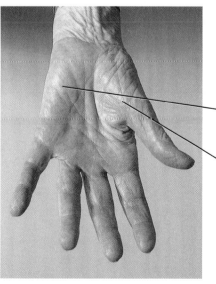

Hypothenar eminence

Flattening of the thenar eminence due to mild atrophy

Hand of a 44-year-old woman   Hand of an 84-year-old woman

Other causes of muscular atrophy include motor neuron diseases, disuse of the muscles, rheumatoid arthritis, and protein-calorie malnutrition.

Be alert for fasciculations in atrophic muscles. If absent, tap on the muscle with a reflex hammer to try to stimulate them.

Fasciculations suggest lower motor neuron disease as a cause of atrophy.

Muscle Tone.   When a normal muscle with an intact nerve supply is relaxed voluntarily, it maintains a slight residual tension known as muscle tone. This can be assessed best by feeling the muscle's resistance to passive stretch. Persuade the patient to relax. Take one hand with yours and, while supporting the elbow, flex and extend the patient's fingers, wrist, and elbow, and put the shoulder through a moderate range of motion. With practice, these actions can be combined into a single smooth movement. On each side, note muscle tone—the resistance offered to your movements. Tense patients may show increased resistance. You will learn the feel of normal resistance only with repeated practice.

Decreased resistance suggests disease of the peripheral nervous system, cerebellar disease, or the acute stages of spinal cord injury. See Table 17-6, Disorders of Muscle Tone (p. 659).

If you suspect decreased resistance, hold the forearm and shake the hand loosely back and forth. Normally the hand moves back and forth freely but is not completely floppy.

Marked floppiness indicates hypotonic or flaccid muscles.

If resistance is increased, determine whether it varies as you move the limb or whether it persists throughout the range of movement and in both directions, for example, during both flexion and extension. Feel for any jerkiness in the resistance.

Increased resistance that varies, commonly worse at the extremes of the range, is called spasticity. Resistance that persists throughout the range and in both directions is called lead-pipe rigidity.

To assess muscle tone in the legs, support the patient's thigh with one hand, grasp the foot with the other, and flex and extend the patient's knee and ankle on each side. Note the resistance to your movements.

Muscle Strength.   Normal individuals vary widely in their strength, and your standard of normal, while admittedly rough, should allow for such variables as age, sex, and muscular training. A person's dominant side is usually slightly stronger than the other side. Keep this difference in mind when you compare sides.

Test muscle strength by asking the patient to move actively against your resistance or to resist your movement. Remember that a muscle is strongest when shortest, and weakest when longest.

Impaired strength is called weakness, or paresis. Absence of strength is called paralysis, or plegia. Hemiparesis refers to weakness of one half of the body; hemiplegia to paralysis of one half of the body. Paraplegia means paralysis of the legs; quadriplegia, paralysis of all four limbs.

If the muscles are too weak to overcome resistance, test them against gravity alone or with gravity eliminated. When the forearm rests in a pronated position, for example, dorsiflexion at the wrist can be tested against gravity alone. When the forearm is midway between pronation and supination, extension at the wrist can be tested with gravity eliminated. Finally, if the patient fails to move the body part, watch or feel for weak muscular contraction.

See Table 17-7, Disorders of the Central and Peripheral Nervous Systems (pp. 660–662).

SCALE FOR GRADING MUSCLE STRENGTH

Muscle strength is graded on a 0 to 5 scale:

0—No muscular contraction detected
1—A barely detectable flicker or trace of contraction
2—Active movement of the body part with gravity eliminated
3—Active movement against gravity
4—Active movement against gravity and some resistance
5—Active movement against full resistance without evident fatigue. This is
    normal muscle strength.

More experienced clinicians make further distinctions by using plus or minus signs toward the stronger end of this scale. Thus 4+ indicates good but not full strength, while 5− means a trace of weakness.

Methods for testing the major muscle groups are described below. The spinal root innervations and the muscles affected are shown in parentheses. To localize lesions in the spinal cord or the peripheral nervous system more precisely, additional testing may be necessary. For these specialized methods, refer to texts of neurology.

Test flexion (C5, C6—biceps) *and extension* (C6, C7, C8—triceps) *at the elbow* by having the patient pull and push against your hand.

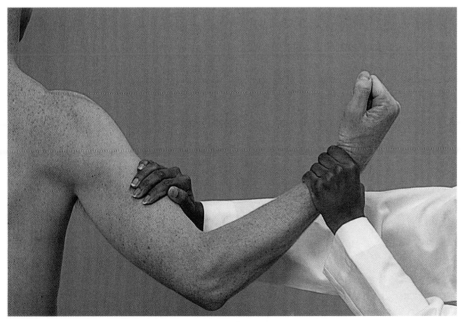

FLEXION AT ELBOW

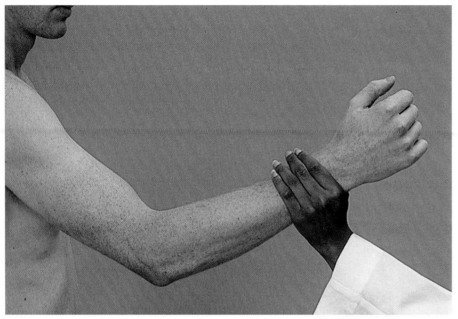

EXTENSION AT ELBOW

Test extension at the wrist (C6, C7, C8, radial nerve) by asking the patient to make a fist and resist your pulling it down.

Weakness of extension is seen in peripheral nerve disease such as radial nerve damage and in central nervous system disease producing hemiplegia, as in stroke or multiple sclerosis.

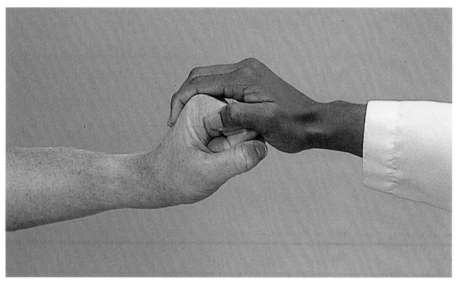

EXTENSION AT WRIST

Test the grip (C7, C8, T1). Ask the patient to squeeze two of your fingers as hard as possible and not let them go. (To avoid getting hurt by hard squeezes, place your own middle finger on top of your index finger.) You should normally have difficulty removing your fingers from the patient's grip. Testing both grips simultaneously with arms extended or in the lap facilitates comparison.

A weak grip may be due to either central or peripheral nervous system disease. It may also result from painful disorders of the hands.

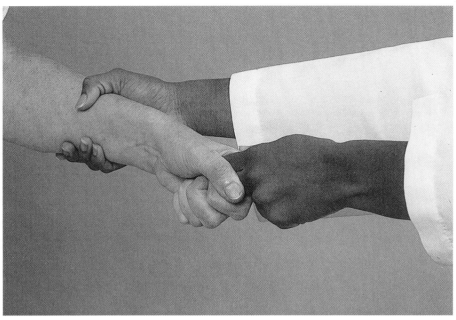

TEST OF GRIP

Test finger abduction (C8, T1, ulnar nerve). Position the patient's hand with palm down and fingers spread. Instructing the patient not to let you move the fingers, try to force them together.

Weak finger abduction in ulnar nerve disorders

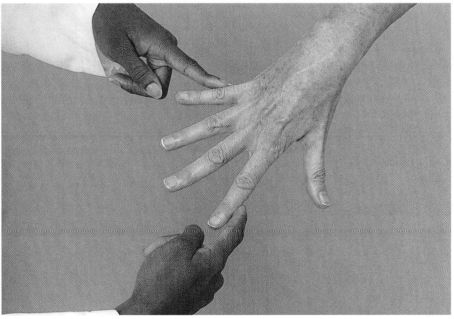

FINGER ABDUCTION

Test opposition of the thumb (C8, T1, median nerve). The patient should try to touch the tip of the little finger with the thumb, against your resistance.

Weak opposition of the thumb in median nerve disorders such as carpal tunnel syndrome

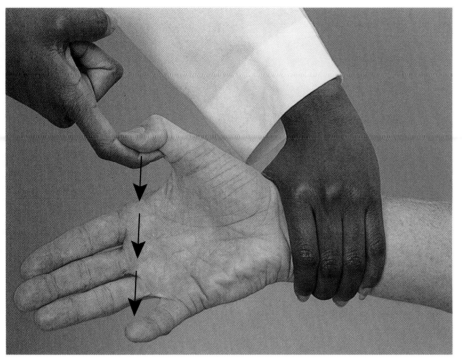

OPPOSITION OF THE THUMB

Assessment of *muscle strength of the trunk* may already have been made in other segments of the examination. It includes:

■ Flexion, extension, and lateral bending of the spine, and

■ Thoracic expansion and diaphragmatic excursion during respiration

Test flexion at the hip (L2, L3, L4—iliopsoas) by placing your hand on the patient's thigh and asking the patient to raise the leg against your hand.

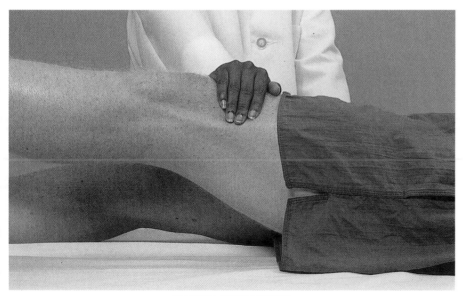

FLEXION OF THE THIGH

Test adduction at the hips (L2, L3, L4—adductors). Place your hands firmly on the bed between the patient's knees. Ask the patient to bring both legs together.

Symmetric weakness of the proximal muscles suggests a *myopathy* or muscle disorder; symmetric weakness of distal muscles suggests a *polyneuropathy,* or disorder of peripheral nerves.

Test abduction at the hips (L4, L5, S1—gluteus medius and minimus). Place your hands firmly on the bed outside the patient's knees. Ask the patient to spread both legs against your hands.

Test extension at the hips (S1—gluteus maximus). Have the patient push the posterior thigh down against your hand.

Test extension at the knee (L2, L3, L4—quadriceps). Support the knee in flexion and ask the patient to straighten the leg against your hand. The quadriceps is the strongest muscle in the body, so expect a forceful response.

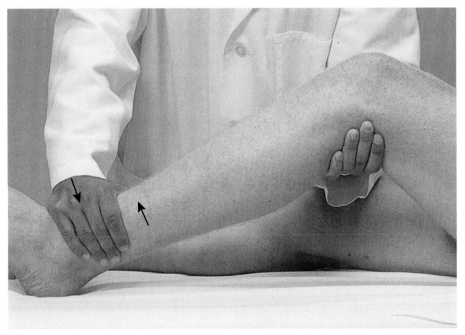

EXTENSION AT THE KNEE

Test flexion at the knee (L4, L5, S1, S2—hamstrings) as shown below. Place the patient's leg so that the knee is flexed with the foot resting on the bed. Tell the patient to keep the foot down as you try to straighten the leg.

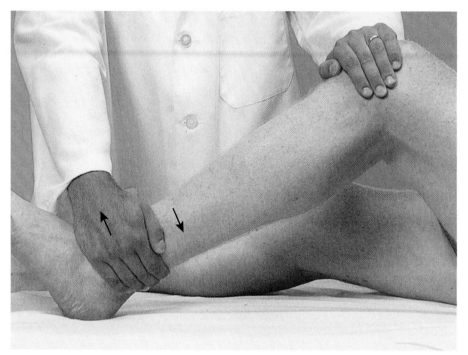

FLEXION AT THE KNEE

Test dorsiflexion (mainly L4, L5) and *plantar flexion* (mainly S1) at the ankle by asking the patient to pull up and push down against your hand.

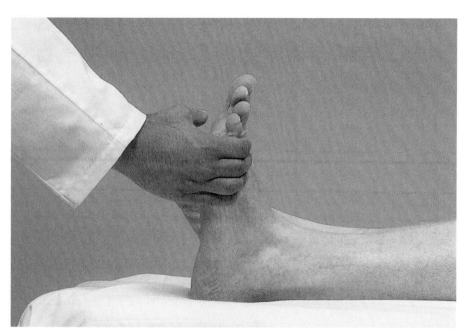

DORSIFLEXION

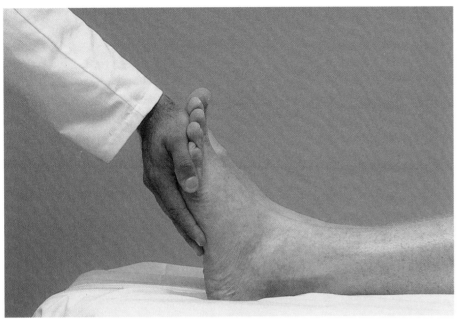

PLANTAR FLEXION

Coordination.   Coordination of muscle movement requires that four areas of the nervous system function in an integrated way:

■ The motor system, for muscle strength

■ The cerebellar system (also part of the motor system), for rhythmic movement and steady posture

■ The vestibular system, for balance and for coordinating eye, head, and body movements

■ The sensory system, for position sense

To assess coordination, observe the patient's performance in:

■ Rapid alternating movements

■ Point-to-point movements

■ Gait and other related body movements

■ Standing in specified ways

Rapid Alternating Movements

ARMS. Show the patient how to strike one hand on the thigh, raise the hand, turn it over, and then strike the back of the hand down on the same place. Urge the patient to repeat these alternating movements as rapidly as possible.

Observe the speed, rhythm, and smoothness of the movements. Repeat with the other hand. The non-dominant hand often performs somewhat less well.

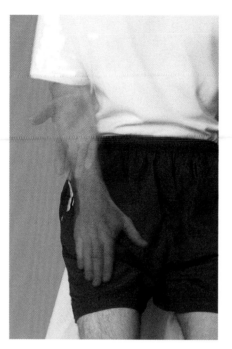

In cerebellar disease, one movement cannot be followed quickly by its opposite and movements are slow, irregular, and clumsy. This abnormality is called *dysdiadochokinesis*. Upper motor neuron weakness and basal ganglia disease may also impair rapid alternating movements, but not in the same manner.

Show the patient how to tap the distal joint of the thumb with the tip of the index finger, again as rapidly as possible. Again, observe the speed, rhythm, and smoothness of the movements. The nondominant side often performs less well.

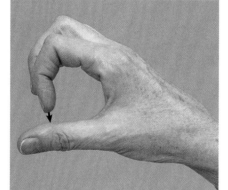

LEGS. Ask the patient to tap your hand as quickly as possible with the ball of each foot in turn. Note any slowness or awkwardness. The feet normally perform less well than the hands.

Dysdiadochokinesis in cerebellar disease

Point-to-Point Movements

ARMS. Ask the patient to touch your index finger and then his or her nose alternately several times. Move your finger about so that the patient has to alter directions and extend the arm fully to reach it. Observe the accuracy and smoothness of movements and watch for any tremor. Normally the patient's movements are smooth and accurate.

In cerebellar disease, movements are clumsy, unsteady, and inappropriately varying in their speed, force, and direction. The finger may initially overshoot its mark, but finally reaches it fairly well. Such movements are termed *dysmetria.* An *intention tremor* may appear toward the end of the movement (see p. 653).

Now hold your finger in one place so that the patient can touch it with one arm and finger outstretched. Ask the patient to raise the arm overhead and lower it again to touch your finger. After several repeats, ask the patient to close both eyes and try several more times. Repeat on the other side. Normally a person can touch the examiner's finger successfully with eyes open or closed. These maneuvers test position sense and the functions of both the labyrinth and the cerebellum.

Cerebellar disease causes incoordination that may get worse with eyes closed. If present, this suggests loss of position sense. Repetitive and consistent deviation to one side, referred to as *past pointing*, worse with the eyes closed, suggests cerebellar or vestibular disease.

LEGS. Ask the patient to place one heel on the opposite knee, and then run it down the shin to the big toe. Note the smoothness and accuracy of the movements. Repetition with the patient's eyes closed tests for position sense. Repeat on the other side.

In cerebellar disease, the heel may overshoot the knee and then oscillate from side to side down the shin. When position sense is lost, the heel is lifted too high and the patient tries to look. With eyes closed, performance is poor.

Gait. Ask the patient to:

Abnormalities of gait increase risk of falls.

■ *Walk across the room* or down the hall, then turn, and come back. Observe posture, balance, swinging of the arms, and movements of the legs. Normally balance is easy, the arms swing at the sides, and turns are accomplished smoothly.

A gait that lacks coordination, with reeling and instability, is called *ataxic.* Ataxia may be due to cerebellar disease, loss of position sense, or intoxication. See Table 17-8, Abnormalities of Gait and Posture (pp. 663–664).

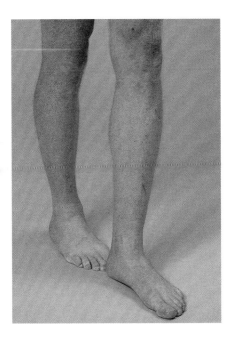

■ *Walk heel-to-toe* in a straight line— a pattern called *tandem walking.*

Tandem walking may reveal an ataxia not previously obvious.

■ *Walk on the toes,* then *on the heels*— sensitive tests, respectively, for plantar flexion and dorsiflexion of the ankles, as well as for balance.

Walking on toes and heels may reveal distal muscular weakness in the legs. Inability to heel-walk is a sensitive test for corticospinal tract weakness.

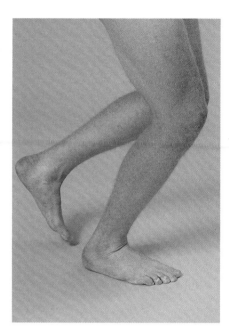

- *Hop in place* on each foot in turn (if the patient is not too ill). Hopping involves the proximal muscles of the legs as well as the distal ones and requires both good position sense and normal cerebellar function.

Difficulty with hopping may be due to weakness, lack of position sense, or cerebellar dysfunction.

- *Do a shallow knee bend,* first on one leg, then on the other. Support the patient's elbow if you think the patient is in danger of falling.

Difficulty here suggests proximal weakness (extensors of the hip), weakness of the quadriceps (the extensor of the knee), or both.

- *Rising from a sitting position* without arm support and *stepping up* on a sturdy stool are more suitable tests than hopping or knee bends when patients are old or less robust.

Proximal muscle weakness involving the pelvic girdle and legs causes difficulty with both of these activities.

Stance. The following two tests can often be performed concurrently. They differ only in the patient's arm position and in what you are looking for. In each case, stand close enough to the patient to prevent a fall.

THE ROMBERG TEST. This is mainly a test of position sense. The patient should first stand with feet together and eyes open and then close both eyes for 20 to 30 seconds without support. Note the patient's ability to maintain an upright posture. Normally only minimal swaying occurs.

In ataxia due to loss of position sense, vision compensates for the sensory loss. The patient stands fairly well with eyes open but loses balance when they are closed, a *positive Romberg sign.* In *cerebellar ataxia,* the patient has difficulty standing with feet together whether the eyes are open or closed.

TEST FOR PRONATOR DRIFT. The patient should stand for 20 to 30 seconds with both arms straight forward, palms up, and with eyes closed. A person who cannot stand may be tested for a pronator drift in the sitting position. In either case, a normal person can hold this arm position well.

The pronation of one forearm suggests a contralateral lesion in the corticospinal tract; downward drift of the arm with flexion of fingers and elbow may also occur. These movements are called *pronator drift,* shown on the next page.

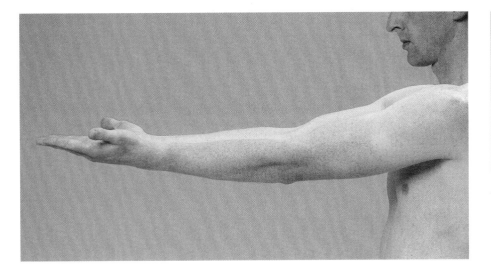

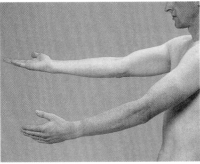

A sideward or upward drift, sometimes with searching, writhing movements of the hands, suggests loss of position sense.

Now, instructing the patient to keep the arms up and eyes shut, as shown above, *tap the arms briskly downward*. The arms normally return smoothly to the horizontal position. This response requires muscular strength, coordination, and a good sense of position.

A weak arm is easily displaced and often remains so. A patient lacking position sense may not recognize the displacement and, if told to correct it, does so poorly. In cerebellar incoordination, the arm returns to its original position but overshoots and bounces.

THE SENSORY SYSTEM

To evaluate the sensory system, you will test several kinds of sensation:

- Pain and temperature (spinothalamic tracts)

- Position and vibration (posterior columns)

- Light touch (both of these pathways)

- Discriminative sensations, which depend on some of the above sensations but also involve the cortex

Familiarize yourself with each kind of test so that you can use it as indicated. When you detect abnormal findings, correlate them with motor and reflex activity. Is the underlying lesion central or peripheral?

See Table 17-7, Disorders of the Central and Peripheral Nervous Systems (pp. 660–662).

Patterns of Testing. Because sensory testing quickly fatigues many patients and then produces unreliable results, conduct the examination as efficiently as possible. Pay special attention to those areas (1) where there are symptoms such as numbness or pain, (2) where there are motor or reflex abnormalities that suggest a lesion of the spinal cord or peripheral nervous system, and (3) where there are trophic changes, such as absent or excessive sweating, atrophic skin, or cutaneous ulceration. Repeated testing at another time is often required to confirm abnormalities.

The following patterns of testing help you to identify sensory deficits accurately and efficiently.

- *Compare symmetric areas* on the two sides of the body, including the arms, legs, and trunk.

- When testing pain, temperature, and touch sensation, also *compare the distal with the proximal areas* of the extremities. Further, scatter the stimuli so as to sample most of the dermatomes and major peripheral nerves (see pp. 605–606). One suggested pattern includes both shoulders (C4), the inner and outer aspects of the forearms (C6 and T1), the thumbs and little fingers (C6 and C8), the fronts of both thighs (L2), the medial and lateral aspects of both calves (L4 and L5), the little toes (S1), and the medial aspect of each buttock (S3).

- When testing vibration and position sensation, first test the fingers and toes. If these are normal, you may safely assume that more proximal areas will also be normal.

- *Vary the pace of your testing.* This is important so that the patient does not merely respond to your repetitive rhythm.

- When you detect an area of sensory loss or hypersensitivity, *map out its boundaries* in detail. Stimulate first at a point of reduced sensation, and move by progressive steps until the patient detects the change. An example is shown at right.

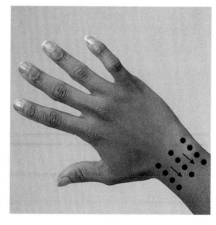

By identifying the distribution of sensory abnormalities and the kinds of sensations affected, you can infer where the causative lesion might be. Any motor deficit or reflex abnormality also helps in this localizing process.

Before each of the following tests, show the patient what you plan to do and what responses you want. Unless otherwise specified, the patient's eyes should be closed during actual testing.

Meticulous sensory mapping helps to establish the level of a spinal cord lesion and to determine whether a more peripheral lesion is in a nerve root, a major peripheral nerve, or one of its branches.

Hemisensory loss due to a lesion in the spinal cord or higher pathways

Symmetric distal sensory loss suggests a *polyneuropathy*, as described in the example on the next page. You may miss this finding unless you compare distal and proximal areas.

Here all sensation in the hand is lost. Repetitive testing in a proximal direction reveals a gradual change to normal sensation at the wrist. This pattern fits neither a peripheral nerve nor a dermatome (see pp. 605–606). If bilateral, it suggests the "glove and stocking" sensory loss of a polyneuropathy, often seen in *alcoholism* and *diabetes*.

Pain.   Use a sharp safety pin, a broken cotton swab, or other suitable tool. Occasionally, substitute the blunt end for the point. Ask the patient, "Is this sharp or dull?" or, when making comparisons, "Does this feel the same as this?" Apply the lightest pressure needed for the stimulus to feel sharp, and try not to draw blood.

To prevent transmitting a blood-borne infection, *discard the pin or other device safely. Do not reuse it on another person.*

Temperature.   (Testing is often omitted if pain sensation is normal, but include it if there is any question.) Use two test tubes, filled with hot and cold water, or a tuning fork heated or cooled by water. Touch the skin and ask the patient to identify "hot" or "cold."

Light Touch.   With a fine wisp of cotton, touch the skin lightly, avoiding pressure. Ask the patient to respond whenever a touch is felt, and to compare one area with another. Calloused skin is normally relatively insensitive and should be avoided.

Vibration.   Use a relatively low-pitched tuning fork of 128 Hz. Tap it on the heel of your hand and place it firmly over a distal interphalangeal joint of the patient's finger, then over the interphalangeal joint of the big toe. Ask what the patient feels. If you are uncertain whether it is pressure or vibration, ask the patient to tell you when the vibration stops, and then touch the fork to stop it. If vibration sense is impaired, proceed to more proximal bony prominences (e.g., wrist, elbow, medial malleolus, patella, anterior superior iliac spine, spinous processes, and clavicles).

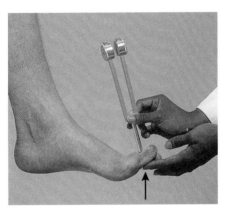

TUNING FORK ON PAD OF LARGE TOE NOT BONE

Position.   Grasp the patient's big toe, *holding it by its sides* between your thumb and index finger, and then pull it away from the other toes. (These precautions prevent extraneous tactile stimuli from revealing position changes that might not otherwise be detected.) Demonstrate "up" and "down" as you move the patient's toe clearly upward and downward. Then, with the patient's eyes closed, ask for a response of "up" or "down" when moving the large toe in a small arc.

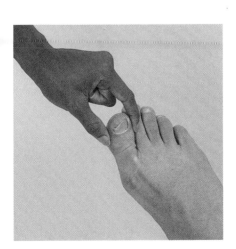

Repeat several times on each side, avoiding simple alternation of the stimuli. If position sense is impaired, move proximally to test it at the

Analgesia refers to absence of pain sensation, *hypalgesia* to decreased sensitivity to pain, and *hyperalgesia* to increased sensitivity.

Anesthesia is absence of touch sensation, *hypesthesia* is decreased sensitivity, and *hyperesthesia* is increased sensitivity.

Vibration sense is often the first sensation to be lost in a peripheral neuropathy. Common causes include *diabetes* and *alcoholism.* Vibration sense is also lost in posterior column disease, as in *tertiary syphilis* or *vitamin B$_{12}$ deficiency.*

Testing vibration sense in the trunk may be useful in estimating the level of a cord lesion.

Loss of position sense, like loss of vibration sense, suggests either posterior column disease or a lesion of the peripheral nerve or root.

ankle joint. In a similar fashion, test position in the fingers, moving proximally if indicated to the metacarpophalangeal joints, wrist, and elbow.

Discriminative Sensations. Several additional techniques test the ability of the sensory cortex to correlate, analyze, and interpret sensations. Because discriminative sensations are dependent on touch and position sense, they are useful only when these sensations are either intact or only slightly impaired.

Screen a patient with *stereognosis,* and proceed to other methods if indicated. The patient's eyes should be closed during all these tests.

- *Stereognosis.* Stereognosis refers to the ability to identify an object by feeling it. Place in the patient's hand a familiar object such as a coin, paper clip, key, pencil, or cotton ball, and ask the patient to tell you what it is. Normally a patient will manipulate it skillfully and identify it correctly. Asking the patient to distinguish "heads" from "tails" on a coin is a sensitive test of stereognosis.

- *Number identification (graphesthesia).* When motor impairment, arthritis, or other conditions prevent the patient from manipulating an object well enough to identify it, test the ability to identify numbers. With the blunt end of a pen or pencil, draw a large number in the patient's palm. A normal person can identify most such numbers.

- *Two-point discrimination.* Using the two ends of an opened paper clip, or the sides of two pins, touch a finger pad in two places simultaneously. Alternate the double stimulus irregularly with a one-point touch. Be careful not to cause pain.

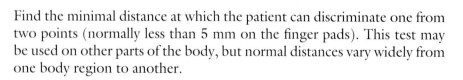

Find the minimal distance at which the patient can discriminate one from two points (normally less than 5 mm on the finger pads). This test may be used on other parts of the body, but normal distances vary widely from one body region to another.

- *Point localization.* Briefly touch a point on the patient's skin. Then ask the patient to open both eyes and point to the place touched. Normally a person can do so accurately. This test, together with the test for extinction, is especially useful on the trunk and the legs.

When touch and position sense are normal or only slightly impaired, a disproportionate decrease in or loss of discriminative sensations suggests disease of the sensory cortex. Stereognosis, number identification, and two-point discrimination are also impaired by posterior column disease.

Astereognosis refers to the inability to recognize objects placed in the hand.

The inability to recognize numbers, like astereognosis, suggests a lesion in the sensory cortex.

Lesions of the sensory cortex increase the distance between two recognizable points.

Lesions of the sensory cortex impair the ability to localize points accurately.

■ *Extinction.* Simultaneously stimulate corresponding areas on both sides of the body. Ask where the patient feels your touch. Normally both stimuli are felt.

With lesions of the sensory cortex, only one stimulus may be recognized. The stimulus on the side opposite the damaged cortex is extinguished.

DEEP TENDON REFLEXES

Eliciting the *deep tendon reflexes* involves a series of examiner skills. Be sure to select a properly weighted reflex hammer. Learn when to use either the pointed or the flat end of the hammer. For example, the pointed end is useful for striking small areas, such as your finger as it overlies the biceps tendon; the flat end causes less discomfort when you test the brachioradialis reflex. Now test the reflexes as follows:

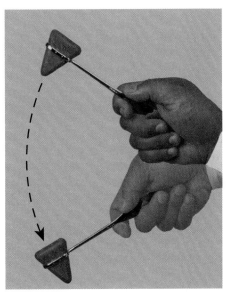

■ Encourage the patient to relax, then position the limbs properly and symmetrically.

■ Hold the reflex hammer loosely between your thumb and index finger so that it swings freely in an arc within the limits set by your palm and other fingers.

■ With your wrist relaxed, strike the tendon briskly using a rapid wrist movement. Your strike should be quick and direct, not glancing.

■ Note the speed, force, and amplitude of the reflex response and grade the response using the scale below. Always compare the response of one side with the other. Reflexes are usually graded on a 0 to 4+ scale.

SCALE FOR GRADING REFLEXES	
4+	Very brisk, hyperactive, with *clonus* (rhythmic oscillations between flexion and extension)
3+	Brisker than average; possibly but not necessarily indicative of disease
2+	Average; normal
1+	Somewhat diminished; low normal
0	No response

Hyperactive reflexes suggest central nervous system disease. Sustained clonus confirms it. Reflexes may be diminished or absent when sensation is lost, when the relevant spinal segments are damaged, or when the peripheral nerves are damaged. Diseases of muscles and neuromuscular junctions may also decrease reflexes.

Reflex response depends partly on the force of your stimulus. Use no more force than you need to provoke a definite response. Differences between sides are usually easier to assess than symmetric changes. Symmetrically diminished or even absent reflexes may be found in normal people.

If the patient's reflexes are symmetrically diminished or absent, use *re-inforcement,* a technique involving isometric contraction of other muscles that may increase reflex activity. In testing arm reflexes, for example, ask the patient to clench his or her teeth or to squeeze one thigh with the opposite hand. If leg reflexes are diminished or absent, reinforce them by asking the patient to lock fingers and pull one hand against the other. Tell the patient to pull just before you strike the tendon.

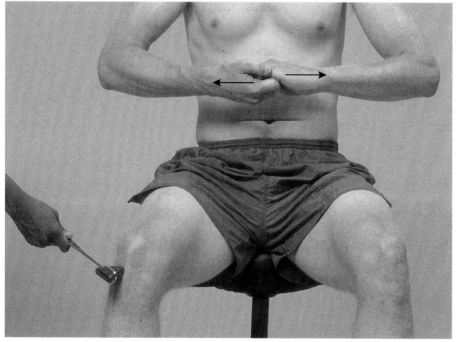

REINFORCEMENT OF KNEE REFLEX

The Biceps Reflex (C5, C6).   The patient's arm should be partially flexed at the elbow with palm down. Place your thumb or finger firmly on the biceps tendon. Strike with the reflex hammer so that the blow is aimed directly through your digit toward the biceps tendon.

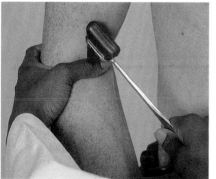

PATIENT SITTING

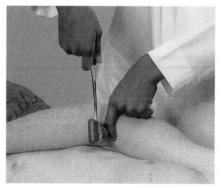

PATIENT LYING DOWN

Observe flexion at the elbow, and watch for and feel the contraction of the biceps muscle.

The Triceps Reflex (C6, C7). The patient may be sitting or supine. Flex the patient's arm at the elbow, with palm toward the body, and pull it slightly across the chest. Strike the triceps tendon above the elbow. Use a direct blow from directly behind it. Watch for contraction of the triceps muscle and extension at the elbow.

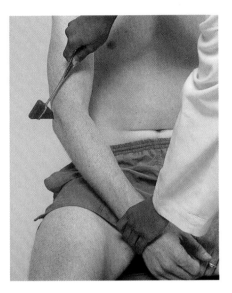 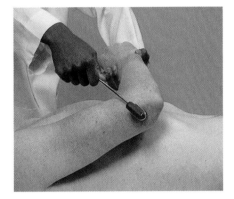

If you have difficulty getting the patient to relax, try supporting the upper arm as illustrated on the right. Ask the patient to let the arm go limp, as if it were "hung up to dry." Then strike the triceps tendon.

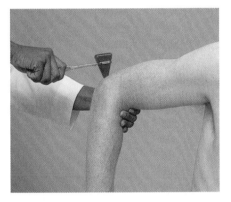

The Supinator or Brachioradialis Reflex (C5, C6). The patient's hand should rest on the abdomen or the lap, with the forearm partly pronated. Strike the radius with the flat edge of the reflex hammer, about 1 to 2 inches above the wrist. Watch for flexion and supination of the forearm.

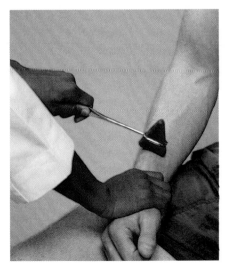

The Abdominal Reflexes. Test the abdominal reflexes by lightly but briskly stroking each side of the abdomen, above (T8, T9, T10) and below (T10, T11, T12) the umbilicus, in the directions illustrated. Use a key, the wooden end of a cotton-tipped applicator, or a tongue blade twisted and split longitudinally. Note the contraction of the abdominal muscles and deviation of the umbilicus toward the stimulus. Obesity may mask an abdominal reflex. In this situation, use your finger to retract the patient's umbilicus away from the side to be stimulated. Feel with your retracting finger for the muscular contraction.

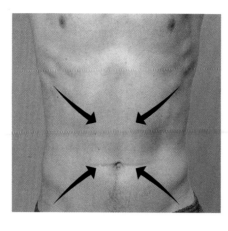

Abdominal reflexes may be absent in both central and peripheral nervous system disorders.

The Knee Reflex (L2, L3, L4). The patient may be either sitting or lying down as long as the knee is flexed. Briskly tap the patellar tendon just below the patella. Note contraction of the quadriceps with extension at the knee. A hand on the patient's anterior thigh lets you feel this reflex.

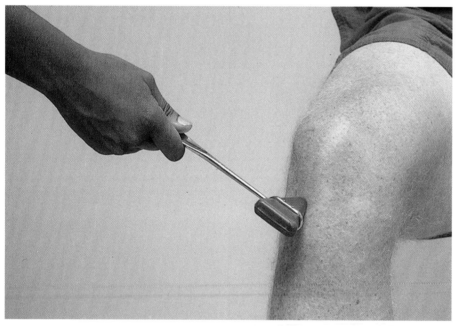

PATIENT SITTING

Two methods are useful when examining the supine patient. Supporting both knees at once, as shown below on the left, allows you to assess small differences between knee reflexes by repeatedly testing one reflex and then the other. Sometimes, however, supporting both legs is uncomfortable for both the examiner and the patient. You may wish to rest your supporting arm under the patient's leg, as shown below on the right. Some patients find it easier to relax with this method.

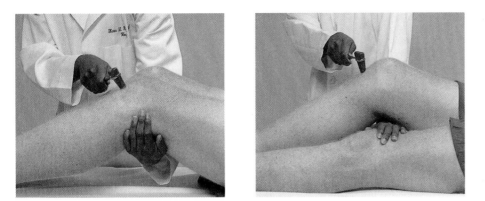

The Ankle Reflex (primarily S1).   If the patient is sitting, dorsiflex the foot at the ankle. Persuade the patient to relax. Strike the Achilles tendon. Watch and feel for plantar flexion at the ankle. Note also the speed of relaxation after muscular contraction.

The slowed relaxation phase of reflexes in *hypothyroidism* is often easily seen and felt in the ankle reflex.

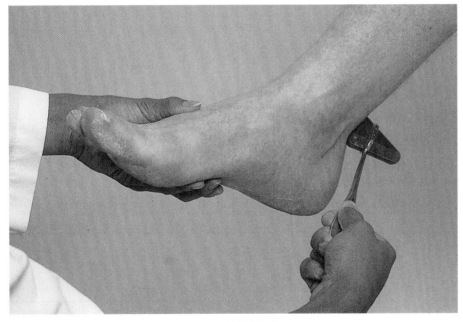

PATIENT SITTING

When the patient is lying down, flex one leg at both hip and knee and rotate it externally so that the lower leg rests across the opposite shin. Then dorsiflex the foot at the ankle and strike the Achilles tendon.

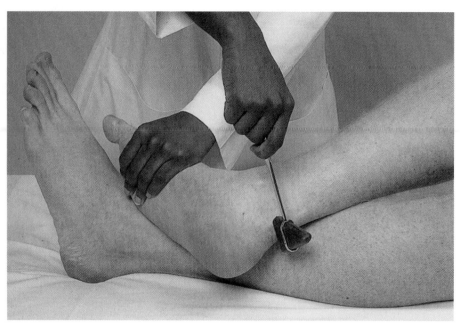

PATIENT LYING DOWN

The Plantar Response (L5, S1). With an object such as a key or the wooden end of an applicator stick, stroke the lateral aspect of the sole from the heel to the ball of the foot, curving medially across the ball. Use the lightest stimulus that will provoke a response, but be increasingly firm if necessary. Note movement of the toes, normally plantar flexion.

Dorsiflexion of the big toe, often accompanied by fanning of the other toes, constitutes a positive Babinski response, suggesting central nervous system lesion in the corticospinal tract.

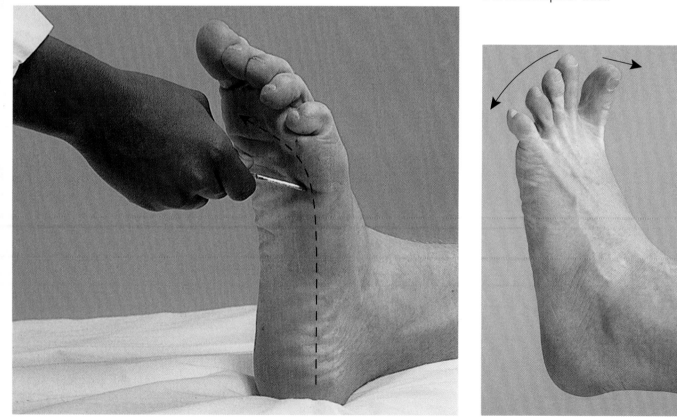

A Babinski response may also be seen in unconscious states due to drug or alcohol intoxication or in the postictal period following a seizure.

Some patients withdraw from this stimulus by flexing the hip and the knee. Hold the ankle, if necessary, to complete your observation. It is sometimes difficult to distinguish withdrawal from a Babinski response.

A marked Babinski response is occasionally accompanied by reflex flexion at hip and knee.

Clonus. If the reflexes seem hyperactive, test for *ankle clonus*. Support the knee in a partly flexed position. With your other hand, dorsiflex and plantar flex the foot a few times while encouraging the patient to relax, and then sharply dorsiflex the foot and maintain it in dorsiflexion. Look and feel for rhythmic oscillations between dorsiflexion and plantar flexion. In most normal people, the ankle does not react to this stimulus. A few clonic beats may be seen and felt, especially when the patient is tense or has exercised.

Sustained clonus indicates central nervous system disease. The ankle plantar flexes and dorsiflexes repetitively and rhythmically.

Clonus may also be elicited at other joints. A sharp downward displacement of the patella, for example, may elicit patellar clonus in the extended knee.

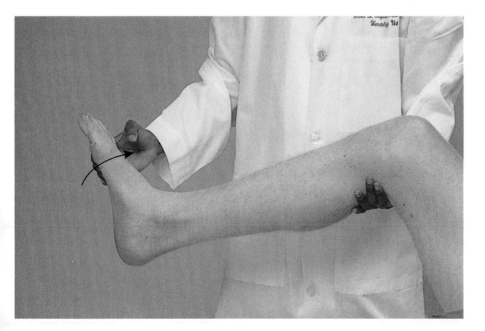

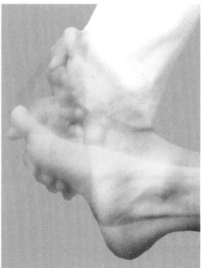

SPECIAL TECHNIQUES

Asterixis. Asterixis helps identify a metabolic encephalopathy in patients whose mental functions are impaired. Ask the patient to "stop traffic" by extending both arms, with hands cocked up and fingers spread. Watch for 1 to 2 minutes, coaxing the patient as necessary to maintain this position.

Sudden, brief, nonrhythmic flexion of the hands and fingers indicates asterixis.

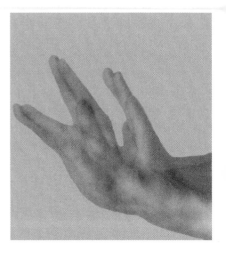

Winging of the Scapula. When the shoulder muscles seem weak or atrophic, look for winging. Ask the patient to extend both arms and push against your hand or against a wall. Observe the scapulae. Normally they lie close to the thorax.

In winging, shown below, the medial border of the scapula juts backward. It suggests weakness of the serratus anterior muscle, as in muscular dystrophy or injury to the long thoracic nerve.

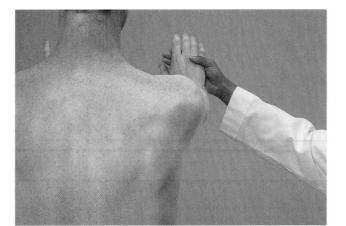

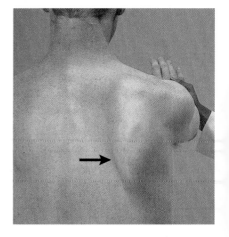

In very thin but normal people, the scapulae may appear "winged" even when the musculature is intact.

Meningeal Signs. Testing for these signs is important if you suspect meningeal inflammation from infection or subarachnoid hemorrhage.

Neck Mobility. First make sure there is no injury to the cervical vertebrae or cervical cord. (In settings of trauma, this may require evaluation by x-ray.) Then, with the patient supine, place your hands behind the patient's head and flex the neck forward, until the chin touches the chest if possible. Normally the neck is supple, and the patient can easily bend the head and neck forward.

Pain in the neck and resistance to flexion can arise from meningeal inflammation, arthritis, or neck injury.

Brudzinski's Sign. As you flex the neck, watch the hips and knees in reaction to your maneuver. Normally they should remain relaxed and motionless.

Flexion of the hips and knees is a *positive Brudzinski's sign* and suggests meningeal inflammation.

Kernig's Sign. Flex the patient's leg at both the hip and the knee, and then straighten the knee. Discomfort behind the knee during full extension occurs in many normal people, but this maneuver should not produce pain.

Pain and increased resistance to extending the knee are a *positive Kernig's sign.* When bilateral, it suggests meningeal irritation.

Compression of a lumbosacral nerve root may also cause resistance, together with pain in the low back and the posterior thigh. Only one leg is usually involved.

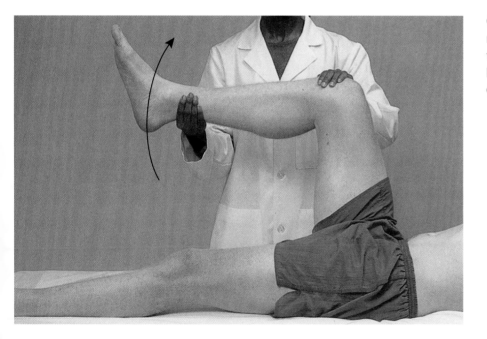

Anal Reflex. Using a dull object, such as a cotton swab, stroke outward in the four quadrants from the anus. Watch for reflex contraction of the anal musculature.

Loss of the anal reflex suggests a lesion in the S2–3–4 reflex arc, as in a cauda equina lesion.

The Stuporous or Comatose Patient. Coma signals a potentially life-threatening event affecting the two hemispheres, the brainstem, or both. The usual sequence of history, physical examination, and laboratory evaluation does not apply. Instead, you must:

See Table 17-9, Metabolic and Structural Coma (p. 665).

- First assess the ABCs (airway, breathing, and circulation)

- Establish the patient's level of consciousness

- Examine the patient neurologically. Look for focal or asymmetric findings, and determine whether impaired consciousness arises from a metabolic or a structural cause.

Interview relatives, friends, or witnesses to establish the speed of onset and duration of unconsciousness, any warning symptoms, precipitating factors, or previous episodes, and the prior appearance and behavior of the patient. Any history of past medical and psychiatric illnesses is also useful.

As you proceed to the examination, remember two cardinal DON'Ts:

1. *Don't* dilate the pupils, the single most important clue to the underlying cause of coma (structural vs. metabolic), and

2. *Don't* flex the neck if there is any question of trauma to the head or neck. Immobilize the cervical spine and get an x-ray first to rule out fractures of the cervical vertebrae that could compress and damage the spinal cord.

Airway, Breathing, and Circulation. Quickly check the patient's color and pattern of breathing. Inspect the posterior pharynx and listen over the trachea for stridor to make sure the airway is clear. If respirations are slowed or shallow, or if the airway is obstructed by secretions, consider intubating the patient as soon as possible while stabilizing the cervical spine.

Assess the remaining vital signs: pulse, blood pressure, and *rectal* temperature. If hypotension or hemorrhage is present, establish intravenous access and begin intravenous fluids. (Further emergency management and laboratory studies are beyond the scope of this text.)

Level of Consciousness. Level of consciousness primarily reflects the patient's capacity for arousal, or wakefulness. It is determined by the level of activity that the patient can be aroused to perform in response to escalating stimuli from the examiner.

Five clinical levels of consciousness are described in the table on the next page, together with related techniques for examination. Increase your stimuli in a stepwise manner, depending on the patient's response.

When you examine patients with an altered level of consciousness, describe and record exactly what you see and hear. Imprecise use of terms such as lethargy, obtundation, stupor, or coma may mislead other examiners.

■ Level of Consciousness (Arousal): Techniques and Patient Response

Level	Technique	Abnormal Response
Alertness	Speak to the patient in a normal tone of voice. An alert patient opens the eyes, looks at you, and responds fully and appropriately to stimuli (arousal intact).	
Lethargy	Speak to the patient in a loud voice. For example, call the patient's name or ask "How are you?"	A lethargic patient appears drowsy but opens the eyes and looks at you, responds to questions, and then falls asleep.
Obtundation	Shake the patient gently as if awakening a sleeper.	An obtunded patient opens the eyes and looks at you, but responds slowly and is somewhat confused. Alertness and interest in the environment are decreased.
Stupor	Apply a painful stimulus. For example, pinch a tendon, rub the sternum, or roll a pencil across a nail bed. (No stronger stimuli needed!)	A stuporous patient arouses from sleep only after painful stimuli. Verbal responses are slow or even absent. The patient lapses into an unresponsive state when the stimulus ceases. There is minimal awareness of self or the environment.
Coma	Apply repeated painful stimuli.	A comatose patient remains unarousable with eyes closed. There is no evident response to inner need or external stimuli.

Neurologic Evaluation

RESPIRATIONS. Observe the rate, rhythm, and pattern of respirations. Because neural structures that govern breathing in the cortex and brainstem overlap those that govern consciousness, abnormalities of respiration often occur in coma.

See Table 17-9, Metabolic and Structural Coma (p. 665), and Table 4-8, Abnormalities in Rate and Rhythm of Breathing (p. 120).

PUPILS. Observe the size and equality of the pupils and test their reaction to light. The presence or absence of the light reaction is one of the most important signs distinguishing structural from metabolic causes of coma. The light reaction often remains intact in metabolic coma.

See Table 17-10, Pupils in Comatose Patients (p. 666).

Structural lesions such as stroke may lead to asymmetrical pupils and loss of light reaction.

OCULAR MOVEMENT. Observe the position of the eyes and eyelids at rest. Check for horizontal deviation of the eyes to one side (*gaze preference*). When the oculomotor pathways are intact, the eyes look straight ahead.

In structural hemispheric lesions, the eyes "look at the lesion" in the affected hemisphere.

In irritative lesions due to epilepsy or early cerebral hemorrhage, the eyes "look away" from the affected hemisphere.

OCULOCEPHALIC REFLEX (DOLL'S EYE MOVEMENTS). This reflex helps to assess brainstem function in a comatose patient. Holding open the upper eyelids so that you can see the eyes, turn the head quickly, first to one side and then to the other. (Make sure the patient has no neck injury before performing this test.)

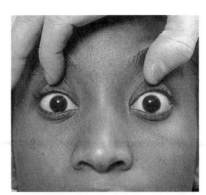

In a comatose patient with an intact brainstem, as the head is turned, the eyes move toward the opposite side (the doll's eye movements). In the adjacent photo, for example, the patient's head has been turned to the right; her eyes have moved to the left. Her eyes still seem to gaze at the camera. The doll's eye movements are intact.

In a comatose patient with absence of doll's eye movements, shown below, the ability to move both eyes to one side is lost, suggesting a lesion of the midbrain or pons.

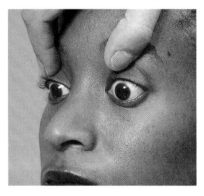

OCULOVESTIBULAR REFLEX (WITH CALORIC STIMULATION). If the oculocephalic reflex is absent and you seek further assessment of brainstem function, test the oculovestibular reflex. Note that this test is almost never performed in an awake patient.

Make sure the eardrums are intact and the canals clear. You must elevate the patient's head to 30° to perform the test accurately. Place a kidney basin under the ear to catch any overflowing water. With a large syringe, inject ice water through a small catheter that is lying in (but not plugging) the ear canal. Watch for deviation of the eyes in the horizontal plane. You may need to use up to 120 ml of ice water to elicit a response. In the comatose patient with an intact brainstem, the eyes drift *toward* the irrigated ear. Repeat on the opposite side, waiting 3 to 5 minutes if necessary for the first response to disappear.

No response to stimulation suggests brainstem injury.

POSTURE AND MUSCLE TONE. Observe the patient's posture. If there is no spontaneous movement, you may need to apply a painful stimulus (see p. 643). Classify the resulting pattern of movement as:

See Table 17-11, Abnormal Postures in the Comatose Patient (p. 667).

■ *Normal–avoidant*—the patient pushes the stimulus away or withdraws.

■ *Stereotypic*—the stimulus evokes abnormal postural responses of the trunk and extremities.

Two stereotypic responses predominate: *decorticate rigidity* and *decerebrate rigidity* (see Table 17-11, Abnormal Postures in the Comatose Patient, p. 667).

■ *Flaccid paralysis or no response*

No response on one side suggests a corticospinal tract lesion.

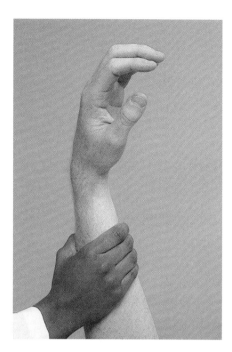

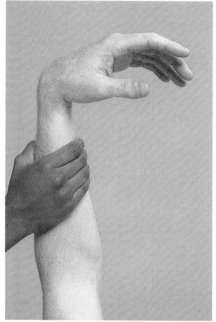

Test muscle tone by grasping each forearm near the wrist and raising it to a vertical position. Note the position of the hand, which is usually only slightly flexed at the wrist.

The hemiplegia of sudden cerebral accidents is usually flaccid at first. The limp hand drops to form a right angle with the wrist.

Then lower the arm to about 12 or 18 inches off the bed and drop it. Watch how it falls. A normal arm drops somewhat slowly.

A flaccid arm drops rapidly, like a flail.

Support the patient's flexed knees. Then extend one leg at a time at the knee and let it fall (see next page). Compare the speed with which each leg falls.

In *acute hemiplegia,* the flaccid leg falls more rapidly

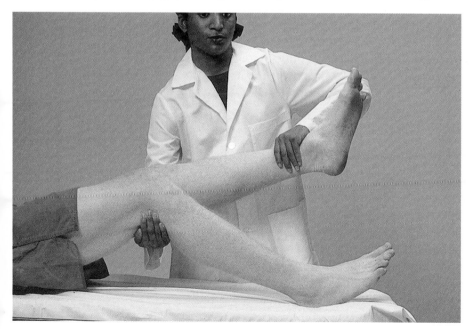

Flex both legs so that the heels rest on the bed and then release them. The normal leg returns slowly to its original extended position.

In acute hemiplegia, the flaccid leg falls rapidly into extension, with external rotation at the hip.

Further Examination

As you complete the neurologic examination, check for facial asymmetry and asymmetries in motor, sensory, and reflex function. Test for meningeal signs if indicated.

Meningitis, subarachnoid hemorrhage

As you proceed to the general physical examination, check for unusual odors.

Alcohol, liver failure, uremia

Look for abnormalities of the skin, including color, moisture, evidence of bleeding disorders, needle marks, and other lesions.

Jaundice, cyanosis, cherry red color of carbon monoxide poisoning

Examine the scalp and skull for signs of trauma.

Bruises, lacerations, swelling

Examine the fundi carefully.

Papilledema, hypertensive retinopathy

Check to make sure the corneal reflexes are intact. (Remember that use of contact lenses may abolish these reflexes.)

Reflex loss in coma and lesions affecting CN V or CN VII

Inspect the ears and nose, and examine the mouth and throat.

Blood or cerebrospinal fluid in the nose or the ears suggests a skull fracture; otitis media suggests a possible brain abscess.

Be sure to evaluate the heart, lungs, and abdomen.

Tongue injury suggests a seizure.

RECORDING YOUR FINDINGS

Note that initially you may use sentences to describe your findings; later you will use phrases. The style below contains phrases appropriate for most write-ups. Note the **five components** of the examination and write-up of the nervous system.

Recording the Examination—The Nervous System

"**Mental Status:** Alert, relaxed, and cooperative. Thought process coherent. Oriented to person, place, and time. Detailed cognitive testing deferred. **Cranial Nerves:** I—not tested; II through XII intact. **Motor:** Good muscle bulk and tone. Strength 5/5 throughout. Cerebellar—Rapid alternating movements (RAMs), finger-to-nose (F→N), heel-to-shin (H→S) intact. Gait with normal base. Romberg—maintains balance with eyes closed. No pronator drift. **Sensory:** Pinprick, light touch, position, and vibration intact. **Reflexes:** 2+ and symmetric with plantar reflexes downgoing."

(continued)

Recording the Examination—The Nervous System (Continued)

OR

"*Mental Status:* The patient is alert and tries to answer questions but has difficulty finding words. *Cranial Nerves:* I—not tested; II—visual acuity intact; visual fields full; III, IV, VI—extraocular movements intact; V motor—temporal and masseter strength intact, sensory corneal reflexes present; VII motor—prominent right facial droop and flattening of right nasolabial fold, left facial movements intact, sensory—taste not tested; VIII—hearing intact bilaterally to whispered voice; IX, X—gag intact; XI—strength of sternomastoid and trapezius muscles 5/5; XII—tongue midline. *Motor:* strength in right biceps, triceps, iliopsoas, gluteals, quadriceps, hamstring, and ankle flexor and extensor muscles 3/5 with good bulk but increased tone and spasticity; strength in comparable muscle groups on the left 5/5 with good bulk and tone. Gait—unable to test. Cerebellar—unable to test on right due to right arm and leg weakness; RAMs, F→N, H→S intact on left. Romberg—unable to test due to right leg weakness. Right pronator drift present. *Sensory:* decreased sensation to pinprick over right face, arm, and leg; intact on the left. Stereognosis and two-point discrimination not tested. *Reflexes* (can record in two ways):

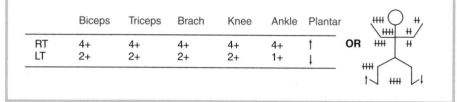

	Biceps	Triceps	Brach	Knee	Ankle	Plantar
RT	4+	4+	4+	4+	4+	↑
LT	2+	2+	2+	2+	1+	↓

OR

Suggest
distribu
cerebral artery,
hemiparesis

BIBLIOGRAPHY

Boyer EW
352(
Buds

Bibliography

CITATIONS

1. Marjama-Lyons JM, Koller WC. Parkinson's disease: update in diagnosis and symptom treatment. Geriatrics 56(8):24–35, 2001.
2. Kistler JP, Furie K, Hakan A. Definition and clinical manifestations of stroke and transient cerebral ischemia. Available at: www.utdol.com. Accessed December 4, 2004.
3. Kidwell CS, Warach S. Acute ischemic cerebrovascular syndrome: diagnostic criteria Stroke 34(12):2995–2998, 2003.
4. Albers GW, Caplan LR, Easton JD, et al. Transient ischemic attack—proposal for a new definition. N Engl J Med 347(21): 1713–1716, 2002.
5. Johnston SC, Gress DR, Browner WS, et al. Short-term prognosis after emergency department diagnosis of TIA. JAMA 284(22):2901–2906, 2000.
6. Douglas JG, Bakris GL, Epstein M, et al. Management of high blood pressure in African Americans: consensus statement of the Hypertension in African Americans Working Group of the International Society on Hypertension in Blacks. Arch Intern Med 163(5):525–541, 2003.
7. Corvol JC, Bouzamondo A, Sirol M, et al. Differential effects of lipid-lowering therapies on stroke prevention: a meta-analysis of randomized trials. Arch Intern Med 163(6):669–676, 2003.
8. Collins R, Armitage J, Parish S, et al. Effects of cholesterol-lowering with simvastatin on stroke and other major vascular events in 20536 people with cerebrovascular disease or other high-risk conditions. Lancet 363(9411):757–767, 2004.
9. Gill JS, Shipley MJ, Tsementzis SA, et al. Alcohol consumption—a risk factor for hemorrhagic and non-hemorrhagic stroke. Am J Med 90(4):489–497, 1991.
10. U.S. Preventive Services Task Force. Aspirin for the primary prevention of cardiovascular events—chemoprevention. January 2002. Available at: www.ahrq.gov/clinic/uspstf/uspsasmi.htm. Accessed December 4, 2004.

ADDITIONAL REFERENCES

Aids to the Examination of the Peripheral Nervous System: Medical Research Council Memorandum No. 45. London, Her Majesty's Stationery Office, 1976.
Booth CN, Boone RH, Tomlinson G, et al. Is this patient dead, vegetative, or severely neurologically impaired? JAMA 291(7): 870–879, 2004.

Shannon M. The serotonin syndrome. N Engl J Med 1(11):1112–1120, 2005.

on AE, Price BH. Memory dysfunction. N Engl J Med 52(7):692–699, 2005.

Campbell WW, DeJong RN, Haerer AF. DeJong's The Neurologic Examination, 6th ed. Philadelphia, Lippincott Williams & Wilkins, 2005.

Elpidoforos SS, Evans JC, Larson MG, et al. Incidence and prognosis of syncope. N Engl J Med 347(12):878–885, 2002.

Gilden DH. Bell's palsy. N Engl J Med 351(13):1323–1331, 2004.

Gilman S, Manter JT, Gatz AJ, et al. Manter and Gatz's Essentials of Clinical Neuroanatomy and Neurophysiology, 10th ed. Philadelphia, FA Davis, 2003.

Goldstein LB, Simel DL. Is this patient having a stroke? JAMA 293(19):2391–2402, 2005.

Griggs RC, Joynt RJ (eds). Baker and Joynt's Clinical Neurology on CD-ROM. Philadelphia, Lippincott Williams & Wilkins, 2003.

Kaniecki R. Headache assessment and management. JAMA 289 (11):1430–1433, 2003.

Katz JN. Carpal tunnel syndrome. N Engl J Med 346(23): 1807–1812, 2002.

Lavan ZP. Stroke prevention through community action. J Community Nurs 19(3):4, 6, 8–10, 2005.

Louis ED. Essential tremor. N Engl J Med 345(12):887–891, 2001.

Mendell JR, Sahenk Z. Painful sensory neuropathy. N. Engl. J Med 348(13):1243–1294, 2003.

Merritt HH, Rowland LP. Merritt's Neurology, 10th ed. Philadelphia, Lippincott Williams & Wilkins, 2000.

Plum F, Posner JB. Diagnosis of Stupor and Coma, 3rd ed. Philadelphia, FA Davis, 1980.

Ropper AH, Adams, RD, Victor, et al. Adams and Victor's Principles of Neurology, 8th ed. New York, McGraw-Hill, 2005.

Saltzman CL, Rashid R, Hayes A, et al. 4.5 Gram monofilament sensation beneath both first metatarsal heads indicates protective foot sensation in diabetic patients. J Bone Joint Surg 86(4): 717–723, 2004.

Siderowf A, Stern M. Update on Parkinson disease. Ann Intern Med 138(8):651–658, 2003.

Van de Beek D, de Gans J, Spanjaard L, et al. Clinical features and prognostic factors in adults with bacterial meningitis. N Engl J Med 351(18):1849–1859.

TABLE 17-1 **Syncope and Similar Disorders**

Problem	Mechanism	Precipitating Factors
Vasodepressor or Vasovagal Syncope *(the common faint)*	Sudden peripheral vasodilatation, especially in the skeletal muscles, without a compensatory rise in cardiac output. Blood pressure falls. Often slow onset, slow offset.	A strong emotion such as fear or pain
Postural *(orthostatic)* **Hypotension**	▪ *Inadequate vasoconstrictor reflexes* in both arterioles and veins, with resultant venous pooling, decreased cardiac output, and low blood pressure	▪ Standing up
	▪ *Hypovolemia,* a diminished blood volume insufficient to maintain cardiac output and blood pressure, especially in the upright position	▪ Standing up after hemorrhage or dehydration
Cough Syncope	Several possible mechanisms associated with increased intrathoracic pressure	Severe paroxysm of coughing
Micturition Syncope	Unclear	Emptying the bladder after getting out of bed to void
Cardiovascular Disorders		
Arrhythmias	Decreased cardiac output secondary to rhythms that are too fast (usually more than 180) or too slow (less than 35–40). Often sudden onset; sudden offset.	A sudden change in rhythm
Aortic Stenosis and Hypertrophic Cardiomyopathy	Vascular resistance falls with exercise, but cardiac output cannot rise.	Exercise
Myocardial Infarction	Sudden arrhythmia or decreased cardiac output	Variable
Massive Pulmonary Embolism	Sudden hypoxia or decreased cardiac output	Variable, including prolonged bed rest and clotting disorders
Disorders Resembling Syncope		
Hypocapnia (decreased carbon dioxide) Due to Hyperventilation	Constriction of cerebral blood vessels secondary to hypocapnia that is induced by hyperventilation	Possibly a stressful situation
Hypoglycemia	Insufficient glucose to maintain cerebral metabolism; secretion of epinephrine contributes to symptoms.	Variable, including fasting
Hysterical Fainting Due to a Conversion Reaction	The symbolic expression of an unacceptable idea through body language. Skin color and vital signs may be normal; sometimes with bizarre and purposive movements; occurrence in the presence of other people.	Stressful situation

(table continues next page)

TABLE 17-1   **Syncope and Similar Disorders** *(Continued)*

Predisposing Factors	Prodromal Manifestations	Postural Associations	Recovery
Fatigue, hunger, a hot humid environment	Restlessness, weakness, pallor, nausea, salivation, sweating, yawning	Usually occurs when standing, possibly when sitting	Prompt return of consciousness when lying down, but pallor, weakness, nausea, and slight confusion may persist for a time.
■ Peripheral neuropathies and disorders affecting the autonomic nervous system; drugs such as antihypertensives and vasodilators; prolonged bed rest	■ Often none	■ Occurs soon after the person stands up	■ Prompt return to normal when lying down
■ Bleeding from the GI tract or trauma, potent diuretics, vomiting, diarrhea, polyuria	■ Lightheadedness and palpitations (tachycardia) on standing up	■ Usually occurs soon after the person stands up	■ Improvement on lying down
Chronic bronchitis in a muscular man	Often none except for cough	May occur in any position	Prompt return to normal
Nocturia, usually in elderly or adult men	Often none	Standing to void	Prompt return to normal
Heart disease and old age decrease tolerance of abnormal rhythms.	Often none	May occur in any position	Prompt return to normal unless brain damage has resulted
Cardiac disorders	Often none. Onset is sudden.	Occurs with or after exercise	Usually a prompt return to normal
Coronary artery disease	Often none	May occur in any position	Variable
Deep vein thrombosis	Often none	May occur in any position	Variable
A predisposition to anxiety attacks and hyperventilation	Dyspnea, palpitations, chest discomfort, numbness and tingling of the hands and around the mouth lasting for several minutes. Consciousness is often maintained.	May occur in any position	Slow improvement as hyperventilation ceases
Insulin therapy and a variety of metabolic disorders	Sweating, tremor, palpitations, hunger; headache, confusion, abnormal behavior, coma. True syncope is uncommon.	May occur in any position	Variable, depending on severity and treatment
Hysterical personality traits	Variable	A slump to the floor, often from a standing position without injury	Variable, may be prolonged, often with fluctuating responsiveness

TABLE 17-2   Seizure Disorders

Partial Seizures

Partial seizures start with focal manifestations. They are further divided into *simple partial seizures,* which do not impair consciousness, and *complex partial seizures,* which do. *Partial seizures may become generalized.* Partial seizures of all kinds usually indicate a structural lesion in the cerebral cortex, such as a scar, tumor, or infarction. The quality of such seizures helps the clinician to localize the causative lesion in the brain.

Problem	Clinical Manifestations	Postictal *(postseizure)* State
Partial Seizures		
Simple Partial Seizures		
■ With motor symptoms		
Jacksonian	Tonic and then clonic movements that start unilaterally in the hand, foot, or face and spread to other body parts on the same side	Normal consciousness
Other motor	Turning of the head and eyes to one side, or tonic and clonic movements of an arm or leg without the Jacksonian spread	Normal consciousness
■ With sensory symptoms	Numbness, tingling; simple visual, auditory, or olfactory hallucinations such as flashing lights, buzzing, or odors	Normal consciousness
■ With autonomic symptoms	A "funny feeling" in the epigastrium, nausea, pallor, flushing, lightheadedness	Normal consciousness
■ With psychiatric symptoms	Anxiety or fear; feelings of familiarity (déjà vu) or unreality; dreamy states; fear or rage; flashback experiences; more complex hallucinations	Normal consciousness
Complex Partial Seizures	The seizure may or may not start with the autonomic or psychic symptoms outlined above. Consciousness is impaired, and the person appears confused. Automatisms include automatic motor behaviors such as chewing, smacking the lips, walking about, and unbuttoning clothes; also more complicated and skilled behaviors such as driving a car.	The patient may remember initial autonomic or psychic symptoms (which are then termed an *aura*), but is amnesic for the rest of the seizure. Temporary confusion and headache may occur.
Partial Seizures That Become Generalized	Partial seizures that become generalized resemble tonic–clonic seizures (see next page). Unfortunately, the patient may not recall the focal onset, and observers may overlook it.	As in a tonic-clonic seizure, described on the next page. Two attributes indicate a partial seizure that has become generalized: (1) the recollection of an *aura,* and (2) a *unilateral* neurologic deficit during the postictal period.

(Source: Commission on Classification and Terminology of the International League Against Epilepsy. Proposal for revised classification of epilepsies and epileptic syndromes. Epilepsia 30:389–399, 1989. See also International League against Epilepsy. A proposed diagnostic scheme for people with epileptic seizures and with epilepsy: report of the ILAE Task Force on Classification and Terminology. (Available at: http://www.ilae-epilepsy.org/Visitors/Centre/ctf/overview.cfm#2. Accessed March 8, 2005.)

TABLE 17-2   Seizure Disorders *(Continued)*

Generalized Seizures and Pseudoseizures

Generalized seizures begin with bilateral body movements, impairment of consciousness, or both. They suggest a widespread, bilateral cortical disturbance that may be either hereditary or acquired. When generalized seizures of the tonic–clonic (grand mal) variety start in childhood or young adulthood, they are often hereditary. When tonic–clonic seizures begin after the age of 30, suspect either a partial seizure that has become generalized or a general seizure caused by a toxic or metabolic disorder. Toxic and metabolic causes include withdrawal from alcohol or other sedative drugs, uremia, hypoglycemia, hyperglycemia, hyponatremia, and bacterial meningitis.

Problem	Clinical Manifestations	Postictal *(postseizure)* State
Generalized Seizures		
Tonic–Clonic Convulsion (grand mal)*	The person loses consciousness suddenly, sometimes with a cry, and the body stiffens into tonic extensor rigidity. Breathing stops, and the person becomes cyanotic. A clonic phase of rhythmic muscular contraction follows. Breathing resumes and is often noisy, with excessive salivation. Injury, tongue biting, and urinary incontinence may occur.	Confusion, drowsiness, fatigue, headache, muscular aching, and sometimes the temporary persistence of bilateral neurologic deficits such as hyperactive reflexes and Babinski responses. The person has amnesia for the seizure and recalls no aura.
Absence	A sudden brief lapse of consciousness, with momentary blinking, staring, or movements of the lips and hands but no falling. Two subtypes are recognized. *Petit mal absences* last less than 10 sec and stop abruptly. *Atypical absences* may last more than 10 sec.	No aura recalled. In petit mal absences, a prompt return to normal; in atypical absences, some postictal confusion
Atonic Seizure, or Drop Attack	Sudden loss of consciousness with falling but no movements. Injury may occur.	Either a prompt return to normal or a brief period of confusion
Myoclonus	Sudden, brief, rapid jerks, involving the trunk or limbs. Associated with a variety of disorders	Variable
Pseudoseizures		
May mimic seizures but are due to a conversion reaction (a psychological disorder)	The movements may have personally symbolic significance and often do not follow a neuroanatomic pattern. Injury is uncommon.	Variable

* *Febrile convulsions* that resemble brief tonic–clonic seizures may occur in infants and young children. They are usually benign but occasionally may be the first manifestation of a seizure disorder.

TABLE 17-3   **Tremors and Involuntary Movements**

Tremors: Tremors are relatively rhythmic oscillatory movements, which may be roughly subdivided into three groups: resting (or static) tremors, postural tremors, and intention tremors.

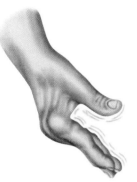

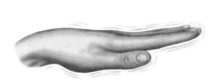

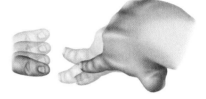

Resting (Static) Tremors

These tremors are most prominent at rest, and may decrease or disappear with voluntary movement. Illustrated is the common, relatively slow, fine, pill-rolling tremor of parkinsonism, about 5 per second.

Postural (Action) Tremors

These tremors appear when the affected part is actively maintaining a posture. Examples include the fine rapid tremor of hyperthyroidism, the tremors of anxiety and fatigue, and benign essential (and sometimes familial) tremor. Tremor may worsen somewhat with intention.

Intention Tremors

Intention tremors, absent at rest, appear with activity and often get worse as the target is neared. Causes include disorders of cerebellar pathways, as in multiple sclerosis.

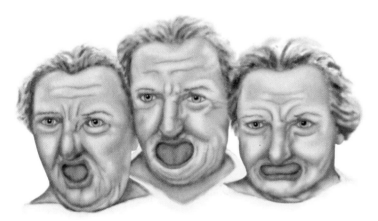

Oral–Facial Dyskinesias

Oral–facial dyskinesias are rhythmic, repetitive, bizarre movements that chiefly involve the face, mouth, jaw, and tongue: grimacing, pursing of the lips, protrusions of the tongue, opening and closing of the mouth, and deviations of the jaw. The limbs and trunk are involved less often. These movements may be a late complication of psychotropic drugs such as phenothiazines, termed *tardive* (late) dyskinesias. They also occur in long-standing psychoses, in some elderly individuals, and in some edentulous persons.

(table continues next page)

TABLE 17-3 **Tremors and Involuntary Movements** *(Continued)*

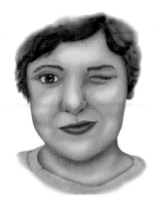

Tics

Tics are brief, repetitive, stereotyped, coordinated movements occurring at irregular intervals. Examples include repetitive winking, grimacing, and shoulder shrugging. Causes include Tourette's syndrome and drugs such as phenothiazines and amphetamines.

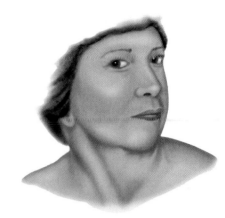

Dystonia

Dystonic movements are somewhat similar to athetoid movements, but often involve larger portions of the body, including the trunk. Grotesque, twisted postures may result. Causes include drugs such as phenothiazines, primary torsion dystonia, and as illustrated, spasmodic torticollis.

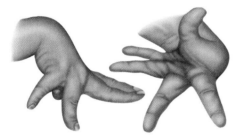

Athetosis

Athetoid movements are slower and more twisting and writhing than choreiform movements, and have a larger amplitude. They most commonly involve the face and the distal extremities. Athetosis is often associated with spasticity. Causes include cerebral palsy.

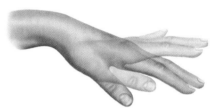

Chorea

Choreiform movements are brief, rapid, jerky, irregular, and unpredictable. They occur at rest or interrupt normal coordinated movements. Unlike tics, they seldom repeat themselves. The face, head, lower arms, and hands are often involved. Causes include Sydenham's chorea (with rheumatic fever) and Huntington's disease.

TABLE 17-4   Nystagmus

Nystagmus is a rhythmic oscillation of the eyes, analogous to a tremor in other parts of the body. Its causes are multiple, including impairment of vision in early life, disorders of the labyrinth and the cerebellar system, and drug toxicity. Nystagmus occurs normally when a person watches a rapidly moving object (e.g., a passing train). Observe the three characteristics of nystagmus listed below and on the following page. Then refer to textbooks of neurology for differential diagnosis.

Direction of the Quick and Slow Components
Example: Left-Beating Nystagmus—a Quick Jerk to the Left in Each Eye, Then a Slow Drift to the Right

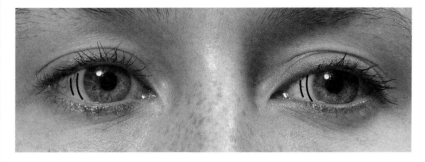

Nystagmus usually has both slow and fast movements, but is defined by its fast phase. For example, if the eyes jerk quickly to the patient's left and drift back slowly to the right, the patient is said to have nystagmus to the left.

Occasionally, nystagmus consists only of coarse oscillations without quick and slow components. It is then said to be *pendular*.

Plane of the Movements
Horizontal Nystagmus

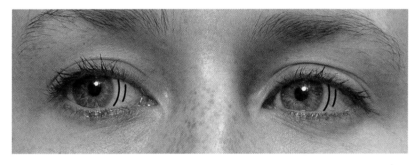

The movements of nystagmus may occur in one or more planes (i.e., horizontal, vertical, or rotary). It is the plane of the movements, not the direction of the gaze, that defines this variable.

Vertical Nystagmus

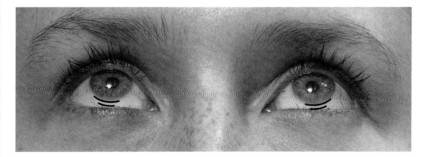

(table continues next page)

TABLE 17-4   **Nystagmus** *(Continued)*

Rotary Nystagmus

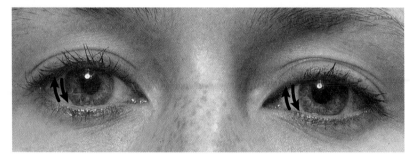

Direction of Gaze in Which Nystagmus Appears
Example: Nystagmus on Right Lateral Gaze

Nystagmus Present (Right Lateral Gaze)

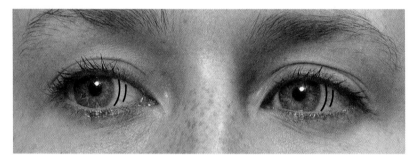

Although nystagmus may be present in all directions of gaze, it may appear or become accentuated only on deviation of the eyes (e.g., to the side or upward). On extreme lateral gaze, the normal person may show a few beats resembling nystagmus. Avoid making assessments in such extreme positions, and *observe for nystagmus only within the field of full binocular vision.*

Nystagmus Not Present (Left Lateral Gaze)

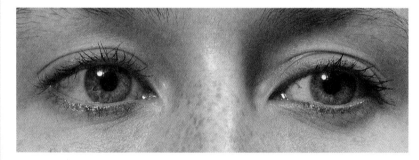

TABLE 17-5   Types of Facial Paralysis

Facial weakness or paralysis may result either (1) from a peripheral lesion of CN VII, the facial nerve, anywhere from its origin in the pons to its periphery in the face, or (2) from a central lesion involving the upper motor neuron system between the cortex and the pons. A peripheral lesion of CN VII, exemplified here by a Bell's palsy, is compared with a central lesion, exemplified by a left hemispheric cerebrovascular accident. These can be distinguished by their different effects on the upper part of the face.

CN VII—Peripheral Lesion

Peripheral nerve damage to CN VII paralyzes the entire right side of the face, including the forehead.

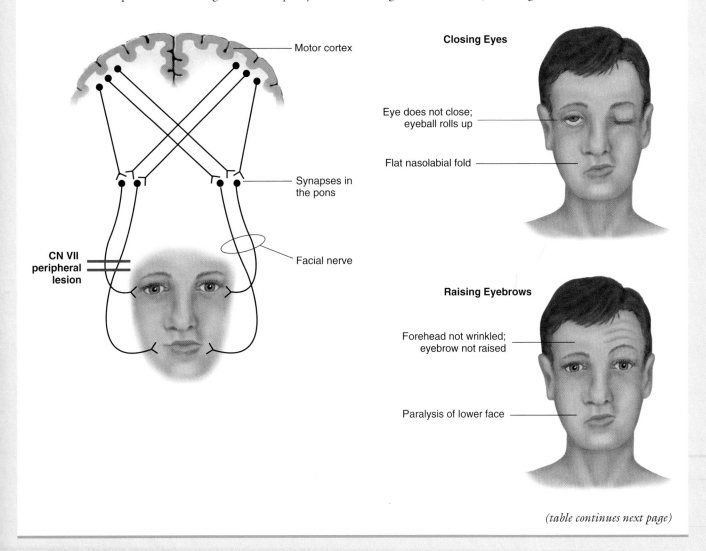

(table continues next page)

TABLE 17-5   **Types of Facial Paralysis** *(Continued)*

CN VII—Central Lesion

The lower part of the face normally is controlled by upper motor neurons located on only one side of the cortex—the opposite side. *Left-sided damage to these pathways, as in a stroke, paralyzes the right lower face.* The upper face, however, is controlled by pathways from both sides of the cortex. Even though the upper motor neurons on the left are destroyed, others on the right remain, and the right upper face continues to function fairly well.

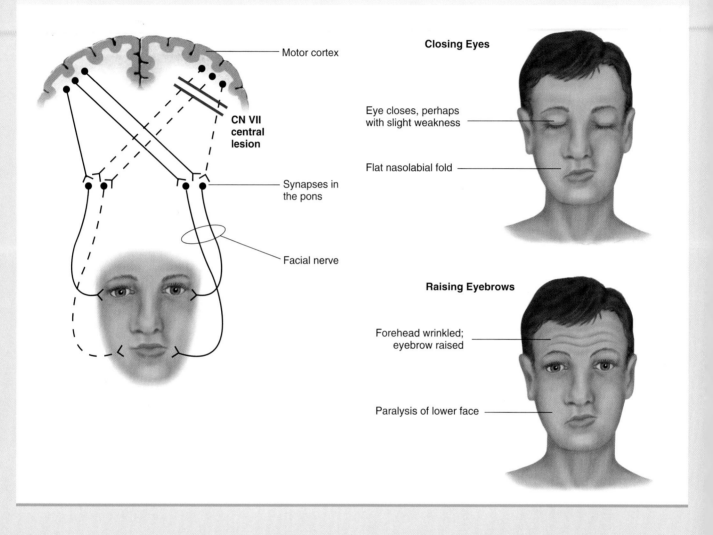

Motor cortex

CN VII central lesion

Synapses in the pons

Facial nerve

Closing Eyes

Eye closes, perhaps with slight weakness

Flat nasolabial fold

Raising Eyebrows

Forehead wrinkled; eyebrow raised

Paralysis of lower face

TABLE 17-6   **Disorders of Muscle Tone**

	Spasticity	Rigidity	Flaccidity	Paratonia
Location of Lesion	Upper motor neuron of the corticospinal tract at any point from the cortex to the spinal cord	Basal ganglia system	Lower motor neuron at any point from the anterior horn cell to the peripheral nerves	Both hemispheres, usually in the frontal lobes
Description	Increased muscle tone (*hypertonia*) that is rate dependent. Tone is greater when passive movement is rapid, and less when passive movement is slow. Tone is also greater at the extremes of the movement arc. During rapid passive movement, initial hypertonia may give way suddenly as the limb relaxes. This spastic "catch" and relaxation is known as "clasp-knife" resistance.	Increased resistance that persists throughout the movement arc, independent of rate of movement, is called *lead-pipe rigidity*. With flexion and extension of the wrist or forearm, a superimposed rachetlike jerkiness is called *cogwheel rigidity*.	Loss of muscle tone (*hypotonia*), causing the limb to be loose or floppy. The affected limbs may be hyperextensible or even flail like.	Sudden changes in tone with passive range of motion. Sudden loss of tone that increases the ease of motion is called *mitgehen* (moving with). Sudden increase in tone making motion more difficult is called *gegenhalten* (holding against).
Common Cause	Stroke, especially late or chronic stage	Parkinsonism	Guillain-Barré syndrome; also initial phase of spinal cord injury (spinal shock) or stroke	Dementia

TABLE 17-7   Disorders of the Central and Peripheral Nervous Systems

Central Nervous System Disorders

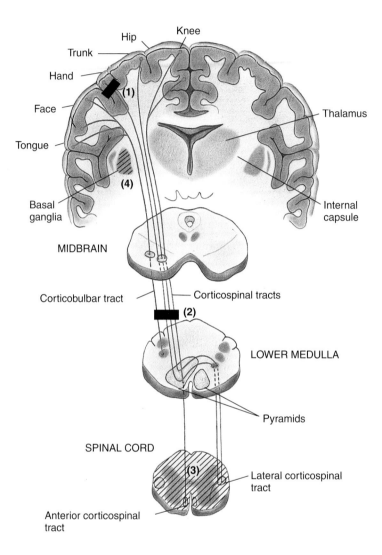

(table continues next page)

Central Nervous System Disorders

Location of Lesion	Typical Findings		Deep Tendon Reflexes	Examples of Cause
	Motor	*Sensory*		
Cerebral Cortex (1)	Chronic contralateral upper motor neuron weakness and spasticity. Flexion is stronger than extension in the arm, plantar flexion is stronger than dorsiflexion in the foot, and the leg is externally rotated at the hip.	Contralateral sensory loss on the limbs and trunk on the same side as the motor deficits	↑	Cortical stroke
Brainstem (2)	Weakness and spasticity as above, plus cranial nerve deficits such as diplopia (from weakness of the extraocular muscles) and dysarthria	Variable. No typical sensory findings	↑	Brainstem stroke, acoustic neuroma
Spinal Cord (3)	Weakness and spasticity as above, but often affecting both sides (when cord damage is bilateral), causing paraplegia or quadriplegia depending on the level of injury	Dermatomal sensory deficit on the trunk bilaterally at the level of the lesion, and sensory loss from tract damage below the level of the lesion	↑	Trauma, causing cord compression
Subcortical Gray Matter: Basal Ganglia (4)	Slowness of movement (bradykinesia), rigidity, and tremor	Sensation not affected	Normal or ↓	Parkinsonism
Cerebellar (not illustrated)	Hypotonia, ataxia, and other abnormal movements, including nystagmus, dysdiadochokinesis, and dysmetria	Sensation not affected	Normal or ↓	Cerebellar stroke, brain tumor

(table continues next page)

Peripheral Nervous System Disorders

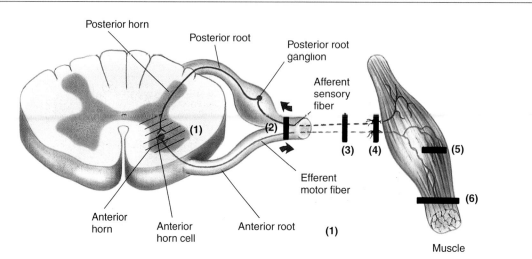

Typical Findings

Location of Lesion	Motor	Sensory	Deep Tendon Reflexes	Examples of Cause
Anterior Horn Cell (1)	Weakness and atrophy in a segmental or focal pattern; fasciculations	Sensation intact	↓	Polio, amyotrophic lateral sclerosis
Spinal Roots and Nerves (2)	Weakness and atrophy in a root-innervated pattern; sometimes with fasciculations	Corresponding dermatomal sensory deficits	↓	Herniated cervical or lumbar disc
Peripheral Nerve— Mononeuropathy (3)	Weakness and atrophy in a peripheral nerve distribution; sometimes with fasciculations	Sensory loss in the pattern of that nerve	↓	Trauma
Peripheral Nerve—Polyneuropathy (4)	Weakness and atrophy more distal than proximal; sometimes with fasciculations	Sensory deficits, commonly in stocking-glove distribution	↓	Peripheral polyneuropathy of alcoholism, diabetes
Neuromuscular Junction (5)	Fatigability more than weakness	Sensation intact	Normal	Myasthenia gravis
Muscle (6)	Weakness usually more proximal than distal; fasciculations rare	Sensation intact	Normal or ↓	Muscular dystrophy

TABLE 17-8	Abnormalities of Gait and Posture

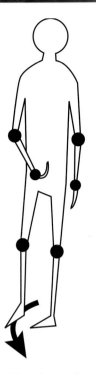 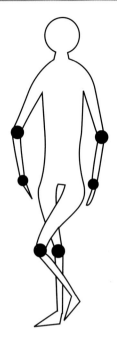 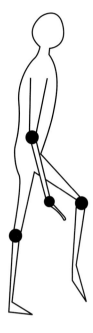

Underlying Defect	Spastic Hemiparesis	Scissors Gait	Steppage Gait
Description	Associated with lesion in corticospinal tract, as with stroke	Associated with bilateral spastic paresis of the legs	Associated with foot drop, usually secondary to lower motor neuron disease
	One arm is held immobile and close to the side, with elbow, wrist, and interphalangeal joints flexed. The leg is extended, with plantar flexion of the foot. On walking, the patient either drags the foot, often scraping the toe, or circles it stiffly outward and forward (*circumduction*).	The gait is stiff. Each leg is advanced slowly, and the thighs tend to cross forward on each other at each step. The steps are short. The patient appears to be walking through water.	These patients either drag their feet or lift them high, with knees flexed, and bring them down with a slap onto the floor, thus appearing to be walking up stairs. They are unable to walk on their heels. The steppage gait may involve one or both sides.

(table continues next page)

TABLE 17-8   **Abnormalities of Gait and Posture** *(Continued)*

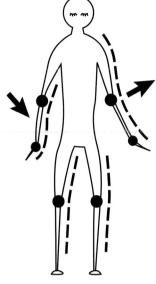
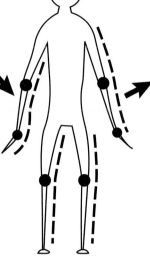
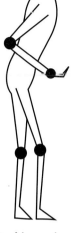

Underlying Defect	**Sensory Ataxia**	**Cerebellar Ataxia**	**Parkinsonian Gait**
	Associated with loss of position sense in the legs, as from polyneuropathy or posterior column damage	Associated with disease of the cerebellum or associated tracts	Associated with the basal ganglia defects of Parkinson's disease
Description	The gait is unsteady and wide based (with feet wide apart). These patients throw their feet forward and outward and bring them down, first on the heels and then on the toes, with a double tapping sound. They watch the ground for guidance while walking. With eyes closed, they cannot stand steadily with feet together (a positive Romberg sign), and the staggering gait worsens.	The gait is staggering, unsteady, and wide based, with exaggerated difficulty on the turns. These patients cannot stand steadily with feet together, whether their eyes are open or closed.	The posture is stooped, with head and neck forward and hips and knees slightly flexed. Arms are flexed at elbows and wrists. The patient is slow in getting started. Steps are short and often shuffling. Arm swings are decreased, and the patient turns around stiffly—"all in one piece."

TABLE 17-9   **Metabolic and Structural Coma**

Although there are many causes of coma, most can be classified as either structural or metabolic. Findings vary widely in individual patients; the features listed are general guidelines rather than strict diagnostic criteria. Remember that psychiatric disorders may mimic coma.

	Toxic–Metabolic	Structural
Pathophysiology	Arousal centers poisoned or critical substrates depleted	Lesion destroys or compresses brainstem arousal areas, either directly or secondary to more distant expanding mass lesions.
Clinical Features		
▪ Respiratory pattern	If regular, may be normal or hyperventilation. If irregular, usually Cheyne-Stokes	Irregular, especially Cheyne-Stokes or ataxic breathing
▪ Pupillary size and reaction	Equal, reactive to light. If *pinpoint* from opiates or cholinergics, you may need a magnifying glass to see the reaction. May be unreactive if *fixed and dilated* from anticholinergics or hypothermia	Unequal or unreactive to light (fixed) *Midposition, fixed*—suggests midbrain compression *Dilated, fixed*—suggests compression of CN III from herniation
▪ Level of consciousness	Changes *after* pupils change	Changes *before* pupils change
Examples of Cause	Uremia, hyperglycemia	Epidural, subdural, or intracerebral hemorrhage
	Alcohol, drugs, liver failure	Cerebral infarct or embolus
	Hypothyroidism, hypoglycemia	Tumor, abscess
	Anoxia, ischemia	Brainstem infarct, tumor, or hemorrhage
	Meningitis, encephalitis	Cerebellar infarct, hemorrhage, tumor, or abscess
	Hyperthermia, hypothermia	

TABLE 17-10   **Pupils in Comatose Patients**

Pupillary size, equality, and light reactions help in assessing the cause of coma and in determining the region of the brain that is impaired. Remember that unrelated pupillary abnormalities, including miotic drops for glaucoma or mydriatic drops for a better view of the ocular fundi, may have preceded the coma.

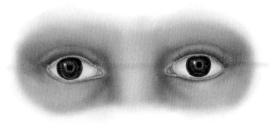

Small or Pinpoint Pupils

Bilaterally small pupils (1–2.5 mm) suggest (1) damage to the sympathetic pathways in the hypothalamus, or (2) metabolic encephalopathy (a diffuse failure of cerebral function that has many causes, including drugs). Light reactions are usually normal.

Pinpoint pupils (< 1 mm) suggest (1) a hemorrhage in the pons, or (2) the effects of morphine, heroin, or other narcotics. The light reactions may be seen with a magnifying glass.

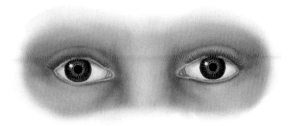

Midposition Fixed Pupils

Pupils that are in the *midposition or slightly dilated* (4–6 mm) and are *fixed to light* suggest structural damage in the midbrain.

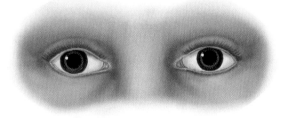

Large Pupils

Bilaterally fixed and dilated pupils may be due to severe anoxia and its sympathomimetic effects, as seen after cardiac arrest. They may also result from atropinelike agents, phenothiazines, or tricyclic antidepressants.

Bilaterally large reactive pupils may be due to cocaine, amphetamine, LSD, or other sympathetic nervous system agonists.

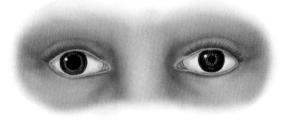

One Large Pupil

A pupil that is *fixed and dilated* warns of herniation of the temporal lobe, causing compression of the oculomotor nerve and midbrain.

TABLE 17-11   Abnormal Postures in Comatose Patients

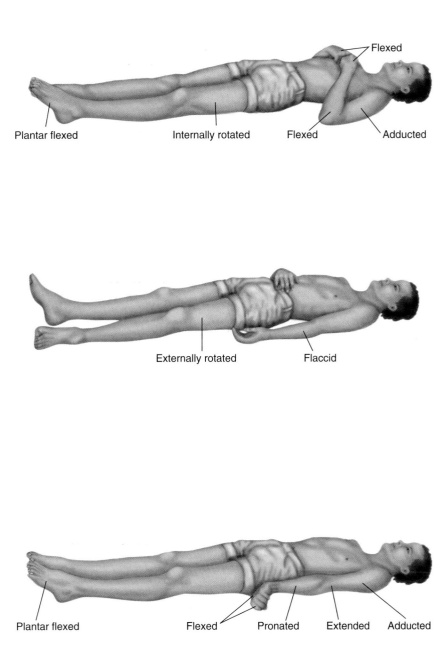

Flexed

Plantar flexed   Internally rotated   Flexed   Adducted

Externally rotated   Flaccid

Plantar flexed   Flexed   Pronated   Extended   Adducted

Decorticate Rigidity (Abnormal Flexor Response)

In decorticate rigidity, the upper arms are held tight to the sides with elbows, wrists, and fingers flexed. The legs are extended and internally rotated. The feet are plantar flexed. This posture implies a destructive lesion of the corticospinal tracts within or very near the cerebral hemispheres. When unilateral, this is the posture of chronic spastic hemiplegia.

Hemiplegia (Early)

Sudden unilateral brain damage involving the corticospinal tract may produce a hemiplegia (one-sided paralysis), which early in its course is flaccid. Spasticity will develop later. The paralyzed arm and leg are slack. They fall loosely and without tone when raised and dropped to the bed. Spontaneous movements or responses to noxious stimuli are limited to the opposite side. The leg may lie externally rotated. One side of the lower face may be paralyzed, and that cheek puffs out on expiration. Both eyes may be turned away from the paralyzed side.

Decerebrate Rigidity (Abnormal Extensor Response)

In decerebrate rigidity, the jaws are clenched and the neck is extended. The arms are adducted and stiffly extended at the elbows, with forearms pronated, wrists and fingers flexed. The legs are stiffly extended at the knees, with the feet plantar flexed. This posture may occur spontaneously or only in response to external stimuli such as light, noise, or pain. It is caused by a lesion in the diencephalon, midbrain, or pons, although severe metabolic disorders such as hypoxia or hypoglycemia may also produce it.

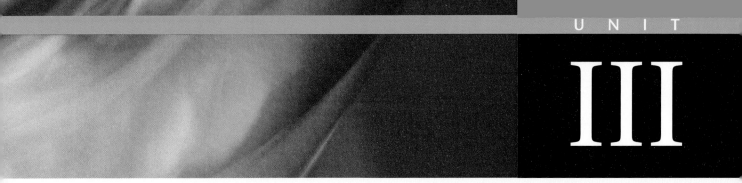

Life Span Examinations

Assessing Children: Infancy Through Adolescence

Peter G. Szilagyi, MD, MPH

When I approach a child, he inspires in me two sentiments: tenderness for what he is, and respect for what he may become.
—*Louis Pasteur*

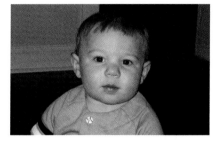

Guide to the Organization of this Chapter

Child Development
Key Principles * Infancy: The First Year of Life * Childhood: 1 Through 10 Years * Adolescence: 11 Through 20 Years

Health Promotion and Counseling

Approach to Examination of Newborns and Infants
Sequence of Examination * Assessing the Newborn * Assessing the Infant

Techniques of Examination for Newborns and Infants
General Survey and Vital Signs * The Skin * The Head * The Neck * The Eye * The Ear * The Nose and Sinuses * The Mouth and Pharynx * The Thorax and Lungs * The Heart * The Breasts * The Abdomen * Male Genitalia * Female Genitalia * Rectal Examination * The Musculoskeletal System * The Nervous System

Approach to Examination of Children
Assessing Early Childhood * Assessing Middle Childhood

Techniques of Examination for Children
General Survey and Vital Signs * The Skin * The Head * The Neck * The Eye * The Ear * The Nose and Sinuses * The Mouth and Pharynx * The Thorax and Lungs * The Heart * The Abdomen * Male Genitalia * Female Genitalia * Rectal Examination * The Musculoskeletal System * The Nervous System

Approach to Examination of Adolescents

Techniques of Examination for Adolescents
General Survey and Vital Signs * Head, Eyes, Ears, Neck, and Throat * The Heart * The Breasts * The Abdomen * Male Genitalia * Female Genitalia * The Musculoskeletal System * The Nervous System

Recording Your Findings

Bibliography

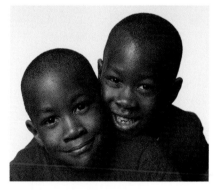

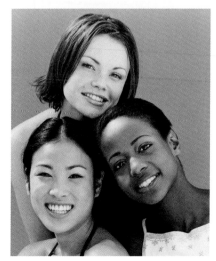

CHILD DEVELOPMENT

KEY PRINCIPLES

Childhood is a period of remarkable physical, cognitive, and social growth, by far the greatest in a person's lifetime. During a few short years, a child will physically increase in size 20-fold, mature into an adult, acquire sophisticated language and reasoning, and develop complex psychosocial interactions. What a journey!

Understanding the normal physical, cognitive, and social development of children will help you tremendously in your interview and physical examination and allow you to distinguish normal from abnormal findings.

Four Principles of Child Development[1]

- Child development proceeds along a predictable pathway governed by the maturing brain.
- The range of normal development is wide.
- Various physical, disease-related, social, and environmental factors affect child development and health.
- The child's developmental level affects the nature of the medical history and physical examination.

The first principle of *child development* is that it *proceeds along a predictable pathway* governed by the maturing brain. You can measure age-specific milestones and characterize a child's development as normal or abnormal according to developmental milestones. Once a milestone is achieved, the

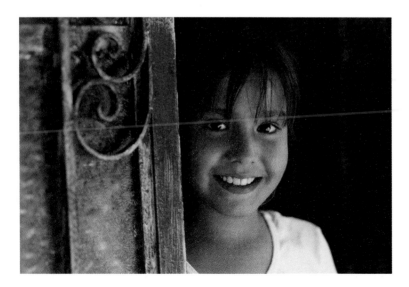

child proceeds to the next. Loss of milestones is concerning. Because your physical examination takes place at one point in time, you need to learn where the child fits along a developmental trajectory.

The second principle is that the *range of normal development is wide.* It is critical to recognize that children mature at different rates. The child's physical, cognitive, and social development should fall within this broad developmental range.

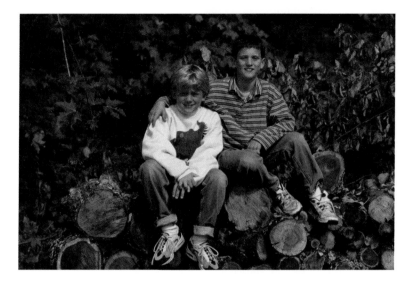

The third principle recognizes that *a variety of physical, disease-related, social, and environmental factors affect child development and health.* For example, chronic diseases and social problems such as child abuse and poverty can result not only in detectable physical abnormalities but also in alterations in the rate and course of developmental advancement. Children with physical or cognitive disabilities may not follow the expected age-specific developmental trajectory. Tailor the physical examination to the child's developmental level.

A fourth principle, specific to the pediatric examination, is that *the child's developmental level affects how you conduct the medical history and physical examination.* For example, interviewing a 5-year-old is fundamentally different from interviewing an adolescent. The physical examination of a rambunctious toddler who is dismantling the examination room has little in common with that of a shy teenager. Both order and style differ from the examination of an adult. You will need to simultaneously adjust your physical examination to the developmental level of the child while attempting to ascertain that developmental level. An understanding of normal child development helps you achieve these tasks. The next section will summarize the physical, cognitive, and social/emotional development of infants, children, and adolescents.[2]

> *Every age has its pleasures, its style of wit, and its own ways.*
> —*Nicholas Boileau-Despreaux*

■ INFANCY: THE FIRST YEAR OF LIFE

Physical Development. The rate of physical growth during the first year of life is the most rapid of any age. By 1 year of age, the child should triple the birth weight and increase in height by 50%. Body proportions change, and the head becomes smaller relative to the body.

The figure on page 675 shows the amazing developmental progression from birth to 1 year of age. Even a newborn has cognitive abilities that may surprise you. For example, a newborn can fix upon and follow a human face and respond to voices. Neurologic development progresses in a central to peripheral direction. Thus, a newborn learns head control before trunk control and use of arms and legs before use of hands and fingers.

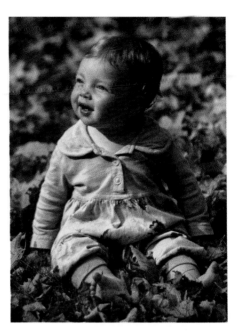

Every child is born a genius.
—*R. Buckminster Fuller*

By 3 months, the normal infant will lift up the head and clasp the hands. By 6 months, the infant will roll over, reach for objects, turn to voices, and possibly sit with support. Learning occurs through activity, exploration, and manipulation of the environment. As peripheral coordination increases, the infant learns to reach for objects, to transfer objects from hand to hand, to crawl, to stand by holding on, and to play with objects by banging and grabbing. A 1-year-old may be standing, exploring the environment, and putting everything in the mouth.[3]

Cognitive and Language Development. With this exploration comes an increased understanding of the self and environment. The infant learns about cause and effect (such as shaking a rattle to produce a sound), the permanence of objects, and the use of tools to explore the environment. By 9 months of age, the child may recognize you as a stranger deserving wary cooperation, seek comfort from parents during the examination, and actively manipulate objects within reach (such as your clothes). Language development proceeds from cooing at 2 months, to babbling at 6 months, to saying 1 to 3 words by 1 year.[4]

Social and Emotional Development. An infant's understanding of self and family also matures. Social tasks include bonding, attachment to caregivers, and trust that loved ones will meet needs. This may result in a reluctance to play with a strange examiner. Temperaments vary greatly. Some infants are predictable, adaptable, and respond positively to new stimuli; others are less adaptable and respond intensely or negatively to new stimuli. Because social development is affected by the environment, observe the child's interactions with caretakers.

Developmental Milestones During Infancy

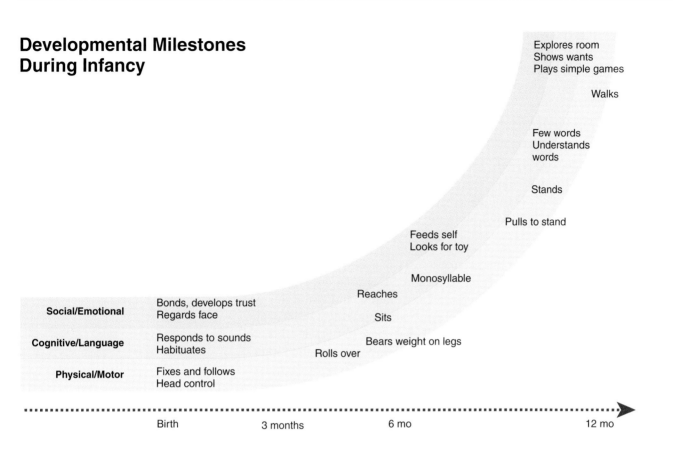

Social/Emotional	Bonds, develops trust Regards face			
Cognitive/Language	Responds to sounds Habituates		Bears weight on legs	
Physical/Motor	Fixes and follows Head control			

Explores room
Shows wants
Plays simple games

Walks

Few words
Understands words

Stands

Pulls to stand

Feeds self
Looks for toy

Monosyllable

Reaches

Sits

Rolls over

Birth | 3 months | 6 mo | 12 mo

CHILDHOOD: 1 THROUGH 10 YEARS

From a developmental perspective, the childhood years are nicely subdivided into early and middle childhood.

EARLY CHILDHOOD: 1 THROUGH 4 YEARS

Physical Development. After 1 year of age, the rate of physical growth slows to half that of infancy. After age 2 years, toddlers gain about 2 to 3 kg and grow 5 cm per year. Growth can proceed in spurts. Physical changes are impressive, and during a few short years, children are transformed from chubby, clumsy toddlers into leaner, more muscular preschoolers. Even more significant are the changes in motor development.

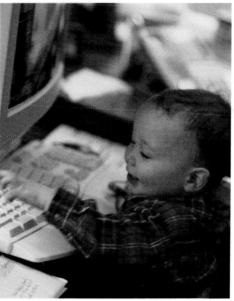

Gross motor skills develop quickly during this period. Most children walk by 15 months, run well by 2 years, and pedal a tricycle and jump around by 3 to 4 years. These new skills make the world a dangerous place for toddlers and pose inherent challenges during your examination. Fine motor skills develop through neurologic maturation and experience with manipulation of the environment. The 18-month-old who scribbles fleetingly develops into a 2-year-old who imitates lines and then a 4-year-old who draws and copies circles.

Cognitive and Language Development. Intellectually, a toddler makes the transition from learning about the environment through touching and looking (sensorimotor learning), to symbolic thinking, solving simple problems, remembering songs, and imitating through play. Take advantage of these changes by making your examination seem like you are playing.

Language develops at extraordinary speed. An 18-month-old with 10 to 20 words emerges as a 2-year-old with two- to three-word sentences, and then a 3-year-old who converses well, asks "why" repeatedly, and entertains you with songs and often uproariously illogical symbolic stories. By 4 years of age, preschoolers form complex sentences. Recall that these ambitious and creative youngsters are still preoperational in thinking and lack sustained logical thought processes.

Social and Emotional Development. The toddler's march to new intellectual pursuits is only surpassed by a new drive for independence. Expect a struggle during parts of your examination. Because toddlers are impulsive, temper tantrums are common. Don't get into a battle of wills with a 2-year-old! Also, don't ask a toddler "May I listen to your chest?" After all, what will you do when the toddler emphatically says "No!"? Just tell the toddler gently what you will do. Note interactions between toddlers and caregivers, assessing both strengths and areas of concern.

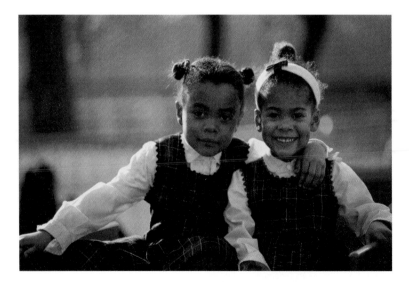

Children are the keys of paradise.
—Richard Stoddard

Developmental Milestones in Early Childhood

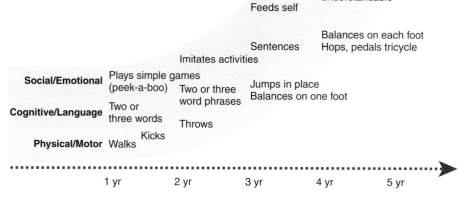

Dresses self
Plays games

Copies figures
Defines words
Some numbers

Skips and
balances
well

Imaginative
Sings, talks
about experiences

Speech all
understandable

Feeds self

Balances on each foot
Sentences   Hops, pedals tricycle

Imitates activities

Social/Emotional Plays simple games
(peek-a-boo)   Two or three   Jumps in place
word phrases Balances on one foot

Cognitive/Language Two or
three words   Throws

Kicks
Physical/Motor Walks

1 yr   2 yr   3 yr   4 yr   5 yr

■ MIDDLE CHILDHOOD: 5 THROUGH 10 YEARS

Despite Freud's viewpoint, the middle childhood years are certainly not latent. Rather, this period is marked by goal-directed exploration of the world, increasing physical and cognitive abilities and achievements, and trials and errors. The physical examination is more straightforward in this age group, but keep in mind the developmental stages and tasks facing these school-age children.

Physical Development. Physically, children in this age group grow steadily but at a slower rate than during the preschool and adolescent periods. Nevertheless, you will see major improvements in strength and coordination, leading to increasing participation in activities. This is also a time when children with physical disabilities or chronic illnesses begin to face their limitations.

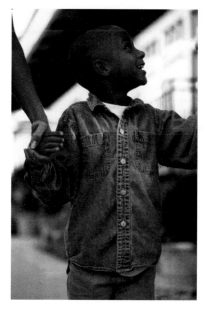

Cognitive and Language Development. Children become "concrete operational"—capable of limited logical thinking and increasingly complicated

learning, yet still rooted in the present, with little ability to understand consequences or abstract issues. A tremendous amount of learning from school and family takes place, and this is greatly influenced by environmental factors. A major developmental task is the achievement of self-efficacy, or the knowledge and ability to thrive in different situations. Moral development remains simple, with a clear sense of "right and wrong." Language becomes increasingly complex during this age period.

> *You know children are growing up when they start asking questions*
> *that have answers.*
> —*John Plomp*

Social and Emotional Development.   School-age children become progressively more independent, initiating their own activities and enjoying their own accomplishments. This is a period of achievements and a critical time for developing self-esteem and an appropriate "fit" within the child's major social structures—the family, the school, and peer activity groups. Guilt and poor self-esteem can also appear. The child's family and environment are crucial to the achievement of a positive self-image. Moral and value systems mature, though they remain relatively simple and concrete.

■ Middle Childhood

Developmental Task	Characteristic	Health Care Needs
Physical	Enhanced strength and coordination	Screening for strengths, assessing problems
	Competence on a variety of tasks and activities	Involvement of parents
		Support for disabilities or problems
		Anticipatory guidance about safety
Cognitive	"Concrete operational": focus on the present	Emphasis on short-term consequences
	Achievement of knowledge and skills, self-efficacy	Support; screening about skills
Social	Achieving good "fit" with family, friends, school	Assessment, support, advice about interactions
	Sustained self-esteem	Support, emphasis on strengths
	Reconciling individuality with conformity	Confidentiality, understanding, advice
	Evolving self-identity	Understanding, support

ADOLESCENCE: 11 THROUGH 20 YEARS

Adolescence can be divided into three stages: early, middle, and late, as shown in the table on p. 680. Your interview and examination techniques will vary widely depending on the adolescent's physical, cognitive, and social–emotional level of development.

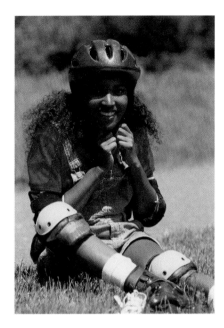

Physical Development. Adolescence is the period of transition from childhood to adulthood. The physical transformation generally occurs over a period of years, beginning at an average age of 10 in girls and 11 in boys. On average, girls end pubertal development with a growth spurt by age 14 and boys by age 16. The age of onset and duration of puberty vary widely, although the stages are predictable. Early adolescents are preoccupied with these physical changes.

A boy becomes an adult three years before his parents think he does, and about two years after he thinks he does.
—Lewis B. Hershey

Cognitive Development. Although not as obvious, cognitive changes during adolescence are as dramatic as changes in physique. Most adolescents progress from concrete to formal operational thinking, acquiring an ability to reason logically and abstractly and to consider future implications of current actions. Although the interview and examination resemble those of adults, keep in mind the wide variability in cognitive development of adolescents and their often erratic and still limited ability to see beyond simple solutions. Moral thinking becomes sophisticated, with lots of time spent debating issues.

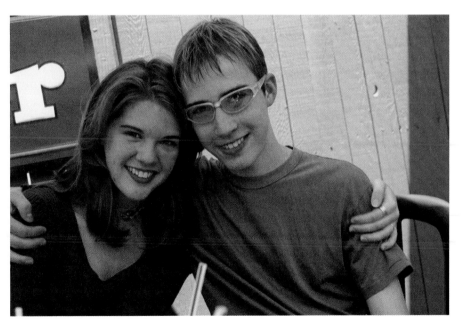

Social and Emotional Development. Adolescence is a tumultuous time, marked by the transition from family-dominated influences to increasing autonomy and peer influence. The struggle for identity, independence, and eventually intimacy leads to much stress, many health-related problems, and, often, high-risk behaviors. This struggle also provides you with an important opportunity for health promotion.

■ *Adolescence*

Developmental Task	Characteristic	Health Care Approaches
Early Adolescence (10–14-year-olds)		
Physical	Puberty (F: 10–14; M: 11–16) variable	Confidentiality; privacy
Cognitive	"Concrete operational"	Emphasis on short-term
Social		
Identity	Am I normal? Peers increasingly important	Reassurance and positive attitude
Independence	Ambivalence (family, self, peers)	Support for growing autonomy
Middle Adolescence (15–16-year-olds)		
Physical	Females more comfortable, males awkward	Support if patient varies from "normal"
Cognitive	Transition; many ideas	Problem solving; decision making
Social		
Identity	Who am I? Much introspection; global issues	Nonjudgmental acceptance
Independence	Limit testing; "experimental" behaviors; dating	Consistency; limit setting
Late Adolescence (17–20-year-olds)		
Physical	Adult appearance	Minimal unless chronic illness
Cognitive	"Formal operational"	Approach as an adult
Social		
Identity	Role with respect to others; sexuality; future	Encouragement of identity to allow growth
Independence	Separation from family; toward real independence	Support, anticipatory guidance

HEALTH PROMOTION AND COUNSELING

An ounce of prevention is worth a pound of cure.
—*Benjamin Franklin*

This sage saying is particularly true for children and adolescents because prevention at a young age can result in improved health outcomes for many decades. Pediatric clinicians dedicate substantial time to health supervision visits and health promotion activities.

Several national and international organizations have identified guidelines for health promotion for children.[5–8] Current concepts of health promotion include not only the detection and prevention of disease but also active promotion of the well-being of children and their families, spanning physical, cognitive, emotional, and social health.

Every interaction with a child and family is an opportunity for health promotion! From your interview to your physical examination, think about your interactions as having two opportunities: the traditional detection of medical problems, and the promotion of health. What a priceless gift!

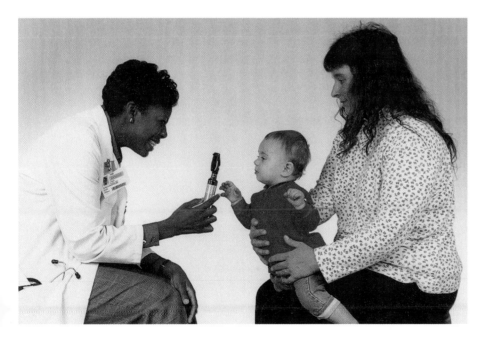

Promotion of development should be age-appropriate and conducted over multiple visits. Promotion regarding development includes suggestions about stimulation (reading, conversing, playing music, optimizing opportunities for gross and fine motor development). Advise parents about upcoming developmental stages and needs of children to help them promote their child's development. Remember, parents are the major agent of health promotion in children, and your advice is implemented through them.

Key components of pediatric health promotion are shown below. Tailor advice to the developmental phase of your patient.

The American Academy of Pediatrics (AAP) publishes guidelines for *health supervision visits* and key age-appropriate components of these visits (see Table 18-3, p. 797). Remember that children and adolescents who have a chronic illness or are from high-risk family or environmental circumstances will probably require more frequent visits and more intensive health promotion.

Integrate explanations of your physical findings with health promotion. For example, provide advice about expected maturational changes or how health behaviors can impact physical findings (e.g., exercise may reduce blood pressure and obesity). It is particularly powerful to demonstrate the relationship between healthy lifestyles and physical health.

Childhood immunizations are a mainstay for health promotion and have been heralded as the most significant medical achievement of public health worldwide. The childhood immunization schedule changes yearly, and updates are published widely and disseminated on Web sites of the Centers for Disease Control and Prevention and the American Academy of Pediatrics (AAP). The figure on p. 683 shows the 2005 Immunization Schedule.

KEY COMPONENTS OF PEDIATRIC HEALTH PROMOTION

1. Age-appropriate developmental achievement of the child
   - Physical (maturation, growth, puberty)
   - Motor (gross and fine motor skills)
   - Cognitive (achievement of milestones, language, school performance)
   - Emotional (self-efficacy and mastery, self-esteem, independence, morality)
   - Social (social competence, self-responsibility, integration with family and community)
2. Health supervision visits
   - Periodic assessment of medical and oral health, per health supervision schedules (see Table 18-3, p. 797)
   - Adjustment of frequency for children or families with special needs
3. Integration of physical examination findings (assure normality, relate findings to healthy lifestyle)
4. Immunizations
5. Screening procedures
6. Anticipatory guidance
   - Healthy habits
   - Nutrition and healthy eating
   - Safety and prevention of injury
   - Sexual development and sexuality
   - Self-responsibility and efficacy
   - Family relationships (interactions, strengths, supports)
   - Emotional and mental health
   - Oral health
   - Prevention or recognition of illness
   - Prevention of risky behaviors
   - School and vocational achievement
   - Peer relationships
   - Community interactions (e.g., school)
7. Partnership between health care provider and child, adolescent, and family

---

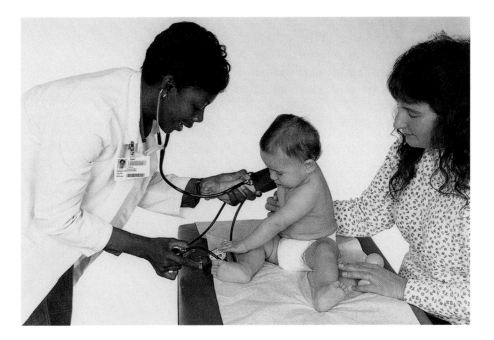

Recommended Childhood and Adolescent Immunization Schedule UNITED STATES • 2005

Vaccine ▼ \ Age ►	Birth	1 mo	2 mos	4 mos	6 mos	12 mos	15 mos	18 mos	24 mos	4-6 yrs	11-12 yrs	13-18 yrs
Hepatitis B	HepB #1	HepB #2				HepB #3				HepB series		
Diphtheria, Tetanus, Pertussis			DTaP	DTaP	DTaP		DTaP			DTaP	Td	Td
Haemophilus influenzae Type b			Hib	Hib	Hib	Hib						
Inactivated Poliovirus			IPV	IPV		IPV				IPV		
Measles, Mumps, Rubella						MMR #1				MMR #2	MMR #2	
Varicella						Varicella				Varicella		
Pneumococcal Conjugate			PCV	PCV	PCV	PCV			PCV		PPV	
Influenza						Influenza (yearly)				Influenza (yearly)		
– – – – Vaccines below this red line are for selected populations												
Hepatitis A										Hepatitis A series		

This schedule indicates the recommended ages for routine administration of currently licensed childhood vaccines, as of December 1, 2004, for children through age 18 years. Any dose not given at the recommended age should be given at any subsequent visit when indicated and feasible.

☐ Indicates age groups that warrant special effort to administer those vaccines not previously given. Additional vaccines may be licensed and recommended during the year. Licensed combination vaccines may be used whenever any components of the combination are indicated and the vaccine's other components are not contraindicated. Providers should consult the manufacturer's package inserts for detailed recommendations. Clinically significant adverse events that follow immunization should be reported to the Vaccine Adverse Event Reporting System (VAERS). Guidance about how to obtain and complete a VAERS form can be found on the Internet: www.vaers.org or by calling 800-822-7967.

☐ range of recommended ages   ☐ only if mother HBsAg(-)

☐ preadolescent assessment   ☐ catch-up immunization

DEPARTMENT OF HEALTH AND HUMAN SERVICES
CENTERS FOR DISEASE CONTROL AND PREVENTION

CDC

The Childhood and Adolescent Immunization Schedule
is approved by:
Advisory Committee on Immunization Practices www.cdc.gov/nip/acip
American Academy of Pediatrics www.aap.org
American Academy of Family Physicians www.aafp.org

More information regarding vaccine administration can be obtained from the websites above or by calling

800-CDC-INFO
ENGLISH & ESPAÑOL
[800-323-4636]

Keep track of your child's immunizations
with the
CDC Childhood
Immunization Scheduler
www.cdc.gov/nip/kidstuff/scheduler.htm

Screening procedures are performed at certain ages. For all children, these include growth parameters and developmental screening at all ages, blood pressure after infancy, and vision and hearing screening at certain key ages. Screening procedures that are particularly recommended for high-risk patients include tests for lead poisoning, tuberculosis exposure, anemia, cholesterol, urinary tract infections, and sexually transmitted diseases. There is variation worldwide in recommendations for screening tests; the AAP recommendations are provided in Table 18-3, p. 797.

Anticipatory guidance is a major component of the pediatric visit. Key areas are shown in the Recommendations for Preventive Pediatric Health Care (p. 797) and cover a broad range of topics, from purely "medical" to social and emotional health. The below examples of anticipatory guidance for a 1-year-old and a 16-year-old highlight key components for two different age groups. The health of children is affected by all of these factors. If we are to achieve a healthier world, we *must* emphasize comprehensive and broadly defined health promotion during childhood. Our children's future depends on it!

EXAMPLES OF ANTICIPATORY GUIDANCE DURING HEALTH SUPERVISION VISITS

1-Year-Old	16-Year-Old
Development	Development
Walking, language, social games	School, social, self, physical
Nutrition	Nutrition
Nutritious snacks	Healthy meals, dieting,
Choking	prevention of obesity
Avoiding overfeeding	
Oral health	Oral health
Brushing	Brushing, dentist
No bottle in bed	Braces
Safety and prevention of injury	Safety and prevention of injury
Safety in home, car, child care	Seat belts, driving and alcohol
Exposures: smoke, drugs	Violence, abuse prevention
Poisonings	Protective gear for activities
Self-efficacy, behavior	Self-efficacy
Praising good behavior	Competence, self-worth, future
Setting limits	Managing stress
Discipline	Mental health, depression
Family relationships	Family relationships
Siblings, spending individual time	Communication
Sharing meals and activities	Separation
Role of other family members	
Community and peer interactions	Community and peer interactions
Playing with other children	Peers, significant others
Assessing child care	Positive activities, financial
Community resources and services	Culture
	Sexuality
	Advice, information, puberty
	Saying no, safer sex, HIV and STDs

APPROACH TO EXAMINATION OF NEWBORNS AND INFANTS

Each child is an adventure into a better life—an opportunity to change the old pattern and make it new.
—Hubert H. Humphrey

Often, neophyte (and some veteran) examiners are intimidated when approaching a tiny baby or a screaming child, especially under the critical eyes of anxious parents. Although it takes a bit of courage, you will come to accept the challenge easily and to enjoy almost all such encounters.

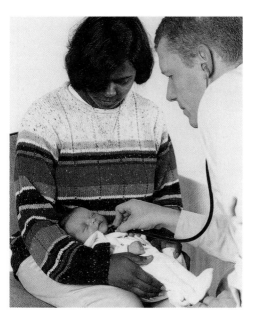

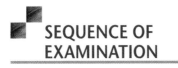

SEQUENCE OF EXAMINATION

Begin by reviewing Chapter 4, Beginning the Physical Examination: General Survey and Vital Signs, for the methods and sequence of examining adults. When examining infants and children, the sequence should vary according to the child's age and comfort level. *Perform nondisturbing maneuvers early on and potentially distressing maneuvers near the end of the examination.* For example, palpate the head and neck and auscultate the heart and lungs early, and examine the ears and mouth and palpate the abdomen near the end. If the child reports pain in one area, examine that part last.

The format of the pediatric medical record is the same as that of the adult record, so although the sequence of the physical examination may vary, you should then convert your written findings back into the traditional format.

The first year of life, infancy, is divided into the neonatal period (the first 28 days) and the postneonatal period (29 days to 1 year).

ASSESSING THE NEWBORN

> ### TIPS FOR EXAMINING NEWBORNS
>
> - Examine the newborn in the presence of the parents.
> - Swaddle and then undress the newborn as the examination proceeds.
> - Dim the lights and rock the baby to encourage the baby's eyes to open.
> - Observe feeding if possible (particularly breast-feeding).
> - Demonstrate calming maneuvers to parents (swaddling, holding techniques).
> - Observe transitions as baby arouses, and teach parents about these transitions.
> - A typical sequence for the examination (for minimal disruption of the baby):
>   Careful observation
>   Head, neck, heart, lungs, abdomen, genitourinary system
>   Lower extremities, back
>   Ears, mouth
>   Eyes, whenever they are spontaneously open
>   Skin, as you go along
>   Neurologic system
>   Hips

Often, the first pediatric examination outside the delivery room is performed in the hospital within 24 hours of birth.

If possible, do the physical examination in front of the parents so that they can interact with you and ask questions. Often parents have specific questions about their baby's physical appearance, so stating normal findings as you go can be quite reassuring. This is also an excellent time to observe parental bonding with the newborn, and to observe how well the breast-feeding baby latches and sucks. To detect problems early, try to observe breast-feeding firsthand. Breast-feeding is physiologically and psychologically optimal, but many mothers will need help and support early on. Early detection of difficulties and anticipatory guidance can promote and sustain healthy breast-feeding.

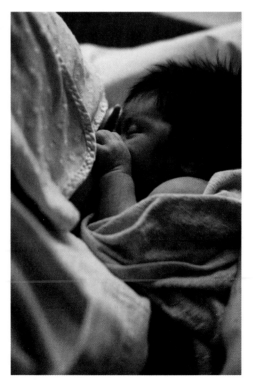

A child is fed with milk and praise.
—*Mary Lamb*

Newborns are most responsive 1 to 2 hours after a feeding, when they are neither too satiated (becoming less responsive) nor too hungry (and often agitated). It is helpful to start with the newborn swaddled and comfortable. Then undress the newborn as the examination proceeds, for gradual stimulation and arousal. If the newborn becomes agitated, use a pacifier or a bottle of formula (if not breast-feeding), or allow the baby to suck on your gloved finger or the baby's own hand. You can also try reswaddling to silence the baby long enough to complete the parts of the examination that require a quiet baby.

IMMEDIATE ASSESSMENT AT BIRTH: ADAPTATION TO EXTRAUTERINE LIFE

Examining newborns immediately after birth is important for determining the general condition, developmental status, abnormalities in gestational development, and any congenital abnormalities. The examination may reveal diseases of cardiac, respiratory, or neurologic origin. Listen to the anterior thorax with your stethoscope, palpate the abdomen, and inspect the head, face, oral cavity, extremities, genitalia, and perineum.

Apgar Score. The Apgar score is the key initial assessment of the baby immediately after birth. It contains five components for classifying the newborn's neurologic recovery from the birth process and immediate adaptation to extrauterine life. Score each newborn according to the following table, at 1 and 5 minutes after birth. Scoring is based on a 3-point scale (0, 1, or 2) for each component. Total scores may range from 0 to 10. Scoring may continue at 5-minute intervals until the score is greater than 7. If the 5-minute Apgar score is 8 or more, proceed to a more complete examination.[9]

■ The Apgar Scoring System

Assigned Score			
Clinical Sign	0	1	2
Heart rate	Absent	<100	>100
Respiratory effort	Absent	Slow and irregular	Good; strong
Muscle tone	Flaccid	Some flexion of the arms and legs	Active movement
Reflex irritability*	No responses	Grimace	Crying vigorously, sneeze, or cough
Color	Blue, pale	Pink body, blue extremities	Pink all over

*Reaction to suction of nares with bulb syringe

1-Minute Apgar Score		5-Minute Apgar Score	
8–10	Normal	8–10	Normal
5–7	Some nervous system depression	0–7	High risk for subsequent central nervous system and other organ system dysfunction
0–4	Severe depression, requiring immediate resuscitation		

Gestational Age and Birth Weight.   Once newborns have successfully adapted to their new environment, it is important to classify them by birth weight and gestational age (maturity). These classifications help predict medical problems and morbidity. Some clinical practice guidelines target infants born below certain gestational age or birth weight.

Gestational age is based on specific neuromuscular signs and physical characteristics that change with gestational maturity. Several scores have been developed to estimate gestational age using these characteristics.

The *Ballard scoring system* estimates gestational age to within 2 weeks, even in extremely premature infants. Table 18-1 (p. 794) includes a complete Ballard scoring system, with instructions for assessing neuromuscular and physical maturity.[10]

CLASSIFICATION BY BIRTH WEIGHT AND GESTATIONAL AGE

Birth Weight

Classification	Weight
■ Extremely low birth weight	<1,000 grams
■ Very low birth weight	<1,500 grams
■ Low birth weight	<2,500 grams
■ Normal birth weight	≥2,500 grams

Gestational Age

Classification	Gestational Age
■ Preterm	<37 wks (<259th day)
■ Term	37–42 wks
■ Postterm	>42 wks (>294th day)

A useful classification, shown on the next page, includes both birth weight and gestational age components, and is based on the birth weight of the newborn on the intrauterine growth curve.

Category	Abbreviation	Percentile
Small for gestational age	SGA	<10th
Appropriate for gestational age	AGA	10–90th
Large for gestational age	LGA	>90th

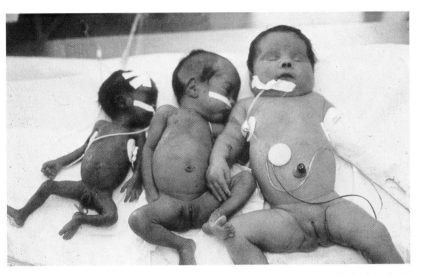

(Reprinted with permission from Korones SB: High-Risk Newborn Infants: The Basis for Intensive Nursing Care, 4th ed. St. Louis, CV Mosby, 1986.)

The figure on the next page shows the intrauterine growth curves for the 10th and 90th percentiles, and depicts the different categories of maturity for newborns based on birth weight and gestational age. The three babies shown above were all born at 32 weeks' gestational age, and weighed 600 g (SGA), 1400 g (AGA), and 2750 g (LGA).

Each of these categories has a different mortality rate, highest for preterm SGA and AGA infants, and lowest for term AGA infants.

Preterm AGA infants are more prone to respiratory distress syndrome, apnea, patent ductus arteriosus with left-to-right shunt, and infection. *Preterm SGA infants* are more likely to experience asphyxia, hypoglycemia, and hypocalcemia.

LGA infants may experience difficulties during birth. Infants of mothers with diabetes are often LGA and may have metabolic abnormalities shortly after birth, as well as congenital anomalies.

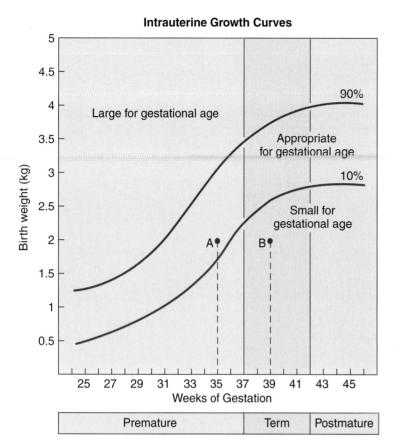

Intrauterine Growth Curves

Level of intrauterine growth based on birth weight and gestational age of liveborn, single, white infants. Point A represents a premature infant, while point B indicates an infant of similar birth weight who is mature but small for gestational age; the growth curves are representative of the 10th and 90th percentiles for all of the newborns in the sampling. (Adapted from Sweet YA. Classification of the low-birth-weight infant. In Klaus MH, Fanaroff AA. Care of the High-Risk Neonate, 3rd ed. Philadelphia, WB Saunders, 1986. Reproduced with permission.)

EXAMINATION SEVERAL HOURS AFTER BIRTH

During the first day of life, and optimally within 8 hours of birth, newborns should have a comprehensive examination. Wait until 1 or 2 hours after a feeding, when the baby is most responsive, and ask the parents to remain in the room.

Observe the baby, first when lying undisturbed and then almost completely undressed if the baby is quiet. Observe the baby's color, size, body proportions, nutritional status, and posture, as well as respirations and movements of the head and extremities.

Most normal, full-term newborns lie in a symmetric position, with the limbs semiflexed and the legs partially abducted at the hip.

In *breech babies,* the legs and head are extended; the legs of a *frank breech baby* are abducted and externally rotated.

Normally there is spontaneous motor activity, with flexion and extension alternating between the arms and legs. The fingers are usually flexed in a tight fist, but may extend in slow, athetoid posturing movements. Brief tremors of the arms, legs, and body are commonly seen for a short time after birth during vigorous crying, and even at rest.

By 4 days after birth, tremors at rest signal central nervous system disease from various possible causes, ranging from *asphyxia* to *drug withdrawal.* Asymmetric movements of the arms or legs at any time suggest *central* or *peripheral neurologic deficits, birth injury* (such as a fractured clavicle or brachial plexus injury), or *congenital anomalies.*

Throughout the examination, and particularly during auscultation and palpation, it is important to have the baby quiet to optimize your examination. Place the tip of your gloved finger in a crying baby's mouth to quiet the baby long enough to complete these portions of the examination. The order of the examination is unimportant.

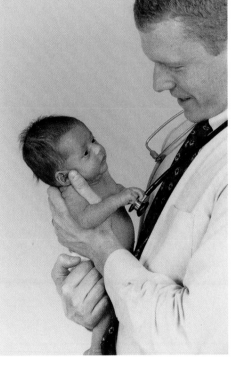

Studies by Dr. T. Berry Brazelton and others have demonstrated the wide range of abilities in newborns.[11] Demonstrating some of the abilities of newborns during your comprehensive examination is both helpful for you and wonderful for the parents. Some of these newborn abilities are described on the following page.

The potential possibilities of any child are the most intriguing and stimulating in all creation.
—*Ray L. Wilbur*

Newborns who cannot perform many of these behaviors may have a neurologic condition, drug withdrawal, or a serious illness.

WHAT A NEWBORN CAN DO: ABILITY FOR COMPLEX BEHAVIOR*

Core Elements

- Newborns can use all five of their senses. For example, they prefer to look at a human face and turn to a parent's voice.
- Newborns are unique individuals, with wide variations in their abilities to interact with their environment. Marked differences exist in temperaments, personality, behavior, and learning.
- Newborns interact dynamically with their caregivers. It is a two-way street! Newborns affect caregivers as much as caregivers influence newborns.

Examples of Complex Newborn Behavior

Habituation	Ability of newborn to selectively and progressively shut out negative stimuli (such as a repetitive sound)
Attachment	A reciprocal, dynamic process of interacting and bonding with the caregiver
State Regulation	A newborn's ability to modulate the level of arousal under different degrees of stimulation (e.g., ability to console self and calm down)
Perception	Newborn's ability to regard faces, turn to voices, quiet in presence of singing, track colorful objects, respond to touch, and recognize familiar scents

*Points from T. Berry Brazelton, MD.

ASSESSING THE INFANT

The key to a successful examination of the infant is using developmentally appropriate methods such as *distraction* and *play*. Because infants usually pay attention to only one thing at a time, it is relatively easy to bring the baby's attention to something other than the examination being performed. Distract the infant with a moving object, a flashing light, a game of peek-a-boo, tickling, or any sort of noise.

If you cannot distract the infant or make the awake infant attend to an object, your face, or a sound, consider a possible *visual* or *hearing deficit*.

TIPS FOR EXAMINING OLDER INFANTS

- Approach the older infant gradually, using a toy or object to distract the infant.
- Do as much of the examination as possible with the infant in the parent's lap.
- Speak softly to the infant or mimic the infant's sounds to attract attention and to keep the infant occupied.
- Ask a parent about the infant's strengths to elicit useful developmental and parenting information.
- If the infant is cranky, make sure he or she is well fed before proceeding with the examination.

GENERAL GUIDELINES

Start the examination with the infant sitting or lying in the parent's lap. If the infant is tired, hungry, or ill, you might ask the parent to hold him against the parent's chest. Make sure there are appropriate toys, a blanket, or other familiar objects nearby. A hungry infant may need to be fed before you can proceed with a complete examination.

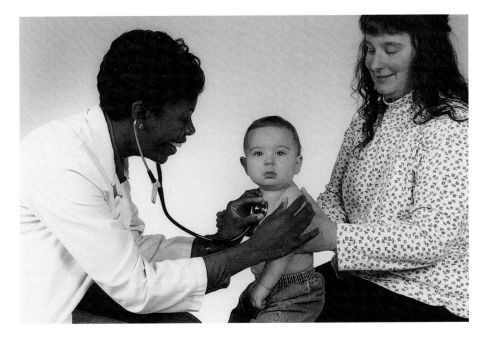

Observe parent–infant interactions. Watch the parent's affect when talking about the infant. Note the parent's manner of holding, moving, and dressing the baby, and response to situations that produce any discomfort for the infant. Assess and comment on positive interactions, such as the obvious pride in the mother's face above.

Infants usually do not object to removal of their clothing. Indeed, most seem to prefer being nude, perhaps because of greater tactile stimulation. To keep yourself and your surroundings dry, it is wise to leave the diaper in place throughout the examination; remove it only to examine the genitals, rectum, lower spine, and hips.

Observation of the infant's communication with the parent can reveal abnormalities such as *developmental delay, language delay, hearing deficits,* or *inadequate parental attachment.* Likewise, observations of the parent–infant interaction may identify maladaptive nurturing patterns that may stem from *maternal depression* or *inadequate social support.*

TESTING FOR DEVELOPMENTAL MILESTONES

Because you'll want to measure the infant's best performance, checking milestones is best at the end of the interview, just before the examination. This "fun and games" interlude also enhances cooperation during the examination. Experienced clinicians can weave the developmental examination into the other parts of the examination. The figure on p. 675 shows some key physical or motor, cognitive or language, and social–emotional milestones during the first year.

One standard for measuring developmental milestones throughout infancy and childhood is the Denver Developmental Screening Test (DDST). It is designed to detect developmental delays in personal–social, fine motor–adaptive, language, and gross motor dimensions from birth through 6 years.

The DDST form is shown on pp. 795–796 in Table 18-2 and includes instructions for recording specific observations. Each test item is represented on the form under the age by a bar, which indicates when 25%, 50%, 75%, and 90% of children attain the milestones depicted. The *DDST is a measure of developmental attainment only in the categories indicated and not a measure of intelligence.*

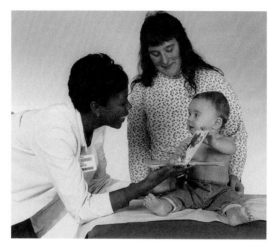

Many disorders cause delays in more than one milestone. For most children with developmental delay, the causes are unknown. Some known causes include *abnormality in embryonic development* (e.g., prenatal insult, chromosomal problem); *hereditary and genetic disorders* (e.g., inborn errors, genetic abnormalities); *environmental and social problems* (e.g., insufficient stimulation); *pregnancy or perinatal problems* (e.g., placental insufficiency, prematurity); and *childhood diseases* (e.g., infection, trauma, chronic illness).

The DDST is a highly specific screening test, but it is not very sensitive. Many children with mild developmental delay score as normal. In particular, the language section is sparse and misses children with mild language delay. Although the DDST is useful, other more sophisticated tests are available to assess motor, language, and social development. Use the DDST as an adjunct to a comprehensive developmental examination. Suspected delays from the general examination or DDST warrant further evaluation. For babies born prematurely, adjust expected developmental milestones for the gestational age up to approximately 12 months.

If a cooperative infant fails items on the DDST, developmental delay is possible, necessitating more precise testing and evaluation.

TECHNIQUES OF EXAMINATION FOR NEWBORNS AND INFANTS

GENERAL SURVEY AND VITAL SIGNS

Important components of the pediatric physical examination include measurement of body size (height, weight, and head circumference) and vital signs (blood pressure, pulse, respiratory rate, and temperature). Tables on the accompanying CD-ROM show norms for blood pressure, height, weight, body mass index (BMI), and head circumference. Deviations from normal may be the first and only indicators of disease (see the tables on the accompanying CD-ROM). Except for body temperature, it is important to compare the child's vital signs or body proportions with age-specific norms, because they change dramatically as children grow older. An increasing number of pediatric practitioners are also assessing pain on a regular basis, using standardized pain scales.

Generally, deviations in measurements beyond two standards for age, or above the 95th percentile or below the 5th percentile, are indications for more detailed evaluation.

SOMATIC GROWTH

Measurement of growth is one of the most important indicators of the health of infants, and deviations from normal may provide an early indication of an underlying problem. To assess growth, it is important to compare a child's growth parameters with respect to

■ Normal values according to age and sex

■ Prior readings on the same child to assess trends

To be clinically meaningful, growth parameters should be measured carefully, using a consistent technique and, optimally, the same scales to measure height and weight.

The most important tools for assessing somatic growth are growth charts, which recently have been modified and published by the National Center for Health Statistics. These charts include height, weight, and head circumference for age, with one set for children up to 36 months and a second set for children ages 2 to 18 years. Charts plotting weight by length are also available. These growth charts have percentile lines indicating the percentage of normal children above and below the child's measurement by chronologic age. Tables on the accompanying CD-ROM display these growth charts.

Failure to thrive is inadequate weight gain for age. Common scenarios are:

■ Growth <5th percentile for age
■ Growth drop >2 quartiles in 6 months
■ Weight for height <5th percentile

Causes include *environmental* or *psychosocial,* and a variety of *gastrointestinal, neurologic, cardiac, endocrine, renal,* and other diseases.

Length. For children younger than 2 years, measure body length by placing the child supine on a measuring board or in a measuring tray, as shown below. Direct measurement of the infant using a tape measure is inaccurate

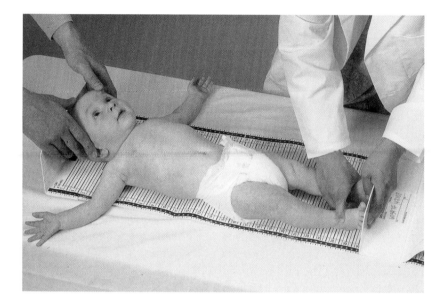

Reduced growth velocity, shown by a drop in height percentile on a growth curve, may signify a chronic condition. Comparison with normal standards is essential, because growth velocity normally is less during the second year than during the first year.

unless an assistant holds the child still with hips and knees extended. Velocity growth curves are helpful in older children, especially those who are suspected of having endocrine disorders.

Weight.   Weigh infants directly with an infant scale; this is more accurate than an indirect method based on weighing the parent and child together and subtracting the weight of the parent from the total weight. Infants should be clothed only in a diaper or weighed naked.

Head Circumference.   The head circumference of infants should be measured during the first 2 years of life, but measurement can be useful at any age to assess growth of the head. The head circumference in infants reflects the rate of growth of the cranium and the brain.

A small head size may be from *premature closure of the sutures* or *microcephaly.* Microcephaly may be familial or the result of various *chromosomal abnormalities, congenital infections, maternal metabolic disorders,* and *neurologic insults.*

An abnormally large head size (>97th percentile or 2 standard deviations above the mean) is *macrocephaly,* which may be from *hydrocephalus, subdural hematoma,* or rare causes like *brain tumor or inherited syndromes. Familial megaloencephaly* (large head) is a benign familial condition with normal brain growth.

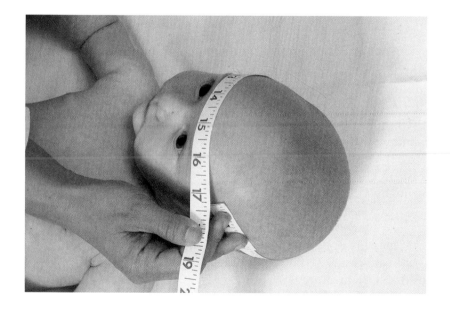

VITAL SIGNS

Blood Pressure.   Although there are special challenges to obtaining accurate blood pressure readings in young infants, this measurement, nevertheless, is important and should be performed at least once in the newborn period.

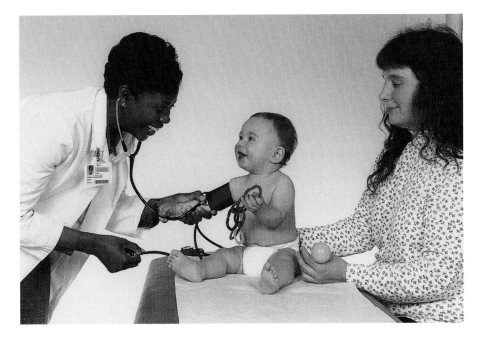

The most easily used measure of the systolic blood pressure of infants is obtained with the *Doppler method,* which detects arterial blood flow vibrations, converts them to systolic blood pressure levels, and transmits them to a digital read-out device. Doppler instruments are expensive, however, and readings tend to be higher than by auscultation.

The systolic blood pressure gradually increases throughout childhood. For example, normal systolic pressure in males is about 70 mm Hg at birth, 85 mm Hg at 1 month, and 90 mm Hg at 6 months. Refer to the tables on the accompanying CD-ROM for normal blood pressure levels by year of life for boys and girls, including percentiles specific to age and height.

Causes of *sustained hypertension* in newborns include renal artery disease (stenosis, thrombosis), congenital renal malformations, and coarctation of the aorta.

Pulse.   The heart rate of infants is quite variable. It is more sensitive to the effects of illness, exercise, and emotion than that of adults. Average heart rates are shown below:

A pulse rate that is too rapid to count (usually >180–200/min) usually indicates *paroxysmal supraventricular tachycardia.*

Age	Average Heart Rate	Range
Birth 0–2	140	90–190
0–6 mo	130	80–180
6–12 mo	115	75–155

You may have trouble obtaining an accurate pulse rate in a squirming infant. The best strategy is to palpate the femoral arteries in the inguinal area or the brachial arteries in the antecubital fossa, or to auscultate the heart.

Bradycardia may be from *drug ingestion, hypoxia, intracranial* or *neurologic conditions,* or, rarely, *cardiac arrhythmia* such as *heart block.*

Respiratory Rate. As with heart rate, compared with that of adults, the respiratory rate in infants has a greater range and is more responsive to illness, exercise, and emotion. The rate of respirations per minute ranges between 30 and 60 in the newborn.

Extremely rapid and shallow respiratory rates are seen in newborns with *cyanotic cardiac disease* who have normal lungs but right-to-left shunting, and in conditions of metabolic acidosis.

The respiratory rate may vary considerably from moment to moment in the newborn, with alternating periods of rapid and slow breathing. The sleeping respiratory rate is most reliable. Respiratory rates during active sleep compared with quiet sleep may be up to 10 breaths per minute faster. The respiratory pattern should be observed for at least 60 seconds. In infancy and early childhood, diaphragmatic breathing is predominant; thoracic excursion is minimal.

Fever can raise respiratory rates in infants. In the absence of pneumonia, an infant's respiratory rate can increase by up to 10 respirations per minute for each degree centigrade of fever.

Commonly accepted cutoffs for defining *tachypnea* are:

Birth–2 months, >60/min
2–12 months, >50/min

Tachypnea and increased respiratory effort in an infant are signs of possible pneumonia.

Temperature. Because fever is so common in children, obtaining an accurate body temperature is helpful whenever you suspect infection, collagen vascular disease, or malignancy. The techniques for obtaining rectal, oral, and auditory canal temperatures in adults are described on pages 112 to 113. Axillary and thermal-tape (temporal artery) skin temperature recordings in infants and children are inaccurate.

Fever (>38.0°C or >100.0°F) in infants <2–3 months may be a sign of *serious infection* or disease. These infants should be evaluated promptly.

The technique for obtaining the *rectal temperature* is relatively simple. One method is illustrated on the next page. Place the infant prone on the examining table, on the parent's lap, or on your own lap. While you separate the buttocks with the thumb and forefinger on one hand, with the other hand gently insert a well-lubricated rectal thermometer, inclined approximately 20° from the table or lap, through the anal sphincter to a depth of approximately 2 to 3 centimeters. Keep the thermometer in place for at least 2 minutes.

Body temperature in infants and children is less constant than in adults. The average rectal temperature is higher in infancy and early childhood, usually not falling below 99.0°F (37.2°C) until after age 3 years. Body temperature may fluctuate as much as 3°F during a single day, approaching 101°F (38.3°C) in normal children, particularly in late afternoon and after vigorous activity.

Anxiety may elevate the body temperature of children. *Excessive bundling* of infants may elevate the skin but not the core temperature.

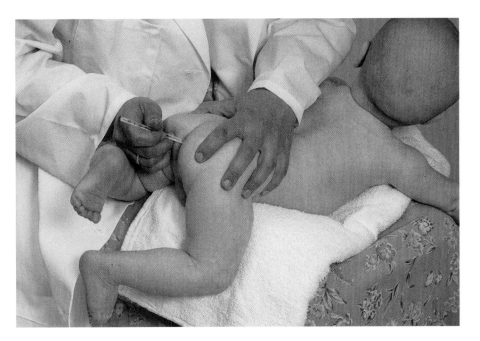

Temperature instability in a newborn may result from sepsis, metabolic abnormality, or other serious conditions. Older infants rarely manifest temperature instability.

THE SKIN

The newborn's skin has a unique characteristic *texture and appearance*. The texture is soft and smooth because it is thinner than the skin of older children. Within the first 10 minutes after birth, a normal newborn progresses from generalized cyanosis to pinkness. In lighter-skinned infants, an erythematous flush, giving the skin the appearance of a "boiled lobster," is common during the first 8 to 24 hours, then the normal pale pink coloring predominates.

Vasomotor changes in the dermis and subcutaneous tissue—a response to cooling or chronic exposure to radiant heat—can produce a lattice-like, bluish mottled appearance (*cutis marmorata*), particularly on the trunk, arms, and legs. This response to cold may last for months in normal infants. *Acrocyanosis*, a blue cast to the hands and feet when exposed to cold (see the photo on the next page), is very common in newborns for the first few days and may recur throughout early infancy. Occasionally in newborns, a striking color change (*harlequin dyschromia*) appears with transient cyanosis of one half of the body or one extremity, presumably from temporary vascular instability.

Cutis marmorata is prominent in *premature infants* and in infants with *congenital hypothyroidism* and *Down syndrome*.

If acrocyanosis does not disappear within 8 hours or with warming, *cyanotic congenital heart disease* should be considered.

The amount of melanin in the skin of newborns varies, affecting *pigmentation*. Black newborns may have a lighter skin color initially than later on, except in the nail beds and genitalia, which are dark at birth. A dark or bluish pigmentation over the buttocks and lower lumbar regions is common in newborns of African, Asian, and Mediterranean descent. These areas, formerly called Mongolian spots, are because of pigmented cells in the deep layers of the skin; they become less noticeable with age and usually disappear during childhood. It is important to document these pigmented areas to avoid later concern about bruising.

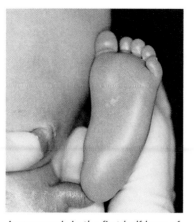

Acrocyanosis in the first half hour of life in a 32-week infant without any underlying heart disease. (From Fletcher M. Physical Diagnosis in Neonatology. Philadelphia, Lippincott-Raven, 1998.)

Central cyanosis in a baby or child of any age should raise suspicion of *congenital heart disease.* The best area to look for central cyanosis is the tongue and oral mucosa, not the nail beds or the extremities.

At birth there is a fine, downy growth of hair called *lanugo* over the entire body, but especially the shoulders and back. This hair is shed within the first few weeks. Lanugo is prominent in premature infants. Hair thickness on the head varies considerably among newborns, and fortunately is not predictive of later hair growth. All of the original hair is shed within months, replaced with a new crop, sometimes of a different color.

Pigmented light-brown lesions (<1–2 cm at birth) are *café-au-lait spots*. Isolated lesions have no significance, but multiple lesions with smooth borders may suggest *neurofibromatosis* (see Table 18-5, p. 799).

INSPECTION

Inspect the newborn closely for a series of common skin conditions. At birth, a cheesy white material called *vernix caseosa,* composed of sebum and desquamated epithelial cells, covers the body. Some newborns have *edema* over their hands, feet, lower legs, pubis, and sacrum; this disappears within a few days. Superficial desquamation of the skin is often noticeable 24 to 36 hours after birth.

Skin desquamation at birth occurs in some normal babies, and frequently in *postterm babies* (>40 wks gestation). Rarely, it is a sign of placental circulatory insufficiency or *congenital ichthyosis.*

You should be able to identify four common dermatologic conditions in newborns. None is clinically significant.

- *Miliaria rubra* consists of scattered vesicles on an erythematous base, usually on the face and trunk, caused by sweat gland duct obstruction; it also disappears spontaneously within weeks.

- *Erythema toxicum,* which usually appears on the second or third day of life, consists of erythematous macules with central pinpoint vesicles scattered diffusely over the entire body, appearing much like flea bites. These lesions are of unknown etiology, but disappear within a week after birth.

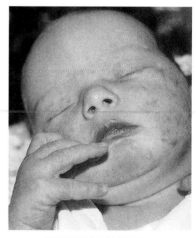

ERYTHEMA TOXICUM

■ *Pustular melanosis,* seen more commonly in black infants, is present at birth as small vesiculopustules over a brown macular base; these can last for several months.

■ *Milia,* pinhead-sized smooth white raised areas without surrounding erythema on the nose, chin, and forehead, is caused by retention of sebum in the openings of the sebaceous glands. Although occasionally present at birth, milia usually appears within the first few weeks and disappears over several weeks.

Note any signs of trauma from the birth process and the use of forceps or suction; these signs disappear but should prompt a careful neurologic examination.

Both erythema toxicum and pustular melanosis may appear similar to the pathologic vesicular rash of *herpes simplex* or *Staphylococcus aureus skin infection,* which are serious infections requiring rapid treatment.

Midline hair tufts over the lumbosacral spine region suggest a *spinal cord defect.*

Jaundice. Normal "physiologic" *jaundice,* which occurs in half of all newborns, appears on the 2nd or 3rd day, peaks at about the 5th day, and usually disappears within a week. Jaundice can best be appreciated in natural daylight rather than artificial light. Newborn jaundice seems to progress from head to toe, with more intense jaundice on the upper body and less intense yellow color in the lower extremities. To detect jaundice, apply pressure to the skin as shown below to press the normal pink or brown color out. Look for the presence of a yellowish "blanching," which indicates jaundice. Another technique is to press a glass slide against the skin to empty the capillary bed and observe for color contrast.

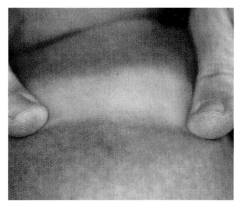

Pressing the red color from the skin allows better recognition of the yellow of jaundice. Infant with no appreciable jaundice at chest level. (From Fletcher M. Physical Diagnosis in Neonatology. Philadelphia, Lippincott-Raven, 1998.)

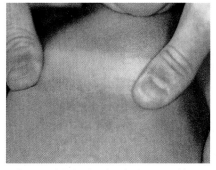

Infant with bilirubin level of 13 mg/dL (222 µmol/L). (From Fletcher M. Physical Diagnosis in Neonatology. Philadelphia, Lippincott-Raven, 1998.)

Jaundice that appears within the first 24 hours of birth is likely to be pathologic jaundice due to *hemolytic disease of the newborn.*

Jaundice that persists beyond 2–3 weeks should raise suspicions of *biliary obstruction* or *liver disease.*

Vascular Markings. A common *vascular marking,* found in 40% of newborns, is the "salmon patch" (also known as *nevus simplex,* telangiectatic nevus, or capillary hemangioma). These flat, irregular, light pink patches are most often seen on the nape of the neck ("stork bite"), upper eyelids, forehead, or upper lip ("angel kisses"). They are not true nevi, but are due to distended dermal capillaries; they almost all disappear by 1 year of age. Darker, purplish lesions on the face or extremities are "port wine stains" and do not fade.

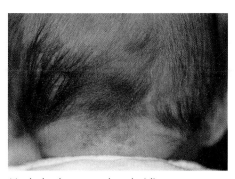

Nuchal salmon patch at hairline. (From Fletcher M. Physical Diagnosis in Neonatology. Philadelphia, Lippincott-Raven, 1998.)

A unilateral port wine stain over the distribution of the ophthalmic branch of the trigeminal nerve may be a sign of *Sturge-Weber syndrome,* which is associated with seizures, hemiparesis, glaucoma, and mental retardation.

Significant edema of the hands and feet of a newborn girl may be suggestive of *Turner's syndrome.*

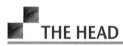

PALPATION

The examination of the skin should include palpation to assess the degree of hydration or *turgor*. Roll a fold of loosely adherent skin on the abdominal wall between your thumb and forefinger to determine its consistency. The skin in well-hydrated infants and children returns to its normal position immediately upon release. Delay in return as shown on the right is a phenomenon called "tenting," and usually occurs in children with significant *dehydration*.

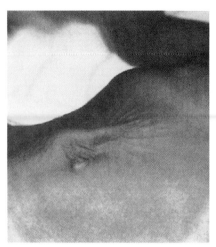

From Zitelli BJ, Davis HW. Atlas of Pediatric Diagnosis, 3rd ed. St. Louis, Mosby–Year Book, 1997.

THE HEAD

At birth, a baby's head may seem relatively large to you. A newborn's head accounts for one fourth of the body length and one third of the body weight; these proportions change, so that by adulthood, the head accounts for one eighth of the body length and about one tenth of the body weight.

Examine the *sutures* and *fontanelles* carefully (see the figure below). The bones of the skull are separated from one another by membranous tissue spaces called *sutures*. The areas where the major sutures intersect in the anterior and posterior portions of the skull are known as *fontanelles*.

On palpation, the sutures feel like ridges and the fontanelles like soft concavities. The *anterior fontanelle* at birth measures 4 cm to 6 cm in diameter and usually closes between 4 and 26 months of age (90% between 7–19 mos). The *posterior fontanelle* measures 1 cm to 2 cm at birth and usually closes by 2 months.

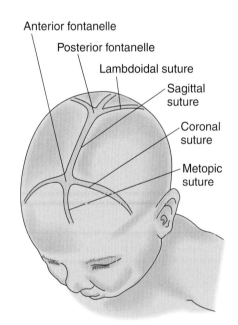

Anterior fontanelle
Posterior fontanelle
Lambdoidal suture
Sagittal suture
Coronal suture
Metopic suture

An enlarged posterior fontanelle may be present in *congenital hypothyroidism.*

A bulging, tense fontanelle is observed in infants with *increased intracranial pressure,* which may be caused by *central nervous system infections, neoplastic disease,* or *hydrocephalus* (obstruction of the circulation of cerebrospinal fluid within the ventricles of the brain).

Careful examination of the fontanelle is important because the fullness of the fontanelle reflects *intracranial pressure*. It is best to palpate the fontanelle while the baby is sitting quietly or being held upright. Experienced pediatric health care providers often palpate the fontanelles at the beginning of the examination. In normal infants, the anterior fontanelle is soft and flat. Increased intracranial pressure produces a bulging, full anterior fontanelle and is seen when a baby cries, vomits, or has underlying pathology. Pulsations of the fontanelle reflect the peripheral pulse.

Inspect the scalp veins carefully to assess for dilatation.

Assess the *symmetry of the skull*. Various conditions can cause asymmetry of the skull in newborns and infants; some are normal or benign, whereas others reflect underlying pathology.

A depressed anterior fontanelle may be a sign of *dehydration*.

Overlap of the cranial bones at the sutures at birth, called *molding*, results from passage of the head through the birth canal; it disappears within 2 days.

Dilated scalp veins are indicative of long-standing *increased intracranial pressure.*

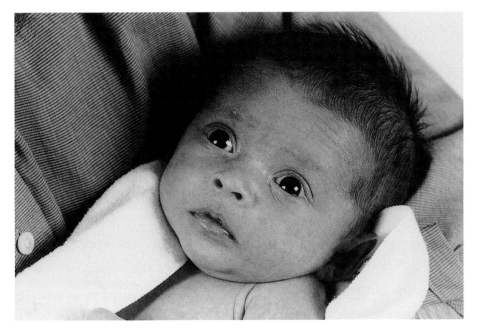

A newborn's scalp is often swollen from localized subcutaneous edema over the occipitoparietal region, called *caput succedaneum*, caused by distention of capillaries and extravasation of blood and fluid resulting from the vacuum effect of rupture of the amniotic sac. This swelling often crosses over suture lines and resolves in 1 to 2 days.

The premature infant's head at birth is relatively long in the occipitofrontal diameter and narrow in the bitemporal diameter (*dolichocephaly*). Usually the skull shape normalizes within 1 to 2 years.

Another type of localized swelling of the scalp is a *cephalohematoma*, caused by subperiosteal hemorrhage from the trauma of birth. This swelling does not cross over suture lines and resolves within 3 weeks. As the hemorrhage resolves and calcifies, there may be a palpable bony rim with a soft center.

Asymmetry of the cranial vault (*plagiocephaly*) occurs when an infant lies mostly on one side, resulting in a flattening of the parieto-occipital region on the dependent side and a prominence of the frontal region on the opposite side. It disappears as the baby becomes more active and spends less time in one position, and symmetry is almost always restored. Interestingly, the current trend to have newborns sleep on their backs to reduce the risk for sudden infant death syndrome has resulted in more cases of plagiocephaly.

Although *plagiocephaly* may result from positioning, it may also reflect pathology such as *torticollis* from injury to the sternocleidomastoid muscle at birth, or *lack of stimulation* of the infant.

Measure the head circumference (p. 696) to detect abnormally large head size (*macrocephaly*) or small head (*microcephaly*), which may signify an underlying disorder affecting the brain.

Premature closure of one or more cranial sutures causes *craniosynostosis,* with an abnormally shaped skull. *Sagittal suture* synostosis causes a narrow head from lack of growth of the parietal bones. Palpation may reveal a raised bony ridge at the suture line.

Palpate the infant's skull with care. The cranial bones usually appear "soft" or pliable; they will normally become firmer with increasing gestational age.

In *craniotabes,* the cranial bones feel pliable and springy, much like a ping-pong ball springs back upon pressure. Craniotabes can result from increased intracranial pressure, as with *hydrocephaly,* metabolic disturbances such as *rickets,* and infection such as *congenital syphilis.*

Auscultation of the skull is not useful in young children because a systolic or continuous bruit may be heard over the temporal areas in many normal children. Older children with significant anemia may have a cranial bruit.

An *arteriovenous fistula* in the brain can produce a loud bruit.

Check the *face* of infants for symmetry. In utero positioning may result in transient facial asymmetries. If the head is flexed on the sternum, a shortened chin (*micrognathia*) may result. Pressure of the shoulder on the jaw may create a temporary lateral displacement of the mandible.

Micrognathia may also be part of a syndrome, such as the *Pierre Robin syndrome.*

Examine the face for an overall impression of the *facies;* it is helpful to compare with the face of the parents. A systematic assessment of a child with abnormal-appearing facies can identify specific syndromes. The box on the next page describes steps for evaluating facies.

Most developmental and genetic syndromes with abnormal facies also have other abnormalities.

EVALUATING A NEWBORN OR CHILD WITH POSSIBLE ABNORMAL FACIES

Carefully review the history, especially:

- Family history
- Pregnancy
- Perinatal history

Note abnormalities on other parts of the physical examination, especially:

- Growth
- Development
- Other dysmorphic somatic features

Perform measurements (and plot percentiles), especially:

- Head circumference
- Height
- Weight

Consider the three mechanisms of facial dysmorphogenesis:

- Deformations due to intrauterine constraint
- Disruptions due to amniotic bands or disruption from fetal tissue
- Malformations due to an intrinsic abnormality in either the face/head or the brain

Examine the parents and siblings:

- Similarity to a parent may be reassuring (e.g., large head) or may represent a familial disorder.

Try to determine whether the facial features fit a recognizable syndrome, comparing with:

- References (including measurements) and pictures of syndromes
- Tables/databases of combinations of features.

A child with abnormal shape or length of palpebral fissures:
    Upslanting (Down syndrome)
    Down-slanting (Noonan's syndrome)
    Short (fetal alcohol effects)

Percussion of the cheek is useful to check for *Chvostek's sign*, which is present in some metabolic disturbances and occasionally in normal infants. Percuss at the top of the cheek just below the zygomatic bone in front of the ear, using the tip of your index or middle finger.

A positive Chvostek's sign produces facial grimacing caused by repeated contractions of the facial muscles. A Chvostek sign is noted in cases of *hypocalcemic tetany, tetanus and tetany due to hyperventilation.*

THE NECK

Palpate the *lymph nodes of the neck* and assess for any additional masses such as *congenital cysts*. Because the necks of infants are short, it is best to palpate the neck while infants are lying supine, whereas older children are best examined while sitting. Check the position of the thyroid cartilage and trachea.

Branchial cleft cysts appear as small dimples or openings anterior to the midportion of the sternocleidomastoid muscle. They may be associated with a sinus tract.

Preauricular cysts and sinuses are common, pinhole-size pits, usually located anterior to the helix of the

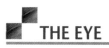

Preauricular

Posterior auricular

Tonsillar

Occipital

Anterior cervical

Posterior cervical

Submandibular

Deep cervical

Submental

Supraclavicular

Epidermoid cyst

Cystic hygroma

2nd branchial cleft cyst

Thyroglossal duct cyst

ear. They are often bilateral and may occasionally be associated with *hearing deficits.*

Thyroglossal duct cysts are located at the midline of the neck, just above the thyroid cartilage. These small, firm, mobile masses move upward with tongue protrusion or with swallowing. They are usually detected after 2 years.

Congenital torticollis, or a "wry neck," is from bleeding into the sternocleidomastoid muscle during the stretching process of birth. A firm fibrous mass is felt within the muscle 2–3 weeks after birth and generally disappears over months.

In newborns, palpate the *clavicles* and look for evidence of a fracture. If present, you may feel a break in the contour of the bone, tenderness, crepitus at the fracture site, and limited movement of the arm on the affected side.

A *fracture of the clavicle* may occur during delivery, particularly during difficult arm or shoulder extractions.

THE EYE

> *We must teach our children to dream with their eyes open.*
> —*Harry Edwards*

Newborns keep their eyes closed except during brief awake periods. If you attempt to separate their eyelids, they will tighten them even more. Bright light causes infants to blink, so use subdued lighting. If you awaken the baby gently, turn down the lights, and support the baby in a sitting position, you will often find that the eyes open. The eyes of many newborns are edematous from the birth process.

A newborn who truly cannot open an eye (even when awake and alert) may have congenital ptosis. Causes include birth trauma, third cranial nerve palsy, and mechanical problems.

You will have to be clever to examine the eyes of infants and young children and use some tricks to get them to cooperate. Small colorful toys are useful as fixation devices in examining the eyes.

Newborns may look at your face and follow a bright light if you catch them during an alert period. You can even get some newborns to follow your face and turn their heads 90° to each side, much to the delight of new parents.

If a newborn fails to gaze at you and follow your face during alert periods, pay particular attention to the rest of the ocular examination. This may still be a normal child, but may indicate *visual impairment.*

The photo below shows one way to examine young infants for *eye movements*. Hold the baby upright, supporting the head. Rotate yourself with the baby slowly in one direction. This usually causes the baby's eyes to open, allowing you to examine the sclerae, pupils, irises, and extraocular movements. The baby's eyes gaze in the direction you are turning. When the rotation stops, the eyes look in the opposite direction, after a few nystagmoid movements.

Nystagmus (wandering or shaking eye movements) persisting after a few days or persisting after the maneuver described on the left may indicate *poor vision* or *central nervous system disease.*

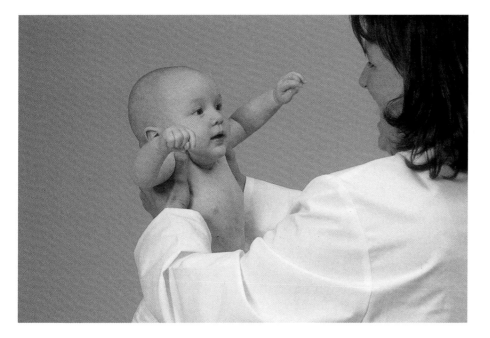

During the first 10 days of life, the eyes may be fixed, staring in one direction if just the head is turned without moving the body (*doll's eye reflex*). During the first few months of life, some infants have intermittent crossed eyes (*intermittent alternating convergent strabismus*, or *esotropia*) or intermittent laterally deviated eyes (*intermittent alternating divergent strabismus*, or *exotropia*).

Alternating convergent or divergent *strabismus* persisting beyond 3 months, or persistent strabismus of any type, may indicate *ocular motor weakness* or another abnormality in the visual system.

Look for abnormalities or congenital problems in the *sclerae* and *pupils*. Subconjunctival hemorrhages are common in newborns.

Colobomas may be seen with the naked eye and represent defects in the iris.

Pupillary reactions can be observed either by response to light or by covering each eye with your hand and then uncovering it. Although there may be some initial asymmetry in the size of the pupils, over time they should be equal in size and reaction to light.

Inspect the irises carefully for abnormalities.

Examine the *conjunctiva* for swelling or redness. Chemical conjunctivitis is common following application of silver nitrate at birth as prophylaxis against gonorrheal conjunctivitis (ophthalmia neonatorum). Most newborn nurseries have switched to using erythromycin ointment because it produces less irritation.

Brushfield spots are a ring of white specks in the iris (see Table 18-11, p. 805). Although sometimes present in normal children, these strongly suggest *Down syndrome.*

You will not be able to measure the *visual acuity* of newborns or infants. You can use visual reflexes to indirectly assess vision: direct and consensual pupillary constriction in response to light, blinking in response to bright light (*optic blink reflex*), and blinking in response to quick movement of an object toward the eyes. During the first year of life, visual acuity sharpens as the ability to focus improves. Infants achieve the following visual milestones:

Persistent ocular discharge and tearing since birth may be from *dacryocystitis* or *nasolacrimal duct obstruction.*

Birth	Blinks, may regard face
1 month	Fixes on objects
1½–2 months	Coordinated eye movements
3 months	Eyes converge, baby reaches
12 months	Acuity around 20/50

Failure to progress along these visual developmental milestones may indicate *delayed visual maturation.*

For the *ophthalmoscopic examination,* with the newborn awake and eyes open, examine the red retinal (fundus) reflex by setting the ophthalmoscope at 0 diopters and viewing the pupil from about 10 inches. Normally, a red or orange color is reflected from the fundus through the pupil.

A thorough ophthalmoscopic examination is difficult in young infants, but may be needed if ocular or neurologic abnormalities are noted. Occasionally, a mydriatic solution may be required to examine the fundus successfully (e.g., using one drop of 2.5% phenylephrine with 0.5% cyclopentolate in each eye); this is usually done with the help of a neurologist or ophthalmologist. The cornea can ordinarily be seen at +20 diopters, the lens at +15 diopters, and the fundus at 0 diopters.

Cloudiness of the cornea may be caused by congenital glaucoma. A dark light reflex can be caused by *cataracts, retinopathy of prematurity,* or other disorders. A white retinal reflex (*leukokoria*) is abnormal, and *cataract, retinal detachment, chorioretinitis,* or *retinoblastoma* should be suspected.

Examine the optic disc area as you would for an adult. In infants, the optic disc is lighter in color. There may be less macular pigmentation, and the foveal light reflection may not be visible. Look carefully for retinal hemorrhages. Papilledema is rare in infants because the fontanelles and open sutures accommodate any increased intracranial pressure, sparing the optic discs.

Small retinal hemorrhages may occur in normal newborns. Extensive hemorrhages may suggest severe *anoxia, subdural hematoma, subarachnoid hemorrhage,* or *severe trauma.*

Pigment changes in the retina can occur in newborns with *congenital toxoplasmosis, cytomegalovirus,* or *rubella.*

THE EAR

The physical examination of the ears of infants is important because many abnormalities can be detected, including structural abnormalities of the ear, otitis media, and hearing loss. This means that you must hone your skills with the otoscope!

The major goals are to determine if the *position, shape,* and *features of the ear* are normal and to detect abnormalities. Note the position of the ears in relation to the eyes. An imaginary line drawn across the inner and outer canthi of the eyes should cross the pinna or auricle; if the pinna is below this line, then the infant has low-set ears.

Examination of the newborn's ear with an otoscope can only detect patency of the *ear canal* because the tympanic membrane is obscured by accumulated vernix caseosa for the first few days of life. In infancy, the ear canal is directed downward from the outside; therefore, you may want to pull the auricle gently downward rather than upward for the best view of the ear drum. Once the tympanic membrane becomes visible, you may note that the light reflex is diffuse and does not become cone-shaped for several months.

The *acoustic blink reflex* is a blinking of the infant's eyes in response to a sudden sharp sound; you can produce this by snapping your fingers or using a bell, beeper, or other noisemaking device about a foot from the infant's ear. Be sure that you are not producing an airstream that may cause the infant to blink. The reflex may be difficult to elicit during the first 2 to 3 days of life. After it is elicited several times within a brief period, the reflex will disappear, a phenomenon known as *habituation*. This is a crude test of hearing, and certainly does not determine normal hearing. Currently, there is an increased movement toward universal hearing screening of all newborns in addition to those at high risk for hearing problems.

Small, deformed, or low-set auricles may indicate associated *congenital defects,* especially renal disease.

A small skin tab, cleft, or pit found just forward of the tragus represents a remnant of the *first branchial cleft* and usually has no significance.

Perinatal problems raising the risk for *hearing defects* include birth weight < 1500 grams, anoxia, treatment with potentially ototoxic medications, congenital infections, severe hyperbilirubinemia, and meningitis.

■ *Signs That an Infant Can Hear*

Age	Sign
0–2 mos	Startle response and blink to a sudden noise
	Calming down with soothing voice or music
2–3 mos	Change in body movements in response to sound
	Change in facial expression to familiar sounds
3–4 mos	Turning eyes and head to sound
6–7 mos	Turning to listen to voices and conversation

Many children with *hearing deficits* are not diagnosed until as old as 2 years. Clues to hearing deficits include parental concern about hearing, delayed speech, and lack of developmental indicators of hearing.

■ THE NOSE AND SINUSES

The most important component of the examination of the nose of newborns is to test for patency of the nasal passages. You can do this by gently occluding each nostril alternately while holding the infant's mouth closed. This will not cause stress in a normal baby because most newborns are nasal breathers. Indeed, some infants are *obligate nasal breathers* and have difficulty breathing through their mouths. Do not occlude both nares simultaneously—this will cause considerable distress!

The nasal passages in newborns may be obstructed in *choanal atresia.* In severe cases, nasal obstruction can be assessed by attempting to pass a No. 8 feeding tube through each nostril into the posterior pharynx.

Inspect the nose to ensure that the nasal septum is midline. You can gently insert a wide nasal speculum of the otoscope into the nose.

At birth, only the ethmoid sinuses are developed. Palpation of the sinuses of newborns is not helpful.

THE MOUTH AND PHARYNX

The face of a child can say it all, especially the mouth part of the face.
—*Jack Handley*

Use both inspection (with a tongue blade and flashlight) and palpation to inspect the mouth and pharynx of newborns. The newborn's mouth is edentulous, and the alveolar mucosa is smooth, with finely serrated borders. Occasionally, pearl-like retention cysts are seen along the alveolar ridges and are easily mistaken for teeth—they disappear within 1 or 2 months. Petechiae are commonly found on the soft palate after birth. Palpate the upper hard palate to make sure it is intact. *Epstein's pearls,* tiny white or yellow, rounded mucous retention cysts, are located along the posterior midline of the hard palate. They disappear within months.

Rarely, *supernumerary teeth* are noted. These are usually dysmorphic and are shed within days but are removed to prevent aspiration.

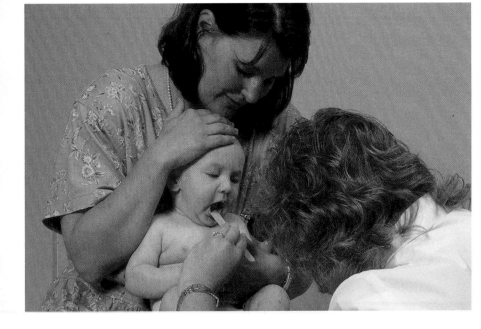

Cysts may be noted on the tongue or mouth. Thyroglossal duct cysts may open under the tongue.

Infants produce little saliva during the first 3 months, but you will note that older infants produce lots of saliva and drool frequently.

Inspect the tongue. The frenulum of the tongue varies, sometimes extending almost to the tip and other times being thick and short, limiting protrusion of the tongue (*ankyloglossia,* or *tongue tie*); these variations rarely interfere with speech or function.

Although unusual, a prominent, protruding tongue may signal *congenital hypothyroidism* or *Down syndrome.*

You will often see a whitish covering on the tongue. If this coating is from milk, it can be easily removed by scraping or wiping it away.

The pharynx of the infant is best seen while the baby is crying. You will likely have difficulty using a tongue blade because it produces a strong gag reflex. Do not expect to be able to visualize the tonsils.

Listen to the quality of the *infant's cry*. Normal infants have a lusty, strong cry. The following box lists some unusual types of infant cries.

Oral candidiasis (thrush) is common in infants. The lesions are difficult to wipe away and have an erythematous raw base (see Table 18-12, Abnormalities of the Mouth and Teeth, p. 806).

Macroglossia is associated with several systemic conditions. If associated with hypoglycemia and omphalocele, the diagnosis is likely Beckwith-Wiedemann's syndrome.

ABNORMAL INFANT CRIES

Type	Possible Related Condition
Shrill or high-pitched	Increased intracranial pressure. Such cries also occur in newborn infants born to narcotic-addicted mothers.
Hoarse	Hypocalcemic tetany or congenital hypothyroidism
Continuous inspiratory and expiratory stridor	Caused by upper airway obstruction due to a variety of lesions (e.g., a polyp or hemangioma), a relatively small larynx (*infantile laryngeal stridor*), or a delay in the development of the cartilage in the tracheal rings (*tracheomalacia*)
Absence of cry	Suggests severe illness, vocal cord paralysis, or profound brain damage

There is a predictable pattern of tooth eruption and also wide variation. A rule of thumb is that a child will have one tooth for each month of age between 6 and 26 months, up to the full complement of 20 primary teeth.

THE THORAX AND LUNGS

The infant's *thorax* is more rounded than that of older children and adults. Also, the chest wall in infancy is thin, with little musculature, and therefore lung and heart sounds are transmitted quite clearly. The bony and cartilaginous rib cage is very soft and pliant. The tip of the xiphoid process is often seen protruding anteriorly immediately beneath the skin at the apex of the costal angle.

Carefully *assess respirations* and the pattern of breathing. Newborn infants, especially those born prematurely, exhibit irregular breathing characterized by periods of breathing at normal rates (30 to 40 per minute) alternating with "periodic breathing," during which the respiratory rate slows markedly and may even cease for 5 to 10 seconds.

Two types of chest wall abnormalities noted in childhood include *pectus excavatum,* or "funnel chest," and *pectus carinatum,* or "chicken breast deformity."

Apnea is defined as cessation of breathing for more than 20 seconds. Apnea is often accompanied by bradycardia and may indicate the presence of a *respiratory disease, central nervous system disease,* or, rarely, a *cardiopulmonary*

An important tip for the examination of the respiratory status of infants and young children is *not* to rush to the stethoscope, but to observe the patient carefully as demonstrated below and in the photograph on the next page. Visual inspection is best done when infants are not crying; thus, work with the parents to settle the child. By observing infants for a significant time (perhaps 1 minute), you can note the general appearance, respiratory rate, color, nasal component of breathing, audible breath sounds, and work of breathing, as described below.

Because infants are obligate nasal breathers, observe their nose as they breathe, looking for *nasal flaring*. Observe the breathing with the infant's mouth closed or with the infant nursing or sucking on a bottle to assess for nasal patency.

Listen to the sounds of the infant's breathing and note any *grunting, audible wheezing*, or *lack of breath sounds (obstruction)*.

It is important to evaluate, by observation, two aspects of the infant: *audible breath sounds* and the *work of breathing*. These are particularly relevant in assessing both upper and lower respiratory illness. Studies in countries that have poor access to chest radiographs have found that these signs are at least as useful as auscultation in assessing both the upper and lower respiratory tract.

condition. Apnea is a high-risk factor for *sudden infant death syndrome (SIDS)*.

In newborns and young infants, nasal flaring may be the result of simply *upper respiratory infections* with subsequent obstruction of their small nares.

■ Observing Respiration—Before You Touch the Child!

Type of Assessment	Specific Observable Pathology
General appearance	Inability to feed or smile Lack of consolability
Respiratory rate	Tachypnea (see p. 698)
Color	Pallor or cyanosis
Nasal component of breathing	Nasal flaring (enlargement of both nasal openings during inspiration)
Audible breath sounds	Grunting (repetitive, short expiratory sound) Wheezing (musical expiratory sound) Stridor (high-pitched, inspiratory noise) Obstruction (lack of breath sounds)

Work of breathing	Nasal flaring (see above)
	Grunting (see above)
	Retractions (or chest indrawing):
	    Supraclavicular (soft tissue above clavicles)
	    Intercostal (indrawing of the skin between ribs)
	    Subcostal (just below the costal margin)

Any of the abnormalities listed at the left should raise concern about underlying respiratory pathology.

Lower respiratory infections, defined as infections below the vocal cords, are common in infants, and include *bronchiolitis* and *pneumonia*.

Acute stridor is a potentially serious condition; causes include *laryngo-tracheo-bronchitis (croup), epiglottitis, bacterial tracheitis, foreign body,* or *a vascular ring*.

In infants, abnormal work of breathing, combined with abnormal findings on auscultation, is the best finding for ruling in *pneumonia*.[12] The best single sign for ruling *out* pneumonia is the absence of tachypnea.

In healthy infants, the ribs do not move much during quiet breathing. If the ribs do move, outward movement is produced by descent of the diaphragm. Descent of the diaphragm compresses the abdominal contents, which in turn shifts the lower ribs outward.

Asymmetric chest movement may indicate a space-occupying lesion. Pulmonary disease causes increased abdominal breathing and can result in *retractions (chest indrawing),* an indicator of pulmonary disease before age 2 years. Chest indrawing is inward movement of the skin between the ribs during inspiration. Movement of the diaphragm primarily affects breathing, with little assistance from the thoracic muscles. As mentioned in the preceding table, three types of retractions can be noted in infants: supraclavicular, intercostal, and subcostal.

Obstructive respiratory disease in infants can result in the *Hoover sign,* or paradoxical (seesaw), breathing in which the abdomen moves outward while the chest moves inward during inspiration.

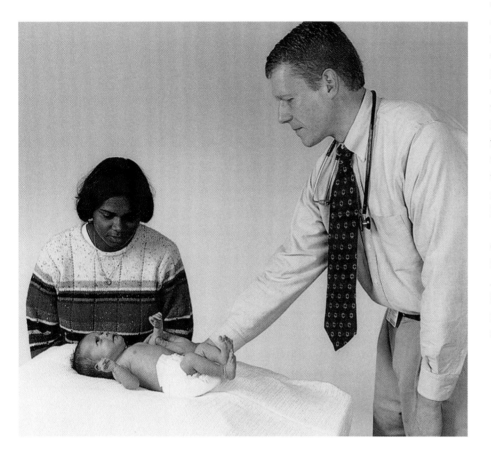

Thoracoabdominal paradox, inward movement of the chest and outward movement of the abdomen during inspiration, is a normal finding in preterm and newborn infants. It continues to persist during active, or REM, sleep even when it is no longer seen during wakefulness or quiet sleep because of the decreased muscle tone of active sleep. As muscle strength increases and chest wall compliance decreases with age and growth, paradox is no longer discernable as a normal finding.

Children with *muscle weakness* may be noted to have thoracoabdominal paradox at several years of age.

Tactile fremitus can be assessed by *palpation.* Place your hand on the chest when the infant cries or makes noise. Place your hand or fingertips over each side of the infant's chest and feel for symmetry in the transmitted vibrations. Percussion is not helpful in infants except in extreme instances. The infant's chest is hyperresonant throughout, and it is difficult to detect abnormalities on percussion.

Because of the excellent transmission of sounds throughout the chest, any abnormalities of tactile fremitus or on percussion suggest severe pathology, such as a large *pneumonic consolidation.*

After performing these maneuvers, you are ready for *auscultation.* Breath sounds are louder and harsher than those of adults because the stethoscope is closer to the origin of the sounds. Also, it is often difficult to distinguish transmitted upper airway sounds from sounds originating in the chest. The

Biphasic sounds imply *severe obstruction from intrathoracic airway narrowing* or *severe obstruction from extrathoracic airway narrowing.*

table below has some useful hints. Upper airway sounds tend to be loud, transmitted symmetrically throughout the chest, and loudest as you move your stethoscope upward toward the neck. They are usually inspiratory, coarse sounds. Lower airway sounds are loudest over the site of pathology, are often asymmetric, and often occur during expiration.

Diminished breath sounds in one side of the chest of a newborn suggest unilateral lesions (e.g., congenital diaphragmatic hernia).

■ Distinguishing Upper Airway From Lower Airway Sounds in Infants

Technique	Upper Airway	Lower Airway
Compare sounds from nose/stethoscope	Same sounds	Often different sounds
Listen to harshness of sounds	Often harsh and loud	Variable
Note symmetry (left/right)	Symmetric	Often asymmetric
Compare sounds at different locations (higher or lower)	Sounds get louder as stethoscope is moved up on the chest	Sounds often louder lower in chest toward abdomen
Inspiratory vs. expiratory	Almost always inspiratory	Often has expiratory phase

Expiratory sounds usually arise from an intrathoracic source. On the other hand, inspiratory sounds typically arise from an extrathoracic airway such as the trachea. During expiration, the diameter of the intrathoracic airways decreases because radial forces from the surrounding lung do not "tether" the airways open as occurs during inspiration. Higher flow rates during inspiration produce turbulent flow, resulting in appreciable sounds.

The characteristics of the breath sounds, such as vesicular and bronchovesicular, and of the adventitious lung sounds, such as crackles, wheezes, and rhonchi, are the same as those for adults, except that they may be more difficult to distinguish in infants and often occur together. Wheezes and rhonchi are common in infants. Wheezes, often audible without the stethoscope, occur more frequently because of the smaller size of the tracheobronchial tree. Rhonchi reflect obstruction of larger airways, or bronchi. Crackles (rales) are discontinuous sounds (see p. 260), near the end of inspiration; they are usually caused by lung disorders and are far less likely to represent cardiac failure in infants than in adults.

Wheezes in infants occur commonly from *asthma* or *bronchiolitis.*

Crackles (rales) can be heard with *pneumonia* and *bronchiolitis.*

THE HEART

The heart is the chief feature of a functioning mind.
—Frank Lloyd Wright

The examination of the heart and vascular systems in infants and children is similar to that in adults, but recognition of their fear, their inability to cooperate, and in many instances, their desire to play, will make the examination easier and more productive. Use your knowledge of the developmental stage of each child. A 2-year-old may be easiest to examine while standing or sitting on the mother's lap, facing her shoulder, as shown on right. Give young children something to hold in each hand. They cannot figure out how to drop the object and therefore have no hand free to push you away. Endless chatter to small children will hold their attention and they will forget you are examining them. Let children move the stethoscope themselves, going back to listen properly. Use your imagination to make the examination work!

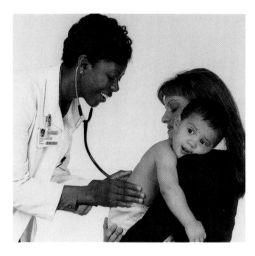

General abnormalities may suggest increased likelihood of congenital cardiac disease, as exemplified by Down syndrome or Turner's syndrome.

INSPECTION

Before examining the heart itself, *observe* the infant carefully for any cyanosis. Acrocyanosis in the newborn is discussed on p. 699. It is important to detect *central cyanosis* (Table 18-14, Cyanosis in Children, p. 808) because it is always abnormal and because many congenital cardiac abnormalities, as well as respiratory diseases, present with cyanosis (see Table 18-15, Congenital Heart Murmurs, pp. 809–810).

Central cyanosis without acute respiratory symptoms suggests cardiac disease.

■ *Cardiac Causes of Central Cyanosis in Children*	
Age of Onset	**Potential Cardiac Cause**
Immediately at birth	Transposition of the great arteries Pulmonary valve atresia Severe pulmonary valve stenosis Possibly Ebstein's malformation

Within a few days after birth	All of the above plus:
	    Total anomalous pulmonary venous return
	    Hypoplastic left heart syndrome
	    Truncus arteriosus (sometimes)
	    Single ventricle variants

Weeks, months, or years of life	All of the above plus:
	    Pulmonary vascular disease with atrial,
	        ventricular, or great vessel shunting

Recognizing minimal degrees of cyanosis requires care. Look inside of the body instead of peering through skin (i.e., the inside of the mouth, the tongue, the conjunctivae, and, to a lesser degree, the nail beds). A true strawberry pink is normal, whereas any hint of raspberry red suggests desaturation.

The distribution of the cyanosis should be evaluated. An oxymetry reading will confirm desaturation.

Observe the infant for *general signs of health*. The infant's nutritional status, responsiveness, happiness, and irritability are all clues that may be useful in evaluating cardiac disease. Note that noncardiac findings can be present in infants with cardiac disease.

Tachypnea, tachycardia, and hepatomegaly in infants suggest congestive heart failure.

COMMON NONCARDIAC FINDINGS IN INFANTS WITH CARDIAC DISEASE

Poor feeding	Tachypnea	Poor overall appearance
Failure to thrive	Hepatomegaly	Weakness
Irritability	Clubbing	

Observation of the respiratory rate and pattern is helpful in distinguishing the degree of illness and cardiac versus pulmonary diseases. An increase in respiratory effort is expected from pulmonary diseases, whereas in cardiac disease, there may be tachypnea, but not increased work of breathing until congestive heart failure becomes significant.

A diffuse bulge outward of the left side of the chest suggests long-standing *cardiomegaly*.

PALPATION

The major branches of the aorta can be assessed by evaluation of the *peripheral pulses*. All neonates should have an evaluation of all pulses at the time of their newborn examination. In neonates and infants, the brachial artery pulse in the antecubital fossa is easier to feel than the radial artery pulse at the wrist. Both temporal arteries should be felt just in front of the ear. It is important to feel the femoral pulses. They lie in the midline just below the inguinal crease, between the iliac crest and the symphysis pubis. Take your time and search for femoral pulses; they are difficult to detect in chubby, squirming infants. If you first flex the infant's thighs on the abdomen, this may overcome the reflex flexion that occurs when you then extend the legs. The dorsalis pedis and posterior tibial pulses in neonates and infants (see the photo on the next page) may be difficult to feel unless there is an abnormality involving aortic run-off. Normal pulses should have a sharp rise and should be firm and well localized.

The absence or diminution of femoral pulses is indicative of *coarctation of the aorta*. If you can't detect femoral pulses, measure blood pressures of the lower and upper extremities. If they are equal or lower in the legs, coarctation is likely to be present.

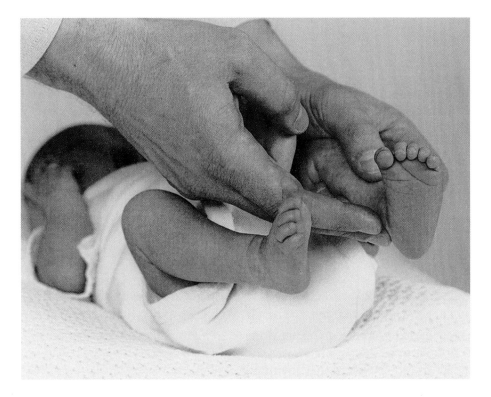

A weak or thready, difficult-to-feel, pulse may reflect *myocardial dysfunction* and *congestive heart failure,* particularly if associated with an unusual degree of tachycardia.

Although the pulses in the feet of neonates and infants are often faint, several conditions can cause full pulses, such as *patent ductus arteriosus* or *truncus arteriosus.*

As discussed on p. 697, carefully measure the *blood pressure* of infants and children as part of the cardiac examination.

The *point of maximal impulse,* or *PMI,* is not always palpable in infants and is affected by respiratory patterns, a full stomach, and the infant's positioning. It is usually an interspace higher than in adults during the first few years of life because the heart lies more horizontally within the chest.

Palpation of the chest wall will allow you to assess volume changes within the heart. For example, a hyperdynamic precordium reflects a big volume change.

Thrills are palpable when there is enough turbulence within the heart or great vessels to be transmitted to the surface. Knowledge of the structures beneath the precordium will allow you to determine the origin of the thrill. Thrills are easiest to feel with your palm or the base of your fingers, not your fingertips. Thrills have a somewhat rough, vibrating quality. The figure on the next page shows locations of thrills from various cardiac abnormalities that occur in infants and children.

A *"rolling"* heave at the left sternal border suggests an *increase in right ventricular work,* whereas the same kind of motion closer to the apex suggests the same thing for the left ventricle.

Aortic valve stenosis

Pulmonary valve stenosis

Severe right ventricular outflow tract obstruction at infundibular level, Tetralogy of Fallot

Ventricular septal defect

LOCATION OF THRILLS

Visible and palpable chest pulsations suggest a hyperdynamic state from either increased metabolic rate or inefficient pumping as a result of an underlying cardiac effect.

AUSCULTATION

The *heart rhythm* is more easily evaluated in infants by listening to the heart than by feeling the peripheral pulses, but in older children can be done either way. Children commonly have a normal sinus dysrhythmia, with the heart rate increasing on inspiration and decreasing on expiration, sometimes quite abruptly. This is a normal finding and can be identified by its repetitive nature, its correlation with respiration, and its involvement of several beats rather than a single beat.

The most common dysrhythmia in children is *paroxysmal supraventricular tachycardia*, or *paroxysmal atrial tachycardia (PSVT, or PAT)*. It can occur at any age, including in utero. It is remarkably well tolerated by some children and is found on examination when the child looks perfectly healthy, may be mildly pale or has tachypnea, but has a rapid, sustained, completely regular heart rate of 240 beats per minute or more. Other children, particularly neonates, appear very ill with this condition. In older children, this dysrhythmia is more likely to be truly paroxysmal, with episodes of varying duration and varying frequency.

Many children, particularly neonates, have premature atrial or ventricular beats that are often appreciated as "skipped" beats. They can usually be eradicated by increasing the intrinsic sinus rate by exercise, such as crying in an infant or jumping in an older child, although they may be more frequent in the postexercise period. In a completely healthy child, they are usually benign and rarely persist.

Pathologic arrhythmias in children can be from *structural cardiac lesions,* but also from other causes such as *drug ingestion, metabolic abnormalities, endocrine disorders, serious infections, and postinfectious states,* or they may be related to conduction disturbances without structural heart disease.

The S₁ and S₂ *heart sounds* should be evaluated carefully. They are normally crisp. The second sounds (S₂) at the base are usually heard separately but should fuse into a single sound in deep expiration. In the neonate, it should be possible to detect a split second sound if the infant is examined when

Distant heart tones suggest *pericardial effusion;* mushy, less distinct heart sounds suggest *myocardial dysfunction.*

completely quiet or asleep; detecting this split eliminates many, but not all, of the more serious congenital cardiac defects.

■ *Characteristics of Normal Variants of Heart Rhythms in Children*

Characteristics	Normal Sinus Arrhythmias	Atrial Premature Contractions (APCs) or Ventricular Premature Contractions (VPCs)
Most common age	After infancy Throughout childhood (less common in adults)	Neonates (but may occur at any time)
Correlation with respiration	Yes: Increases on inspiration Decreases on expiration	No
Effect of exercise on tachycardia	Disappears	Eradicated by exercise May be more frequent postexercise
Characteristic of rhythm	Gradually faster with inspiration Often suddenly slower on expiration	Skipped or missed beat Irregularly occurring
Number of beats	Several beats, usually in repetitive cycles	Usually single abnormal beats
Severity	Benign (by definition)	Usually benign

Although VPCs generally occur in otherwise healthy infants, they can occur with underlying cardiac disease, particularly cardiomyopathies and congenital heart disorders. Electrolyte or metabolic disturbances are additional causes.

In addition to trying to detect splitting of the second heart sound, listen for the intensity of A_2 and P_2. The aortic, or first component of the second sound at the base, is normally louder than the pulmonic, or second component.

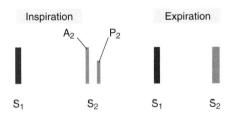

A louder-than-normal pulmonic component, particularly when louder than the aortic sound, suggests *pulmonary hypertension.*

Persistent splitting of S_2 may indicate a right ventricular volume load such as *atrial septal defect, anomalies of pulmonary venous return,* or *chronic anemia.*

Third heart sounds, which are low-pitched, early diastolic sounds best heard at the lower left sternal border, or apex, are frequently heard in children and are normal. They reflect rapid ventricular filling.

The third heart sound S_3 should be differentiated from the higher intensity third heart sound gallop, which is a sign of underlying pathology.

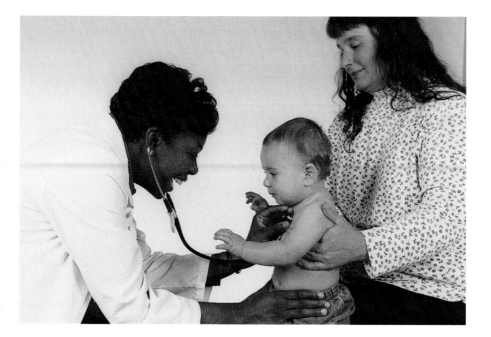

Fourth heart sounds (S₄), which are not often heard in children, are low-frequency, late diastolic sounds, occurring just before the first heart sound.

Fourth heart sounds represent decreased ventricular compliance and are associated with *congestive heart failure.*

An *apparent gallop,* in the presence of a normal heart rate and rhythm, is a frequent finding in normal children and does not represent pathology.

A *gallop rhythm*—tachycardia plus a loud S₃, S₄, or both—is pathologic and indicates *congestive heart failure* and *poor ventricular function.*

One of the most challenging aspects to the cardiac examination in children is the evaluation of *heart murmurs.* In addition to the task of trying to listen to a squirming, perhaps uncooperative child, a major challenge is to distinguish common benign murmurs from unusual or pathologic ones. Heart murmurs in children must be characterized by specific location (e.g., left upper sternal border, not just left sternal border), timing, intensity, and quality. If each murmur is delineated that completely, the diagnosis is usually made, and all that is needed is confirmation and amplification with laboratory tools such as ECG, chest x-ray, and echocardiography.

An important rule of thumb is that, by definition, *benign murmurs in children have no associated abnormal findings.* Many (but not all) children with serious cardiac malformations have signs and symptoms other than a heart murmur obtainable on careful history or examination. Many have other, noncardiac signs and symptoms as well, including evidence of genetic defects that may offer helpful diagnostic clues.

Any of the *noncardiac findings* that frequently accompany cardiac disease in children markedly raises the possibility that a murmur that appears benign is really pathologic.

Most children (indeed, some say nearly all) will have one or more *functional, or benign, heart murmur* before reaching adulthood.[13] It is important to

Many *pathologic murmurs of congenital heart disease* are present at

identify functional murmurs by their specific qualities rather than by their intensity. The common functional murmurs of infancy and childhood should be easily recognized by the practitioner and under most circumstances do not require evaluation.

The figure below characterizes two *benign* heart murmurs in infants according to their location and key characteristics.

birth. Others are not apparent until later, depending on their severity, drop in pulmonary vascular resistance following birth, or changes associated with growth of the child. Table 18-15, on pp. 809–810 shows examples of pathologic murmurs of childhood.

■ *Benign Murmurs in Infants*

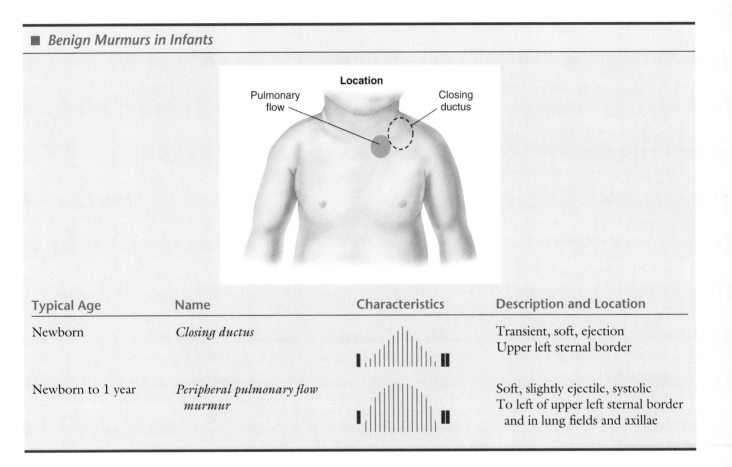

Typical Age	Name	Characteristics	Description and Location
Newborn	*Closing ductus*		Transient, soft, ejection Upper left sternal border
Newborn to 1 year	*Peripheral pulmonary flow murmur*		Soft, slightly ejectile, systolic To left of upper left sternal border and in lung fields and axillae

Some neonates and infants will have a soft, somewhat ejectile murmur heard, not over the precordium, but over the lung fields, particularly in the axillae. This represents peripheral pulmonary artery flow and is partly the result of inadequate pulmonary artery growth in utero (when there is little pulmonary blood flow) and the sharp angle at which the pulmonary artery curves backward. In the absence of any physical findings to suggest additional underlying diseases, this *peripheral pulmonary flow murmur* can be considered benign and usually disappears by the age of 1 year.

A pulmonary flow murmur in the newborn who has signs of other disease is more likely to be pathologic. Diseases may include *Williams syndrome, congenital rubella syndrome,* and *Alagille syndrome.*

PHYSIOLOGIC BASIS FOR SOME PATHOLOGIC HEART MURMURS

Change in Pulmonary Vascular Resistance

Heart murmurs that are dependent on a postnatal drop in pulmonary vascular resistance, allowing turbulent flow from the high-pressure systemic circuit to the lower-pressure pulmonary circuit, are not audible until such a drop has occurred. Therefore, except in premature infants, murmurs of a *ventricular septal defect* or *patent ductus arteriosus* are not expected in the first few days of life and usually become audible after a week to 10 days.

Obstructive Lesions

Obstructive lesions, such as *pulmonic and aortic stenosis,* are caused by normal blood flow through two small valves and, therefore, are not dependent on a drop in pulmonary vascular resistance and are audible at birth.

Pressure Gradient Differences

Murmurs of *atrioventricular valve regurgitation* are audible at birth because of the high pressure gradient between the ventricle and its atrium.

Changes Associated With Growth of Children

Some murmurs do not follow the rules above, but are audible due to alterations in normal blood flow and occur or change with growth. For example, even though it is an obstructive defect, *aortic stenosis* may not be audible until considerable growth has occurred and, indeed, is frequently not heard until adulthood, although a congenitally abnormal valve is responsible. Similarly, the pulmonary flow murmur of an *atrial septal defect* may not be heard for a year or more because right ventricular compliance gradually increases and the shunt becomes larger, eventually producing a murmur caused by too much blood flow across a normal pulmonic valve.

A newborn with a heart murmur and central cyanosis likely has congenital heart disease and requires urgent cardiac evaluation.

When you detect any murmur in children, note all of the qualities as described in Chapter 8, The Cardiovascular System, to help you distinguish *pathologic murmurs* from the benign murmurs just described. Heart murmurs that reflect underlying structural heart disease are easier to evaluate if you have a good knowledge of intrathoracic anatomy and the functional cardiac changes following birth and if you understand the physiologic basis for heart murmurs. Understanding these physiologic changes can help you to distinguish pathologic murmurs from benign heart murmurs in children.

Characteristics of specific pathologic heart murmurs in children are described in Table 18-15 on pp. 809–810.

THE BREASTS

The breasts of the newborn in both males and females are often enlarged from maternal estrogen effect; this may last several months. The breasts may also be engorged with a white liquid, sometimes colloquially called "witch's milk," which may last 1 or 2 weeks.

In *premature thelarche,* breast development occurs, most often between 6 months and 2 years. Other signs of puberty or hormonal abnormalities are not present.

THE ABDOMEN

Inspect the abdomen with the infant lying supine, optimally while asleep. The infant's abdomen is protuberant from poorly developed abdominal musculature. You will easily notice abdominal wall blood vessels and intestinal peristalsis.

Inspect the newborn's *umbilical cord* to detect abnormalities. Normally, there are two thick-walled umbilical arteries and one larger but thin-walled umbilical vein, which is usually located at the 12-o'clock position.

A *single umbilical artery* may be associated with congenital anomalies but also occurs in normal infants as an isolated anomaly.

The umbilicus in the newborn may have a long cutaneous portion (*umbilicus cutis*), which is covered with skin, or an amniotic portion (*umbilicus amnioticus*), which is covered by a firm gelatinous substance. The amniotic portion dries up and falls off within 2 weeks, whereas the cutaneous portion retracts to be flush with the abdominal wall.

An *umbilical granuloma* at the base of the navel is the development of pink granulation tissue formed during the healing process.

Inspect the area around the umbilicus for redness or swelling. *Umbilical hernias* are detectable at a few weeks of age.

Umbilical hernias in infants are caused by a defect in the abdominal wall, and can be up to 6 cm in diameter and quite protuberant when intra-abdominal pressure is increased. Most disappear by 1 year, nearly all by 5 years.

A *diastasis recti* may be noted in normal infants. This involves separation of the two rectus abdominis muscles, causing a midline ridge, most apparent on contraction of the abdominal muscles. A benign condition in most cases, it resolves during early childhood. Chronic abdominal distention may also predispose to this condition.

Auscultation of a quiet infant's abdomen is easy. Don't be surprised if you hear an orchestra of musical tinkling bowel sounds every 10 to 30 seconds.

An increase in pitch or frequency of bowel sounds is heard with *gastroenteritis* or, rarely, with *intestinal obstruction*.

A palpable liver without hepatomegaly (i.e., normal span) can be normal or may result from lung pathology, producing downward displacement of the right hemidiaphragm.

■ *Expected Liver Span of Infants*		
	Mean Estimated Liver Span (cm)	
Age	*Males*	*Females*
6 mos	2.4	2.8
12 mos	2.8	3.1

You can *percuss* an infant's abdomen as you would an adult's, but be prepared to note greater tympanic sounds because of the infant's propensity to swallow air. Percussion is useful for determining the size of organs and abdominal masses.

A silent, tympanic, distended abdomen suggests *peritonitis.*

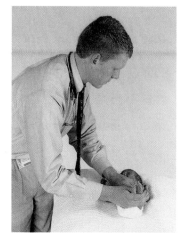

You will find it easy to *palpate* an infant's abdomen because he likes being touched. A useful technique to relax the infant, shown here, is to hold the legs flexed at the knees and hips with one hand and palpate the abdomen with the other. You may also want to use a pacifier or bottle to quiet the infant in this position.

Start gently palpating the liver of infants low in the abdomen, moving upward with your fingers. This technique helps you avoid missing an extremely enlarged liver that extends down into the pelvis. With a careful examination, you can feel the liver edge in most infants, 1 to 2 cm below the right costal margin.

An enlarged, tender liver may be due to *congestive heart failure* or to *storage diseases.* Among newborns, causes of hepatomegaly include hepatitis, storage diseases, vascular congestion, and biliary obstruction.

The *spleen,* like the liver, is felt easily in most children. It too is soft with a sharp edge, and it projects downward like a tongue from under the left costal margin. The spleen is moveable and rarely extends more than 1 cm to 2 cm below the costal margin.

Splenomegaly can be caused by several diseases, including *infections, hematologic disorders* such as *hemolytic anemias, infiltrative disorders,* and *inflammatory* or *autoimmune diseases,* as well as congestion from *portal hypertension.*

Palpate the *other abdominal structures.* You will commonly note pulsations in the epigastrium caused by the aorta. This is felt most easily to the left of the midline, on deep palpation.

Similarly, you can usually palpate the spleen tip. In fact, you may be able to palpate the kidneys of infants by carefully placing the fingers of one hand in front of and those of the other behind each kidney. The descending colon is a sausage-like mass in the left lower quadrant.

Abnormal abdominal masses in infants can be associated with the kidney (e.g., *hydronephrosis*), bladder (e.g., *urethral obstruction*), bowel (e.g., *Hirschsprung's disease,* or *intussusception*), and tumors.

Once you have identified the normal structures in the infant's abdomen, use palpation to identify abnormal masses.

In *pyloric stenosis,* deep palpation in the right upper quadrant or midline can reveal an "olive," or a 2-cm firm pyloric mass. While feeding, some infants with this condition will have visible peristaltic waves pass across their abdomen, followed by projectile vomiting.

MALE GENITALIA

Inspect the male genitalia with the infant in the supine position, noting the appearance of the penis, testes, and scrotum. The *foreskin* completely covers the glans penis. It is nonretractable at birth, though you may be able to retract it enough to visualize the external urethral meatus. Retraction of the foreskin in the uncircumcised male occurs months to years later. The rate of circumcision has declined recently in North America and varies worldwide, depending on cultural practices.

Inspect the shaft of the penis, noting any abnormalities on the ventral surface. Make sure the penis appears straight.

Scrotal edema may be present for several days following delivery because of the effect of maternal estrogens.

Inspect the scrotum, noting rugae, which should be present by 40 weeks' gestation. Palpate the testes in the scrotal sacs, proceeding downward from the external inguinal ring to the scrotum. If you feel a testis up in the inguinal canal, gently milk it downward into the scrotum. The newborn's testes should be about 10 mm in width and 15 mm in length and should lie in the scrotal sacs most of the time.

In 3% of neonates, one or both testes cannot be felt in the scrotum or inguinal canal. This raises concern of *cryptorchidism*. In two thirds of these cases, both testes are descended by 1 year of age.

Examine the testes for swelling within the scrotal sac and over the inguinal ring. If you detect swelling in the scrotal sac, try to differentiate it from the testis. Note whether the size changes when the infant increases abdominal pressure by crying. See if your fingers can get above the mass, trapping it in the scrotal sac. Apply gentle pressure to try to reduce the size of the mass and note any tenderness. Note whether it transilluminates.

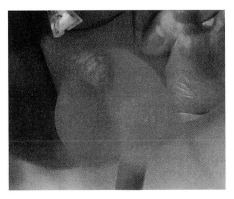

From Fletcher M. Physical Diagnosis in Neonatology. Philadelphia, Lippincott-Raven, 1998.

A *hypospadias* is present when the urethral orifice appears at some point along the ventral surface of the glans or shaft of the penis (see Table 18-18, The Male Genitourinary System, p. 813). The foreskin is incompletely formed ventrally.

A fixed, downward bowing of the penis is a *chordee;* this may accompany a hypospadias.

In newborns with an *undescended testicle* (*cryptorchidism*), the scrotum often appears underdeveloped and tight, and palpation reveals an absence of scrotal contents (see Table 18-18, The Male Genitourinary System, p. 813).

Two common scrotal masses in newborns are *hydroceles* and *inguinal hernias;* frequently both coexist, and both are more common on the right side. Hydroceles overlie the testes and the spermatic cord, are not reducible, and can be transilluminated (see photo at left). Most resolve by 18 months. Hernias are separate from the testes, are usually reducible, and often do not transilluminate. They do not resolve. Sometimes a thickened spermatic cord is noted (called the *silk sign*).

FEMALE GENITALIA

Every health care provider should be familiar with the anatomy of a normal female. It is difficult to identify an abnormality unless you know what normal is. The challenge is to determine the actual anatomy of the female infant's genitalia. Therefore, anatomical structures are depicted on the next page on both a figure of newborn female genitalia and a close-up photograph.

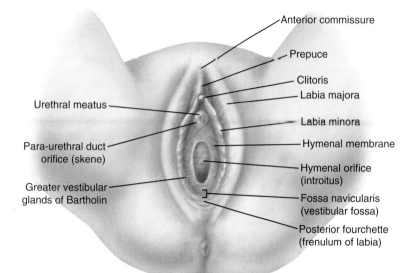

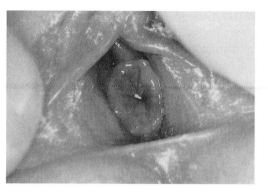

In the newborn female, the genitalia will be prominent from the effects of maternal estrogen. The labia majora and minora have a dull pink color in light-skinned infants and may be hyperpigmented in dark-skinned infants. During the first few weeks of life, there is often a milky white discharge that may be blood tinged. This estrogenized appearance of the genitalia decreases during the first year of life.

Ambiguous genitalia, involving masculinization of the female external genitalia, is a rare condition caused by endocrine disorders such as *congenital adrenal hyperplasia.*

Examine the female genitalia with the infant in the supine position.

Examine the different structures systematically, including the size of the clitoris, the color and size of the labia majora, and any rashes, bruises, or external lesions. Next, separate the labia majora at their midpoint with the thumb of each hand for young infants, or as shown in the diagrams on p. 767 for early and late childhood. Infants will not mind the examination because they are used to having their diapers changed and their bodies washed.

An imperforate hymen may be noted at birth. Labial adhesions are more common, tend to be paper thin, and often disappear without treatment.

Inspect the urethral orifice and the labia minora. Assess the hymen, which in newborns and infants is a thickened, avascular structure with a central orifice, covering the vaginal opening. You should note a vaginal opening, although the hymen will be thickened and redundant. Note any discharge.

RECTAL EXAMINATION

The rectal examination generally is not performed unless there is question of patency of the anus or an abdominal mass. In such cases, flex the infant's hips and fold the legs to the head. Use your lubricated and gloved pinky.

◢ THE MUSCULOSKELETAL SYSTEM

Enormous changes in the musculoskeletal system occur during infancy. Much of the newborn musculoskeletal examination focuses on detection of congenital abnormalities, particularly in the hands, spine, hips, legs, and feet. With a little practice, you will be able to combine the musculoskeletal examination with the neurologic and developmental examination.

The *newborn's hands* are clenched. Because of the palmar grasp reflex (see the discussion on the nervous system), you will need to help the infant extend the fingers. Inspect the fingers carefully, noting any defects.

Palpate along the *clavicle* of the newborn, noting any lumps, tenderness, or crepitus; these may indicate a fracture.

Inspect the *spine* carefully. Although major defects of the spine such as *meningomyelocele* are obvious and often detected by ultrasound before birth, subtle abnormalities may include pigmented spots, hairy patches, or deep pits. These abnormalities, if present within 1 cm or so of the midline, may overlie external openings of sinus tracts that extend to the spinal canal. Do not probe sinus tracts because of the potential risk for infection. Palpate the spine, particularly in the lumbosacral region, noting any deformities of the vertebrae.

Examine the newborn and infant's *hips* carefully at each examination for signs of dislocation.[14] The following photos demonstrate the two major techniques, one to test for the presence of a posteriorly dislocated hip (*Ortolani test*), and the second to test for the ability to sublux or dislocate an intact but unstable hip (*Barlow test*).

Careful inspection can reveal gross deformities such as dwarfism, congenital abnormalities of the extremities or digits, and annular bands that constrict an extremity.

Skin tags, remnants of digits, polydactyly (extra fingers), or *syndactyly* (webbed fingers) are congenital defects noted at birth.

A *fracture of the clavicle* can occur during a difficult delivery.

Spina bifida occulta (a defect of the vertebral bodies) may be associated with defects of the spinal cord, which can cause severe neurologic dysfunction.

A soft audible "click" heard with these maneuvers does not prove a dislocated hip, but should prompt a careful examination.

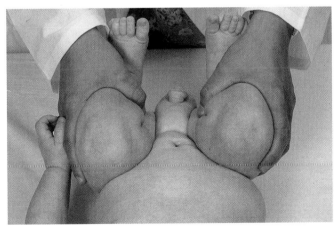

ORTOLANI TEST

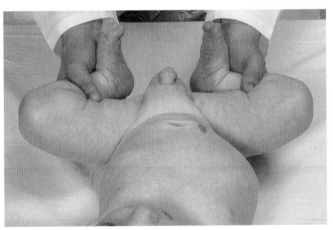

BARLOW TEST

Make sure the baby is relaxed for the next two techniques, using a bottle or pacifier if appropriate. For the *Ortolani test,* place the baby supine with the legs pointing toward you. Flex the legs to form right angles at the hips and knees, placing your index fingers over the greater trochanter of each femur and your thumbs over the lesser trochanters. Abduct both hips simultaneously until the lateral aspect of each knee touches the examining table. A palpable movement of the femoral head back into place constitutes a *positive Ortolani sign.*

With a *hip dysplasia,* you feel a "clunk" as the femoral head, which lies posterior to the acetabulum, enters the acetabulum.

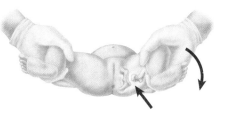

Congenital hip dysplasia is important to detect: Early appropriate treatment has excellent outcomes.

For the *Barlow test,* place your hands in the same position as for the Ortolani test. This time, press in the opposite direction with your thumbs moving down toward the table and outward. Feel for any movement of the head of the femur laterally. Normally there is no movement and the hip feels "stable." If you feel the head of the femur slipping out onto the posterior lip of the acetabulum, this constitutes a *positive Barlow's sign.* If you do feel this dislocation movement, abduct the hip by pressing with your index and middle fingers back inward and feel for the movement of the femoral head as it returns to the hip socket.

A positive Barlow's sign is not diagnostic of a *dysplastic hip,* but it indicates laxity and a dislocatable hip progressively, and the baby needs to be reexamined in the future.

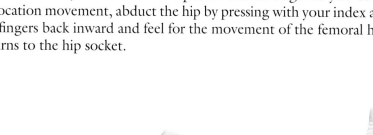
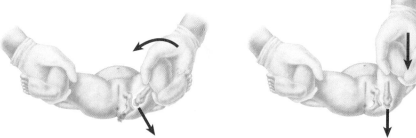

Children older than 3 months may have a negative Ortolani or Barlow sign and still have a *dislocated hip* due to tightening of the hip muscles and ligaments.

In addition to examining the hips, it is important to examine a newborn or infant's *legs and feet* to detect developmental abnormalities. Assess symmetry, bowing, and torsion of the legs. There should be no discrepancy in leg length. It is common for normal infants to have asymmetric thigh skin folds, but if you do detect asymmetry, make sure you perform the instability tests because dislocated hips are commonly associated with this finding.

Most newborns are *bowlegged,* reflecting their curled up intrauterine position.

Another finding after 3 months of age is apparent femoral shortening (*positive Galeazzi* or *Alice test*). The picture below demonstrates this technique. Place the feet together and note any difference in knee heights.

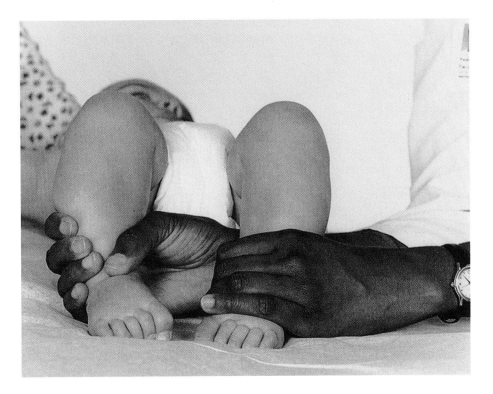

Some normal infants exhibit twisting or *torsion of the tibia* inwardly or outwardly on its longitudinal axis. Parents may be concerned about a toeing in or toeing out of the foot and an awkward gait, all of which are usually normal. Tibial torsion corrects itself during the second year of life after months of weight bearing.

Pathologic tibial torsion occurs only in association with *deformities of the feet or hips.*

Now examine the feet of newborns and infants. At birth, the feet may appear deformed from retaining their intrauterine positioning, often turned inward as shown on the following page. Manipulate the affected foot—a normal foot should be easy to correct to the neutral and even to an overcorrected position. Also, you can scratch or stroke along the outer edge to see if the foot assumes a normal position.

True *deformities of the feet* do not return to the neutral position even with manipulation.

The normal newborn's foot has several benign features that may initially concern you. The newborn's foot appears flat because of a plantar fat pad. There is often inversion of the foot, elevating the medial margin. Other babies will have adduction of the forefoot without inversion, called *metatarsus adductus.* Still others will have adduction of the entire foot. Finally, most toddlers have some pronation during early stages of weight bearing, with eversion of the foot. In all of these normal variants, the abnormal position can be easily overcorrected past midline. They all tend to resolve within 1 or 2 years.

The most common severe congenital foot deformity is talipes equinovarus (talipes calcaneovalgus), or *clubfoot.*

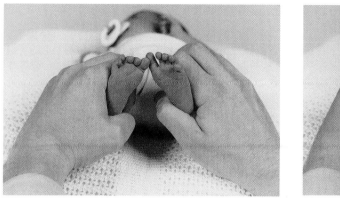 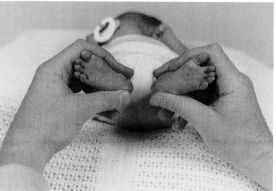

THE NERVOUS SYSTEM

The examination of the nervous system in infants includes techniques that are highly specific to this particular age. Testing primitive reflexes is important in infants; they are only present at certain ages, and then disappear. Absent reflexes or retention of these reflexes may signify abnormalities.

Although many neurologic abnormalities in adults produce asymmetric localized findings, neurologic abnormalities in infants often present as developmental abnormalities such as failure to do age-appropriate tasks. Therefore, the neurologic and developmental examinations need to proceed hand in hand. Finding a developmental abnormality should prompt you to pay particular attention to the neurologic examination.

The neurologic screening examination of all newborns should include assessment of mental status, gross and fine motor function, tone, cry, deep tendon reflexes, and primitive reflexes. More detailed examination of cranial nerve function, sensory function, and less common primitive reflexes are indicated if you suspect any abnormalities from the history or screening.[15] The neurologic examination can reveal extensive disease but will not pinpoint specific functional deficits or minute lesions.

Assess the *mental status* of newborns by observing many of the newborn activities discussed on pp. 690–692 ("What newborns can do"). Make sure you test the newborn during alert periods and, if possible, return at a later time if the baby is transiently too drowsy.

Assess the *motor tone* of newborns and infants, first by carefully watching their position at rest and testing their resistance to passive movement.

Signs of severe neurologic disease include *extreme irritability; persistent asymmetry of posture; persistent extension of extremities; constant turning of head to one side; marked extension of head, neck,* and *extremities (opisthotonus); severe flaccidity;* and *limited response to pain.*

Persistent irritability in the newborn may be a sign of *neurologic insult,* or may reflect a variety of *metabolic, infectious,* or other *constitutional abnormalities,* or environmental conditions such as *drug withdrawal.*

Then assess *tone* as you move each major joint through its range of motion, noting any spasticity or flaccidity. Hold the baby in your hands, as shown below, to determine whether the tone is normal, increased, or decreased. Either increased or decreased tone may indicate intracranial disease, although such disease is usually accompanied by a number of other signs.

You can only test for *sensory function* of the newborn in a limited way. Test for pain sensation by flicking the infant's palm or sole with your finger. Observe for withdrawal, arousal, and change in facial expression. Do not use a pin to test for pain.

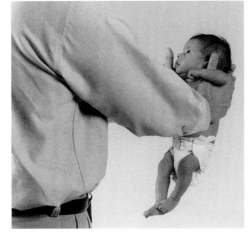

The *cranial nerves* of the newborn or infant can be tested, although you will have to open your bag of tricks for special methods that differ from those used for the older child or adult. The table on the next page provides some useful strategies.

The *deep tendon reflexes* are variable in newborns and infants because the corticospinal pathways are not fully developed. Thus, their exaggerated presence or their absence has little diagnostic significance unless this response is different from results of previous testing, or extreme responses are observed.

Newborns with *hypotonia* often lie in a frog-leg position, with arms flexed and hands near the ears. Hypotonia can be caused by a variety of *central nervous system abnormalities* and *disorders of the motor unit.*

If changes in facial expression or cry follow a painful stimulus but no withdrawal occurs, *paralysis* may be present.

A progressive increase in deep tendon reflexes during the first year of life may indicate central nervous system disease such as *cerebral palsy*, especially if it is coupled with increased tone.

■ *Strategies to Assess Cranial Nerves in Newborns and Infants*

Cranial Nerve		Strategy
I	Olfactory	Difficult to test
II	Visual acuity	Have baby regard your face and look for facial response and tracking.
II, III	Response to light	Darken room, raise baby to sitting position to open eyes. Use light and test for *optic blink reflex* (blinking in response to light). Use the otoscope (without a speculum) to assess papillary responses.
III, IV, VI	Extraocular movements	Observe tracking as the baby regards your smiling face move side to side. Use light if needed.
V	Motor	Test rooting reflex. Test sucking reflex (watch baby suck breast, bottle, or possibly pacifier).
VII	Facial	Observe baby crying and smiling, note symmetry of face and forehead.
VIII	Acoustic	Test acoustic blink reflex (blinking of both eyes in response to loud noise). Observe tracking in response to sound.
IX, X	Swallow	Observe coordination during swallowing.
	Gag	Test for gag reflex.
XI	Spinal accessory	Observe symmetry of shoulders.
XII	Hypoglossal	Observe coordination of swallowing, sucking, and tongue thrusting. Pinch nostrils, observe reflex opening of mouth with tip of tongue to midline.

Abnormalities in the cranial nerves suggest an intracranial lesion such as hemorrhage or congenital malformation.

Use the same techniques to elicit deep tendon reflexes as you would for an adult. You can substitute your index or middle finger for the neurologic hammer, as shown below.

As in adults, asymmetric reflexes suggest a lesion of the peripheral nerves or spinal segment.

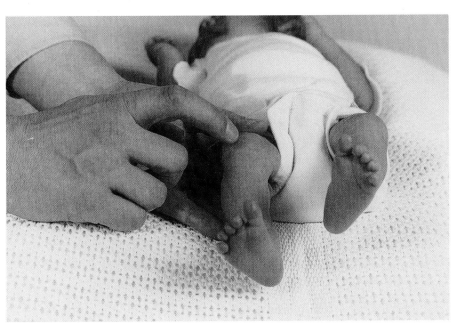

The triceps, brachioradialis, and abdominal reflexes are difficult to elicit before 6 months of age. The *anal reflex* is present at birth and important to elicit if a spinal cord lesion is suspected.

An absent anal reflex suggests loss of innervation of the external sphincter muscle caused by a spinal cord abnormality such as a congenital anomaly (e.g., *spina bifida*), *tumor*, or *injury*.

Although a normal flexion plantar response is obtained in 90% of infants, a *positive Babinski response* to plantar stimulation (dorsiflexion of big toe and fanning of other toes) can be elicited in some normal babies until 2 years of age.

You can try to elicit the ankle reflex as for adults by tapping on the Achilles tendon but often will not get a response. Another method shown on the next page is to grasp the infant's malleolus with one hand and abruptly dorsiflex the ankle. Don't be surprised if you note rapid, rhythmic plantar flexion of the newborn's foot (*ankle clonus*) in response to this maneuver. Up to 10 beats are normal in newborns and young infants; this is *unsustained ankle clonus*.

When the contractions are continuous (*sustained ankle clonus*), *central nervous system disease* should be suspected.

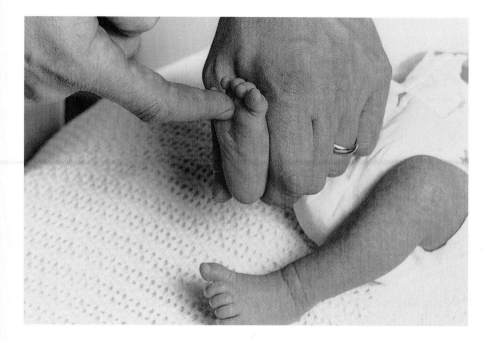

The newborn and infant's developing central nervous system can be evaluated by assessing *infantile automatisms,* called *primitive reflexes.* These develop during gestation, are generally demonstrable at birth, and disappear at defined ages. Abnormalities in these primitive reflexes suggest neurologic disease and merit more intensive investigation. The most important primitive reflexes are illustrated on the next page.

Additional primitive reflexes shown on p. 736 are not usually used in the general examination but helpful in a more extensive evaluation of an infant with abnormal neurologic findings.

Refer to the developmental milestones on pages 674 to 675 and to the DDST on pages 795 to 796 to learn which age-specific developmental tasks to evaluate. By observation and play with the infant, you can do both a developmental screening examination and an assessment for gross and fine motor achievement. Specifically, look for *weakness* by observing sitting, standing, and transitions. Note *station,* or the posture of sitting or standing. Carefully observe the *gait* of the toddler, including balance and fluidity of movements. Fine motor development can be assessed in a similar way, combining the neurologic and developmental exam. Again, refer to the milestones on pages 674 to 675. Key milestones include the development of the pincer grasp, ability to manipulate objects with the hands, and more precise tasks, such as building a tower of cubes or scribbling, as fine motor development progresses in a proximal to distal direction.

Cognitive and social–emotional development should also be assessed as you proceed with the comprehensive neurologic and developmental examination. Some neurologic abnormalities produce deficits or slowing in cognitive and social development. As stated, infants who have developmental

A *neurologic* or *developmental abnormality* is suspected if primitive reflexes are
- Absent at appropriate age
- Present longer than normal
- Asymmetric
- Associated with posturing or twitching

■ Primitive Reflexes That Should Be Part of the Routine Neurologic Examination of Infants

Primitive Reflex		Maneuver	Ages	
Palmar Grasp Reflex		Place your fingers into the baby's hands and press against the palmar surfaces. The baby will flex all fingers to grasp your fingers.	Birth to 3–4 mos	Persistence beyond 4 mos suggests cerebral dysfunction. Persistence of clenched hand beyond 2 mos suggests central nervous system damage, especially if fingers overlap thumb.
Plantar Grasp Reflex		Touch the sole at the base of the toes. The toes curl.	Birth to 6–8 mos	Persistence beyond 8 mos suggests cerebral dysfunction.
Moro Reflex (Startle Reflex)		Hold the baby supine, supporting the head, back, and legs. Abruptly lower the entire body about 2 feet. The arms abduct and extend, hands open, and legs flex. Baby may cry.	Birth to 4 mos	Persistence beyond 4 mos suggests neurologic disease; beyond 6 mos strongly suggests it. Asymmetric response suggests fracture of clavicle or humerus or brachial plexus injury.
Asymmetric Tonic Neck Reflex		With baby supine, turn head to one side, holding jaw over shoulder. The arms/legs on side to which head is turned extend while the opposite arm/leg flex. Repeat on other side.	Birth to 2 mos	Persistence beyond 2 mos suggests neurologic disease.
Positive Support Reflex		Hold the baby around the trunk and lower until the feet touch a flat surface. The hips, knees, and ankles extend, the baby stands up, partially bearing weight, sags after 20–30 seconds.	Birth or 2 mos until 6 mos	Lack of reflex suggests hypotonia or flaccidity. Fixed extension and adduction of legs (scissoring) suggests spasticity due to neurologic disease.

■ **Additional Primitive Reflexes That Should Be Tested If Neurologic Abnormality Is Suspected**

Primitive Reflex	Maneuver	Ages	
Rooting Reflex	Stroke the perioral skin at the corners of the mouth. The mouth will open and baby will turn the head toward the stimulated side and suck.	Birth to 3–4 mos	Absence of rooting indicates severe generalized or central nervous system disease.
Trunk Incurvation (Galant's) Reflex	Support the baby prone with one hand, and stroke one side of the back 1 cm from midline, from shoulder to buttocks. The spine will curve toward the stimulated side.	Birth to 2 mos	Absence suggests a transverse spinal cord lesion or injury. Persistence may indicate delayed development.
Placing and Stepping Reflexes	Hold baby upright from behind as in positive support reflex. Have one sole touch the tabletop. The hip and knee of that foot will flex and the other foot will step forward. Alternate stepping will occur.	Birth (best after 4 days). Variable age to disappear	Absence of placing may indicate paralysis. Babies born by breech delivery may not have placing reflex.
Landau Reflex	Suspend the baby prone with one hand. The head will lift up, and the spine will straighten.	Birth to 6 mos	Persistence may indicate delayed development.
Parachute Reflex	Suspend the baby prone and slowly lower the head toward a surface. The arms and legs will extend in a protective fashion.	4–6 mos and does not disappear	Delay in appearance may predict future delays in voluntary motor development.

delay may have abnormal findings on the neurologic examination because much of the examination is based on age-specific norms.

A normative measure of development is the developmental quotient, which is shown here:

$$\text{Developmental quotient} = \frac{\text{Developmental age}}{\text{Chronologic age}} \times 100$$

The development of an infant or child can be assessed using standard scales such as the DDST for each type of development. For example, you can assign to a child a gross motor developmental quotient, a fine motor developmental quotient, a cognitive developmental quotient, and so forth.

DEVELOPMENTAL QUOTIENTS

>85	Normal
70–85	Possibly delayed; follow-up needed
<70	Delayed

CASE EXAMPLES OF GROSS AND FINE MOTOR DEVELOPMENT

Gross Motor Development

A 12-month-old child who is just pulling to stand (gross motor developmental age of 9 mos), cruising (10 mos), and walking when both hands are held (10 mos) has a gross motor developmental age of 10 months. This child's gross motor developmental quotient is:

$$\left(\tfrac{10}{12} \times 100\right) = 83$$

This child is in the gray zone, is likely to do well without intervention, but requires close follow-up.

Fine Motor Development

A 12-month-old child can transfer objects from hand to hand (a fine motor developmental age of 6 mos), rake objects into his palm (7 mos), and pull things (7 mos). He cannot hold blocks in each hand and does not have thumb and finger grasp (8–9 mos).

He has normal primitive reflexes (most absent), increased tone, scissoring of legs when held, spasticity, and delays on the gross motor part of the DDST.

This child's fine motor developmental quotient is:

$$\left(\tfrac{7}{12} \times 100\right) = 58$$

This child is delayed in fine motor development and has signs of *cerebral palsy.*

APPROACH TO EXAMINATION OF CHILDREN

> *All kids are gifted; some just open their packages earlier than others.*
> —*Michael Carr*

An important and unique aspect of examining children is that parents are usually watching and taking part in the interaction, providing you the opportunity to observe the parent–child interaction. Note whether the child displays age-appropriate behaviors. Assess the "goodness of fit" between parents and child. Although some abnormal interactions may be from the unnatural setting of the examination room, others may be the result of interactional problems. Careful *observation* of the child's interactions with parents and the child's unstructured play in the examination room can reveal *abnormalities in physical, cognitive, and social development.*

Normal toddlers are occasionally terrified, more commonly angry at the examiner, and often completely uncooperative. Most eventually warm up. If this behavior continues and is not developmentally appropriate (e.g., stranger anxiety of the infant or shyness of the early adolescent), there may be an *underlying behavioral* or *developmental abnormality.*

SOME TIPS FOR EXAMINING YOUNG CHILDREN (1–4-YEAR-OLDS)

Useful Strategies for Examination	*Useful Toys and Aids*
Examine a child sitting on parent's lap. Try to be at the child's eye level.	"Blow out" the otoscope light.
First examine the child's toy or teddy bear, then the child.	"Beep" the stethoscope on your nose.
Let the child do some of the exam (e.g., move the stethoscope). Then go back and "get the places we missed."	Make tongue-depressor puppets.
Ask the toddler who keeps pushing you away to "hold your hand." Then have the toddler "help you" with the exam.	Use the child's own toys for play.
Some toddlers believe that if they can't see you, then you aren't there. Perform the exam while the child stands on the parent's lap, facing the parent.	Jingle your keys to test for hearing.
If 2-year-olds are holding something in each hand (such as tongue depressors), they can't fight or resist!	Shine the otoscope through the tip of your finger, "lighting it up," and then examine the child's ears with it.

THE "POWER OF OBSERVATION": ABNORMALITIES THAT CAN BE DETECTED WHILE OBSERVING PLAY

Behavioral Problems*

Poor parent–child interactions
Sibling rivalry
Inappropriate parental discipline
"Difficult temperament"

Developmental Delay (see DDST)

Gross motor delay
Fine motor delay
Language delay (expressive, receptive)
Delay in social or emotional tasks

Social or Environmental Problems

Parental problem, e.g., stress, depression
Risk for abuse or neglect

Neurologic Problems

Weakness
Abnormal posture
Spasticity
Clumsiness
Attentional problems and hyper-activity
Autistic features
Musculoskeletal abnormalities
    Foot deformities
    Gait problems

Specific Systems

The initial paragraphs of each section in this chapter describe components of the examination that can be accomplished by observation alone.

*Note: The child's behavior during the visit may not represent typical behavior, but your observations may serve as a springboard for discussion with parents.

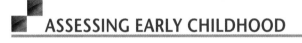

ASSESSING EARLY CHILDHOOD

One of the most difficult challenges facing the clinician examining children in this age group is avoiding a physical struggle, a crying child, or a distraught parent. Accomplishing this successfully is satisfying to all and is one aspect of the "art of medicine" in the practice of pediatrics.

Gaining the child's confidence and allaying the child's fears begin at the start of the encounter. The approach varies with the circumstances of the visit. A health supervision visit for a well child allows greater rapport than a visit when the child is acutely ill.

Letting the child remain dressed during the interview makes her less apprehensive. It also allows you to interact more naturally and observe the child playing, interacting with her parents, and undressing and dressing.

Toddlers who are 9 to 15 months may have *stranger anxiety,* a fear of strangers that is developmentally normal. It signals the infant's growing awareness that the stranger is "new." You should not approach these infants quickly. Make sure they remain solidly in their parent's lap throughout much of the examination.

Engage children in conversation appropriate to their ages, and then ask simple questions about themselves, their illness, or their toys. It is helpful to compliment them about their appearance or behavior, tell a story, or play a simple game or trick to "break the ice." If a child is shy and reticent, turn your attention to the parent to allow the child to warm up to you gradually.

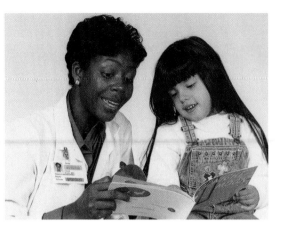

You can observe a lot just by watching.
—*Yogi Berra*

The physical examination, with certain exceptions, does not need to take place on the examining table; it can occur on the floor or with the child sitting on the parent's lap. The key is to engage the child's cooperation. For the few young children who resist undressing, expose only the part of the body being examined. When examining two or more siblings, it is wise to begin with the older one, who is more likely to cooperate and set a good example.

Your approach to the child should be pleasant. Explain each step of the examination as you are performing it. Keep up a running conversation with the parent or the child during the examination to provide distraction.

Plan the order of the examination so that you do the least distressing procedures first and the most distressing (which tend to involve the throat and ears) last. Start with the parts that can be accomplished while the child is sitting—for example, examination of the eyes, palpation of the neck, percussion, and auscultation.

TIPS FOR EXAMINING THE YOUNG CHILD

Let the child see and touch the tools you will be using during the examination.

Use a reassuring voice throughout the examination.

Avoid asking permission to examine a body part because you will do the examination anyway. Instead, ask the child which ear or which part of the body he or she would like you to examine "first."

Examine an apprehensive child in the parent's lap, and let the parent undress the child.

If unable to console the child, complete the examination expediently or give the child a short break.

Make a game out of the examination! For example, "Let's see how big your tongue is!" or "Is Barney in your ear? Let's see!"

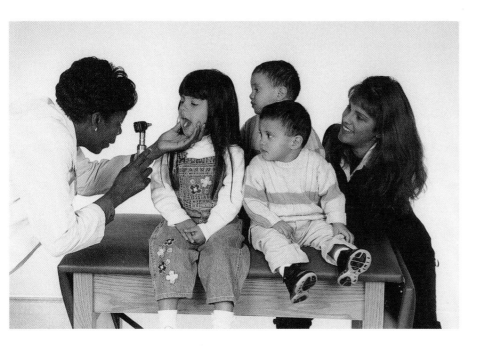

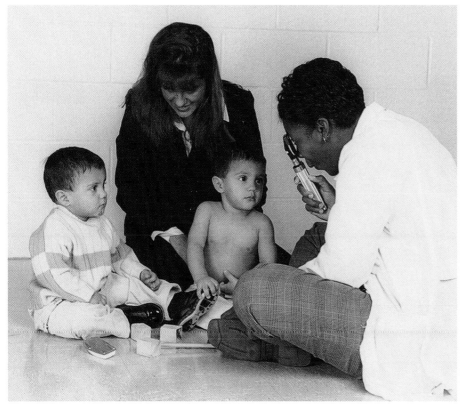

Lying down may make the child feel vulnerable and likely to resist further examination, so make this change with care. Once the child is supine, examine the abdomen first, saving either the throat and ears or genitalia for last.

Remember that the physical examination is designed to gather essential information, and an incomplete examination is frustrating for both you and the parents. Thus, patience, distraction, play, flexibility in the order of the examination, and a caring but firm and gentle approach are all keys to successfully examining the young child.

Usually, resistance to the examination is developmentally appropriate. Many toddlers will strive to stay upright and seek the comfort of their parents. In these cases, avoid conveying frustration and reassure the parents that this behavior is normal. Some parents become embarrassed and scold the child, compounding the problem. Involve the parent in the examination (by removing diapers or palpating the abdomen) and play with the child. If needed, pause to allow the child to recover. Learn which techniques work best for you and which approach you find most comfortable. It is not unusual to require a parent's help to restrain the child for examination of the ears or throat. However, use of formal restraints is not appropriate.

ASSESSING MIDDLE CHILDHOOD

Usually you will find little difficulty in examining children after they reach school age. Although some may have unpleasant memories of previous clinical encounters, most children will respond well when the examiner is attuned to their level of development.

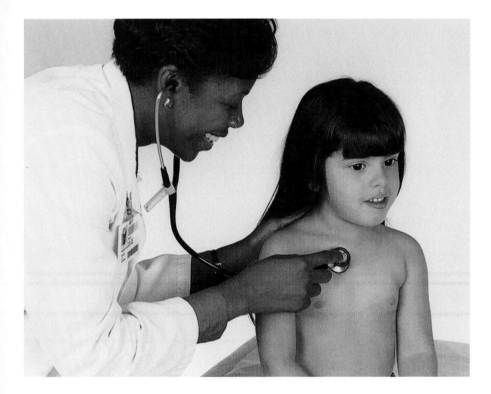

Many children at this age are modest. It is wise to provide gowns and to leave underwear in place until removal is required. It is also helpful to have children disrobe behind a curtain. Consider leaving the room when the children change with parents' help. Some children may prefer that siblings of the opposite sex depart, but most prefer to have a parent of either sex remain in the room, and parents of children younger than 11 years should remain with them.

Children usually are accompanied by a parent or caregiver. Even when alone, they are often seeking health care at the request of their parents—indeed, the parent is usually sitting in the waiting room. When interviewing a child, you need to consider the needs and perspectives of both the child and the caregivers. In addition, the dictates of "well child care" may preset the clinician's agenda toward immunizations, anticipatory guidance, or developmental assessment.

Establishing Rapport. Begin the interview by greeting and establishing rapport with each person present. Refer to the child by name rather than by "him" or "her." Clarify the role or relationship of all of the adults and children. "Now, are you Jimmy's grandmother?" "Please help me by telling me Jimmy's relationship to everyone here." Address the parents as "Mr. Smith" and "Ms. Smith" rather than by their first names or "Mom" or "Dad." When the family structure is not immediately clear, you may avoid embarrassment by asking directly about other members. "Who else lives in the home?" "Who is Jimmy's father?" "Do you live together?" Do not assume that just because parents are separated, only one parent is actively involved in the child's life.

To establish rapport, meet children on their own level. Use your personal experiences with children to guide how you interact in a health care setting. Eye contact on their level (e.g., sit on the floor if needed), participating in playful engagement, and talking about what interests them are always good strategies. Ask children about their clothes, one of their toys, what book or TV show they like, or their adult companion in an enthusiastic but gentle style. Spending time at the beginning of the interview to calm down and connect with an anxious child can put both the child and the caregiver at ease.

Working With Families. One challenge when several people are present is deciding to whom to direct your questions. While eventually you need to get information from both the child and the parent, it is useful to start with the child. Asking simple open-ended questions like "Are you sick? . . . Tell me about it," followed by more specific questions often provides much of the clinical data. The parents can then verify the information, add details that give you the larger context, and identify other issues you need to address. Characterize symptom attributes the same way you do with adults. Sometimes children are embarrassed to begin, but once the parent has started the conversation, you can direct questions back to the child:

> Your mother tells me that you get a lot of stomach aches. Tell me about them.
> Show me where you get the pain. What does it feel like?
> Is it sharp like a pin prick, or does it ache?
> Does it stay in the same spot, or does it move around?
> What helps make it go away?

What makes it worse?

What do you think causes it?

How about missing school a lot?

The presence of family members also provides a rich opportunity to observe how they interact with the child. An older child may be able to sit still or may get restless and start fidgeting. Watch how the parents set limits with the child or fail to set limits when needed.

Multiple Agendas.   Each individual in the room, including the clinician, may have a different idea about the nature of the problem and what needs to be done about it. It is your job to discover as many of these perspectives and agendas as possible. Family members who are not present (the absent parent or grandparent) may also have concerns. It is a good idea to ask about those concerns, too. "If Suzie's father were here today, what questions or concerns would he have?" "Have you, Mrs. Jones, discussed this with your mother or anyone else?" "What does she think?" Mrs. Jones brings Suzie in for abdominal pain because she is worried that Suzie may have an ulcer. She is also worried about Suzie's eating habits. Suzie is not worried about the belly pain—it rarely interferes with what she wants to do. She is uneasy about the changes in her body, especially her belief that she is getting fat. Mr. Jones thinks that Suzie's school work is not getting enough attention. You, as the clinician, need to balance these concerns with what you see as a healthy 12-year-old girl in early puberty with some mild functional abdominal pain. Your goals need to include helping the family to be realistic about the range of "normal" and uncovering the concerns of Mr. and Mrs. Jones and Suzie.

The Family as a Resource.   Much of the information you obtain about a child comes from the family. In general, family members provide most of the care and are your natural allies in promoting the child's health. Being open to a wide range of parenting behaviors helps to make this alliance. Raising a child reflects cultural, socioeconomic, and family practices. It is important to respect the tremendous variation in these practices. A good strategy is to view the parents as experts in the care of their child and yourself as their consultant. This demonstrates respect for the parents' care and minimizes their likelihood of discounting or ignoring your advice. Most parents face many challenges raising children, so practitioners need to be supportive, not judgmental. Comments like, "Why didn't you bring him in sooner?" or "What did you do that for!" do not improve your rapport with the parent. Statements acknowledging the hard work of parenting and praising successes are always appreciated. "Mr. Smith, you are doing such a wonderful job with Bobby. Being a parent takes so much work and Bobby's behavior here today clearly shows your efforts." Or to the child, "Bobby you are so lucky to have such a wonderful Dad."

Hidden Agendas.   Finally, as with adults, the chief complaint may not relate to the real reason the parent has brought the child to see you. The complaint may be a "ticket to care" or bridge to concerns that may not seem quite legitimate as a reason to go to the doctor. Try to create a trusting atmosphere that allows parents to be open about all their concerns. Ask facilitating questions like:

Do you have any other concerns about Randy that you would like to tell me about?

What did you hope I would be able to do for you today?

Was there anything else that you wanted to tell/ask me today?

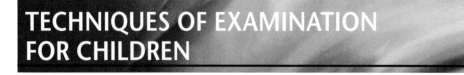

TECHNIQUES OF EXAMINATION FOR CHILDREN

The order of the examination now begins to follow that used for adults. As at any age, examine painful areas last, and forewarn children about areas you are going to examine. If a child resists part of the examination, you can return to it at the end.

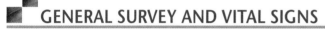

GENERAL SURVEY AND VITAL SIGNS

SOMATIC GROWTH

Height.   For children older than 2 years, measure standing height, optimally using wall-mounted stadiometers. Have the child stand with heels, back, and head against a wall or the back of the stadiometer. If using a wall

Reduced growth in height may indicate *endocrine disease*, other causes of *short stature*, or, if weight is also low, other *chronic diseases*.

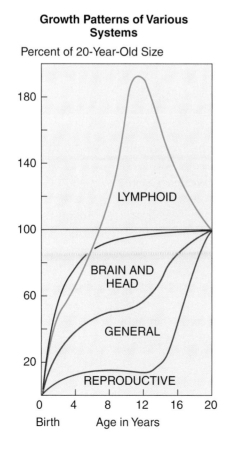

Growth Patterns of Various Systems

Percent of 20-Year-Old Size

with a marked ruler, make sure to place a flat board or surface against the top of the child's head and at right angles to the ruler. Stand-up weight scales with a height attachment are not very accurate.

Rule of thumb on height: After age 2 years, children should grow at least 5 centimeters per year.

Short stature, defined as subnormal height for age, can be a normal variant or from endocrine or other diseases. Normal variants include *familial short stature* and *constitutional delay.* Chronic diseases include *growth hormone deficiency,* other endocrine diseases, *gastrointestinal disease* (e.g., inflammatory bowel disease or celiac disease), *renal* or *metabolic disease,* and *genetic syndromes.*

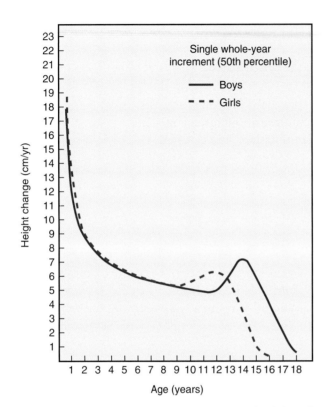

Velocity curves for length and height for boys and girls based on intervals of 1 year. (From Lowrey GH. Growth and development of children, 8th ed. Chicago, Mosby, 1986.)

Weight. Young children who can stand and school-age children should be weighed in their underpants or in a gown on a stand-up scale. Although initially nervous, most young children can be coaxed onto such scales. Use the same scales if possible.

Although failure to thrive often is considered a condition of infancy, young children can have inadequate weight and eventually height if caloric intake for need is insufficient. Common etiologies include *psychosocial, interactional, gastrointestinal, and endocrine disorders.*

Head Circumference. In older children, head size is affected by genetic factors, and it may be useful to measure the head circumference of parents when children have abnormal head sizes.

Body Mass Index for Age. Age-and sex-specific charts are now available to assess BMI in children (see the following table). BMI in children is associated with body fat, related to subsequent health risks for obesity. BMI measurements are helpful for early detection of obesity in children older than 2 years. Obesity is now a major childhood epidemic, and it often begins before 6 to 8 years. Consequences of childhood obesity include hypertension, diabetes, metabolic syndrome, and poor self-esteem. Childhood obesity often leads to adult obesity and shortened lifespan.

Most children with exogenous obesity are also tall for their age. Endocrine causes of childhood obesity tend to involve short stature.

■ Interpreting BMI in Children

Group	BMI-for-Age
Underweight	<5th percentile
At risk of overweight	≥85th percentile
Overweight	≥95th percentile

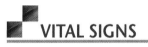

VITAL SIGNS

Blood Pressure. Hypertension during childhood is more common than previously thought, and it is important to recognize, confirm, and appropriately manage it.

Children have elevated blood pressure during exercise, crying, and anxiety. Although young children may be anxious at first, when the procedure is explained and demonstrated beforehand, most children are cooperative. If the blood pressure is initially elevated, you can perform blood pressure readings again at the end of the examination; one trick is to leave the cuff on the arm (deflated) and repeat the reading later. Elevated readings must always be confirmed by subsequent measurements.

The most frequent "cause" of an elevated blood pressure in children is probably an *improperly performed examination,* often due to an incorrect cuff size.

Select the blood pressure cuff as you would in adults. It should be wide enough to cover two thirds of the upper arm or leg. A narrower cuff falsely elevates the blood pressure reading, whereas a wider cuff lowers it and may interfere with proper placement of the stethoscope diaphragm over the artery. *Thus, a proper cuff size is essential for accurate determinations of blood pressure in children.*

In children, as in adults, blood pressure readings from the thigh are approximately 10 mm Hg higher than those from the upper arm. If they are the same or lower, *coarctation of the aorta* should be suspected.

With children, as with adults, the point at which the Korotkoff sounds disappear constitutes the diastolic pressure. At times, especially among chubby young children, the Korotkoff sounds are not easily heard. In such instances, you can use palpation to determine the systolic blood pressure, remembering that the systolic pressure is approximately 10 mm Hg lower by palpation than by auscultation.

A relatively inaccurate means is to use "inspection." Watch for the needle to bounce about 10 mm Hg higher than it does in auscultation. Although this technique is suboptimal, in squirming children it is sometimes all you can get.

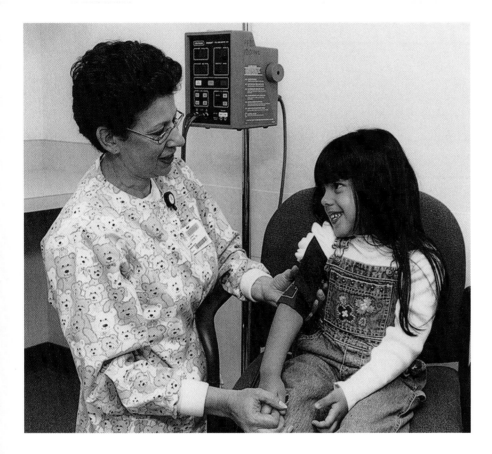

In 1995, the National Heart, Lung, and Blood Institute's National High Blood Pressure Working Group on Hypertension Control in Children and Adolescents defined normal, high-normal, and high blood pressure as follows, with measurements on at least three separate occasions:

Causes of *sustained hypertension* in childhood include renal parenchymal or artery disease, coarctation of the aorta, and primary hypertension

Blood Pressure Category	Average Systolic and/or Diastolic Blood Pressure for Age, Sex, and Height
Normal	<90th percentile
High-normal	90th–95th percentile
High	≥95th percentile

Children who have hypertension should be evaluated extensively to determine the cause. For infants and young children, a specific cause can usually be found. An increasing proportion of older children and adolescents, however, have essential or primary hypertension. In all cases, it is important to repeat measurements to reduce the possibility that the elevation reflects anxiety. Sometimes repeating measurements in school is a way to obtain readings in a more relaxed environment.

It is also important not to *falsely label* a child or adolescent as having hypertension, because of the stigma of labeling, potential limitations to activities, and possible side effects of treatment.

Pulse.   Rates are shown in the table below:

■ Average Heart Rate of Children at Rest

Age	Average Rate	Range (Two Standard Deviations)
1–2 years	110	70–150
2–6 years	103	68–138
6–10 years	95	65–125

Sinus bradycardia is a heart rate <100 beats per minute in children younger than 3 years, and <60 beats per minute in children 3 to 9 years.

> *To measure the man, measure his heart.*
> —*Malcolm Stevenson Forbes*

Respiratory Rate.   The rate of respirations per minute ranges from 20 to 40 during early childhood, and 15 to 25 during late childhood, reaching adult levels at age 15 years.

For young children, observe the movements of the chest wall for two 30-second intervals or over 1 minute, preferably before stimulating them. Direct auscultation of the chest or placing the stethoscope in front of the mouth is also useful for counting respirations, but the measurement may be falsely elevated if the child becomes agitated. For older children, use the same technique as used for adults.

Children with respiratory diseases such as *bronchiolitis* or *pneumonia* have rapid respirations (up to 80–90/min), but *also* increased work of breathing such as grunting, nasal flaring, or use of accessory muscles.

The commonly accepted cutoff for tachypnea in children older than 1 year is a respiratory rate greater than 40 breaths per minute.

The best single physical finding for ruling out *pneumonia* is an absence of tachypnea

Temperature.   In children, auditory canal temperature recordings are preferable because they can be obtained quickly with essentially no discomfort.

Young children with infections can have extremely high fevers (up to 104°F or 40°C). Children younger than 3 years, who appear very ill with a fever, should be evaluated for possible sepsis, urinary tract infection, pneumonia, or other infectious etiology.

THE SKIN

After a child's first year of life, the techniques of examination are the same as those for the adult (see Chap. 5, The Skin, Hair, and Nails.)

THE HEAD

In examining the head and neck, tailor your examination to the child's stage of growth and development.

Even before touching the child, carefully observe the shape of the head, its symmetry, and the presence of abnormal facies. Abnormal facies may not be apparent until later in childhood; therefore, carefully examine the face as well as the head of all children.

There are diagnostic facies in childhood (Table 18-10, pp. 803–804 shows several) that reflect chromosomal abnormalities, endocrine defects, chronic illness, and other disorders.

THE NECK

Beyond infancy, the techniques for examining the neck are the same as for adults.

Lymphadenopathy is usually from viral or bacterial infections (see Table 18-13, Abnormalities of the Neck and Pharynx, p. 807).

Lymphadenopathy is unusual during infancy but very common during childhood. As shown on p. 745, the child's lymphatic system reaches its zenith of growth at 12 years, and cervical or tonsillar lymph nodes reach their peak size between 8 and 16 years. The vast majority of enlarged lymph nodes in children are due to infections (mostly viral but frequently bacterial) and not to malignant disease, even though the latter is a concern for many parents. It is important to differentiate normal lymph nodes from abnormal ones or from congenital cysts of the neck. The figure on page 706 demonstrates the typical anatomical locations of lymph nodes and congenital cysts of the neck.

Malignancy is more likely if the node is greater than 2 cm, is hard or fixed to the skin or underlying tissues (i.e., not mobile), is accompanied by serious systemic signs such as weight loss, and, in the case of cervical lymph nodes, if the chest x-ray findings are abnormal.

In young children with small necks, it may be difficult to differentiate low posterior cervical lymph nodes from *supraclavicular lymph nodes* (which are always abnormal and raise suspicion for malignancy).

Check for *neck mobility*. It is important to ensure that the neck of all children is supple and easily mobile in all directions. This is particularly important when the patient is holding the head in an asymmetric manner, and when central nervous system disease such as meningitis is suspected.

In children, the presence of nuchal rigidity is a more reliable indicator of meningeal irritation than *Brudzinski's sign* or *Kernig's sign*. To detect nuchal rigidity in older children, ask the child to sit with legs extended on the examining table. Normally, children should be able to sit upright and touch their chins to their chests. Younger children can be persuaded to flex their necks by having them follow a small toy or light beam. You also can test for nuchal rigidity with the child lying on the examining table, as shown below. Nearly all children with nuchal rigidity will be extremely sick, irritable, and difficult to examine. In developed countries, incidence of bacterial meningitis has plummeted because of vaccinations.

Nuchal rigidity is marked resistance to movement of the head in any direction. It suggests meningeal irritation due to *meningitis, bleeding, tumor,* or *other causes.* These children are extremely irritable and difficult to console and may have "paradoxical irritability"— increased irritability when being held.

When meningeal irritation is present, the child assumes the *tripod position* and is unable to assume a full upright position to perform the chin-to-chest maneuver.

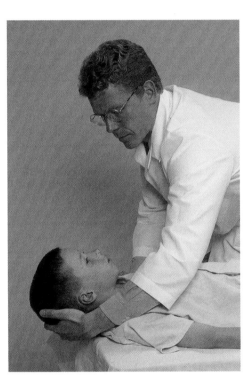

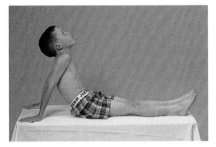

THE EYE

The two most important aspects of the eye examination for young children are to determine whether the gaze is conjugate or symmetric and to test visual acuity in each eye.

Strabismus (see Table 18-11, p. 805) in children requires treatment by an ophthalmologist.

Use the methods described in Chapter 6 for adults to assess *conjugate gaze,* or the *position and alignment of the eyes,* and the function of the extraocular muscles. The corneal light reflex test and the cover–uncover test are particularly useful in young children.

You can perform the cover–uncover test as a game by having the young child watch your nose or tell you if you are smiling or not while you cover one of the child's eyes.

Both *ocular strabismus* and *anisometropia* (eyes with significantly different refractive errors) can result in *amblyopia,* or reduced vision in an otherwise normal eye. *Amblyopia* can lead to a "lazy eye," with permanently reduced visual acuity if not corrected early (generally by 6 years).

It may not be possible to measure the *visual acuity* of children younger than 3 years who cannot identify pictures on an eye chart. For these children, the simplest examination is to assess for fixation preference by alternately covering one eye; the child with normal vision will not object, but a child with poor vision in one eye will object to having the good eye covered. In all tests of visual acuity, it is important that both eyes show the same result.

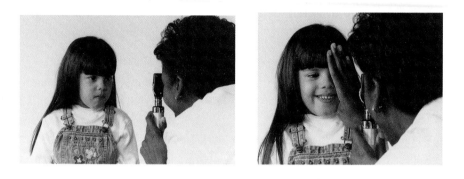

Age	Acuity
3 months	Eyes converge, baby reaches
12 months	~20/200
Less than 4 years	20/40
4 years and older	20/30

Any difference in visual acuity between the eyes (e.g., 20/20 on the left and 20/30 on the right) is abnormal, and the patient should be referred to an ophthalmologist.

As shown on the next page, visual acuity in children 3 years and older can usually be formally tested using an eye chart with one of a variety of optotypes (characters or symbols). A child who does not know letters or numbers reliably can be tested using pictures, symbols, or the "E" chart. Using the "E" chart, most children will cooperate by telling you in which direction the "E" is pointing.

The *visual fields* can be examined in infants and young children with the child sitting on the parent's lap. One eye should be tested at a time with the other eye covered. Hold the child's head in the midline while bringing an object such as a toy into the field of vision from behind the child. The overall method is the same as that for adults, except that you will have to make this into a game for your patient.

The most common visual disorder of childhood is myopia, which can be easily detected using this examination technique.

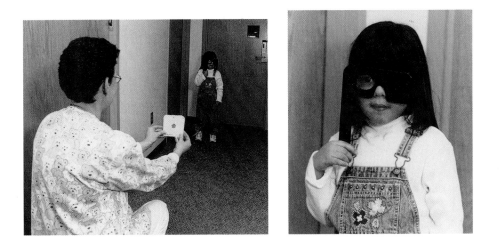

THE EAR

You may feel as if you need 10 hands and a bag of tricks to examine the ears of toddlers and young children, who are sensitive to *examining the ear canal and drum* and fearful because they cannot observe the procedure. With a little practice you can master this technique. Unfortunately, many young children will need to be briefly restrained during this part of the examination, which is why you may want to leave it for the end.

If the child is not too fearful, you may be able to do the examination while the child is sitting on his parent's lap. It is helpful to make a game out of the otoscopic examination, such as finding an imaginary object in the child's ear, or talking playfully throughout the examination to allay any fears. It is sometimes helpful to place the otoscopic speculum gently into the external auditory canal of one ear and then withdraw it to have the child get used to the procedure, before performing the actual examination. Ask the parent for a preference regarding the positioning of the child for the examination.

There are two common positions—the child lying down and restrained, and the child sitting in the parent's lap. If the child is being held supine, have the parent hold the arms either extended or close to the sides to limit motions. You can hold the head and retract the tragus with one hand while you hold the otoscope with your other hand. If the child is on the parent's lap, the child's legs should be between the parent's legs. The parent could help with gentle restraint by placing one arm around the child's body and a second arm to steady the head.

Many students have difficulty even visualizing a child's tympanic membrane. In young children, the external auditory canal is directed upward and backward from the outside, and the auricle must be pulled upward, outward, and backward to afford the best view. Hold the child's head with one hand (your left hand if you are right-handed), and with that same hand pull up on the auricle. With your other hand, position the otoscope.

TIPS FOR CONDUCTING THE OTOSCOPIC EXAMINATION

Use the best angle of the otoscope.
Use the largest possible speculum.
   A larger speculum will allow you to visualize the tympanic membrane better.
   A small speculum may not provide a seal for pneumatic otoscopy.
Don't apply too much pressure.
   Too much pressure will cause the child to cry and may cause false-positive results on pneumatic otoscopy.
Insert the speculum ¼ to ½ inch into the canal.
First find the landmarks.
   Sometimes the ear canal resembles the tympanic membrane—don't be fooled!
Note whether the tympanic membrane is abnormal.
Remove cerumen if it is blocking your view, using
   Special plastic curettes
   A moistened microtipped cotton swab
   Flushing of ears for older children
   Special instruments that can also be purchased.

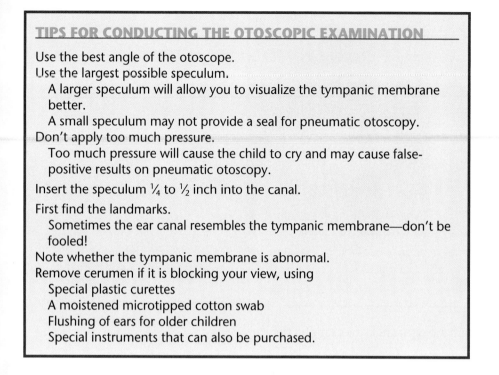

Not only are there two positions for the child lying down or sitting, there are two ways to hold the otoscope, as illustrated by the following photos:

- The first is the method generally used in adults, with the otoscope handle pointing upward or laterally while you pull up on the auricle. Hold the lateral aspect of your hand that has the otoscope against the child's head to provide a buffer against sudden movements by the patient.

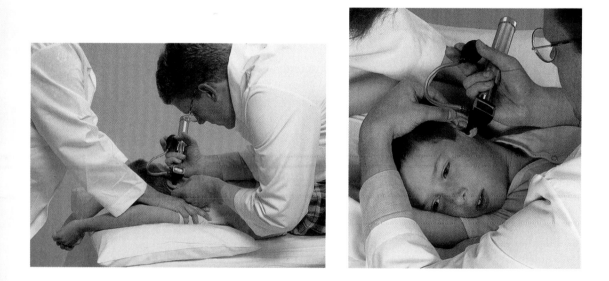

- The second technique is used by many pediatricians because of the different angle of the auditory canal in children. This involves holding the otoscope with the handle pointing down toward the child's feet while you pull up on the auricle. Hold the head and pull up on the auricle with one hand, while you hold the otoscope with the other hand.

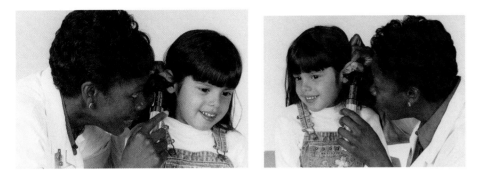

Learn to use a *pneumatic otoscope* to improve your accuracy of diagnosis of otitis media in children. This allows you to assess the mobility of the tympanic membrane as you increase or decrease the pressure in the external auditory canal by squeezing the rubber bulb of the pneumatic otoscope.

First, check the pneumatic otoscope for leaks by placing your finger over the tip of the speculum and squeezing the bulb. Note the pressure on the bulb. Then insert the speculum, obtaining a proper seal; this is critical because failure to obtain a seal can produce a false-positive finding (lack of movement of the tympanic membrane).

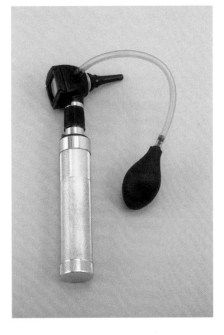

When air is introduced into the normal ear canal, the tympanic membrane and its light reflex move inward. When air is removed, the tympanic membrane moves outward, toward you. This to-and-fro movement of the tympanic membrane has been likened to the luffing of a sail. If the tympanic membrane fails to move perceptibly as you introduce positive or negative pressure, then the child is likely to have a middle ear effusion. A child with acute otitis media may flinch because of pain due to the air pressure.

Gently move and pull on the *pinna* before or during your otoscopic examination. Carefully inspect the area behind the pinna, over the mastoid bone.

Acute otitis media is a common condition of childhood. A symptomatic child has a red, bulging tympanic membrane, with a dull or absent light reflex and diminished movement on pneumatic otoscopy. Purulent material may also be seen behind the tympanic membrane. See Table 18-11, Abnormalities of the Eyes and Ears, p. 805.

This movement of the tympanic membrane is absent in middle ear effusion (*otitis media with effusion*).

Significant, temporary hearing loss for several months can accompany otitis media with effusion.

With *otitis externa* (but not otitis media), movement of the pinna elicits pain.

With acute *mastoiditis,* the auricle may protrude forward, and the area over the mastoid bone will be red, swollen, and tender.

Although formal hearing testing is necessary for accurate detection of hearing deficits in young children, you can grossly *test for hearing* by whispering at a distance of 8 feet, asking the child questions or giving simple commands. All children older than 4 years should have a full-scale acoustic screening test using standardized equipment, as illustrated here.

Younger children who fail these screening maneuvers or who have speech delay should have audiometric testing.

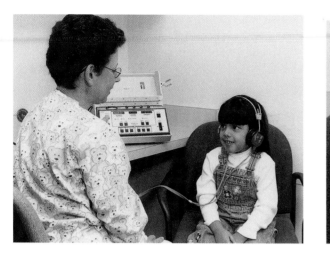
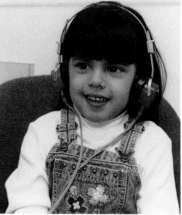

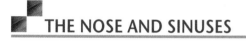

THE NOSE AND SINUSES

You can inspect the anterior portion of the nose by using a large speculum on your otoscope. Inspect the nasal mucous membranes, noting their color and condition. Look for nasal septal deviation and the presence of polyps.

Pale, boggy nasal mucous membranes are found in children with *chronic (perennial) allergic rhinitis.*

Purulent rhinitis is common in viral infections, but may be part of the constellation of symptoms of *sinusitis.*

Foul-smelling purulent, unilateral discharge from the nose may be due to a *foreign body* in the nose. This is particularly common among young preschool children who tend to stick objects into any body orifice.

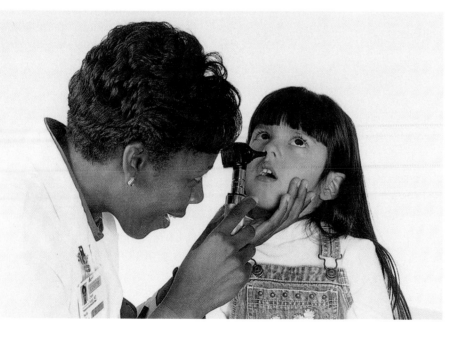

Maxillary sinuses are noted on x-rays by age 4 years, sphenoid sinuses by age 6, and frontal sinuses by age 6 to 7. The sinuses of older children can be palpated as in adults, looking for tenderness. Transillumination of the paranasal sinuses of younger children has poor sensitivity and specificity for diagnosing sinusitis or fluid in the sinuses.

THE MOUTH AND PHARYNX

For anxious or young children, you may want to leave this part of the examination toward the end, because it may require parental restraint. The young, cooperative child may be more comfortable sitting in the parent's lap, as shown below.

The following figure demonstrates some tricks to getting children to open their mouths. The child who can say "ahhh" will usually offer a sufficient (albeit

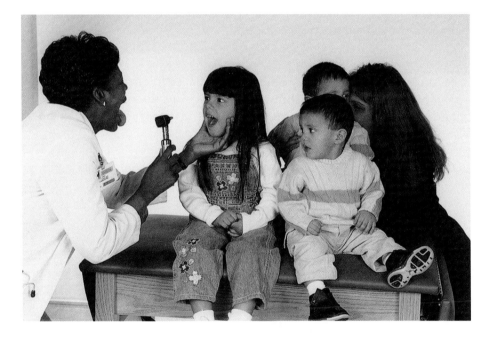

**HOW TO GET CHILDREN TO OPEN THEIR MOUTHS
(AKA, "WOULD YOU *PLEASE* SAY 'AHHH'?")**

- Turn it into a game.
  - "Now let's see what's in your mouth."
  - "Can you stick out your *whole tongue*?"
  - "I bet you can't open your mouth *really wide*!"
  - "Let me see the inside of your teeth."
  - "Is Barney stuck in there?"
- Don't show a tongue blade unless really necessary.
- Demonstrate first on an older sibling (or even the parent).
- Offer enthusiastic praise for opening their mouths a little and encourage them to open even wider!

---

brief) view of the posterior pharynx so that a tongue blade is unnecessary. Healthy children are more likely to cooperate with this examination than sick children, especially if the sick child sees the tongue blade or has had previous experience with throat cultures.

If you need to use the tongue blade, the best technique is to push down and pull slightly forward toward yourself while the child says "ahhh," being careful not to place the blade too far posteriorly, eliciting a gag reflex. Sometimes young and anxious children will need to be restrained and will clamp their teeth and purse their lips. In these cases, you will need to carefully slip the tongue depressor between the teeth and onto the tongue. This will either allow you to push down on the tongue or elicit a gag reflex, which should permit a brief look at the posterior pharynx and tonsils. Remember, an unplanned, direct frontal assault on the front teeth will only meet with failure and a splintered tongue blade; careful planning and parental help are needed.

Examine the *teeth* for the timing and sequence of eruption, number, character, condition, and position. Abnormalities of the enamel may reflect local or general disease.

Carefully inspect the inside of the upper teeth, as shown in the figure below. This is a common location for *nursing-bottle caries*. The technique shown in the photo, called "lift the lip," can facilitate visualization of dental caries.

Dental caries are caused by bacterial activity. Caries are more likely among young children who have prolonged bottle-feeding ("nursing-bottle caries"). See Table 18-12, Abnormalities of the Mouth and Teeth, p. 806, for different stages of caries.

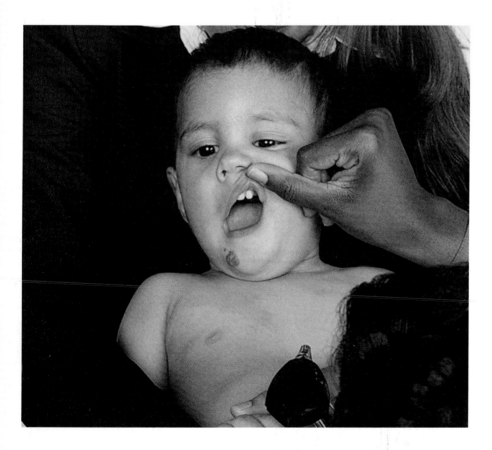

The table below displays a common pattern of teeth eruption. In general, lower teeth erupt a bit earlier than upper teeth.

Staining of the teeth may be intrinsic or extrinsic. Intrinsic stains may be from tetracycline use before 8 years (yellow, gray, or brown stain). Iron preparation (black stain) is an example of extrinsic stain. Extrinsic stains can be polished off; intrinsic stains cannot (see Table 18-12, Abnormalities of the Mouth and Teeth, p. 806).

■ Tooth Types and Age of Eruption

Tooth Type	Approximate Age of Eruption	
	Primary (mos)	Permanent (yrs)
Central incisor	5–8	6–8
Lateral incisor	5–11	7–9
Cuspids	24–30	11–12
First bicuspids	—	10–12
Second bicuspids	—	10–12
First molars	16–20	6–7
Second molars	24–30	11–13
Third molars	—	17–22

Look for abnormalities of the position of the teeth. These include malocclusion, maxillary protrusion (*overbite*), and mandibular protrusion (*underbite*). You can demonstrate the latter two by asking the child to bite down hard and part the lips. Observe the true bite. In normal children, the lower teeth are contained within the arch formed by the upper teeth.

Malocclusion and misalignment of teeth are often from excessive thumb sucking and are reversible if the habit is arrested by 6 or 7 years. Malocclusion can also be a hereditary condition, or from premature loss of primary teeth.

Carefully inspect the *tongue,* including the underside. Most children will happily stick their tongue out at you, move it from side to side, and demonstrate its color (the blue tongue below is from eating candy!).

Common abnormalities include *coated tongue* in viral infections, *congenital geographic tongue,* and *strawberry tongue* found in scarlet fever.

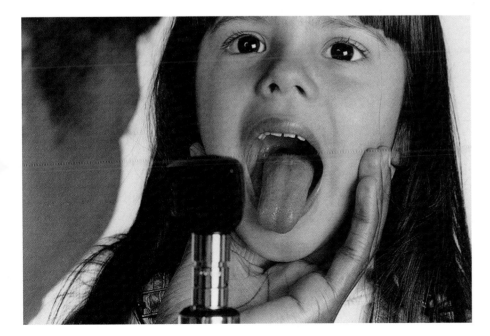

Note the size, position, symmetry, and appearance of the *tonsils*. The peak growth of tonsillar tissue is between 8 and 16 years (see figure on p. 745). The size of the tonsils varies considerably in children and is often categorized on a scale of 1+ to 4+, with 1+ being easy visibility of the gap between the tonsils, and 4+ being tonsils that touch in the midline with the mouth wide open. The tonsils in children often appear more obstructive than they really are.

Streptococcal pharyngitis typically produces a strawberry tongue, white exudates on the tonsils, beefy-red uvula, and palatal petechiae.

Tonsils in children usually have deep crypts on their surfaces, which often have white concretions or food particles protruding from their depths. This does not indicate disease.

A *peritonsillar abscess* is suggested by asymmetric enlargement of the tonsils and lateral displacement of the uvula.

Look for clues of a submucosal cleft palate, such as notching of the posterior margin of the hard palate or a bifid *uvula*. Because the mucosa is intact, the underlying defect is easily missed.

There is one condition—*acute epiglottitis*—now thankfully rare in the United States due to immunization against *Haemophilus influenzae* type B, which is a contraindication to examination of the throat because of potential gagging and laryngeal obstruction.

Note the quality of the child's voice. Certain abnormalities can change the pitch and quality.

■ Voice Changes—Clues to Underlying Abnormalities

Voice Change	Possible Abnormality
Hypernasal speech	Submucosal cleft palate
Nasal voice plus snoring	Adenoidal hypertrophy
Hoarse voice plus cough	Viral infection (croup)
"Rocks in mouth"	Tonsillitis

You may note an abnormal breath odor, which may help lead to a diagnosis.

Halitosis in a young child often is caused by upper respiratory, pharyngeal, or mouth infection; other causes include foreign body in the nose, dental disease, and gastroesophageal reflux.

THE THORAX AND LUNGS

As children become older, the examination of the lungs begins to approach that used in adults. Again, it is critical for children to cooperate with this examination. Auscultation is often best accomplished when the child is barely aware of the examination (as when he is in his parent's lap). If a toddler seems fearful of your stethoscope, you might let the child play with it before touching the chest.

In examining children, assess the relative proportion of time spent on inspiration versus expiration. Normally, this ratio is about 1:1.

If you ask young children to "take deep breaths," they will often hold their breath, making it even more difficult for you to auscultate the lungs. Thus it is easier, for preschool children, to let them breathe normally. For older children, you can demonstrate how to take nice, quiet, deep breaths, and make a game out of it. A forced expiratory maneuver can be accomplished by asking the child to blow out the candles on an imaginary birthday cake.

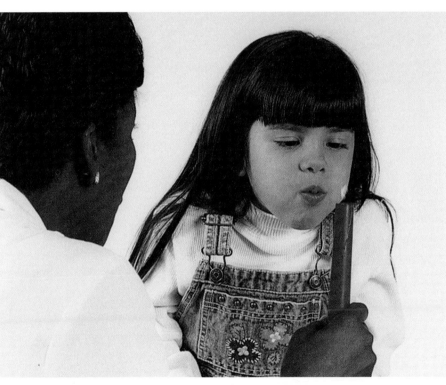

Older children will be cooperative for the respiratory examination and can even go through the maneuvers of assessing fremitus or listening to "E to A" changes (see p. 261). As children grow, the evaluation by observation discussed on the previous page, such as assessing the work of breathing, nasal flaring, and grunting, becomes less helpful in evaluating for respiratory pathology, and palpation, percussion, and auscultation achieve greater importance in a careful examination of the thorax and lungs.

In the presence of upper airway obstruction such as croup, inspiration is prolonged and accompanied by other signs such as stridor, cough, or rhonchi. In the presence of lower airway obstruction such as asthma, expiration is prolonged and often accompanied by audible wheezing.

Pneumonia in young children generally is manifested by fever, tachypnea, and dyspnea.

Childhood asthma is an extremely common condition throughout the world. Children with acute asthma present with varying severity and often have increased work of breathing. Expiratory wheezing and a prolonged expiratory phase, caused by reversible bronchospasm, can be heard without the stethoscope and are apparent on auscultation.

◼ THE HEART

It may be helpful to measure the blood pressure in both arms and one leg at one time around age 3 to 4 years to check for possible *coarctation of the aorta*. Thereafter, only the right arm blood pressure needs to be measured.

Preschool and school-aged children often have benign murmurs. The most common (*Still's murmur*) is a grade I–II/VI, musical, vibratory, early and midsystolic murmur with multiple overtones, located over the mid or lower left sternal border, but also frequently heard over the carotid arteries. Carotid artery compression will usually cause the precordial murmur to disappear. This murmur may be extremely variable and may be accentuated when cardiac output is increased, as occurs with fever or exercise.

◼ *Location and Characteristics of Benign Heart Murmurs in Children*

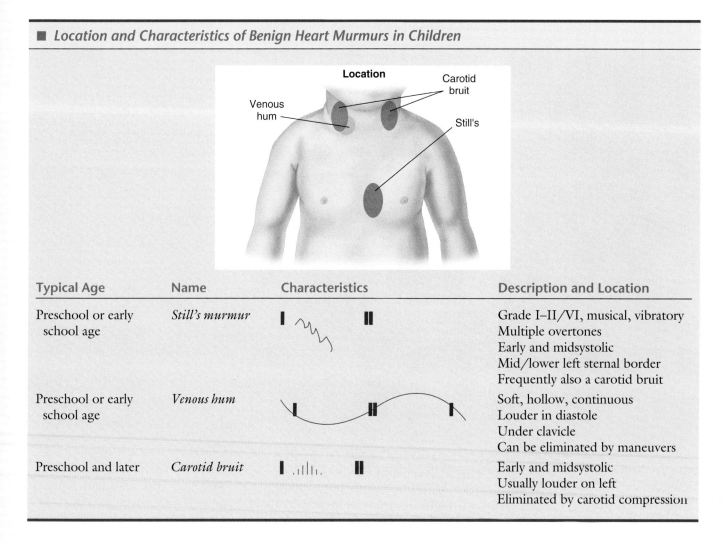

Typical Age	Name	Characteristics	Description and Location
Preschool or early school age	*Still's murmur*		Grade I–II/VI, musical, vibratory Multiple overtones Early and midsystolic Mid/lower left sternal border Frequently also a carotid bruit
Preschool or early school age	*Venous hum*		Soft, hollow, continuous Louder in diastole Under clavicle Can be eliminated by maneuvers
Preschool and later	*Carotid bruit*		Early and midsystolic Usually louder on left Eliminated by carotid compression

The murmur heard in the carotid area or just above the clavicles is known as a *carotid bruit*. It is early and midsystolic, with a slightly harsh quality. It is usually louder on the left and may be heard alone or in combination with the Still's murmur, as noted above. It may be completely eradicated by carotid artery compression.

Also in preschool or school-age children, you may detect a *venous hum*. This is a soft, hollow, continuous sound, louder in diastole, heard just below the right clavicle. It can be completely eliminated by maneuvers that affect venous return, such as lying supine, changing head position, or jugular venous compression. It has the same quality as breath sounds and therefore is frequently overlooked.

Among young children, murmurs without the recognizable features of the three common benign murmurs on the previous page may signify underlying heart disease and should be evaluated thoroughly.

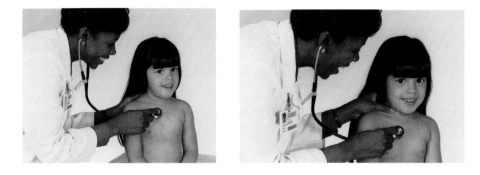

THE ABDOMEN

Toddlers and young children commonly have protuberant abdomens, most apparent when they are upright. The examination can follow the same order as for adults, except that you may need to open your bag of tricks to distract the child during the examination.

An exaggerated "pot-belly appearance" may indicate malabsorption due to *celiac disease, cystic fibrosis,* or *constipation* or *aerophagia.*

Most children are ticklish when you first place your hand on their abdomens for *palpation*. This reaction tends to disappear, particularly if you distract the child with conversation and place your whole hand flush on the abdominal surface for a few moments without probing. For children who are particularly sensitive and who tighten their abdominal muscles, you can start by placing the child's hand under yours as shown in the following photo. Eventually you will be able to remove the child's hand and palpate the abdomen freely.

You can also try flexing the knees and hips to relax the child's abdominal wall. Palpate lightly in all areas, then deeply, leaving a site of potential pathology to the end.

■ *Expected Liver Span of Children by Percussion*

Age in Years	Mean Estimated Liver Span (cm)	
	Males	Females
2	3.5	3.6
3	4.0	4.0
4	4.4	4.3
5	4.8	4.5
6	5.1	4.8
8	5.6	5.1
10	6.1	5.4

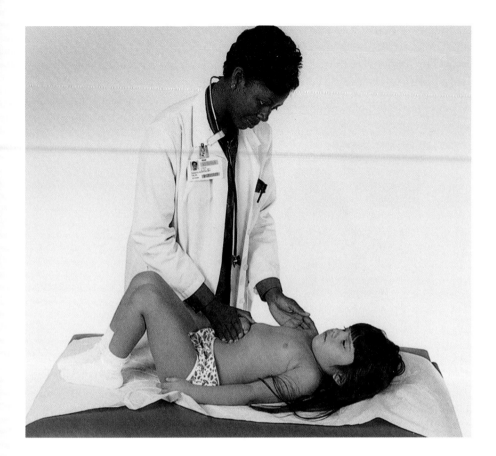

One method to determine the lower border of the liver involves the *scratch test*, shown in the figure below. Place the diaphragm of your stethoscope just above the right costal margin at the midclavicular line. With your fingernail, lightly scratch the skin of the abdomen along the midclavicular line, moving from below the umbilicus toward the costal margin. When your scratching finger reaches the liver's edge, you will hear a change in the scratching sound as it passes through the liver to your stethoscope.

Hepatomegaly in young children is unusual. It can be caused by cystic fibrosis, protein malabsorption, parasites, and tumors.

If hepatomegaly is accompanied by splenomegaly, portal hypertension, storage diseases, chronic infections, and malignancy should be considered.

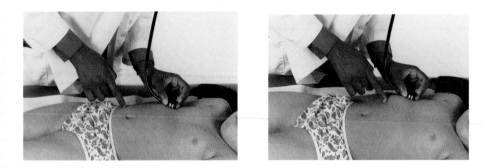

The *spleen*, like the liver, is felt easily in most children. It too is soft with a sharp edge, and it projects downward like a tongue from under the left costal margin. The spleen is moveable and rarely extends more than 1 cm to 2 cm below the costal margin.

Splenomegaly can be caused by a variety of diseases, including *infections, hematologic disorders* such as *hemolytic anemias, infiltra-*

Palpate the *other abdominal structures.* You will commonly note pulsations in the epigastrium caused by the aorta. This is felt most easily to the left of the midline, on deep palpation.

Palpating for abdominal tenderness in an older child is the same as for the adult; however, the causes of abdominal pain are often different, encompassing a wide spectrum of acute and chronic diseases. Localization of tenderness may help you pinpoint the abdominal structures most likely to be causing the abdominal pain.

tive disorders, and *inflammatory* or *autoimmune diseases,* as well as congestion from *portal hypertension.*

In a child with an acute abdomen, as in *acute appendicitis,* special techniques are helpful, such as checking for involuntary rigidity, rebound tenderness, a Rovsing's sign, or a positive psoas or obturator sign (see p. 388).

MALE GENITALIA

Inspect the penis. The size in prepubertal children has little significance unless it is abnormally large. In obese boys, the fat pad over the symphysis pubis may obscure the penis.

There is an art to *palpation* of the young boy's scrotum and testes because many have an extremely active cremasteric reflex that may cause the testis to retract upward into the inguinal canal and thereby appear to be undescended. Examine the child when he is relaxed because anxiety stimulates the cremasteric reflex. With warm hands, palpate the lower abdomen, working your way downward toward the scrotum along the inguinal canal. This will minimize retraction of the testes into the canal.

In *precocious puberty,* the penis and testes are enlarged, with signs of pubertal changes. This is caused by a variety of conditions associated with excess androgens, including *adrenal or pituitary tumors.* Other pubertal changes also occur.

A useful technique is to have the boy sit cross-legged on the examining table, as shown here. You can also give him a balloon to inflate or an object to lift to increase intra-abdominal pressure. If you can detect the testis in the scrotum, it is descended even if it spends much time in the inguinal canal.

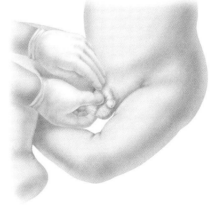

The cremasteric reflex can be tested by scratching the medial aspect of the thigh. The testis on the side being scratched will move upward.

Cryptorchidism may be noted at this age. It requires surgical correction. It should be differentiated from a retractible testis.

A painful testicle requires rapid treatment; common causes include infection such as *epididymitis* or *orchitis, torsion of the testicle,* or *torsion of the appendix testis.*

Examine the inguinal canal as you would for adults, noting any swelling that may reflect an *inguinal hernia.*

Inguinal hernias in older boys present as they do in adult men, with swelling in the inguinal canal, particularly following a Valsalva maneuver.

FEMALE GENITALIA

The genital examination can be anxiety provoking for the older child and adolescent (especially if you are of the opposite sex), for parents, and for you; however, if not performed, a significant finding may be missed. Depending on the child's developmental stage, explain what parts of the body you will check, and that this is part of the routine examination.

After infancy, the labia majora and minora flatten out, and the hymenal membrane becomes thin, translucent, and vascular, with the edges easily identified.

The genital examination is the same for all ages of children, from late infancy until adolescence. Use a calm, gentle approach, including a developmentally appropriate explanation as you do the examination. A bright light source is essential. Most children can be examined in the supine, frog-leg position.

If the child seems reluctant, it may be helpful to have the parent sit on the examination table with the child; alternatively, the exam may be performed while the child sits in the parent's lap. Do not use stirrups as these may frighten the child. The following diagram demonstrates a 5-year-old child sitting on her parent's lap with the parent holding her knees outstretched.

The appearance of pubic hair before the age of 7 years should be considered *precocious puberty* and requires evaluation to determine the cause.

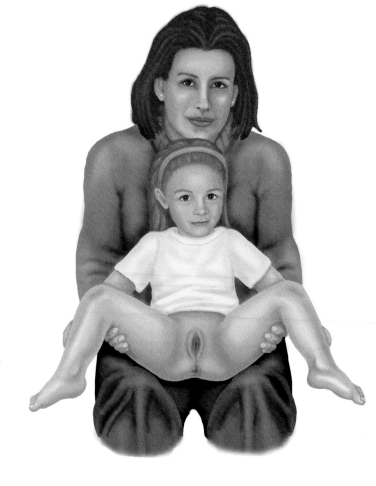

Examine the genitalia in an efficient and systematic manner. Inspect the external genitalia for the presence of pubic hair, the size of the clitoris, the color and size of the labia majora, and the presence of rashes, bruises, or other lesions.

Next, visualize the structures by separating the labia with your fingers as shown at the left on the following page. You can also apply gentle traction by grasping the labia between your thumb and index finger of each hand, and separating the labia majora laterally and posteriorly to examine the inner structures, as shown below. *Labial adhesions,* or fusion of the labia minora, may be noted in prepubertal children and can obscure the vaginal and urethral orifices. They may be a normal variant.

A *vaginal discharge* in early childhood can be from *perineal irritation* (e.g., bubble baths or soaps), *foreign body, vaginitis,* or a *sexually transmitted disease* from sexual abuse.

Vaginal bleeding is always concerning. Etiologies include *vaginal irritation, accidental trauma, sexual abuse, foreign body,* and *tumors. Precocious puberty* from many causes can induce menses in a young girl.

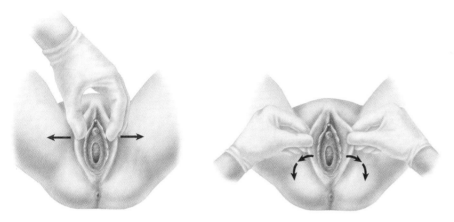

Purulent, profuse, malodorous, and blood-tinged discharge should be evaluated for the presence of *infiltration, foreign body,* or *trauma.*

Note the condition of the labia minora, urethra, hymen, and proximal vagina. If you are unable to visualize the edges of the hymen, ask the child to take a deep breath to relax the abdominal muscles. Another useful technique is to position her in the knee-chest position, as shown on the right and on the next page. These maneuvers will often open the hymen. You can also use saline drops to make the edges of the hymen less sticky.

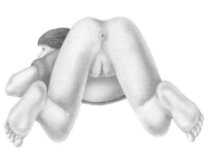

Avoid touching the hymenal edges because the hymen is exquisitely tender without the protective effects of hormones. Examine for discharge, labial adhesions, lesions, estrogenization (indicating onset of puberty), hymenal variations (such as imperforate or septate hymen, which is rare), and hygiene. A thin, white discharge (leukorrhea) is often present. A speculum examination of the vagina and cervix is not necessary in a prepubertal child unless there is suspicion of severe trauma or foreign body.

Abrasions or signs of trauma of the external genitalia can be from benign causes such as masturbation, irritants, or accidental trauma, but should also raise the possibility of *sexual abuse.*

The normal hymen in infants and young children can have a variety of configurations, as shown in Table 18-16 on page 811.

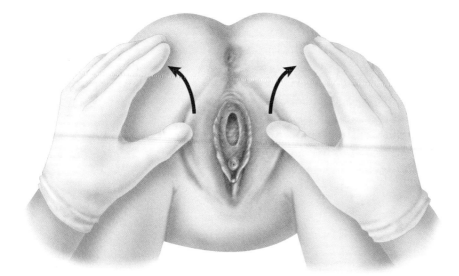

The physical examination may reveal signs that suggest *sexual abuse,* and the exam is particularly important if there are suspicious clues in the history. Bear in mind that, even with known abuse, the great majority of examinations will be unremarkable; thus, a normal genital examination does not rule out sexual abuse. Mounds, notches, and tags on the hymen may all be normal variants. The size of the orifice can vary with age and the examination technique.

PHYSICAL SIGNS OF SEXUAL ABUSE IN CHILDREN*

Possible Indications

1. Marked and immediate dilatation of the anus in knee–chest position, with no constipation, stool in the vault, or neurologic disorders
2. Hymenal notch or cleft that extends greater than 50% of the inferior hymenal rim (confirmed in knee–chest position)
3. Condyloma acuminata in a child older than 3 years
4. Bruising, abrasions, lacerations, or bite marks of labia or perihymenal tissue
5. Herpes of the anogenital area beyond the neonatal period
6. Purulent or malodorous vaginal discharge in a young girl (all discharges should be cultured and viewed under a microscope for evidence of a sexually transmitted disease)

Strong Indications*

1. Lacerations, ecchymoses, and newly healed scars of the hymen or the posterior fourchette
2. Absence of hymenal tissue from 3 to 9 o'clock (confirmed in various positions)
3. Healed hymenal transections, especially between 3 and 9 o'clock (complete cleft)
4. Perianal lacerations extending to external sphincter

A child with concerning physical signs must be evaluated by a sexual abuse expert for a complete history and sexual abuse examination.

*Any physical sign must be evaluated in light of the entire history, other parts of the physical examination, and laboratory data.

If the hymenal edges are smooth and without interruption in the inferior half, then the hymen is probably normal. Certain physical findings, however, suggest the possibility of sexual abuse and require more complete evaluation by an expert in the field.

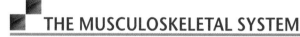

THE RECTAL EXAMINATION

The rectal examination is not part of the routine pediatric examination, but should be done whenever intra-abdominal, pelvic, or perirectal disease is suspected.

The rectal examination of the young child can be performed with the child either in the side-lying or lithotomy position. For many young children, the lithotomy position is less threatening and easier to perform. Have the child lie on the back with the knees and hips flexed and the legs abducted. Drape the child from the waist down. Provide frequent reassurance during the examination, and ask the child to breathe in and out through the mouth to relax. Spread the buttocks and observe the anus. You can use your lubricated gloved index finger, even in small children. Palpate the abdomen with your other hand, both to distract the child and to note the abdominal structures between your hands. The prostate gland is not palpable in young boys.

Anal skin tags are present in *inflammatory bowel disease,* but are more often an incidental finding.

Tenderness noted on rectal examination of a child usually indicates an infectious or inflammatory cause, such as an *abscess,* or *appendicitis.*

THE MUSCULOSKELETAL SYSTEM

In older children, abnormalities of the upper extremities are rare in the absence of injury.

Toddlers may acquire *nursemaid's elbow* or subluxation of the radial head due to a tugging injury.

The normal young child has increased lumbar concavity and decreased thoracic convexity compared with the adult, and often a protuberant abdomen.

Observe the child standing and walking barefoot. You can also ask the child to touch the toes, rise from a sitting position, run a short distance, and pick up objects. You will detect most abnormalities by watching carefully from both front and behind. To indirectly assess the gait pattern of the child, you can also note the soles of the shoes to see which side of the soles is worn down.

During early infancy, there is a common and normal progression of increased bowlegged growth (as shown below, left), which begins to disappear at about 18 months of age, often followed by transition toward knock-knees. The *knock-knee pattern* (as shown below, right), is usually maximal by age 3 to 4 years, and gradually corrects by age 9 or 10 years.

Severe bowing of the legs (genu varum) may still be physiologic bowing and will spontaneously resolve. Extreme bowing or unilateral bowing may be from pathologic causes such as *rickets* or *tibia vara* (*Blount's disease*).

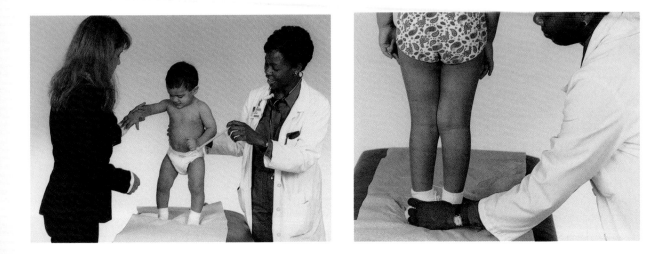

The presence of tibial torsion can be assessed in several ways; one method is shown above. Have the toddler lie prone on the examination table, with the knees flexed to 90°, as shown. Note the thigh–foot axis. Usually there is ±10° of internal or external rotation noted by a foot pointing off in a direction.

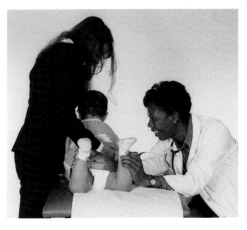

Children may *toe in* when they begin to walk. This may increase up to 4 years and then gradually disappear by about 10 years of age.

Inspect any child who can stand for *scoliosis* using techniques described under "Adolescents."

Test for severe hip disease, with its associated weakness of the gluteus medius muscle—observe the child from behind as the child shifts weight from one leg to the other. The pelvis should remain level when the weight is borne on the unaffected side, called a *negative Trendelenburg's sign*, as shown on the following page.

In *severe hip disease,* the pelvis tilts toward the unaffected hip when weight is borne on the affected side (an abnormal *positive Trendelenburg's sign,* as shown on the following page).

Determine any *leg shortening* that may accompany hip disease by comparing the distance from the anterior superior spine of the ilium with the medial malleolus on each side. First, straighten out the child by gently pulling on the legs, and then compare the levels of the medial malleoli with each other. You can also put a small ink dot over the prominent malleoli and touch them together to give you a contact point to measure.

Also, have the child stand straight and place your hands horizontally over the iliac crests from behind. Small discrepancies in leg length can be appreciated. If such a discrepancy is noted, a clever trick is to place a book under the shorter leg; this should eliminate the discrepancy.

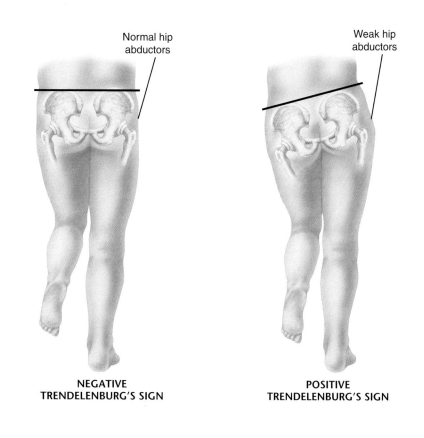

NEGATIVE
TRENDELENBURG'S SIGN

POSITIVE
TRENDELENBURG'S SIGN

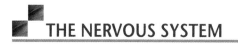 ## THE NERVOUS SYSTEM

Beyond infancy, when the primitive reflexes have disappeared, the neurologic examination includes the components evaluated in adults. Again, you should combine the neurologic and developmental assessment and will need to turn this into a game with the child. The goal is to assess optimal development and neurologic performance, and this requires the child to be cooperative.

Perform the DDST as described and shown on pp. 795–796. Children usually enjoy this component, and you can too. Remember that the DDST is better at detecting delays in motor skills than in language or cognitive milestones.

Cranial Nerves. The cranial nerves can be assessed quite well using developmentally appropriate strategies, as shown in the following table:

Children with *spastic diplegias* will often have hypotonia as infants and then excessive tone with spasticity, scissoring, and perhaps clenched fists as toddlers and young children.

Localizing neurologic signs are rare in children but can be from trauma, brain tumor, intracranial bleed, or infection.

■ Strategies to Assess Cranial Nerves in Young Children		
Cranial Nerve		Strategy
I	Olfactory	Testable in older children.
II	Visual acuity	Use Snellen chart after age 3 years. Test visual fields as for an adult. A parent may need to hold the child's head.
		(continued)

■ Strategies to Assess Cranial Nerves in Young Children (Continued)

Cranial Nerve		Strategy
III, IV, VI	Extraocular movements	Have the child track a light or an object (a toy is preferable). A parent may need to hold the child's head.
V	Motor	Play a game with a soft cotton ball to test sensation. Have the child clench the teeth and chew or swallow some food.
VII	Facial	Have the child "make faces" or imitate you as you make faces (including moving your eyebrows), and observe symmetry and facial movements.
VIII	Acoustic	Perform auditory testing after age 4 years. Whisper a word or command behind the child's back and have the child repeat it.
IX, X	Swallow and gag	Have the child stick the "whole tongue out" or "say 'ah'." Observe movement of the uvula and soft palate. Test the gag reflex.
XI	Spinal accessory	Have the child push your hand away with his head. Have the child shrug his shoulders while you push down with your hands to "see how strong you are."
XII	Hypoglossal	Ask the child to "stick out your tongue all the way."

Gait, Strength, and Coordination.   An important part of the motor examination is to observe the child's gait while the child is walking and, optimally, running. Note any asymmetries, weakness, undue tripping, or clumsiness. Follow the DDST examination milestones to test for appropriate maneuvers such as heel-to-toe walking (photo on the next page), hopping, and jumping. Use a toy to test for coordination and strength of the upper extremities.

In children with uncoordinated gait, be sure to distinguish *orthopedic causes* such as positional deformities of the hip, knee, or foot from *neurologic abnormalities* such as *cerebral palsy, ataxia, neuromuscular conditions* producing weakness, or *degenerative diseases.*

If you are concerned about the child's strength, have the child lie on the floor and then stand up, and closely observe the stages. Most normal children will first sit up, then flex the knees and extend the arms to the side to push off from the floor and stand up.

Hand preference is demonstrated in most children by age 2 and rarely before 18 months of age.

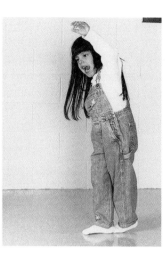

In certain forms of *muscular dystrophy* with weakness of the pelvic girdle muscles, children will rise to standing by rolling over prone and pushing off the floor with the arms while the legs remain extended (*Gower's sign*).

Sensation. The sensory examination can be performed using a cotton ball or tickling the child. This is best performed with the child's eyes closed. Do not use pin pricks to evaluate sensation or else you will have a very uncooperative and unhappy patient!

Deep Tendon Reflexes. Deep tendon reflexes can be tested as in adults. First demonstrate the use of the reflex hammer on the child's hand, assuring the child that it will not hurt. Children love to feel their legs bounce when you test their patellar reflexes. You will need to have the child cooperate and keep the eyes closed during some of this examination because tensing will disrupt the results.

You can ask children older than 3 years to draw a picture, copy objects as is done in the DDST, and then discuss their pictures to test simultaneously for fine motor coordination, cognition, and language.

The cerebellar examination can be tested using finger-to-nose and rapid alternating movements of the hands or fingers. Children enjoy this game. Children older than 5 years should be able to tell right from left, so you can assign them right–left discrimination tasks, as is done in the adult patient.

It is important to distinguish between isolated delays in one aspect of development (e.g., coordination or language) and more generalized delays that occur in several components. The latter is more likely to reflect global neurologic disorders such as *mental retardation* that can be caused by a large number of etiologies.

Use the expected milestones on the DDST and on pages 675–678 to test for language, cognitive, and social and emotional development. Remember that the neurologic and developmental examinations require a cooperative child, so be patient, have fun, and don't be embarrassed to play and innovate as you refine your examination skills to the developmental level of your pediatric patient.

Some children who have *attention deficit disorder with hyperactivity (ADHD)* will have a great deal of difficulty cooperating with your neurologic and developmental examination because of problems focusing. These children often have high energy levels, cannot stay still for extended periods, and have a history of difficulty in school or structured situations.

APPROACH TO EXAMINATION OF ADOLESCENTS

The key to successfully examining adolescents is a comfortable, confidential environment. This makes the examination more relaxed and informative. Consider the cognitive and social development of the adolescent when deciding issues of privacy, parental involvement, and confidentiality.

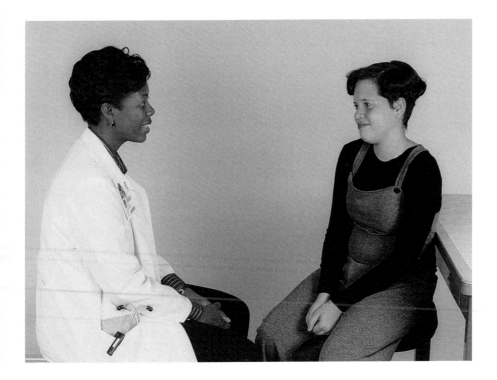

Adolescents, like most other people, usually respond positively to anyone demonstrating a genuine interest in them. It is important to show interest early and then sustain the connection if communication is to be effective. Adolescents are more likely to open up when the interview is focused on them rather than on their problems. In contrast to most other interviews, *start with specific focused questions* to build trust and rapport and get the conversation going. You may have to do more talking than usual, at the beginning. A good way to start is to chat informally about friends, school, hobbies, and family. Using silence in an attempt to get adolescents to talk or asking about feelings directly is usually not a good idea. It is particularly important to use summarization and transitional statements and to explain what you are going to do during the physical examination. The physical examination can also be an opportunity to get the young person talking. Once you have established rapport, return to more open-ended questions. At that point, make sure to ask what concerns or questions the adolescent may have.

Remember also that adolescents' behavior is related to their developmental stage, and not necessarily to chronologic age or physical maturation. Their age and appearance may fool you into assuming that they are functioning on a more future-oriented and realistic level. The reverse can also be true, especially in teens with delayed puberty or chronic illness.

Issues of *confidentiality* are important in adolescence. Explain to both parents and adolescents that the best health care allows adolescents some degree of independence and confidentiality. It helps if the clinician starts asking the parent to leave the room for part of the interview when the child is age 10 or 11 years. This prepares both caregivers and young people for future visits when the patient spends time alone with the clinician.

Before the parent leaves the room, get any relevant medical history from the parent, for example, certain elements of Past History, and clarify the parent's agenda for the visit. Also discuss the need for confidentiality. Explain that the purpose of confidentiality is to improve health care, not to keep secrets. Adolescents need to know that you will hold in confidence what they discuss with you. However, never make confidentiality unlimited. Always state explicitly that you may need to act on information that makes you concerned about safety: "I will not tell your parents what we talk about unless you give me permission or I am concerned about your safety—for example, if you were to talk to me about killing yourself and I thought that you really were at risk to follow through, I would need to discuss it with others."

Your goal is to help adolescents bring their concerns or questions to their parents. Encourage adolescents to discuss sensitive issues with their parents and offer to be present or help. Although young people may believe that their parents would "kill them if they only knew," you may be able to promote more open dialogue. This entails a careful assessment of the parents' perspective and the full and explicit consent of the young person. Sometimes the adolescent is correct in their assessment of parental reaction.

As in middle childhood, modesty is important. The patient should remain dressed until the examination begins, and you should leave the room while the patient gowns. Most adolescents older than age 13 prefer to be examined without a parent in the room, but this depends on the patient's developmental level, familiarity with the examiner, relationship with the parent, and medical issues. For younger adolescents, ask the adolescent and parent their preferences. While the examination of the adolescent can be anxiety provoking for the novice clinician, with practice, these interactions can be very rewarding for both the adolescent and the clinician.

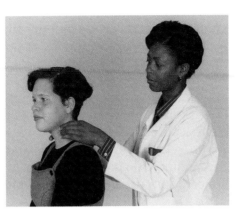

TECHNIQUES OF EXAMINATION FOR ADOLESCENTS

The sequence and content of the physical examination of the adolescent are similar to those in the adult. The examiner must keep in mind, however, particular issues unique to adolescents, such as puberty, growth, development, family and peer relationships, sexuality, decision making, and risk behaviors.

The sections below outline modifications to specific regional examinations that are needed when working with adolescents. For more details on techniques of examination, the reader should refer to the corresponding chapter for the regional examination of interest or concern.

■ GENERAL SURVEY AND VITAL SIGNS

SOMATIC GROWTH

Adolescents should wear gowns to be weighed. This is particularly important for adolescent girls being evaluated for underweight problems. Ideally, serial weights (and heights) should use the same scales.

VITAL SIGNS

Ongoing evaluations of blood pressure are important for adolescents.

Causes of sustained hypertension for this age group include *primary hypertension, renal parenchymal disease,* and *drug use.*

The average heart rate from age 10 to 14 years is 85 beats per minute, with a range of 55 to 115 beats per minute considered normal. Average heart rate for those 15 years and older is 60 to 100 beats per minute.

HEAD, EARS, EYES, NECK, AND THROAT

The examination is generally the same as for adults.

The methods used to examine the eye, including testing for visual acuity, are the same as those for adults. Refractive errors become common, and it is important to test visual acuity monocularly at regular intervals, such as during the annual health supervision visit.

As the child grows, the ease and techniques of examining the ears and testing the hearing approach the methods used for adults. There are no ear abnormalities or variations of normal unique to this age group. Of course, parents of older children routinely refer to the normal condition of "selective deafness," defined as choosing to hear what the adolescent wishes to hear.

THE HEART

The technique and sequence of examination are the same as those for adults. Murmurs are a continued cardiovascular issue for evaluation. The *pulmonary flow murmur* is a common benign murmur in adolescents.

■ *Location and Characteristics of Benign Heart Murmurs in Adolescents*

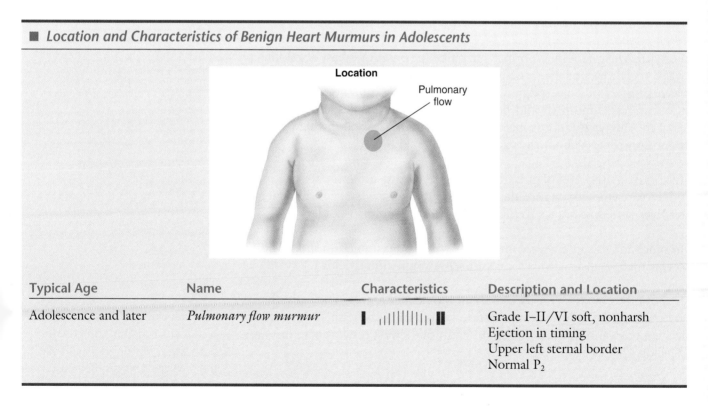

Typical Age	Name	Characteristics	Description and Location
Adolescence and later	*Pulmonary flow murmur*	I ⦙⦙⦙⦙⦙⦙ II	Grade I–II/VI soft, nonharsh Ejection in timing Upper left sternal border Normal P$_2$

The *pulmonary flow murmur* is a grade I–II/VI soft, nonharsh murmur with the timing characteristics of an ejection murmur, beginning after the first sound and ending before the second sound but without the marked crescendo–decrescendo quality of an organic ejection murmur. If you hear

A pulmonary flow murmur accompanied by a fixed split-second heart sound suggests right-heart volume load such as an *atrial septal defect.*

this murmur, make sure to evaluate whether the pulmonary closure sound is of normal intensity and whether splitting of the second heart sound is eliminated during expiration. An adolescent with a benign pulmonary ejection murmur will have normal intensity and normally split second heart sounds.

This pulmonary flow murmur may also be heard in the presence of volume overload from any reason, such as chronic anemia, and following exercise. It may persist into adulthood.

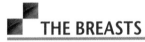

THE BREASTS

Physical changes in a young girl's breasts are one of the first signs of puberty. As in most developmental changes, there is a systematic progression of maturational changes. Generally, over a 4-year period, the breasts progress through five stages, called Tanner stages or Tanner sex maturity rating (SMR) stages, as shown on the next page. These progress from a preadolescent stage, to the appearance of breast buds, to subsequent enlargement and change in the contour of the breasts and areola. These stages are accompanied by the development of pubic hair and other secondary sexual characteristics, as shown on page 783. Menarche usually occurs when a girl is in breast stage 3 or 4, and by then she has passed her peak growth spurt (see the figure on p. 782).

For years the established normal age range for onset of breast development was 8 to 13 years of age (average age of 11 years), with breast development occurring before 8 years being abnormal. Some recent studies suggest that the lower age cutoff should be 7 years for white females and 6 years for African American (and probably Hispanic) females, though there remains some controversy about the exact age.

In approximately 10% of girls, the breasts develop at different rates, and considerable asymmetry may result in either size or Tanner stage. This generally resolves, and reassurance to the patient is most helpful.

In older adolescent girls, a comprehensive breast examination should be accompanied by instructions for breast self-examination (p. 351).

In boys, the breasts consist of a small nipple and areola. During puberty, about one third of boys develop a firm button of breast tissue 2 cm or more in diameter, and these are often noted in one breast only. Obese boys can develop substantial breast tissue.

Masses or nodules in the breasts of adolescent girls should be examined carefully. They are usually *benign fibroadenomas* or *cysts;* less likely etiologies include *abscesses* or *lipomas.* Breast carcinoma is extremely rare in adolescence, and nearly always occurs in families with a strong family history of the disease.

A substantial number of adolescent boys develop *gynecomastia,* or breast enlargement, on one or both sides. Although usually slight, the enlargement can be substantial and quite embarrassing. It generally resolves within a few years.

SEX MATURITY RATINGS IN GIRLS: BREASTS

Stage 1

Preadolescent. Elevation of nipple only

Stage 2

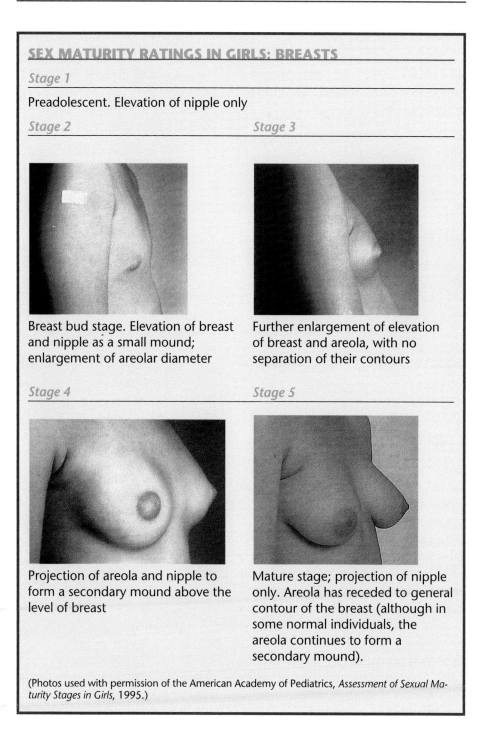

Breast bud stage. Elevation of breast and nipple as a small mound; enlargement of areolar diameter

Stage 3

Further enlargement of elevation of breast and areola, with no separation of their contours

Stage 4

Projection of areola and nipple to form a secondary mound above the level of breast

Stage 5

Mature stage; projection of nipple only. Areola has receded to general contour of the breast (although in some normal individuals, the areola continues to form a secondary mound).

(Photos used with permission of the American Academy of Pediatrics, *Assessment of Sexual Maturity Stages in Girls*, 1995.)

THE ABDOMEN

Techniques of abdominal examination are the same as for adults. See the table below for estimated liver span in adolescents according to age and sex.

Hepatomegaly in teens may be from infections such as hepatitis or infectious mononucleosis, inflammatory bowel disease, or tumors.

■ *Expected Liver Span of Adolescents*		
	Mean Estimated Liver Span (cm)	
Age in Years	*Males*	*Females*
12	6.5	5.6
14	6.8	5.8
16	7.1	6.0
18	7.4	6.1
20	7.7	6.3

MALE GENITALIA

The genital examination of the adolescent boy proceeds like the examination of the adult male. Be particularly aware of the embarrassment of many boys regarding this aspect of the examination.

Important anatomical changes in the male genitalia accompany puberty and help to define its progress. The first reliable sign of puberty, starting between ages 9 and 13.5 years, is an increase in the size of the testes. Next, pubic hair appears, along with progressive enlargement of the penis. The complete change from preadolescent to adult anatomy requires about 3 years, with a range of 1.8 to 5 years.

Delayed puberty is suspected in boys who have no signs of pubertal development by 14 years of age.

An important goal when examining the adolescent male is to assign a sexual maturity rating. The five stages of sexual development, first described by Tanner, are outlined and illustrated on the next page.[16] These involve changes in the penis, testes, and scrotum. In addition, in about 80% of men, pubic hair spreads farther up the abdomen in a triangular pattern pointing toward the umbilicus; this phase is not completed until the 20s.

The most common cause of delayed puberty in males is *constitutional delay,* frequently a familial condition involving delayed bone and physical maturation but normal hormonal levels.

An important developmental principle is that physical pubertal changes progress along a well-established sequence, as diagrammed on page 782. Although there are wide age ranges for the start and completion, the sequence for each boy is nevertheless the same. This is helpful in counseling an anxious adolescent regarding his current and future maturation, and regarding the normality of pubertal changes along a wide age range. It is also helpful for detecting abnormal physical changes.

Although nocturnal or daytime ejaculation tends to begin around Sexual Maturity Rating 3, a finding on either history or physical examination of penile discharge may indicate a *sexually transmitted disease.*

■ Sex Maturity Ratings in Boys

In assigning SMRs in boys, observe each of the three characteristics separately because they may develop at different rates. Record two separate ratings: pubic hair and genital. If the penis and testes differ in their stages, average the two into a single figure for the genital rating.

	Pubic Hair	Penis	Testes and Scrotum
Stage 1	Preadolescent—no pubic hair except for the fine body hair (vellus hair) similar to that on the abdomen	Preadolescent—same size and proportions as in childhood	Preadolescent—same size and proportions as in childhood
Stage 2	Sparse growth of long, slightly pigmented, downy hair, straight or only slightly curled, chiefly at the base of the penis	Slight or no enlargement	Testes larger; scrotum larger, somewhat reddened, and altered in texture
Stage 3	Darker, coarser, curlier hair spreading sparsely over the pubic symphysis	Larger, especially in length	Further enlarged
Stage 4	Coarse and curly hair, as in the adult; area covered greater than in stage 3 but not as great as in the adult and not yet including the thighs	Further enlarged in length and breadth, with development of the glans	Further enlarged; scrotal skin darkened
Stage 5	Hair adult in quantity and quality, spread to the medial surfaces of the thighs but not up over the abdomen	Adult in size and shape	Adult in size and shape

(Photos reprinted from *Pediatric Endocrinology and Growth*, 2nd ed., Wales & Wit, 2003, with permission from Elsevier.)

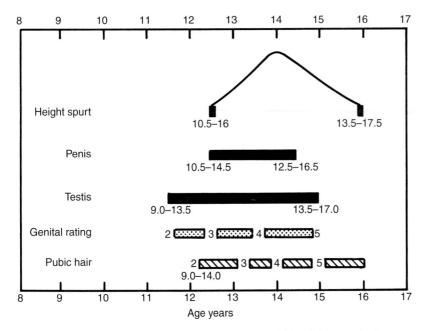

Numbers below the bars indicate the ranges in age within which certain changes occur. (Redrawn from Marshall WA, Tanner JM. Variations in the patterns of pubertal changes in boys. Arch Dis Child 45:22, 1970.)

■ FEMALE GENITALIA

The external examination of adolescent female genitalia proceeds in the same manner as for the school-age child. If it is necessary to complete a full pelvic exam on an adolescent, the actual technique is the same as that used for an adult including the rectal examination. A full explanation of the steps of the examination, demonstration of the instruments, and a gentle, reassuring approach is necessary because the adolescent is usually quite anxious. An adolescent's first pelvic examination should be performed by an experienced health care provider. A chaperone (parent or nurse) must be present.

The presence of a *vaginal discharge* in a young adolescent should be treated as in the adult. Causes include *physiologic* leukorrhea, *sexually transmitted diseases* from consensual sexual activity or *sexual abuse, bacterial vaginosis, foreign body,* and *external irritants.*

You should assign a sexual maturity rating to every female, irrespective of chronologic age. The assessment of sexual maturity in girls is based on both growth of pubic hair and the development of breasts.[17] The assessment (Tanner staging) of pubic hair growth is shown in the figure illustrating the five Tanner stages of sexual maturity, on page 783. See page 779 for breast development assessment.

Although there is a wide variation in the age of onset and completion of puberty, remember that the stages occur in a predictable sequence, as shown next.

Delayed puberty in an adolescent female below the 3rd percentile in height may be from Turner's syndrome or chronic disease. The two most common causes of delayed sexual development in an extremely thin adolescent girl are anorexia nervosa and chronic disease.

SEX MATURITY RATINGS IN GIRLS: PUBIC HAIR

Stage 1

Preadolescent—no pubic hair except for the fine body hair (vellus hair) similar to that on the abdomen

Stage 2

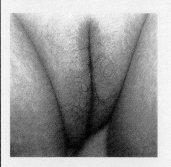

Sparse growth of long, slightly pigmented, downy hair, straight or only slightly curled, chiefly along the labia

Stage 3

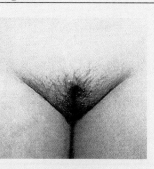

Darker, coarser, curlier hair, spreading sparsely over the pubic symphysis

Stage 4

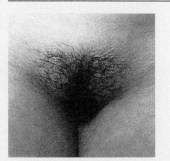

Coarse and curly hair as in adults; area covered greater than in stage 3 but not as great as in the adult and not yet including the thighs

Stage 5

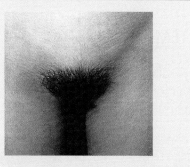

Hair adult in quantity and quality, spread on the medial surfaces of the thighs but not up over the abdomen

(Photos used with permission of the American Academy of Pediatrics, *Assessment of Sexual Maturity Stages in Girls*, 1995.)

It is helpful to counsel girls about this sequence and their current maturational stage. A girl's initial signs of puberty are hymenal changes secondary to estrogen, widening of the hips, and beginning of a height spurt, although these changes are difficult to detect. The first easily detectable sign of puberty is usually the appearance of breast buds, although pubic hair sometimes appears earlier. The average age of the appearance of pubic hair has decreased in recent years, and current consensus is that the appearance of pubic hair as early as 7 years can be normal, particularly in dark-skinned girls who develop secondary sexual characteristics at an earlier age.

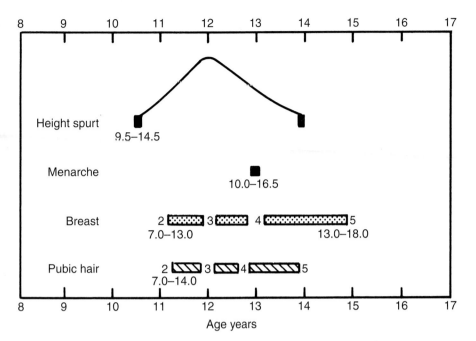

Numbers below the bars indicate the ranges in age within which certain changes occur. (Redrawn from Marshall WA, Tanner JM. Variations in the pattern of pubertal changes in girls. Arch Dis Child 45:22, 1970.)

THE MUSCULOSKELETAL SYSTEM

Evaluations for scoliosis and screening for participation in sports (pp. 786–788) remain common components of examination in adolescents. Other segments of the musculoskeletal examination are the same as for adults.

Assessing for Scoliosis.   Make sure to have the child bend forward with the knees straight (*Adams' bend test*). Evaluate any asymmetry in positioning or gait. Scoliosis in a young child is unusual and abnormal; mild scoliosis in an older child is not uncommon.

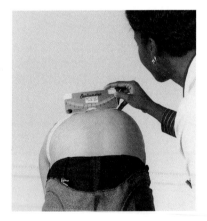

If you detect scoliosis, you can use a *scoliometer* to test for the degree of scoliosis. With the child standing, look for asymmetry of the shoulder blades or gluteal folds. Have the child bend forward as described. Look for prominence of the posterior ribs. Place the scoliometer over the spine at a point of maximum prominence, making sure that the spine is parallel to the floor at that point, as shown above. Have the child bend fully forward to assess lumbar scoliosis, and less so to assess thoracic scoliosis.

Several types of *scoliosis* may present during childhood. Idiopathic scoliosis (75% of cases), seen mostly in girls, is usually detected in early adolescence.

You can also use a *plumb line,* a string with a weight attached, to assess symmetry of the back. Place the top of the plumb line at C-7 and have the child stand straight. The plumb line should extend to the gluteal crease (not shown here).

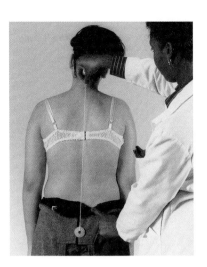

The Sports Preparticipation Screening Musculoskeletal Examination. More than 25 million children and adolescents in the United States and a large number in other countries participate in organized sports and often require "medical clearance." Start the exam with a thorough medical history, focusing on cardiovascular risk factors, prior surgeries, prior injuries, other medical problems, and a family history. The preparticipation physical exam is often the only time a healthy adolescent will see a medical professional, so it is important to include some screening questions and anticipatory guidance (see the discussion in Health Promotion and Counseling). Finally, perform a general physical, with special attention to the cardiac and lung exams and a vision and hearing screen. The preparticipation exam should then include a focused, thorough musculoskeletal exam, looking for weakness, limited range of motion, and evidence of previous injury.

A 2-minute preparticipation screening musculoskeletal examination has been recommended.[18,19] See an illustrated version of this examination on pages 786 to 788.

Important risk factors for sudden cardiovascular death during sports include episodes of *dizziness or palpitations, prior syncope* (particularly if associated with exercise), or family history of *sudden death* in young or middle-aged relatives.

During the preparticipation sports physical, assess carefully for *cardiac murmurs* and *wheezing* in the lungs.

■ Screening Musculoskeletal Examination for Children Participating in Sports

Specific Components of the Musculoskeletal Examination		Common Abnormalities
Positioning	Instructions to Patients	Due to Prior Injury

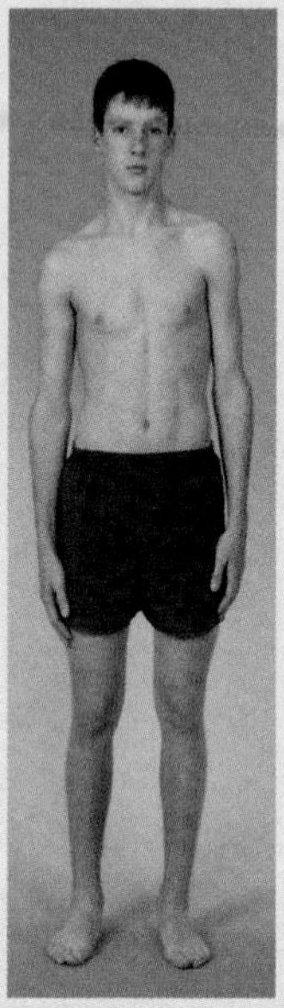

Step 1

1. Stand straight, facing you.

Asymmetry, swelling of joints

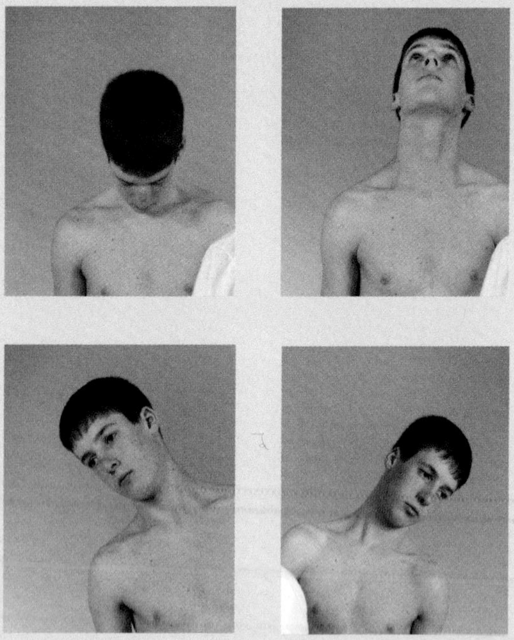

Step 2

2. Move neck in all directions—look at the ceiling and floor, touch ears to shoulders.

Loss of range of motion

(continued)

■ *Screening Musculoskeletal Examination for Children Participating in Sports* (Continued)

Specific Components of the Musculoskeletal Examination		Common Abnormalities Due to Prior Injury
Positioning	*Instructions to Patients*	

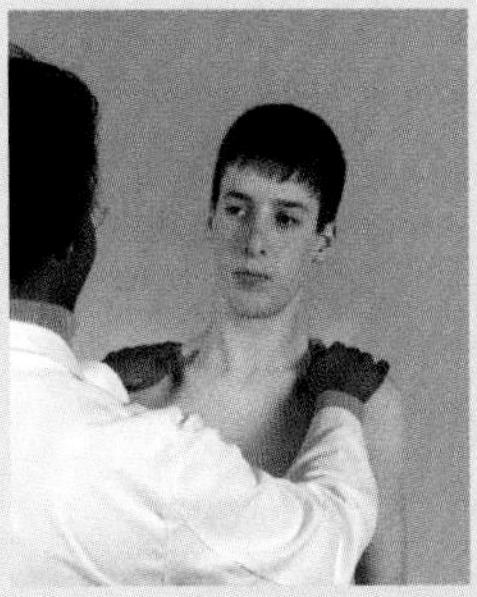

Step 3   **Step 4**

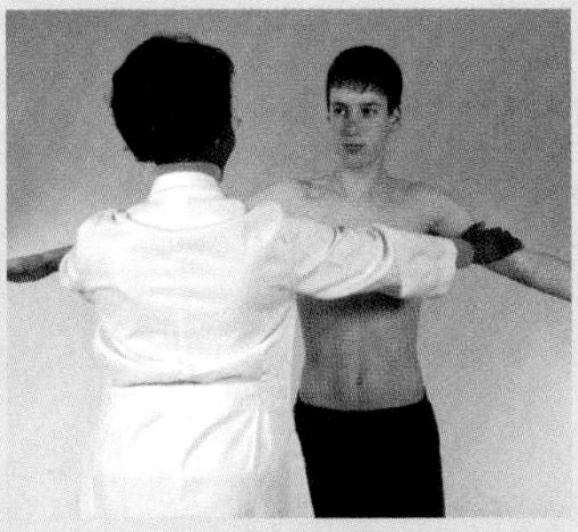

3. Shrug shoulders while you hold them down.

Weakness of shoulder, neck, or trapezius muscles

4. Hold arms out to side and lift arms while you press down.

Loss of strength of deltoid muscle

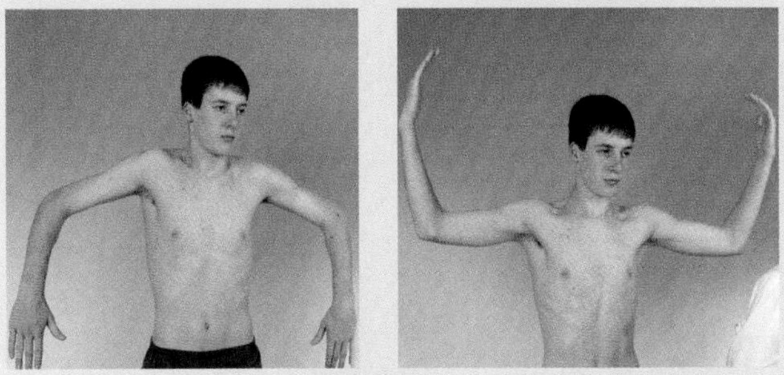

Step 5

5. Hold arms out to side with elbows bent 90°, raise and lower arms.

Loss of external rotation and injury to glenohumeral joint

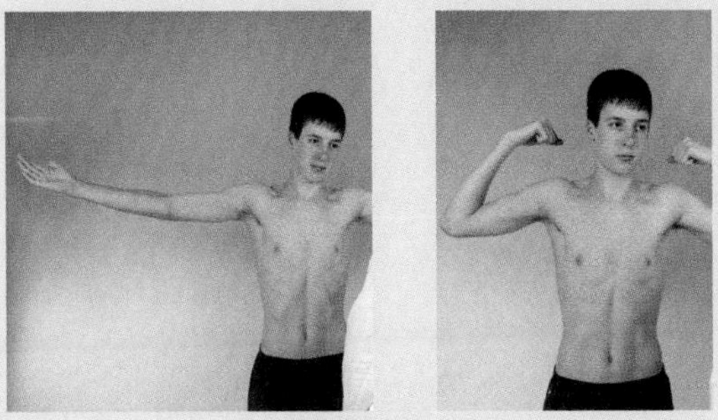

Step 6

6. Hold arms out, completely bend and straighten elbows.

Reduced range of motion of elbow

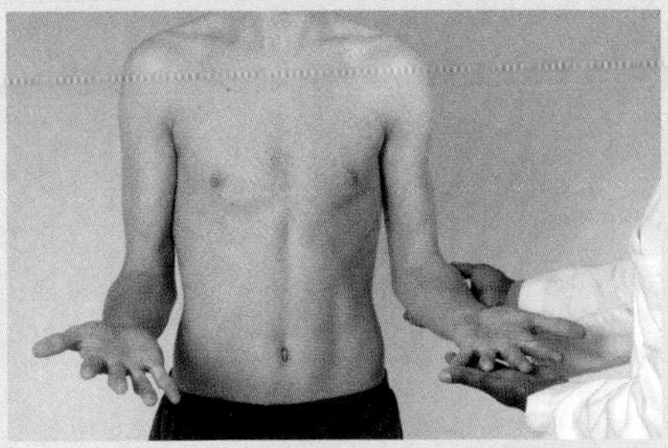

Step 7

7. Hold arms down, bend elbows 90°, and pronate and supinate forearm.

Reduced range of motion from injury to forearm, elbow, or wrist

(continued)

■ *Screening Musculoskeletal Examination for Children Participating in Sports* (Continued)

Specific Components of the Musculoskeletal Examination		Common Abnormalities Due to Prior Injury
Positioning	*Instructions to Patients*	

Step 8

8. Make a fist, clench and then spread fingers.

Protruding knuckle, reduced range of motion of fingers from prior sprain or fracture

Step 9   **Step 10**

9. Squat and duck-walk for four steps toward you.

Inability to fully flex knees and difficulty standing up due to prior knee or ankle injury

10. Stand straight with arms at sides, back to you.

Asymmetry from scoliosis, or leg-length discrepancy, or weakness from injury

Step 11   **Step 12**

11. Bend forward with knees straight and touch toes.

Asymmetry from scoliosis, and twisting of back from low back pain

12. Stand on heels and rise to the toes.

Wasting of calf muscles from ankle or Achilles tendon injury

◼ THE NERVOUS SYSTEM

The neurologic examination of the adolescent and the adult is the same. Still, it is important to assess the adolescent's developmental achievement according to age-specific milestones as described on pages 678–680.

RECORDING YOUR FINDINGS

Note that initially you may use sentences to describe your findings; later you will use phrases. The style here contains phrases appropriate for most write-ups. As you read through this write-up, you will notice some atypical findings. Try to test yourself. See if you can interpret these findings in the context of all you have learned about the examination of pediatric clients. You also will note the modifications necessary to accommodate reports from the small child's parent, rather than from the child himself or herself.

Recording the Examination: The Pediatric Patient

2/1/06

Brian is an active, rambunctious 26-month-old boy accompanied by his mother for concern about his development and behavior.

Referral. None

Source and Reliability. Mother (Mom), who seems extremely tuned into Brian.

Chief Complaint: Slow development and difficult behavior.

Present Illness: Brian appears to be developing more slowly than his older sister did. He uses only single words and simple phrases, rarely combines words, and appears frustrated with not being able to communicate. People understand approximately 25% of his speech. Physical development seems normal; he can throw a ball, kick, scribble, and dress himself well. He has had no head trauma, chronic illnesses, seizures, or regression in his milestones.

Mom also is concerned about his behavior. Brian is extremely stubborn, frequently has tantrums, gets angry easily (especially with his older sister), throws objects, bites, and physically strikes others when he doesn't get his way. His behavior seems worse around Mom, with reports of him being "fine" at his childcare center. He moves from one activity to another with an inability to sit still to read or play a game.

He is an extremely picky eater who eats a large quantity of junk food and little else. He will not eat fruits or vegetables and drinks enormous quantities of juice and soda. His mother has tried everything to get him to eat healthy food, to no avail.

(continued)

The family has been under substantial stress during the past year from Brian's father being unemployed. Although Brian now has Medicaid insurance, the parents are uninsured.

Medications. One multivitamin daily.

Past History

Pregnancy.   Uneventful. Mom reduced her tobacco intake to a half-pack a day and drank alcohol at times. She denies use of other drugs or having infections.

Newborn Period.   Born vaginally at 40 weeks; left the hospital in 2 days. Birth weight 2.5 kg (5 lbs, 8 oz). Mom does not know why Brian was small at birth.

Illnesses.   Only minor illnesses; no hospitalizations.

Accidents.   Required sutures last year for a facial laceration secondary to a fall on the road.

Preventive Care.   Brian has had regular preventive check-ups. At the last appointment 6 months ago, his regular physician said that Brian was a bit behind on some developmental milestones and suggested a childcare center that he knew was excellent, as well as increased parental attention to reading, speaking, playing, and stimulation. Immunizations are current. Lead level was elevated mildly last year; he had "low blood," which Mom thinks is called anemia. His physician recommended iron supplements and foods high in iron, but Brian really won't eat them.

Family History

Strong family history of diabetes (two grandparents, none with diabetes as children) and hypertension. No family history of childhood developmental, psychiatric, or chronic illnesses.

Developmental History: Sat up at 6 months, crawled at 9 months, and walked at 13 months. First words ("mama" and "car") said at approximately 1 year.

Personal and Social History: Parents are married and live with the two children in a rented apartment. Dad has not had a steady job for 1 year but has worked intermittently in construction. Mom works as a waitress part-time while Brian is in childcare.

Mom had depression during Brian's first year and attended some counseling sessions, but stopped because she could not pay for them or medications. She gets support from her mother who lives 30 minutes away, and many friends, some of whom baby sit occasionally.

Despite substantial family stress, Mom describes a loving and intact family. They try to eat dinner together daily, limit television, read to both children (although Brian won't sit still), and go to the nearby park regularly to play.

Environmental Exposures. Both parents smoke, although generally outside the house.

Safety. Mom reports this as a major concern: she can barely leave Brian out of her sight without him getting into something. She fears he will run under a car; the family is thinking of fencing in their small yard. Brian sits in his car seat most of the time; smoke detectors work in the home. Dad's guns are locked; medications are in a cabinet in the parents' bedroom.

Review of Systems

General.   No major illnesses.

Skin.   Dry and itchy. Last year he was prescribed hydrocortisone for it.

Head, Eyes, Ears, Nose, and Throat (HEENT).   *Head*: No trauma. *Eyes*: Vision fine. *Ears*: Multiple infections in the past year. Frequently ignores parents' requests; they can't tell if this is purposeful. *Nose*: Often runny; Mom wonders about allergies. *Mouth*: No dentist visit yet. Brushes teeth sometimes (a frequent source of dispute).

Neck.   No lumps. Glands in neck seem large.

Respiratory.   Frequent cough and whistle in chest. Mom cannot tell what triggers it; it tends to go away. He can run around all day without seeming to get tired.

Cardiovascular.   No known heart disease. He had a murmur when younger, but it went away.

Gastrointestinal.   Appetite and eating habits described above. Regular bowel movements. He is in the process of toilet training and wears pull-ups at night, but not at childcare.

Urinary.   Good stream. No prior urinary tract infections.

Genital.   Normal.

Musculoskeletal.   He is "all boy" and never gets tired. Minor bumps and bruises occasionally.

Neurologic.   Walks and runs well; seems coordinated for age. No stiffness, seizures, or fainting. Mom says his memory seems great, but his attention span is terrible.

Psychiatric.   Generally seems happy. Cries easily; bounces back and forth from trying to be independent to needing cuddling and comforting.

Physical Examination

Brian is a chubby, active, and energetic toddler. He plays with the reflex hammer, pretending it is a truck. He appears closely bonded with his mother, looking at her occasionally for comfort. She seems concerned that Brian will break something. His clothes are clean.

Vital Signs.   Ht 90 cm (90th percentile). Wt 16 kg (>95th percentile). BMI 19.8 (>95th percentile). Head circumference 50 cm (75th percentile). BP 108/58. Heart rate 90 and regular. Respiratory rate 30; varies with activity. Temperature (ear) 37.5°C. Obviously no pain.

Skin.   Normal except for bruises on legs, and patchy, dry skin over external surface of elbows.

HEENT.   *Head:* Normocephalic; no lesions. *Eyes:* Difficult to examine because he won't sit still. Symmetric with normal extraocular movements. Pupils 4 to 5 mm constricting. Discs difficult to visualize; no hemorrhages noted. *Ears:* Normal pinna; no external abnormalities. Normal external canals and tympanic membranes (TMs). *Nose:* Normal nares; septum midline. *Mouth:* Several darkened teeth on inside surface of upper incisors. One clear cavity on upper right incisor. Tongue normal. Cobblestoning of posterior pharynx; no exudates. Tonsils large but adequate gap (1.5 cm) between them.

(continued)

Neck.   Supple, midline trachea, no thyroid palpable.

Lymph Nodes.   Easily palpable (1.5 to 2 cm) tonsillar lymph nodes bilaterally. Small (0.5 cm) nodes in inguinal canal bilaterally. All lymph nodes mobile and nontender.

Lungs.   Good expansion. No tachypnea or dyspnea. Congestion audible, but seems to be upper airway (louder near mouth, symmetric). No rhonchi, rales, or wheezes. Clear to auscultation.

Cardiovascular.   PMI in 4th or 5th interspace and midsternal line. Normal S_1 and S_2. No murmurs or abnormal heart sounds. Normal femoral pulses; dorsalis pedis pulses palpable bilaterally.

Breasts.   Normal, with some fat under both.

Abdomen.   Protuberant but soft; no masses or tenderness. Liver span 2 cm below right costal margin (RCM) and not tender. Spleen and kidneys not palpable.

Genitalia.   Tanner I circumcised penis; no pubic hair, lesions, or discharge. Testes descended, difficult to palpate because of active cremasteric reflex. Normal scrotum both sides.

Musculoskeletal.   Normal range of motion of upper and lower extremities and all joints. Spine straight. Gait normal.

Neurologic.   *Mental Status:* Happy, cooperative child. *Developmental (DDST):* Gross motor—Jumps and throws objects. Fine motor—Imitates vertical line. Language—Does not combine words; single words only, three to four noted during examination. Personal-social—Washes face, brushes teeth, and puts on shirt. Overall—Normal, except for language, which appears delayed. *Cranial Nerves:* Intact, although several difficult to elicit. *Cerebellar:* Normal gait; good balance. *Deep tendon reflexes (DTRs):* Normal and symmetric throughout with downgoing toes. *Sensory:* Deferred.

Bibliography

CITATIONS

1. Levine MD, Carey WB, Crocker AC: Developmental–Behavioral Pediatrics, 3rd ed. Philadelphia, WB Saunders, 2002.
2. Johnson, CP, Blasco PA: Infant growth and development. Pediatr in Rev 18(7):224–242, 1997.
3. Colson ER, Dworkin PH: Toddler development. Pediatr in Rev 18(8):255–259, 1997.
4. Copelan J: Normal speech and development. Pediatr in Rev 18:91–100, 1995.
5. American Academy of Pediatrics: Guidelines for Health Supervision III, Rev ed. Elk Grove Village, IL, Author, 2002.
6. American Academy of Pediatrics: Bright Futures. Available at: http://brightfutures.aap.org/web/aboutBrightFutures.asp. Accessed August 30, 2005.
7. American Medical Association: Guidelines for Adolescent Preventive Services (GAPS). Available at: http://www.ama-assn.org/ama/upload/mm/39/gapsmono.pdf. Accessed August 30, 2005.
8. United States Department of Health and Human Services: U.S. Preventive Services Task Force (USPSTF). Available at: http://www.ahrq.gov/clinic/uspstfix.htm. Accessed August 30, 2005.
9. American Academy of Pediatrics and American College of Obstetricians and Gynecologists: Guidelines for Perinatal Care, 4th ed. Elk Grove Village, IL and Washington, DC, 1997.
10. Ballard JL, Khoury JC, Wedig K, et al: New Ballard score, expanded to include extremely premature infants. Journal of Pediatrics 119(3):417–423, 1991.
11. Brazelton TB. Working with families: Opportunities for early intervention. Pediatric Clinics of North America 42(1):1–9, 1995.
12. Margolis P, Gadomski A: Does this infant have pneumonia? JAMA 279(4):308–313, 1998.
13. Gessner IH: What makes a heart murmur innocent? Pediatric Annals 26(2):82–84, 87–88, 90–91, 1997.
14. Goldberg MJ: Early detection of developmental hip dysplasia: synopsis of the AAP Clinical Practice Guideline. Pediatr in Rev 22(4):131–134, 2001.
15. Zafeiriou DI: Primitive reflexes and postural reactions in the neurodevelopmental examination. Pediatric Neurology 31(1):1–8, 2004.

BIBLIOGRAPHY

16. Herman-Giddens ME, Wang L, Koch G: Secondary sexual characteristics in boys: estimates from the national health and nutrition examination survey III, 1988–1994. Arch Pediatr & Adolesc Med 155(9):1022–1028, 2001.

17. Herman-Giddens ME, Slora EJ, Wasserman RC, et al: Secondary sexual characteristics and menses in young girls seen in office practice: a study from the Pediatric Research in Office Settings Network. Pediatrics 99(4):505–512, 1997.

18. Metzl JD: Preparticipation examination of the adolescent athlete: part 1. Pediatr in Rev 22(6):199–204, 2001.

19. Metzl JD: Preparticipation examination of the adolescent athlete: part 2. Pediatr in Rev 22(7):227–239, 2001.

20. Botash AS: Examination for sexual abuse in prepubertal children: an update. Pediatric Annals 26(5):312–320, 1997.

ADDITIONAL REFERENCES

Allen HD, Moss AJ, Adams FH: Moss and Adams' Heart Disease in Infants, Children, and Adolescents, 6th ed. Philadelphia, Lippincott Williams & Wilkins, 2001.

American Academy of Family Physicians: Preparticipation Examination. Appendix. Available at: http://www.aafp.org/afp/20000501/2696.html. Accessed January 29, 2002.

American Academy of Pediatrics: Recommendations for Preventive Pediatric Health Care. Available at: http://www.aap.org/policy/re9939.html. Accessed January 29, 2002.

Blake J: Gynecologic examination of the teenager and young child. Obstet Gynecol Clin North Am 19:27, 1992.

Cohen ME, Duffer PK: Weiner and Levitt's Pediatric Neurology, 4th ed. Philadelphia, Lippincott Williams & Wilkins, 2003.

Coupey SM: Interviewing adolescents. Pediatr Clin of North Am 44(6): 1349–1364, 1997

Emmanouilides GC, et al (eds): Heart Disease of Infants, Children and Adolescents, including the Fetus and Young Adult, 5th ed. Baltimore, Williams & Wilkins, 1994.

Fanaroff AA, Martin RJ: Neonatal–Perinatal Medicine: Diseases of the Fetus and Infants, 7th ed. St. Louis, Mosby, 2002.

Fletcher MA: Physical Diagnosis in Neonatology. Philadelphia, Lippincott-Raven, 1997.

Goodheart HP: A Photoguide of Common Skin Disorders: Diagnosis and Management. Philadelphia, Lippincott Williams & Wilkins, 1999.

Green M: Bright Futures: Guidelines for Health Supervision of Infants, Children, and Adolescents. Arlington, VA, National Center for Education in Maternal and Child Health. 2000.

Harlan WR, Grillo GP, Comoni-Huntley J, et al: Secondary sex characteristics of boys 12 to 17 years of age. The U.S. Health Examination Survey. J Pediatr 95:293, 1979.

Harlan WR, Harlan EA, Grillo GP: Secondary sex characteristics of girls 12 to 17 years of age. The U.S. Health Examination Survey. J Pediatr 96:1074, 1980.

Harris JP: Consultation with the specialist. Evaluation of heart murmurs. Pediatr in Rev 15(12):490–494, 1994.

Herring JA, Tachdjian MO: Tachdjian's Pediatric Orthopedics, 3rd ed. (3 vols). Philadelphia, WB Saunders, 2002.

Hoekelman RA, et al (eds): Primary Pediatric Care, 4th ed. St. Louis, Mosby–Year Book, 2001.

Kreipe RE, McAnarney ER: Adolescent growth and development. In Behrman RE and Kliegman R: Nelson Essentials of Pediatrics, 4th ed. Philadelphia, WB Saunders. 2002.

Levine MD, Carey WB, Crocker AC: Developmental–Behavioral Pediatrics, 3rd ed. Philadelphia, WB Saunders, 2002.

McAnarney ER, Kreipe RE, Orr DP, et al: Textbook of Adolescent Medicine. Philadelphia, WB Saunders, 1992.

Myers GJ, McBride MC: Clinical neurologic examination of the preterm and term neonate. Semin Neurol 13(1): 1993.

Nelson LB, Calhoun JH, Harley RD: Pediatric Ophthalmology, 3rd ed. Philadelphia, WB Saunders, 1991.

Park MK: Pediatric Cardiology for Practitioners. 4th ed. St Louis, Mosby, 2002.

Piper MC, Darrah J: Motor Assessment of the Developing Infant. Philadelphia, WB Saunders, 1994.

Pizzutillo PD: Practical Orthopaedics in Primary Practice. New York, McGraw-Hill, 1997.

Reece RM, Ludwig S: Child Abuse: Medical Diagnosis and Management. 2nd ed. Philadelphia, Lippincott Williams & Wilkins, 2001.

Smith DM, Kovan JR, Rich BSE, et al: Preparticipation Physical Evaluation, 2nd ed. Minneapolis, McGraw-Hill Co., 1997.

Swaiman KF, Ashwal S: Pediatric Neurology: Principles and Practice, 3rd ed, (2 vols). St. Louis, Mosby–Year Book, 1999.

Tanner JM: Growth at Adolescence, 2nd ed. Oxford, Blackwell Scientific Publications, 1962.

Neuromuscular Maturity

	-1	0	1	2	3	4	5
Posture							
Square Window (wrist)	>90°	90°	60°	45°	30°	0°	
Arm Recoil		180°	140°-180°	110°-140°	90°-110°	<90°	
Popliteal Angle	180°	160°	140°	120°	100°	90°	<90°
Scarf Sign							
Heel to Ear							

Physical Maturity

Skin	sticky friable transparent	gelatinous red, translucent	smooth pink, visible veins	superficial peeling &/or rash. few veins	cracking pale areas rare veins	parchment deep cracking no vessels	leathery cracked wrinkled
Lanugo	none	sparse	abundant	thinning	bald areas	mostly bald	
Plantar Surface	heel-toe 40-50mm:-1 <40mm:-2	>50mm no crease	faint red marks	anterior transverse crease only	creases ant. 2/3	creases over entire sole	
Breast	imperceptible	barely perceptible	flat areola no bud	stippled areola 1-2mm bud	raised areola 3-4mm bud	full areola 5-10mm bud	
Eye/Ear	lids fused loosely:-1 tightly:-2	lids open pinna flat stays folded	sl. curved pinna; soft; slow recoil	well-curved pinna; soft but ready recoil	formed &firm instant recoil	thick cartilage ear stiff	
Genitals male	scrotum flat, smooth	scrotum empty faint rugae	testes in upper canal rare rugae	testes descending few rugae	testes down good rugae	testes pendulous deep rugae	
Genitals female	clitoris prominent labia flat	prominent clitoris small labia minora	prominent clitoris enlarging minora	majora & minora equally prominent	majora large minora small	majora cover clitoris & minora	

Maturity Rating

score	weeks
-10	20
-5	22
0	24
5	26
10	28
15	30
20	32
25	34
30	36
35	38
40	40
45	42
50	44

The Neuromuscular Maturity Criteria are depicted in the top half of the figure. Asphyxiated neonates or neonates obtunded by anesthetic agents or drugs will score lower on neuromuscular maturity criteria. In such instances, scoring should be repeated at 24 to 48 hours of age. The Physical Maturity Criteria are shown in the bottom half of the figure and are self-explanatory. The scores for each criterion are again the numbers at the top of the columns. The sum of the scores for all of the neuromuscular and physical maturity items provides an estimate of gestational age in weeks, using the maturity rating scale at the lower right portion of the figure. (Figure from Ballard JL, et. al. J. Pediatr 119:417, 1991.)

TABLE 18-2 Denver Developmental Screening Test

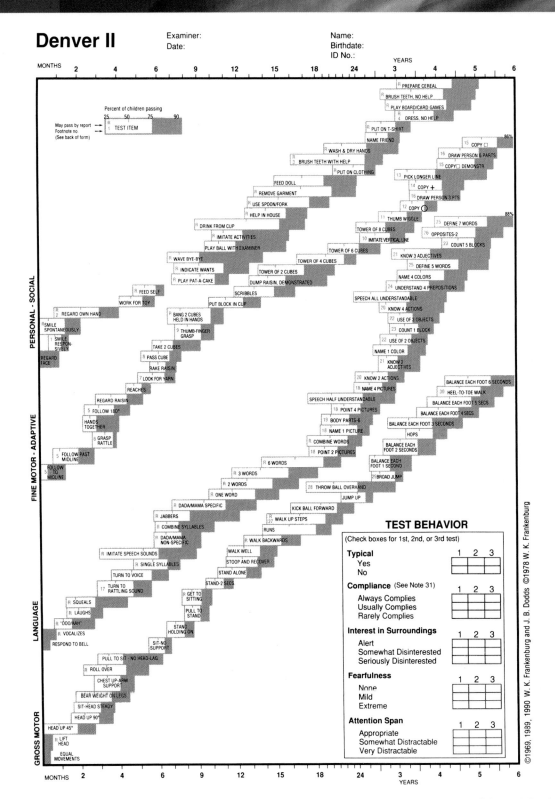

Denver II

(table continues next page)

TABLE 18-2   **Denver Developmental Screening Test** (Continued)

DIRECTIONS FOR ADMINISTRATION

1. Try to get child to smile by smiling, talking or waving. Do not touch him/her.
2. Child must stare at hand several seconds.
3. Parent may help guide toothbrush and put toothpaste on brush.
4. Child does not have to be able to tie shoes or button/zip in the back.
5. Move yarn slowly in an arc from one side to the other, about 8 above child's face.
6. Pass if child grasps rattle when it is touched to the backs or tips of fingers.
7. Pass if child tries to see where yarn went. Yarn should be dropped quickly from sight from tester's hand without arm movement.
8. Child must transfer cube from hand to hand without help of body, mouth, or table.
9. Pass if child picks up raisin with any part of thumb and finger.
10. Line can vary only 30 degrees or less from tester's line. /
11. Make a fist with thumb pointing upward and wiggle only the thumb. Pass if child imitates and does not move any fingers other than the thumb.

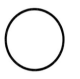

12. Pass any enclosed form. Fail continuous round motions.

13. Which line is longer? (Not bigger.) Turn paper upside down and repeat. (pass 3 of 3 or 5 of 6)

14. Pass any lines crossing near midpoint.

15. Have child copy first. If failed, demonstrate.

When giving items 12, 14, and 15, do not name the forms. Do not demonstrate 12 and 14.

16. When scoring, each pair (2 arms, 2 legs, etc.) counts as one part.
17. Place one cube in cup and shake gently near child's ear, but out of sight. Repeat for other ear.
18. Point to picture and have child name it. (No credit is given for sounds only.)
    If less than 4 pictures are named correctly, have child point to picture as each is named by tester.

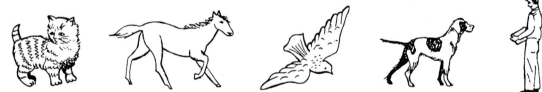

19. Using doll, tell child: Show me the nose, eyes, ears, mouth, hands, feet, tummy, hair. Pass 6 of 8.
20. Using pictures, ask child: Which one flies?... says meow?... talks?... barks?... gallops? Pass 2 of 5, 4 of 5.
21. Ask child: What do you do when you are cold?... tired?... hungry? Pass 2 of 3.
22. Ask child: What do you do with a cup? What is a chair used for? What is a pencil used for? Action words must be included in answers.
23. Pass if child correctly places <u>and</u> says how many blocks are on paper. (1, 5)
24. Tell child: Put block **on** table; **under** table; **in front of** me, **behind** me. Pass 4 of 4. (Do not help child by pointing, moving head or eyes.)
25. Ask child: What is a ball?... lake?... desk?... house?... banana?... curtain?... fence?... ceiling? Pass if defined in terms of use, shape, what it is made of, or general category (such as banana is fruit, not just yellow). Pass 5 of 8, 7 of 8.
26. Ask child: If a horse is big, a mouse is __? If fire is hot, ice is __? If the sun shines during the day, the moon shines during the __? Pass 2 of 3.
27. Child may use wall or rail only, not person. May not crawl.
28. Child must throw ball overhand 3 feet to within arm's reach of tester.
29. Child must perform standing broad jump over width of test sheet (8½ inches).
30. Tell child to walk forward, ⚭⚭⚭➤ heel within 1 inch of toe. Tester may demonstrate. Child must walk 4 consecutive steps.
31. In the second year, half of normal children are noncompliant.

OBSERVATIONS:

Instructions printed on the back of the DDST form for administering some of the items contained in the Denver Developmental Screening Test. (Reprinted with permission from William K. Frankenburg, M.D.)

TABLE 18-3 Recommendations for Preventive Pediatric Health Care

Each child and family is unique; therefore, these recommendations are designed for the care of children who are receiving competent parenting, have no manifestations of any important health problems, and are growing and developing in satisfactory fashion. Additional visits may become necessary if circumstances suggest variations from normal.

	Infancy								Early Childhood				
AGE	2–4 days¹	By 1 mo	2 mo	4 mo	6 mo	8 mo	10 mo	12 mo	15 mo	18 mo	24 mo	3 y	4 y
HISTORY													
Initial/Interval	●	●	●	●	●	●	●	●	●	●	●	●	●
MEASUREMENTS													
Height and Weight	●	●	●	●	●	●	●	●	●	●	●	●	●
Head Circumference	●	●	●	●	●	●	●	●	●	●	●		
Blood Pressure												●	●
SENSORY SCREENING													
Vision	S	S	S	S	S	S	S	S	S	S	S	O	O
Hearing	S	S	S	S	S	S	S	S	S	S	S	S	O
DEVELOPMENTAL/ BEHAVIORAL ASSESSMENT²	●	●	●	●	●	●	●	●	●	●	●	●	●
PHYSICAL EXAMINATION³	●	●	●	●	●	●	●	●	●	●	●	●	●

	Middle Childhood				Adolescence									
AGE	5 y	6 y	8 y	10 y	11 y	12 y	13 y	14 y	15 y	16 y	17 y	18 y	19 y	20 y+
HISTORY														
Initial/Interval	●	●	●	●	●	●	●	●	●	●	●	●	●	●
MEASUREMENTS														
Height and Weight	●	●	●	●	●	●	●	●	●	●	●	●	●	●
Head Circumference														
Blood Pressure	●	●	●	●	●	●	●	●	●	●	●	●	●	●
SENSORY SCREENING														
Vision	O	O	O	O	S	O	S	S	O	S	S	O	S	S
Hearing	O	O	O	O	S	O	S	S	O	S	S	O	S	S
DEVELOPMENTAL/ BEHAVIORAL ASSESSMENT²	●	●	●	●	●	●	●	●	●	●	●	●		●
PHYSICAL EXAMINATION³	●	●	●	●	●	●	●	●	●	●	●	●		●

1. For newborns discharged in less than 48 hours after delivery
2. By history and appropriate physical examination: if suspicious, by specific objective development testing
3. At each visit, a complete physical examination is essential, with infant totally unclothed, older child undressed and suitably draped

Key: ● = to be performed   S = subjective, by history   O = objective, by a standard testing method

Adapted from Recommendations For Preventive Pediatric Health Care promulgated by the American Academy of Pediatrics Committee on Practice and Ambulatory Medicine. Pediatrics 96:373, 1995. Additional recommendations made by the Committee regarding screening for metabolic disorders, tuberculosis, anemia, and urinary tract diseases, administration of immunizations, provision of anticipatory guidance, and initial dental referral are not included in the above summation.

TABLE 18-4   Abnormalities in Heart Rhythm and Blood Pressure

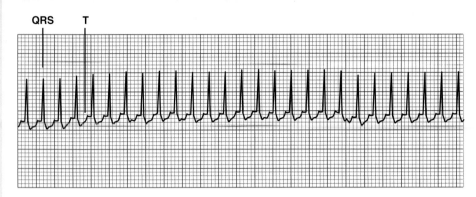

Supraventricular Tachycardia

Paroxysmal supraventricular tachycardia (SVT) is the most common dysrhythmia in children. Some infants with SVT look quite well or may be somewhat pale with tachypnea, but have a heart rate of 240 beats per minute or greater. Others are quite ill and in cardiovascular collapse.

SVT in infants is usually sustained, requiring medical therapy for conversion to a normal rate and rhythm. In older children, it is more likely to be truly paroxysmal, with episodes of varying duration and frequency.

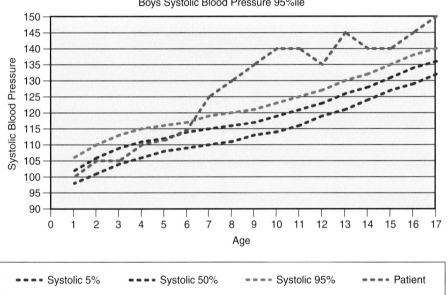

Hypertension in Childhood—A Typical Example

Hypertension can start in childhood. While young children with elevated blood pressure are more likely to have a renal, cardiac, or endocrine cause, adolescents with hypertension are most likely to have primary or essential hypertension.

This child developed hypertension during adolescence, and it "tracked" into adulthood. Children tend to remain in the same percentile for blood pressure as they grow. This tracking of blood pressure continues into adulthood, supporting the concept that adult essential hypertension begins during childhood.

The consequences of untreated hypertension can be severe.

You will need to differentiate common, benign birthmarks from uncommon but neurologically significant neurocutaneous syndromes.

Benign Birthmarks

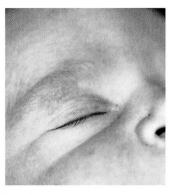

Eyelid Patch. This birthmark fades, usually in the first year.

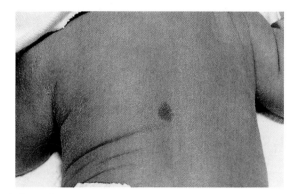

Café-au-lait spots. These light-brown pigmented lesions usually have ragged borders and are uniform. They are noted in more than 10% of black infants.

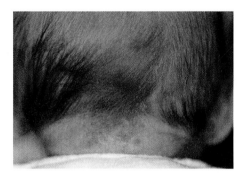

Salmon Patch. Also called "stork bite," this splotchy pink mark fades with age.

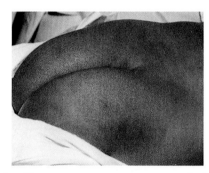

Mongolian Spots. These are more common among dark-skinned babies. It is important to note them so that they are not mistaken for bruises.

Neurocutaneous Syndromes

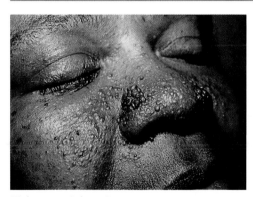

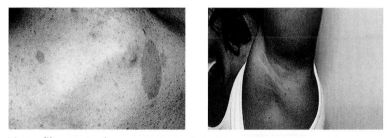

Neurofibromatosis. Characteristic features include more than 5 café-au-lait spots and axillary freckling, both shown above. Later findings include neurofibromas and Lish nodules (not shown).

Tuberous Sclerosis. Findings in young children include adenoma sebaceum as shown here (angiofibromas surrounding sweat glands). Older children may have oval, depigmented ash-leaf spots (not shown).

(Sources of photos: *Café-au-lait Spots, Salmon Patch, Eyelid Patch, Mongolian Spots*—Fletcher M. Physical Diagnosis in Neonatology. Philadelphia, Lippincott-Raven, 1998; *Neurofibromatosis*—Goodheart H. A Photoguide of Common Skin Disorders. Baltimore, Williams & Wilkins, 1999; *Tuberous Sclerosis*—Hall J. Sauer's Manual of Skin Diseases, 8th ed. Philadelphia, Lippincott Williams & Wilkins, 2000.)

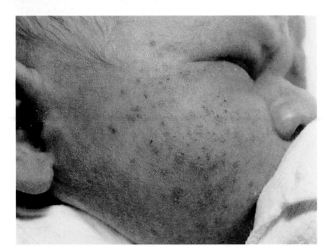

Erythema Toxicum

These yellow or white pustules are surrounded by a red base and are commonly noted in normal newborns.

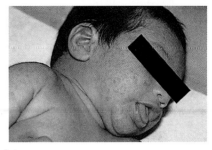

Neonatal Acne

Red pustules and papules are most prominent over the cheeks and nose of some normal newborns.

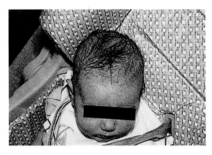

Seborrhea

The salmon red, scaly eruption often involves the face, neck, axilla, diaper area, and behind the ears.

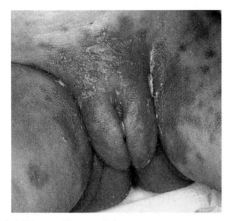

Candidal Diaper Dermatitis

This bright red rash involves the intertriginous folds, with small "satellite lesions" along the edges.

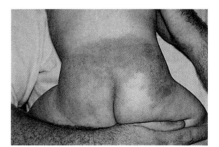

Contact Diaper Dermatitis

This irritant rash is secondary to diarrhea or irritation and is noted along contact areas (here, the area touching the diaper).

(Sources of photos: *Erythema Toxicum, Candidal Diaper Dermatitis*—Fletcher M. Physical Diagnosis in Neonatology. Philadelphia, Lippincott Raven, 1998; *Neonatal Acne, Seborrhea, Contact Diaper Dermatitis*—Goodheart H. A Photoguide of Common Skin Disorders. Baltimore, Williams & Wilkins, 1999.)

TABLE 18-7	Warts, Lesions That Resemble Warts, and Other Raised Lesions

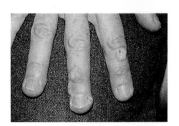

Verruca Vulgaris
Dry, rough warts on hands

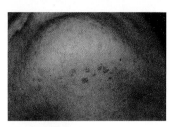

Verruca Plana
Small, flat warts

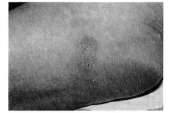

Plantar Warts
Tender warts on feet

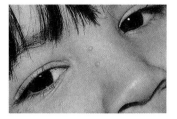

Molluscum Contagiosum
Dome-shaped, fleshy lesions

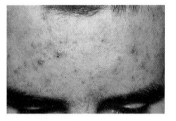

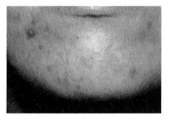

Adolescent Acne
You will frequently note acne in adolescents. Differentiate between open comedones (blackheads) and closed comedones (whiteheads) shown at the left, and inflamed pustules (right).

(Source of photos: Goodheart H. A Photoguide of Common Skin Disorders. Baltimore, Williams & Wilkins, 1999.)

TABLE 18-8	Common Skin Lesions During Childhood

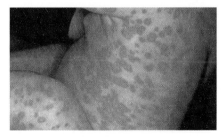

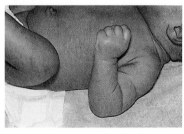

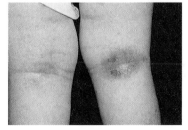

Urticaria (Hives)
This pruritic, allergic sensitivity reaction changes shape quickly.

Atopic Dermatitis (Eczema)
Erythema, scaling, dry skin, and intense itching characterize this condition in children.

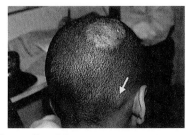

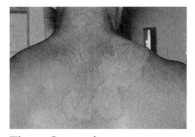

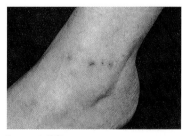

Tinea Capitis
Scaling, crusting, and hair loss are seen in the scalp, along with a painful plaque (kerion) and occipital lymph node (*arrow*).

Tinea Corporis
This annular lesion has central clearing and papules along the border.

Insect Bites
Intensely pruritic, red, distinct papules characterize these lesions.

(Source of all photos except *Urticaria*—Goodheart H. A Photoguide of Common Skin Disorders. Baltimore, Williams & Wilkins, 1999.)

TABLE 18-9   **Abnormalities of the Head**

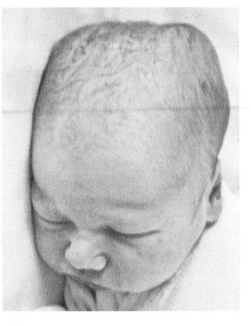

Cephalohematoma

Although not present at birth, cephalohematomas appear within the first 24 hours and are due to subperiosteal hemorrhage involving the outer table of one of the cranial bones. The swelling, as above, does not extend across a suture, though it is occasionally bilateral following a difficult delivery. The swelling is initially soft, then develops a raised bony margin within a few days due to calcium deposits at the edge of the periosteum, and tends to resolve within several weeks.

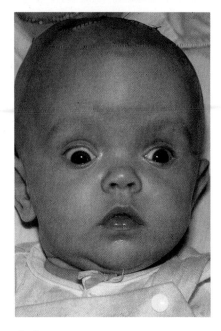

Hydrocephalus

In hydrocephaly, the anterior fontanelle is bulging, and the eyes may be deviated downward, revealing the upper scleras and creating the *setting sun* sign, as shown in the figure above. The setting sun sign is also seen briefly in some normal newborns. (From Zitelli BJ, Davis HW. Atlas of Pediatric Physical Diagnosis, 3rd ed. St. Louis, Mosby–Year Book, 1997. Courtesy of Dr. Albert Briglan, Children's Hospital of Pittsburgh.)

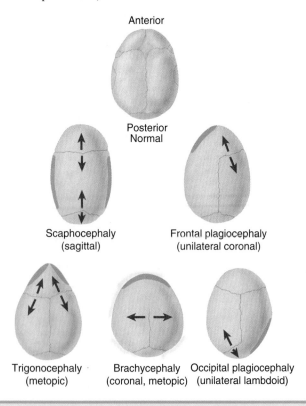

Anterior

Posterior
Normal

Scaphocephaly
(sagittal)

Frontal plagiocephaly
(unilateral coronal)

Trigonocephaly
(metopic)

Brachycephaly
(coronal, metopic)

Occipital plagiocephaly
(unilateral lambdoid)

Craniosynostosis

Craniosynostosis is a condition of premature closure of one or more sutures of the skull. This results in an abnormal growth and shape of the skull because growth will occur across sutures that are not affected but not across sutures that are affected. The figures above demonstrate different skull shapes associated with the various types of craniosynostosis. Scaphocephaly and frontal plagiocephaly are the more common types. The *blue shading* shows areas of maximal flattening. The *red arrows* show the direction of continued growth across the sutures, which is normal.

TABLE 18-10   **Diagnostic Facies in Infancy and Childhood**

Fetal Alcohol Syndrome

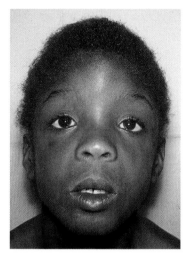

Babies born to women who are chronic alcoholics are at increased risk for growth deficiency, microcephaly, and mental retardation. Facial characteristics shown here include short palpebral fissures, a wide and flattened philtrum (the vertical groove in the midline of the upper lip), and thin lips.

Congenital Syphilis

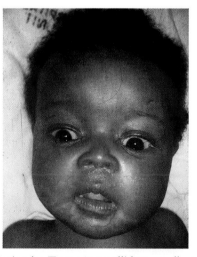

In utero infection by *Treponema pallidum* usually occurs after the 16th week of gestation and affects virtually all fetal organs. If it is not treated, 25% of infected babies will die before birth and another 30% shortly thereafter. Signs of illness appear in survivors within the first month of life. Facial stigmata shown here include bulging of the frontal bones and nasal bridge depression (*saddle nose*), both due to periostitis; rhinitis from weeping nasal mucosal lesions (*snuffles*); and a circumoral rash. Mucocutaneous inflammation and fissuring of the mouth and lips (*rhagades*), not shown here, may also occur as stigmata of congenital syphilis, as may craniotabes tibial periostitis (*saber shins*) and dental dysplasia (*Hutchinson's teeth*—see p. 236).

Congenital Hypothyroidism

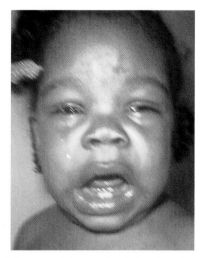

The child with congenital hypothyroidism (cretinism) has coarse facial features, a low-set hair line, sparse eyebrows, and an enlarged tongue. Associated features include a hoarse cry, umbilical hernia, dry and cold extremities, myxedema, mottled skin, and mental retardation. It is important to note that the majority of infants with congenital hypothyroidism have no physical stigmata; this has led to screening of all newborns in the United States and in most other developed countries for depressed thyroxine or elevated thyroid-stimulating hormone levels.

Facial Nerve Palsy

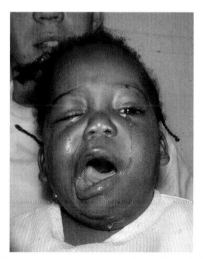

Peripheral (lower motor neuron) paralysis of the facial nerve may be due to (1) an injury to the nerve from pressure during labor and delivery, (2) inflammation of the middle ear branch of the nerve during episodes of acute or chronic otitis media, or (3) unknown causes (Bell's palsy). The nasolabial fold on the affected left side is flattened, and the eye does not close. This is accentuated during crying, as shown here. Full recovery occurs in ≥ 90% of those affected, usually within a few weeks. *(table continues next page)*

TABLE 18-10   Diagnostic Facies in Infancy and Childhood (Continued)

Down Syndrome

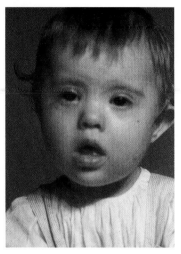

The child with Down syndrome (trisomy 21) usually has a small, rounded head, a flattened nasal bridge, oblique palpebral fissures, prominent epicanthal folds, small, low-set, shell-like ears, and a relatively large tongue. Associated features include generalized hypotonia, transverse palmar creases (*simian lines*), shortening and incurving of the 5th fingers (*clinodactyly*), Brushfield's spots (see p. 805), and mental retardation.

Battered Child Syndrome

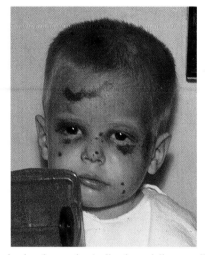

The child who has been physically abused (battered) may have old *and* fresh bruises about the head and face and may either look sad and forlorn or be actively seeking to please, sometimes even particularly involved with and attentive to the abusing parent. Other stigmata include bruises in areas (axilla and groin) not usually subject to injury rather than the bony prominences; x-ray evidence of fractures of the skull, ribs, and long bones in various stages of healing; and skin lesions that are morphologically similar to implements used to inflict trauma (hand, belt buckle, strap, rope, coat hanger, or lighted cigarette).

Perennial Allergic Rhinitis

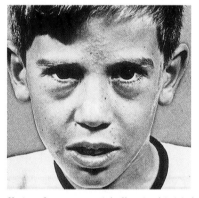

The child suffering from perennial allergic rhinitis has an open mouth (cannot breathe through the nose) and edema and discoloration of the lower orbitopalpebral grooves ("allergic shiners"). Such a child is often seen to push the nose upward and backward with a hand ("allergic salute") and to grimace (wrinkle the nose and mouth) to relieve nasal itching and obstruction. (Photograph reproduced with permission from Marks MB. Allergic shiners: dark circles under the eyes in children. Clin Pediatr 5:656, 1966.)

Hyperthyroidism

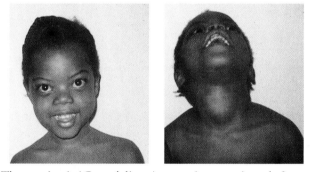

Thyrotoxicosis (*Graves' disease*) occurs in approximately 2 per 1,000 children under the age of 10 years. Affected children exhibit hypermetabolism and accelerated linear growth. Facial characteristics shown in this 6-year-old girl are "staring" eyes (not true exophthalmos, which is rare in children) and an enlarged thyroid gland (*goiter*). See p. 239.

TABLE 18-11   Abnormalities of the Eyes and Ears

Eye Abnormalities

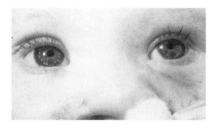

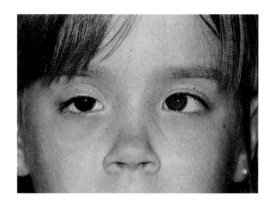

Brushfield's Spots
These abnormal speckling spots on the iris suggest Down syndrome.

Strabismus
Strabismus, or misalignment of the eyes, can lead to visual impairment. Esotropia, shown here, is an inward deviation.

Ear Abnormalities

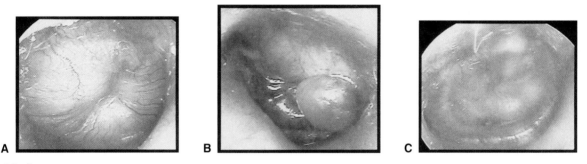

Otitis Media
Otitis media is one of the most common conditions in young children. The spectrum of otitis media is shown here. **(A)** Typical acute otitis media with a red, distorted, bulging tympanic membrane in a highly symptomatic child. **(B)** Acute otitis media with bullae formation and fluid visible behind the tympanic membrane. **(C)** Otitis media with effusion, showing a yellowish fluid behind a retracted and thickened tympanic membrane.

(Source of photos: *Otitis Media*—Courtesy of Alejandro Hoberman, Children's Hospital of Pittsburgh, University of Pittsburgh.)

TABLE 18-12 Abnormalities of the Mouth and Teeth

Mouth Abnormalities

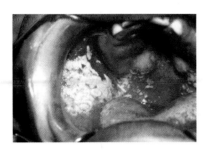

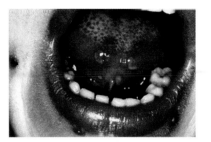

Oral Candidiasis ("thrush")
This infection is common in infants.
The white plaques do not rub off.

Herpetic Stomatitis
Tender ulcerations on the oral
mucosa are surrounded by erythema.

Dental Abnormalities

Dental Caries

Dental caries is a major public health and pediatric problem throughout the world. The photographs below show different characteristics of caries.

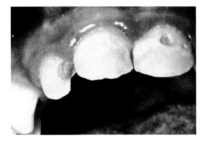

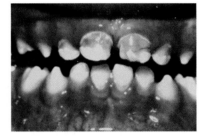

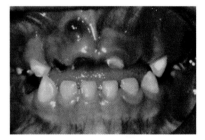

Nursing-bottle caries   Erosion of teeth   Severe erosion

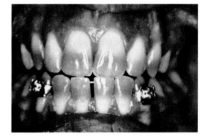

Staining of the Teeth
The teeth of children can become stained from a variety of
causes, including intrinsic stains such as tetracycline (right)
or extrinsic stains such as poor oral hygiene (not shown).
Extrinsic stains can be removed.

(Photos courtesy of American Academy of Pediatrics.)

TABLE 18-13 **Abnormalities of the Neck and Pharynx**

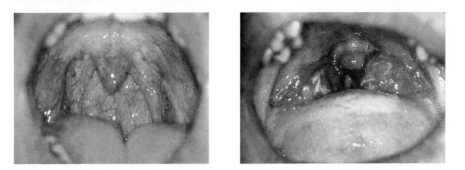

Streptococcal Pharyngitis ("strep throat")
This common childhood infection has a classic presentation of erythema of the
posterior pharynx and palatal petechiae (*left*). A foul-smelling exudate (*right*) is also
commonly noted.

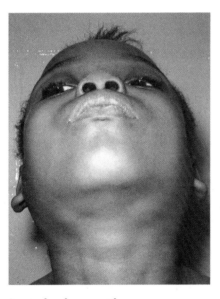

Lymphadenopathy
Enlarged and tender cervical lymph
nodes are common in children. The
most likely causes are viral and bacterial
infections. Lymph node enlargement
can be bilateral, as shown above.

(Source of photo: *Lymphadenitis and Abscess*—Fleisher G, Ludwig S. Textbook of Pediatric Emergency Medicine, 4th ed. Philadelphia, Lippincott
Williams & Wilkins, 2000.)

TABLE 18-14   Cyanosis in Children

It is important for you to be able to recognize cyanosis. The best location to examine is the mucous membranes. Cyanosis is a "raspberry" color, whereas normal mucous membranes should have a "strawberry color." Try to identify the cyanosis in these photographs before reading the captions.

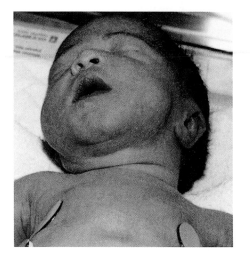

Generalized Cyanosis
This baby has total anomalous pulmonary venous return and an oxygen saturation level of 80%.

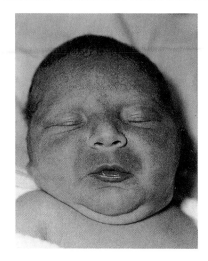

Perioral Cyanosis
This baby has mild cyanosis above the lips, but the mucous membranes remain pink.

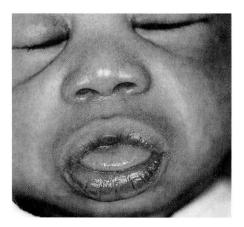

Bluish Lips, Giving Appearance of Cyanosis
Normal pigment deposition in the vermilion border of the lips gives them a bluish hue, but the mucous membranes are pink.

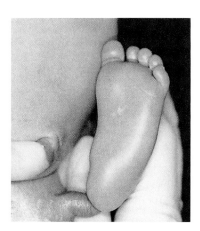

Acrocyanosis
This commonly appears on the feet and hands of babies shortly after birth. This infant is a 32-week newborn.

(Source of photos: Fletcher M. Physical Diagnosis in Neonatology. Philadelphia, Lippincott-Raven, 1998.)

TABLE 18-15   Congenital Heart Murmurs

Some heart murmurs reflect underlying heart disease. If you understand their physiologic causes, you will more readily be able to identify them and distinguish them from innocent heart murmurs. Obstructive lesions are caused by normal blood flow through valves that are too small. Because this problem is not dependent on the drop in pulmonary vascular resistance following birth, these murmurs are audible at birth. Defects with left-to-right shunts, on the other hand, are dependent on the drop in pulmonary vascular resistance. In the case of high-pressured shunts such as ventricular septal defect, patent ductus arteriosus, and persistent truncus arteriosus, they are not heard until 1 week or more after birth. Low-pressured left-to-right shunts, such as in atrial septal defects, may not be heard for considerably longer, usually first being noted at 1 year or more of age. Many children with congenital cardiac defects have combinations of defects or variations of abnormalities, so that findings on cardiac examination will not follow these classic patterns. This table shows a limited selection of the more common defects.

Congenital Defect and Mechanism	Characteristics of the Murmur	Associated Findings
Pulmonary Valve Stenosis Usually a normal valve anulus with fusion of some or most of the valve leaflets, restricting flow across the valve *Mild* 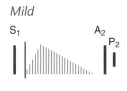 *Severe* 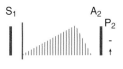	*Location.* Upper left sternal border *Radiation.* In mild degrees of stenosis, the murmur may be heard over the course of the pulmonary arteries in the lung fields. *Intensity.* Increases in intensity and duration as the degree of obstruction increases *Quality.* Ejection, peaking later in systole as the obstruction increases	Usually a prominent ejection click in early systole Pulmonary component of the second sounds at the base (P2) becomes delayed and softer, disappearing as obstruction increases. Inspiration may increase murmur; expiration may increase click. Growth is usually normal. Newborns with severe stenosis may be cyanotic from right-to-left atrial shunting and rapidly develop congestive heart failure.
Aortic Valve Stenosis Usually a bicuspid valve with progressive obstruction, but there may be a dysplastic valve or damage from rheumatic fever or degenerative disease. 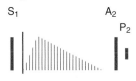	*Location.* Midsternum, upper right sternal border *Radiation.* To the carotid arteries and suprasternal notch; may also be a thrill *Intensity.* Varies, louder with increasingly severe obstruction *Quality.* An ejection, often harsh, systolic murmur	May be an associated ejection click The aortic closure sound may be increased in intensity. There may be a diastolic murmur of aortic valve regurgitation. Newborns with severe stenosis may have weak or absent pulses and severe congestive heart failure. May not be audible until adulthood even though the valve is congenitally abnormal
Tetralogy of Fallot Complex defect with ventricular septal defect, infundibular and usually valvular right ventricular outflow obstruction, malrotation of the aorta, and right-to-left shunting at ventricular septal level. *With Pulmonic Stenosis* *With Pulmonic Atresia* 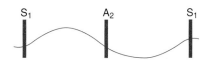	*General.* Variable cyanosis, increasing with activity *Location.* Mid-to-upper left sternal border. If pulmonary atresia, there is no systolic murmur but the continuous murmur of ductus arteriosus flow at upper left sternal border or in the back. *Radiation.* Little, to upper left sternal border, occasionally to lung fields *Intensity.* Usually grade III–IV *Quality.* Midpeaking, systolic ejection murmur	Normal pulses The pulmonary closure sound is usually not heard. May have abrupt hypercyanotic spells with sudden increase in cyanosis, air hunger, altered level of awareness Failure to gain weight with persistent and increasingly severe cyanosis Long-term persistence of cyanosis accompanied by clubbing of fingers and toes Persistent hypoxemia leads to polycythemia, which will accentuate the cyanosis.

(table continues next page)

TABLE 18-15   **Congenital Heart Murmurs** *(Continued)*

Congenital Defect and Mechanism	Characteristics of the Murmur	Associated Findings
Transposition of the Great Arteries A severe defect with failure of rotation of the great vessels, leaving the aorta to arise from the right ventricle and the pulmonary artery from the left ventricle	*General.* Intense generalized cyanosis *Location.* No characteristic murmur. If is present, it may reflect an associated defect such as VSD. *Radiation and Quality.* Depends on associated abnormalities	Single loud second sound of the anterior aortic valve Frequent rapid development of congestive heart failure Frequent associated defects as described at the left
Ventricular Septal Defect Blood going from a high-pressured left ventricle through a defect in the septum to the lower-pressured right ventricle creates turbulence, usually throughout systole. *Small to Moderate* 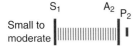	*Location.* Lower left sternal border *Radiation.* Little *Intensity.* Variable, only partially determined by the size of the shunt. Small shunts with a high pressure gradient may have very loud murmurs. Large defects with elevated pulmonary vascular resistance may have no murmur. Grade II–IV/VI with a thrill if grade IV/VI or higher. *Quality.* Pansystolic, usually harsh, may obscure S_1 and S_2 if loud enough	With large shunts, there may be a low-pitched middiastolic murmur of relative mitral stenosis at the apex. As pulmonary artery pressure increases, the pulmonic component of the second sounds at the base increases in intensity. When pulmonary artery pressure equals aortic pressure, there may be no murmur, and P_2 will be very loud. In low-volume shunts, growth is normal. In larger shunts, congestive heart failure may occur by 6–8 weeks; poor weight gain. Associated defects are frequent.
Patent Ductus Arteriosus Continuous flow from aorta to pulmonary artery throughout the cardiac cycle when ductus arteriosus does not close after birth *Small to Moderate* 	*Location.* Upper left sternal border and to left *Radiation.* Sometimes to the back *Intensity.* Varies depending on size of the shunt, usually grade II–III/VI. *Quality.* A rather hollow, sometimes machinery-like murmur that is continuous throughout the cardiac cycle, although occasionally almost inaudible in late diastole, uninterrupted by the heart sounds, louder in systole	Full to bounding pulses Noticed at birth in the premature infant who may have bounding pulses, a hyperdynamic precordium, and an atypical murmur Noticed later in the full-term infant as pulmonary vascular resistance falls May develop congestive heart failure at 4–6 weeks if large shunt Poor weight gain related to size of shunt Pulmonary hypertension affects murmur as above.
Atrial Septal Defect Left-to-right shunt through an opening in the atrial septum, possible at various levels 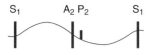	*Location.* Upper left sternal border *Radiation.* To the back *Intensity.* Variable, usually grade II–III/VI *Quality.* Ejection but without the harsh quality	Widely split second sounds throughout all phases of respiration, normal intensity Usually not heard until after age of 1 year Gradual decrease in weight gain as shunt increases Decreased exercise tolerance, subtle, not dramatic Congestive heart failure is rare.

TABLE 18-16

Normal Configurations of the Hymen in Prepubertal and Adolescent Females

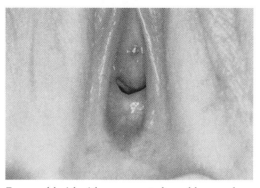

7-year-old girl with a crescent-shaped hymenal orifice

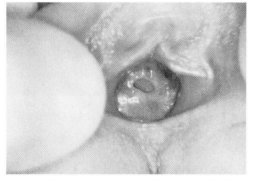

2-year-old with an annular orifice, located off-center, visible with labial traction

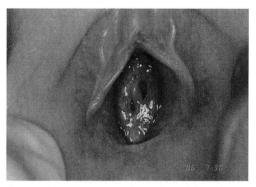

6-year-old with a septate hymen causing two orifices. Traction is needed to visualize the two openings.

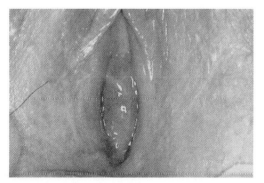

9-year-old girl with redundant labial tissue. Greater traction or a knee–chest position would reveal a normal orifice.

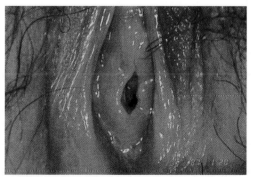

12-year-old girl with annular-shaped orifice and hormonal influence of puberty, causing thickened, pink tissue

(Source of photos: Reece R, Ludwig S (eds). Child Abuse: Medical Diagnosis and Management, 2nd ed. Philadelphia, Lippincott Williams & Wilkins, 2001.)

TABLE 18-17   Physical Signs of Sexual Abuse in Girls

Sexual Abuse

Because sexual abuse is all too common, you will need to recognize genital abnormalities associated with sexual abuse. These include:

(**A**) Acute hemorrhage and ecchymoses of tissues (10-mo old)
(**B**) Erythema and superficial abrasions to the labia minora (5-yr old)
(**C**) Healed interruption of hymenal membrane at 9 o'clock (4-yr old)
(**D**) Narrowed posterior ring continuous with floor of vagina (12-yr old)
(**E**) Copious vaginal discharge and erythema (9-yr old)
(**F**) Extensive condylomata around the anus (2-yr old)

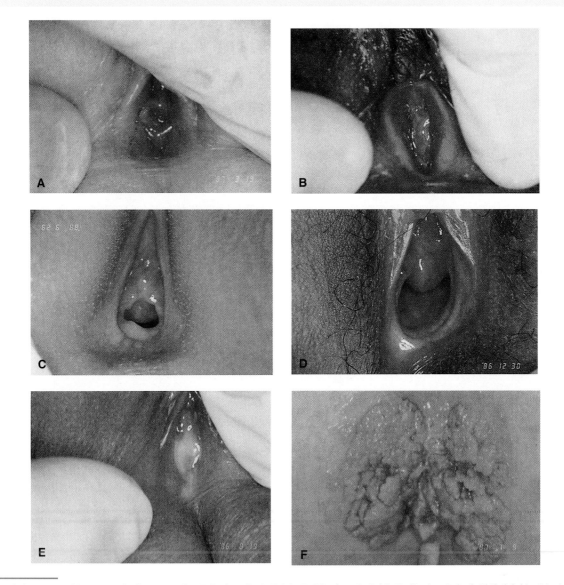

(Sources of photos: *Ambiguous Genitalia*—McMillan J, DeAngelis C, Feigin R, Warshaw J. Oski's Pediatrics, 3rd ed. Philadelphia, Lippincott Williams & Wilkins, 1999; *Sexual Abuse, (A), (B), (C), (D), (E), (F)*—Reece R, Ludwig S (eds.). Child Abuse Medical Diagnosis and Management, 2nd ed. Philadelphia, Lippincott Williams & Wilkins, 2001.)

TABLE 18-18   **The Male Genitourinary System**

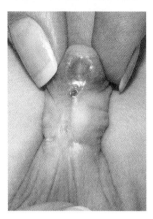

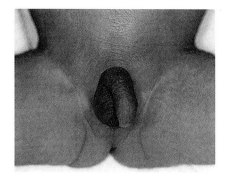

Hypospadius

Hypospadius is the most common congenital penile abnormality. The urethral meatus opens abnormally on the ventral surface of the penis. One form is shown above; more severe forms involve openings on the lower shaft or scrotum.

Undescended Testicle

You should distinguish between undescended testes, shown above (with testes in the inguinal canals), from highly retractile testes due to an active cremasteric reflex.

(Source of photos: *Hypospadius*—Courtesy of Warren Snodgrass, MD, UT–Southwestern Medical Center at Dallas; *Undescended Testicle*—Fletcher M. Physical Diagnosis in Neonatology. Philadelphia, Lippincott-Raven, 1998.)

TABLE 18-19   **Common Musculoskeletal Findings in Young Children**

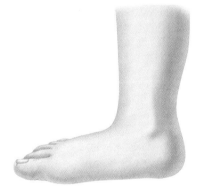

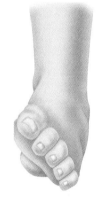

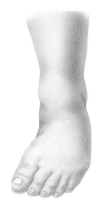

Flat feet or *pes planus* due to laxity of the soft tissue structures of the foot

Inversion of the foot (*varus*)

Metatarsus adductus in a child. The forefoot is adducted and not inverted.

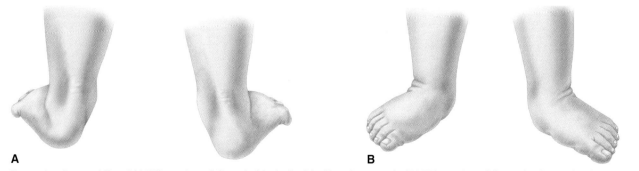

A   **B**

Pronation in a toddler. (**A**) When viewed from behind, the hindfoot is everted. (**B**) When viewed from the front, the forefoot is everted and abducted.

TABLE 18-20	The Gower Maneuver

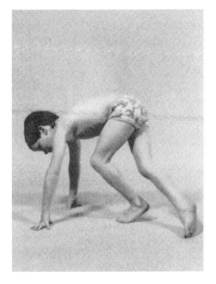
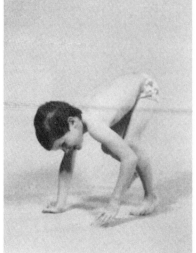
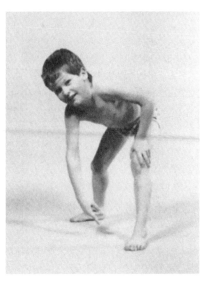
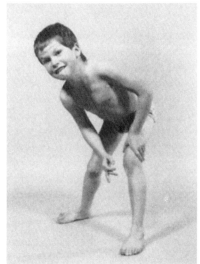
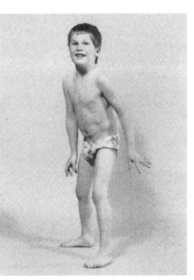

Certain forms of muscular dystrophy involve weakness of the pelvic girdle muscles. Children with this disease rise from a supine to a standing position in a characteristic manner, by rolling over to a prone position, pushing off the floor with the arms, bringing the legs to a flexed position under the trunk, and extending the legs with help of the hands.

TABLE 18-21

The Power of Prevention: Vaccine-Preventable Diseases

This table shows photographs of children with vaccine-preventable diseases. Childhood vaccines have been named the single most important medical intervention in the world from the standpoint of impact on public health. Because of vaccinations, we hope you will never see many of these conditions, but you should be able to identify them. Try to identify the diseases before reading the captions.

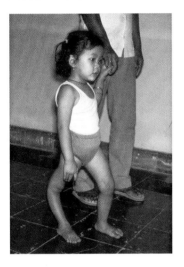

Polio
The deformed leg of this child is due to polio.

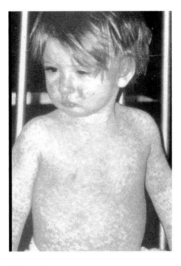

Measles
Characteristic rash of measles

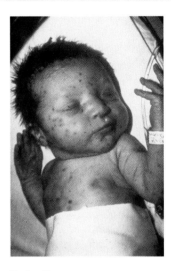

Rubella
Infant born with congenital rubella syndrome

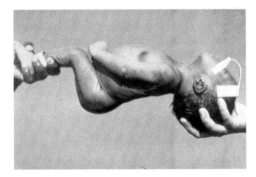

Tetanus
Rigid newborn with neonatal tetanus

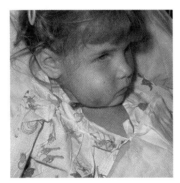

***Haemophilus influenzae* Type b**
Periorbital cellulitis due to this invasive bacterial disease

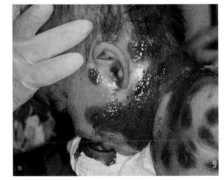

Varicella
An infant with a severe form of varicella

(Sources of photos: *Polio*—Courtesy of World Health Organization; *Haemophilus influenzae*—Courtesy of American Academy of Pediatrics; *Varicella*—Courtesy of Barbara Watson, MD, Albert Einstein Medical Center and Division of Disease Control, Philadelphia Department of Health; all others courtesy of Centers for Disease Control and Prevention.)

The Pregnant Woman

This chapter focuses on history taking and physical examination of the healthy adult woman during pregnancy. The techniques of examination are similar to those of the nonpregnant woman; however, the clinician must distinguish the changes in anatomy and physiology arising from pregnancy from findings that are abnormal. This chapter emphasizes common changes in anatomy and physiology that evolve throughout pregnancy; special concerns when eliciting the health history; and recommendations for nutrition, exercise, and screening for domestic violence. Then follow techniques of examination basic to prenatal care.

ANATOMY AND PHYSIOLOGY

Hormonal Changes.   During pregnancy, hormonal changes lead to extensive anatomical and physiologic changes in every major organ system. Many of the endocrine and metabolic changes of pregnancy are driven by increasing levels of estradiol and progesterone and by the placental hormones, especially human chorionic gonadotropin (HCG). These many complex changes can only be summarized here in brief:

- Estradiol appears to stimulate lactotrophs in the *anterior lobe of the pituitary gland*. These cells may triple in size as increasing prolactin output readies the breast tissue for lactation.[1]

- The *posterior pituitary gland* stores oxytocin and antidiuretic hormone (ADH)—HCG appears to reset the receptors for thirst and ADH release, leading to decreases in serum sodium concentration and, in some women, polyuria.

- The *thyroid gland* remains normal in size; however, estrogen effects on thyroxine-binding globulin and HCG stimulation of the thyrotropin (TSH) receptor lead to fluctuations in free T4 and T3 levels and in TSH, usually within the normal range.[2]

■ *Placental hormones* contribute to increased *insulin resistance* in later pregnancy and a shift from carbohydrate to fat metabolism. Insulin resistance is linked to transient hyperglycemia after meals, but between meals, fasting glucose levels fall, partly because of the demands of fetal growth and increased peripheral use of glucose.[3]

■ At the end of pregnancy, increases in placental corticotrophin-releasing factor and in adrenal adrenocorticotropic hormone produce "a state of *relative hypercortisolism*" that may be a trigger for labor.[1,4]

■ Rising *progesterone* levels have several effects. Although respiratory rate does not change, tidal volume and minute ventilation increase, sometimes leading to complaints of dyspnea. Progesterone and estradiol lower esophageal sphincter tone, contributing to symptoms of reflux and heartburn. Progesterone also relaxes tone and contraction in the ureters, causing hydronephrosis, and in the bladder, increasing risk for bacteriuria.

■ *Cardiovascular changes* in pregnancy are significant. Plasma volume increases up to 50% by the end of pregnancy, causing a dilutional but physiologic anemia. Cardiac output increases, and systemic vascular resistance and blood pressure fall.

■ Finally, *musculoskeletal changes* ensue from weight gain and *relaxin,* a hormone secreted in the corpus luteum and placenta: lumbar lordosis as the gravid uterus enlarges, contributing to mechanical low back discomfort, and ligamentous laxity in the sacroiliac joints and the pubic symphysis, to ease passage of the baby through the birth canal.

Changes in the Breasts and Pelvis.   Changes in the breasts and uterus are the most visible signs of pregnancy. To refresh your understanding of basic anatomy and physiology of the breasts and pelvis, review those sections of Chapter 9, The Breasts and Axillae, and Chapter 12, Female Genitalia.

The breasts undergo moderate enlargement as a result of hormone stimulation, increased vascularity, and hyperplasia of glandular tissue. There may be tenderness and tingling in the breasts that make them more sensitive during examination. By the third month of gestation, the breasts become more nodular. You will need to palpate carefully to avoid discomfort as you examine for any breast masses. The nipples become larger and more erectile. From mid- to late pregnancy, *colostrum,* a thick yellowish secretion rich in nutrients, may be expressed from the nipples. The areolae darken, and Montgomery's glands are more pronounced. The venous pattern over the breasts becomes increasingly visible as pregnancy progresses.

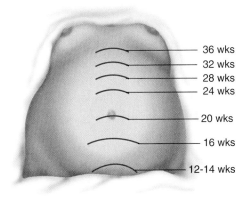

EXPECTED HEIGHT OF THE UTERINE FUNDUS BY MONTH OF PREGNANCY

36 wks
32 wks
28 wks
24 wks
20 wks
16 wks
12-14 wks

The abdomen becomes increasingly prominent to accommodate the growing uterus and fetus. You may detect early distention from fluid retention and relaxation of the abdominal muscle even before the uterus expands into the abdominal cavity at approximately 12 to 14 weeks' gestation. The expected growth patterns of the gravid uterus are illustrated on the left, and the standing contours of the primigravid abdomen in each trimester of pregnancy are shown to the right.[5]

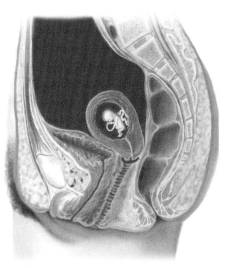

FIRST TRIMESTER

The early diagnosis of pregnancy is based in part on changes in the vagina and the uterus. With the increased vascularity throughout the pelvic region, the vagina takes on a bluish or violet color, known as *Chadwick's sign*. The vaginal walls appear thicker and deeply rugated because of increased thickness of the mucosa, loosening of the connective tissue, and hypertrophy of smooth muscle cells. Vaginal secretions are thick, white, and more profuse. Vaginal pH often becomes more acidic from the action of *Lactobacillus acidophilus* on the increased levels of glycogen stored in the vaginal epithelium.[6] This change in pH helps protect the woman against some vaginal infections, but increased glycogen may contribute to higher rates of vaginal candidiasis (see p. 454).

Early in pregnancy, the uterus loses the firmness and resistance of the nonpregnant organ. The palpable softening at the isthmus, called *Hegar's sign*, is an early diagnostic sign of pregnancy, and is illustrated on the right.

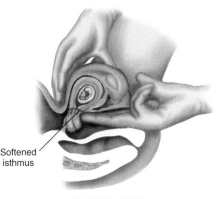

Softened isthmus

HEGAR'S SIGN

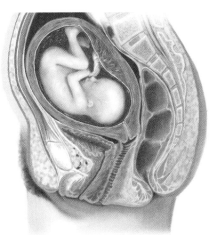

SECOND TRIMESTER

With advancing pregnancy, uterine weight increases from 50 to 70 grams to 800 to 1200 grams, and its volume expands from approximately 10 ml to 5 liters. Contributing to these changes are muscle cell hypertrophy, more extensive fibrous and elastic tissue, and considerable increases in the size and number of blood vessels and lymphatics.

As the uterus grows, it changes shape and position. The nongravid uterus may be anteverted, retroverted, or retroflexed. Until up to 12 weeks of gestation, the gravid uterus is still a pelvic organ. Regardless of its initial posi-

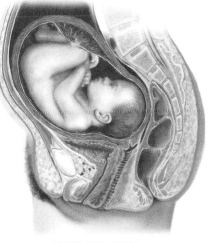

THIRD TRIMESTER

tioning, the enlarging uterus becomes anteverted and quickly fills space usually occupied by the bladder, triggering frequent voiding. By 12 weeks' gestation, the uterus straightens and rises out of the pelvis and can be felt when palpating the abdomen.

The enlarging uterus pushes the intestinal contents laterally and superiorly and stretches its supporting ligaments, sometimes causing "round ligament pain" in the lower quadrants, more typically on the right. The uterus adapts to fetal growth and positions, and tends to rotate to the right to accommodate to the rectosigmoid structures on the left side of the pelvis.

The cervix also looks and feels quite different. *Chadwick's sign,* the early softening and cyanosis of the cervix, continues throughout pregnancy. The cervical canal fills with a tenacious *mucous plug,* thought to protect the developing fetus from infection. Red velvety mucosa, termed *cervical erosion* or *eversion,* also commonly appears on the cervix and is considered normal.

The ovaries and fallopian tubes undergo changes as well, but few are noticeable during physical examination. Early in pregnancy, the *corpus luteum,* the ovarian follicle that has discharged its ovum, may be sufficiently prominent to be felt on the affected ovary as a small nodule, but it disappears by mid-pregnancy.

As the skin over the abdomen stretches to adapt to the growing fetus, purplish striae may appear, and a *linea nigra,* a brownish black pigmented line along the midline may become visible.

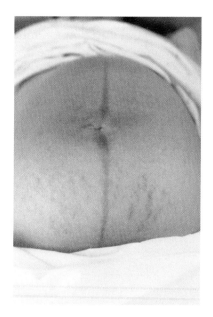

As muscle tone diminishes with advancing pregnancy, the rectus abdominis muscles may separate at the midline, termed *diastasis recti.* If diastasis is severe, as in some multiparous women, only a layer of skin, fascia, and peritoneum covers most of the anterior uterine wall. The fetus is easily palpable through this muscular gap.[7]

The anatomy and physiology of common concerns in pregnancy are provided in the following table.

■ Common Concerns During Pregnancy and Their Explanations

Common Concerns	Time in Pregnancy	Explanation
No menses (*amenorrhea*)	Throughout	Continued high levels of estrogen, progesterone, and human chorionic gonadotropin following fertilization of the ovum build up the endometrium to support the developing pregnancy, averting menses and shedding of the endometrial lining.
Nausea with or without vomiting	1st trimester	Possible causes include hormonal changes of pregnancy leading to slowed peristalsis throughout the GI tract, changes in taste and smell, the growing uterus, or emotional factors. Women may have a modest (2–5 lb) weight loss in the first trimester.[8]
Breast tenderness, tingling	1st trimester	The hormones of pregnancy stimulate the growth of breast tissue. As the breasts enlarge throughout pregnancy, women may experience upper backache from their increased weight. There is also increased blood flow throughout the breasts, and delicate veins become visible beneath the skin.
Weight loss	1st trimester	If a woman experiences nausea and vomiting, she may not be eating normally in early pregnancy (see nausea above).
Groin/lower abdominal pain	2nd trimester: 14–20 weeks	Rapid uterine growth early in second trimester causes tension and stretching of round ligaments, causing spasm with sudden movement or change of position.
Urinary frequency	1st/3rd trimesters	There is increased blood volume and increased filtration rate in the kidneys with increased urine production. As a result of less space for the bladder from pressure from the growing uterus (first trimester) or from the descent of the fetal head (third trimester), the woman needs to empty her bladder more frequently.
Fatigue	1st/3rd trimesters	Rapid change in energy requirements; hormonal changes (progesterone has a sedative effect); in third trimester, weight gain, changes in mechanics of movement, and sleep disturbances contribute.
Edema	3rd trimester	There is increased venous pressure in the legs, obstruction of lymphatic flow, and reduced plasma colloid osmotic pressure.
Heartburn, constipation	Throughout	Relaxation of the lower esophageal sphincter allows stomach contents to back up into the lower esophagus. The decreased GI motility caused by pregnancy hormones slows peristalsis and causes constipation. Constipation may cause or aggravate existing hemorrhoids.
Backache	Throughout	Hormonally induced relaxation of joints and ligaments and the minor lordosis required to balance the growing uterus sometimes result in a lower backache. Pathologic causes must be ruled out.
Leukorrhea	Throughout	Increased secretions from the cervix and the vaginal epithelium, due to the hormones and vasocongestion of pregnancy, result in an asymptomatic milky white vaginal discharge.

THE HEALTH HISTORY

Common Concerns

- Symptoms of pregnancy
- Smoking, alcohol, use of illicit drugs, domestic violence
- Prior complications of pregnancy
- Chronic illnesses and family history
- Determining weeks of gestation by date and expected date of delivery

Focus prenatal care on providing optimal health for mother and baby over the course of pregnancy, while minimizing risk to the mother. During the *initial prenatal visit,* your goals will be threefold: confirming the pregnancy, assessing the health status of the mother and any risks for complications, and counseling to ensure a healthy pregnancy.

- Ask about *symptoms of pregnancy:* absence of menses, breast fullness or tenderness, nausea or vomiting, fatigue, and urinary frequency (see table on p. 821). Explain that serum or urine testing for beta HCG offers the best confirmation of pregnancy.

- Assess the *current state of health* and any risk factors that could adversely affect the mother or fetus or cause any complications during the pregnancy. Review the mother's attitude toward the pregnancy, and if she plans to continue to term. Ask about her eating patterns and assess the quality of her nutrition. Does she smoke, drink alcohol, or use any illicit drugs? Does she take any medications? Or have any exposures to toxic substances? What about her income and her social support network? Are there any sources of unusual stress at home or in the workplace? Is there any history of physical abuse or domestic violence?

- Assess the *past obstetric history.* What about prior pregnancies because past obstetric problems tend to recur? Has she had any past complications during labor and delivery? Ask about the birth weights of prior children. Has she had a premature or growth-retarded infant, or a baby large for gestational age? Also, has there been a prior fetal demise?

- Ask about the *past medical history.* A thorough inquiry into acute or chronic illnesses in the major organ systems is in order. Ask especially about hypertension, diabetes, cardiac conditions, asthma, systemic lupus erythematosis (SLE), seizures, and any history of sexually transmitted diseases, exposure to diethylstilbestrol in utero, or HIV infection.

- Also review any *family history* of chronic illnesses or genetically transmitted diseases such as sickle cell anemia, cystic fibrosis, or muscular dystrophy.

You will need to elicit features of the current pregnancy that enable you to calculate the *expected weeks of gestation by dates* and the *expected date of delivery* (EDD). To establish *expected weeks of gestation,* count in weeks from either (1) the first day of the last menstrual period (LMP), known as *menstrual age;* or (2) the date of conception if this is known, or *conception age.* Menstrual age is the most frequently used method of calculation. The expected weeks of gestation can help with later assessment of uterine size, but this assumes that the LMP was normal, the dates were remembered accurately, and conception actually occurred. During the examination, you will compare your estimate of expected uterine size with the palpable size of the uterus if still within the pelvic cavity, or by the height of the fundus if above the symphysis pubis. If there are discrepancies, you will need to investigate possible causes.

The first day of the LMP is also used to calculate the *expected date of delivery,* or the time projected to term labor and delivery assuming regular 28- to 30-day menstrual cycles. Using *Naegele's rule,* estimate the EDD by adding 7 days to the first day of the LMP, subtract 3 months, and add 1 year. This date may be one of the first questions the mother asks you.

Accurate dating of the pregnancy is best done early and improves decision making in the event of later delays in fetal growth, preterm labor, or pregnancy beyond 42 weeks of gestation. If the patient cannot remember her LMP or has irregular menstrual cycles, or if the dating is uncertain, vaginal probe ultrasound is used to confirm dating in the first trimester.

Establish the desired frequency of *follow-up visits* based on the patient's needs. These visits will include measurement of blood pressure and weight, palpation of the uterine fundus to assess fetal growth, verification of fetal heart tones, and determination of fetal presentation and activity. Many clinicians also check for urinary protein and glucose. Additional laboratory tests will be needed in the second and third trimesters.

HEALTH PROMOTION AND COUNSELING

Important Topics for Health Promotion and Counseling

- Nutrition
- Weight gain
- Exercise
- Smoking cessation
- Screening for domestic violence

Counseling about *nutrition* and *weight gain* helps protect the health of the pregnant woman and baby. Evaluate the nutritional status of the mother during the first prenatal visit, including a diet history; measurement of height, weight, and body mass index (BMI); and a hematocrit to screen for anemia. Be sure to explore the mother's habits and attitudes about eating and weight gain, as well as her use of needed vitamin and mineral supplements. Develop a nutrition plan appropriate to the woman's cultural preferences. Three meals each day consisting of a balanced diet with increased intake of calories and protein are generally sufficient. Advise the pregnant woman to increase her diet each day by the following amounts: 300 additional kilocalories; 5 to 6 grams of protein; 15 milligrams of iron; 250 mg of calcium; and 400 to 800 micrograms of folic acid.[9] Determine whether prenatal multivitamin and mineral supplements are warranted because of inadequate diet or conditions such as multiple gestation, smoking, or vegetarian diet. At the same time, counsel the pregnant woman to beware of ingesting excess amounts of vitamin A, which can become toxic; fish with mercury exposure such as sharks, swordfish, or even canned tuna; caffeine, which increases risk for spontaneous abortion; unpasteurized dairy products; and undercooked meats.[10]

Ideal weight gain during pregnancy follows a pattern: very little gain the first trimester, rapid increase in the second trimester, and mild slowing of the increase in the third trimester. Average weight gain is approximately 28 lbs, or approximately 10 kilograms. Women should be weighed at each visit, with the results plotted on a graph for the patient and provider to review and discuss. Recommended weight gain ranges from the Institute of Medicine (1992), displayed below, are still current.

■ *Recommended Total Weight Gain Ranges for Pregnant Women*		
Prepregnancy Weight-for-Height Category	**Recommended Total Gain**	
	lbs	*kg*
Low—BMI <19.8	28–40	12.5–18
Normal—BMI 19.8 to 26.0	25–35	11.5–16
High—BMI 26.0 to 29.0	15–25	7.0–11.5
Obese—BMI >29.0	~15	~7.0

Figures are for single pregnancies. The range for women carrying twins is 35 to 45 lb (16 to 20 kg). Young adolescents (<2 years after menarche) should strive for gains at the upper end of the range. Short women (<62 in or <157 cm) should strive for gains at the lower end of the range.

(Source: Institute of Medicine. Nutrition During Pregnancy and Lactation: An Implementation Guideline. Washington, DC, National Academy Press, 1992.)

Exercise is important to the health and lifestyle of pregnant women. The 2002 guidelines for the American College of Obstetricians and Gynecologists recommend that in conjunction with their physician, and in the absence of contraindications, pregnant women should engage in moderate exercise for

30 minutes or more on most days of the week.[11] Women exercising regularly before pregnancy can continue mild to moderate exercise, preferably for short periods three times a week. Women initiating exercise during pregnancy should be more cautious, and consider programs developed specifically for pregnant women. After the first trimester, women should avoid exercise in the supine position, which can compress the inferior vena cava and decrease blood flow to the placenta. The pregnant woman should stop exercise when she feels fatigued or uncomfortable and avoid overheating and dehydration. Because the center of gravity shifts in the third trimester, advise her that exercises that could cause loss of balance are unwise.

Any *smoking* should be discontinued. Smoking has been linked to complications of labor such as placental abruption and placenta previa, and to preterm deliveries, low-birthweight babies, and even perinatal death.

Pregnancy may be a time when women are more likely to be abused by an intimate partner or when patterns of abuse may intensify, increasing the risk for delayed prenatal care, miscarriage, and low-birthweight babies. The prevalence of abuse during pregnancy ranges from 7% to 20%, depending on the setting, and may result in femicide, or murder of the mother and child.[12,13] The American College of Obstetricians and Gynecologists recommends universal assessment of all women for any history of *domestic violence* that may escalate during the pregnancy.[14,15] Clues to domestic violence include frequent changes in appointments at the last minute, behavior during the interview, chronic headache or abdominal pain, and bruises and other signs of injury.

Clinicians can overcome barriers to screening by adopting direct questioning in a nonjudgmental manner in a private setting at each prenatal visit.[16,17] For example, you may ask "Since you've been pregnant, have you been hit or slapped or otherwise physically hurt by anyone?" Women may need multiple opportunities to discuss abuse because of fears about safety and reprisal. Validate positive responses and mark the area of injury on a body diagram. Above all, in situations of admitted abuse, ask the woman how you might help her. Offer information on safe shelters, counseling centers, hotline telephone numbers, and other sources of assistance when she is ready to pursue these. Assess the patient's safety and make any necessary referrals. Learn about any requirements for mandatory reporting.

NATIONAL DOMESTIC VIOLENCE HOTLINE

- Website: www.ncvh.org/index.html
- 1-800-799-SAFE (7233)
- TTY for hearing impaired: 1-800-787-3224

TECHNIQUES OF EXAMINATION

As you begin the examination, show respect for the patient's comfort and need for privacy and for her individual needs and sensitivities. If this is a first visit, take the history before asking her to change into a gown. Ask if she has ever had a complete pelvic examination. If not, take the time to explain what is involved and seek her cooperation with each of its components. This will strengthen rapport and help her understand the changes in her body in response to pregnancy. Note that if she has ever experienced a sexual assault, this may lead her to resist the examination of the pelvis.

Now instruct her to put on the gown with the opening in the front. This will ease examination of the breasts and the pregnant abdomen. Have the needed equipment readily at hand.

Positioning.   Take a few minutes to adjust the positioning of the pregnant woman because you will need to give added time and attention to palpating the uterus and listening to the fetal heart. The semi-sitting position with the knees bent, as shown below, affords the greatest comfort and reduces the weight of the gravid uterus on the abdominal organs and vessels, especially in the later trimesters.

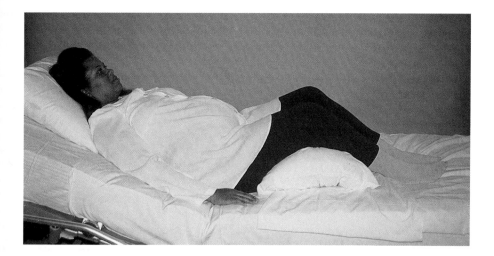

Avoid asking the pregnant woman to spend prolonged periods lying on her back. In this position, the uterus lies directly on the woman's vertebral column and may compress the descending aorta and inferior vena cava, interfering with the return of venous blood from the lower extremities and the pelvic vessels. Therefore, make your abdominal palpation efficient in time and results.

Encourage the woman to sit again briefly before proceeding to the pelvic evaluation. This pause also provides time for the woman to empty her bladder again. However, make sure that she is acclimated to sitting before allow-

Supine hypotensive syndrome after approximately 20 weeks is a form of this diminished circulation and may lead the woman to feel dizzy and faint, especially when lying down.

ing her to stand up. The pelvic examination should likewise be relatively quick. All other examination procedures should be done in the sitting or left-side–lying position.

Equipment.   The examiner's hands are the primary means of examination. They should be warm and firm, yet gentle in palpation. Whenever possible the fingers should be together and flat against the abdominal or pelvic tissue to minimize discomfort. Likewise, all touching and palpation should be done with smooth continuous contact against the skin rather than kneading or abrupt motion. The palmar surfaces of the ends of the fingers are the most sensitive.

The gynecologic speculum is used for inspecting the cervix and the vagina before taking specimens for cytologic or bacteriologic study. Because the vaginal walls are relaxed during pregnancy and may fall medially, obscuring your view, a speculum of larger than expected size may be needed. The relaxation of perineal and vulvar structures minimizes any discomfort. Because of the increased vascularity of the vaginal and cervical structures, insert and open the speculum gently. This will help avoid tissue trauma and bleeding, which interfere with the interpretation of Pap smears.

The Ayre wooden spatula or cotton-tipped applicator is generally used to obtain the Pap smear. In pregnant women, the cervical brush may cause bleeding.

Review Chapter 12 for instruments and techniques used to take cervical smears (pp. 441–445).

GENERAL INSPECTION

Observe the overall health, emotional state, nutritional status, and neuromuscular coordination as the woman walks into the room and climbs on the examination table. Discussion of the woman's priorities for the examination, her responses to pregnancy, and her general health provide useful information and help to put the woman at ease.

VITAL SIGNS, HEIGHT, AND WEIGHT

Take the blood pressure. A baseline reading helps to determine the woman's usual range. In midpregnancy, blood pressure is normally lower than in the nonpregnant state.

Gestational hypertension is systolic blood pressure (SBP) ≥ 140 and diastolic blood pressure (DBP) ≥ 90, first occurring after week 20 and *without proteinuria.*

Chronic hypertension is SBP ≥ 140 and DBP ≥ 90 before pregnancy, before week 20, and after 12 weeks postpartum.

Preeclampsia is SBP ≥ 140 and DBP ≥ 90 after week 20 and *with proteinuria.*[18]

Measure the height and weight. Calculate the BMI using standard tables and considering 19 to 25 as normal for the prepregnant state (see p. 91).

Note that first-trimester weight loss related to nausea and vomiting is common but should not exceed 5% of prepartum weight.

Weight loss of more than 5% during the first trimester may be due to excessive vomiting, or *hyperemesis*.[19]

HEAD AND NECK

Stand facing the seated woman and observe the head and neck, including the following features:

- *Face.* The mask of pregnancy, *chloasma,* is normal. It consists of irregular brownish patches around the forehead and cheeks, across the nose, or along the jaw.

  Facial edema after 24 weeks of gestation may suggest gestational hypertension.

- *Hair,* including texture, moisture, and distribution. Dryness, oiliness, and sometimes minor generalized hair loss may be noted.

  Localized patches of hair loss should not be attributed to pregnancy (though hair loss is common postpartum).

- *Eyes.* Note the conjunctival color.

  Anemia of pregnancy may cause pallor.

- *Nose,* including the mucous membranes and the septum. Nasal congestion is common during pregnancy.

  Nosebleeds are more common during pregnancy. The nasal septum can show signs of cocaine use.

- *Mouth,* especially the gums and teeth.

  Gingival enlargement with bleeding (p. 235) is common during pregnancy.

- *Thyroid gland.* Inspect and palpate the gland. Modest symmetric enlargement is expected.[15]

  Significant enlargement is abnormal and should be investigated.

THORAX AND LUNGS

Inspect the thorax for contours and pattern of breathing. Elevation of the diaphragms and an increase in chest diameter may be seen as early as the first trimester. Tidal volume and alveolar minute ventilation increase, but respiratory rate remains constant. These changes sometimes lead to subjective complaints of shortness of breath. Expect a respiratory alkalosis.[20]

Pursue complaints of dyspnea accompanied by cough or respiratory distress for possible infection, asthma, or pulmonary embolus.

HEART

Palpate the apical impulse. In advanced pregnancy, it may be slightly higher than normal in the 4th intercostal space, because of transverse and leftward rotation of the heart from the higher diaphragm.

Auscultate the heart. A venous hum and systolic or continuous mammary souffle (see p. 335) are common during pregnancy, reflecting increased blood flow in normal vessels.[21] Listen for a mammary souffle (pronounced *soo-fl*), late in pregnancy and during lactation. It is most easily heard in the second or third interspace in the parasternal areas and is typically both systolic and diastolic. Only the systolic component may be audible.

Murmurs may also accompany anemia. New diastolic murmurs should be investigated.

BREASTS

Inspect the breasts and nipples for symmetry and color. The venous pattern may be marked, the nipples and areolae are dark, and Montgomery's glands are prominent.

An inverted nipple needs attention if breast-feeding is planned.

Palpate for masses. During pregnancy, breasts are tender and nodular.

A pathologic mass may be difficult to isolate.

Compress each nipple between your index finger and thumb. This maneuver may express colostrum from the nipples.

A bloody or purulent discharge should not be attributed to pregnancy.

ABDOMEN

Position the pregnant woman in a semi-sitting position with her knees flexed (see p. 826).

Inspect any scars or striae, the shape and contour of the abdomen, and the fundal height. Purplish striae and linea nigra are normal in pregnancy. The shape and contour may indicate pregnancy size (see figures on p. 819).

Scars may confirm the type of prior surgery, especially cesarean section.

Palpate the abdomen for:

■ *Organs or masses.* The mass of pregnancy is expected.

■ *Fetal movements.* These can usually be felt by the examiner after 24 weeks (and by the mother at 18–20 weeks).

If movements cannot be felt after 24 weeks, consider error in calculating gestation, fetal death or morbidity, or false pregnancy.

■ *Uterine contractility.* Irregular uterine contractions occur after 12 weeks, and often in response to palpation during the third trimester. The abdomen then feels tense or firm to the examiner, and it is difficult to feel fetal parts. If the hand is left resting on the fundal portion of the uterus, the fingers will sense the relaxation of the uterine muscle.

Before 37 weeks, regular uterine contractions with or without pain or bleeding are abnormal, suggesting preterm labor.

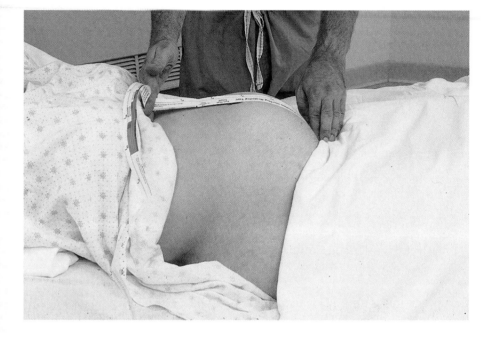

Measure the fundal height with a tape measure if the woman is more than 20 weeks' pregnant. Holding the tape as illustrated and following the midline of the abdomen, measure from the top of the symphysis pubis to the top of the uterine fundus. Although subject to error, for weeks 20 to 32, measurement in centimeters should roughly equal the weeks of gestation.[22,23]

If fundal height is more than 4 cm higher than expected, consider multiple gestation, a big baby, extra amniotic fluid, or uterine leiomyoma. If it is lower than expected by more than 4 cm, consider missed abortion, transverse lie, growth retardation, or false pregnancy.

Auscultate the fetal heart, noting its rate (FHR), location, and rhythm. A doptone will detect the FHR after approximately 10 weeks. The FHR is audible with a fetoscope after approximately 18 weeks, although this instrument is now used less commonly.

Lack of an audible fetal heart may indicate pregnancy of fewer weeks than expected, fetal demise, or false pregnancy.

Palpate the *left and right adnexa*. The corpus luteum may feel like a small nodule on the affected ovary during the first few weeks after conception. Late in pregnancy, adnexal masses may be difficult to feel.

Early in pregnancy, it is important to rule out a tubal (*ectopic*) pregnancy. See Table 12-9, Adnexal Masses, p. 457.

Palpate for *pelvic muscle strength* as you withdraw your examining fingers.

Do a *rectovaginal examination* if you need to confirm uterine size or the integrity of the rectovaginal septum. A pregnancy of less than 10 weeks in a retroverted and retroflexed uterus lies totally in the posterior pelvis. Only this examination confirms its size.

EXTREMITIES

General inspection may be done with the woman seated or lying on her left side.

Inspect the legs for *varicose veins*.

Varicose veins may begin or worsen during pregnancy.

Inspect the hands and legs for *edema*. Palpate for pretibial, ankle, and pedal edema. Edema is rated on a 0 to 4+ scale. Physiologic edema is more common in advanced pregnancy, during hot weather, and in women who stand for long periods.

Check knee and ankle *reflexes*.

SPECIAL TECHNIQUES

MODIFIED LEOPOLD'S MANEUVERS

These maneuvers are important adjuncts to palpation of the pregnant abdomen beginning at 28 weeks of gestation. They help determine where the fetus is lying in relation to the woman's back (longitudinal or transverse), what end of the fetus is presenting at the pelvic inlet (head or buttocks), where the fetal back is located, how far the presenting part of the fetus has descended into the maternal pelvis, and the estimated weight of the fetus. This information is necessary to assess the adequacy of fetal growth and the probability of successful vaginal birth.

Interpretation
Common deviations include *breech presentation* (the fetal buttocks presenting at the outlet of the maternal pelvis) and absence of the presenting part well down into the maternal pelvis at term. Neither situation necessarily precludes vaginal birth. The most serious findings are a *transverse lie* close to term and slowed fetal growth that could represent *intrauterine growth retardation (IUGR)*.

First Maneuver (Upper Pole). Stand at the woman's side facing her head. Keeping the fingers of both examining hands together, palpate gently with the fingertips to determine what part of the fetus is in the upper pole of the uterine fundus.

The fetal buttocks are usually at the upper pole. They feel firm but irregular, and less globular than the head. The fetal head feels firm, round, and smooth.

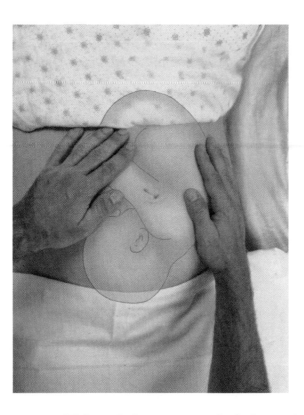

Second Maneuver (Sides of the Maternal Abdomen). Place one hand on each side of the woman's abdomen, aiming to capture the body of the fetus between them. Use one hand to steady the uterus and the other to palpate the fetus.

The hand on the fetal back feels a smooth, firm surface the length of the hand (or longer) by 32 weeks of gestation. The hand on the fetal arms and legs feels irregular bumps, and also perhaps kicking if the fetus is awake and active.

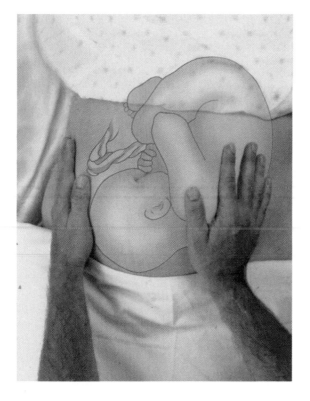

Third Maneuver (Lower Pole). Turn and face the woman's feet. Using the flat palmar surfaces of the fingers of both hands and, at the start, touching the fingertips together, palpate the area just above the symphysis pubis. Note whether the hands diverge with downward pressure or stay together. This tells you whether or not the presenting part of the fetus, head or buttocks, is descending into the pelvic inlet.

If the fetal head is presenting, the fingers feel a smooth, firm, rounded surface on both sides.

If the hands diverge, the presenting part is descending into the pelvic inlet, as illustrated.

If the hands stay together and you can gently depress the tissue over the bladder without touching the fetus, the presenting part is above your hands.

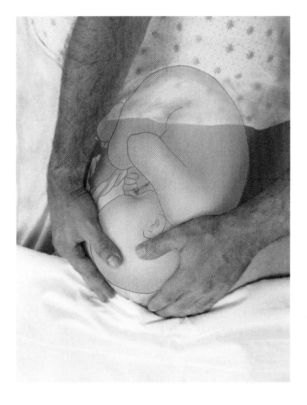

If the presenting fetal part is descending, palpate its texture and firmness. If not, gently move your hands up the lower abdomen and capture the presenting part between your hands.

The fetal head feels smooth, firm, and rounded; the buttocks, firm but irregular.

Fourth Maneuver (Confirmation of the Presenting Part).   With your dominant hand, grasp the part of the fetus in the lower pole, and with your nondominant hand, the part of the fetus in the upper pole. With this maneuver, you may be able to distinguish between the head and the buttocks.

The head is usually in the lower pole, and the fetal buttocks are in the upper pole. If the head is above the pelvic inlet, it moves somewhat independently of the rest of the fetal body.

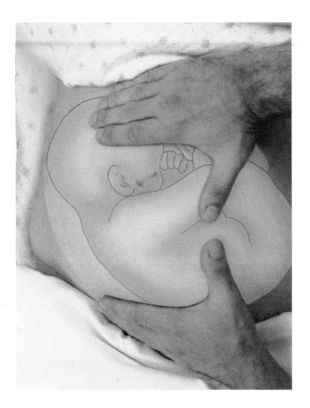

CONCLUDING THE VISIT

Once you have completed the examination and the woman is dressed, review your findings with her. If further data are necessary to confirm pregnancy, discuss next steps for obtaining them. Reinforce the importance of prenatal care. Record all your findings on the prenatal record.

RECORDING YOUR FINDINGS

Note that initially you may use sentences to describe your findings; later you will use phrases. The style below contains phrases appropriate for most write-ups.

Recording the Physical Examination— The Pregnant Woman

"*Abdomen*: No surgical scars. Active bowel sounds. Soft, nontender; no palpable hepatosplenomegaly or masses. Fundus palpable 2 fingerbreadths below the umbilicus; shape is ovoid and smooth. Fetal heart rate 144. No inguinal adenopathy. *External genitalia*: midline episiotomy scar present. No lesions, discharge, or signs of infection. Bimanual examination: cervix midline, soft; external os admits fingertip, internal os closed. No pain elicited on movement of cervix; no adnexal masses. Fundus enlarged to 20 weeks' size, midline, smooth; vaginal tone reduced."

OR

"*Abdomen*: Low transverse surgical scar. Active bowel sounds. Soft, nontender; no palpable hepatosplenomegaly or masses. Fundus: barely palpable above symphysis pubis. Fetal heart rate not heard. No inguinal adenopathy. *Bimanual examination*: cervix midline, soft, internal os closed. No pain on movement of cervix. Right ovary palpable, left nonpalpable; no other adnexal masses. Fundus anteverted, enlarged to 14–16 weeks' size; moderate vaginal tone."

Describes examination of healthy pregnant woman at 16 weeks' gestation, third pregnancy

Describes examination of healthy pregnant woman reporting dates of 20-week gestation but with examination consistent with 14-week gestation

Bibliography

CITATIONS

1. Petraglia F, D'Antona Donato D. Maternal endocrine and metabolic adaptation to pregnancy. Available at www.utdol.com. Accessed December 17, 2004.
2. Berghout A, Wiersinga W. Thyroid size and function during pregnancy: an analysis. Eur J Endocrinol 138:536–542, 1998.
3. Boden G. Fuel metabolism in pregnancy and in gestational diabetes mellitus. Obstet Gynecol Clin North Am 23:1–10, 1996.
4. Mazjoub JA, McGregor JA, Lockwood CJ, et al. A central theory of preterm and term labor: putative role for corticotrophin-releasing hormone. Am J Obstet Gynecol 180:S232–S241, 1999.
5. Andersen HF, Johnson TR, Barclay ML, et al. Gestational age assessment. I. Analysis of individual clinical observations. Am J Obstet Gynecol 139(2):173–177, 1981.
6. Hillier SL, Krohn MA, Rabe LK, et al. The normal vaginal flora, H2O2-producing lactobacilli, and bacterial vaginosis in pregnant women. Clin Infect Dis 16(Suppl 4):S273–S281, 1994.
7. Boisonnault JS, Blaschak MJ. Incidence of diastasis rectus abdominis during the childbearing year. Phys Ther 68(7): 1082–1086, 1988.
8. American College of Obstetricians and Gynecologists (ACOG). Nausea and vomiting of pregnancy. Practice Bulletin No. 52. Obstet Gynecol 104(4):803–814, 2004.
9. Institute of Medicine. Nutrition during Pregnancy and Lactation: An Implementation Guideline, p. 14. Washington, DC: National Academy Press, 1992.
10. Gillen-Goldstein J, Funai EF, Roque H. Nutrition in pregnancy. Available at www.utdol.com. Accessed December 19, 2004.
11. American College of Obstetrics and Gynecology (ACOG). Exercise during pregnancy and the postpartum period. ACOG Committee Opinion, No. 267, January 2002.

12. Gazmararian JA, Lazorick S, Spitz AM, et al. Prevalence of violence against pregnant women. JAMA 275:1915–1920, 1996.

13. Martin SL, Mackie L, Kupper LL, et al. Physical abuse of women before, during, and after pregnancy. JAMA 85(12):1581–1584, 2001.

14. American College of Obstetrics and Gynecology (ACOG). Psychosocial risk factors: perinatal screening and intervention. No. 255, 1999.

15. American College of Obstetricians and Gynecologists (ACOG). Guidelines for Women's Health Care, 2nd ed. Washington, DC, ACOG, 2002.

16. Elliott L, Nerney M, Jones T, et al. Barriers to screening for domestic violence. J Gen Intern Med 17:112–116, 2002.

17. Friedman LS, Samet JH, Roberts MS, et al. Inquiry about victimization experiences: a survey of patient preferences and physician practices. Arch Intern Med 152:1186–1190, 1992.

18. American College of Obstetrics and Gynecology (ACOG). Chronic hypertension in pregnancy. No. 29. Obstet Gynecol 98(1):S177–S185, 2001.

19. Goodwin TM, Montoro M, Mestman JH. Transient hyperthyroidism and hyperemesis gravidarum: clinical aspects. Am J Obstet Gynecol 167(3):648–652, 1992.

20. Elkus R, Popovich J. Respiratory physiology in pregnancy. Clin Chest Med 13:555–565, 1992.

21. Foley MR. Maternal cardiovascular adaptation to pregnancy. Available at: www.updol.com. Accessed December 16, 2004.

22. Belizan JM, Villar J, Nardin JC, et al. Diagnosis of intrauterine growth retardation by a simple clinical method: measurement of uterine height. Am J Obstet Gynecol 131(6):643–646, 1978.

23. Persson B, Stangenberg M, Lunell NO, et al. Prediction of size of infants at birth by measurement of symphysis fundus height. Br J Obstet Gynaecol 93(3):206–211, 1986.

ADDITIONAL REFERENCES

American Diabetes Association. Preconception care of women with diabetes. Diabetes Care 25(suppl 1):S82–S84, 2002.

Cunningham FG, Williams JW. Williams Obstetrics, 22nd ed. New York, McGraw-Hill, Medical Pub Division, 2005.

Enkin M. A Guide to Effective Care in Pregnancy and Childbirth, 3rd ed. New York, Oxford University Press, 2000.

Fraser DC, Cooper MA, Myles MF. Myles Textbook for Midwives, 14th ed. New York, Churchill Livingstone, 2003.

Gabbe SG, Graves CR. Management of diabetes mellitus complicating pregnancy. Obstet Gynecol 102(4):857–868, 2003.

Kirkham C, Harris S, Grzybowski S. Evidence-based prenatal care: Part I. General prenatal care and counseling issues. Am Fam Physician 71(7):1307–1316, 2005.

Pick ME, Edwards M, Moreau D, et al. Assessment of diet quality in pregnant women using the Healthy Eating Index. J Am Diet Assoc 105(2):240–246, 2005.

Read JS, American Academy of Pediatrics Committee on Pediatric AIDS. Human milk, breastfeeding, and transmission of human immunodeficiency virus type 1 in the United States. American Academy of Pediatrics Committee on Pediatric AIDS. Pediatrics 112(5):1196–1205, 2003.

United Nations Population Fund (UNFPA). A practical approach to gender-based violence: a programme guide for health care providers and managers. New York, UNFPA, 2001.

Varney, HK, Kriebs JM, Gegor CL. Varney's Midwifery, 4th ed. Sudbury, MA, Jones and Bartlett Publishers, 2004.

Villar J, Bergsjo P. Scientific basis for the content of routine antenatal care. I. Philosophy, recent studies, and power to eliminate or alleviate adverse maternal outcomes. Acta Obstet Gynecol Scand 76:1–14, 1997.

Wisner KL, Parry BL, Piontek CM. Postpartum depression. N Engl J Med 347(3):194–199, 2002.

The Older Adult

Older adults now number more than 25 million people in the United States and are expected to reach 80 million by 2050.[1] These seniors will live longer than previous generations: life span at birth is currently 79 years for women and 74 years for men. Those older than 85 years are projected to increase to 5% of the U.S. population within 40 years. Hence, the "demographic imperative" is to maximize not only the life span but also the "health span" of our older population, so that seniors maintain full function for as long as possible, enjoying rich and active lives in their homes and communities.

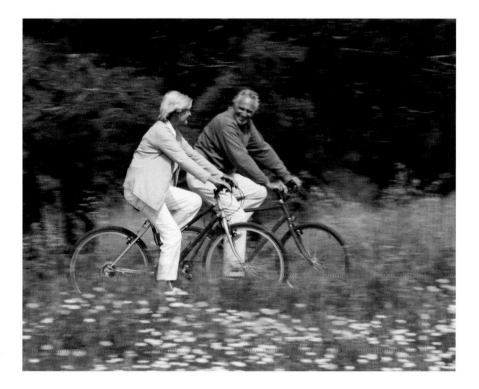

Clinicians now recognize frailty as one of society's common myths about aging—more than 95% of Americans older than 65 years live in the community, and only 5% reside in long-term care facilities.[1,2] Over the past 20 years, seniors actually have become more active and less disabled. These changes call for new goals for clinical care—"an informed activated patient interacting with a prepared proactive team, resulting in high quality satisfying encounters and improved outcomes"[3]—and a distinct set of clinical attitudes and skills.

Assessing the older adult presents special opportunities and special challenges. Many of these are quite different from the disease-oriented approach of history taking and physical examination for younger patients: the focus on healthy or "successful" aging; the need to understand and mobilize family, social, and community supports; the importance of skills directed to functional assessment, "the sixth vital sign"; and the opportunities for promoting the older adult's long-term health and safety.

In this chapter, we review the physiologic changes of aging in *Anatomy and Physiology*, as well as the heterogeneity of the aging process and the challenges of distinguishing normal from abnormal physical findings. Then follows *The Health History*, which begins with the Approach to the Patient. This section discusses how to adjust the office environment and adapt the content and pace of the interview to the older patient; the varying meanings and significance of symptoms in older adults, especially when linked to one of the geriatric syndromes; and the cultural dimensions of aging. The next section, Special Areas of Concern when Assessing Common or Concerning Symptoms, explores the importance of assessing activities of daily living, medications, nutrition, acute and chronic pain, lifestyle behaviors such as alcohol use and smoking, and advance directives and palliative care. *Health Promotion and Counseling* provides guidelines for health screening in older adults, including recommendations for topics such as vision and hearing, exercise, immunizations, household safety, cancer, depression, dementia, and elder mistreatment. *Techniques of Examination* discusses Functional Assessment: The "Sixth Vital Sign," and provides an efficient tool for office evaluation, the 10-Minute Geriatric Screener. Then follows the Physical Examination of the Older Adult, which builds on the techniques you already have learned for physical examinations in general, but highlights special aspects for older patients when surveying general appearance, measuring vital signs, and completing each regional examination. *Recording Your Findings* contains a sample of the written history and physical examination of the older adult.

ANATOMY AND PHYSIOLOGY

Primary aging reflects changes in physiologic reserves over time that are independent of and not induced by any disease. These changes are especially likely to appear during periods of stress, such as exposure to fluctuating temperatures, dehydration, or even shock. Decreased cutaneous vasoconstriction and sweat production can impair responses to heat; declines in thirst may delay recovery from dehydration; and the physiologic drops in maximum cardiac output, left ventricular filling, and maximum heart rate seen with aging may impair the response to shock.

At the same time, the aging population displays marked heterogeneity. Investigators have identified vast differences in how people age and have distinguished "usual" aging, with its complex of diseases and impairments, from "successful" aging. "Successful aging" occurs in those people who escape debilitating disease entirely and maintain healthy lives late into their 80s and 90s. Studies of centenarians show that genes account for approximately 20% of the probability of living to 100, with healthy lifestyles accounting for approximately 20% to 30%.[4–6]

These findings provide compelling evidence for promoting optimal nutrition, strength training and exercise, and daily function for older adults to delay unnecessary depletion of physiologic reserves.

Vital Signs

Blood Pressure.   In Western societies, systolic blood pressure tends to rise from childhood through old age. The aorta and large arteries stiffen and become atherosclerotic. As the aorta becomes less distensible, a given stroke volume causes a greater rise in systolic blood pressure; *systolic hypertension* with a *widened pulse pressure* often ensue. Diastolic blood pressure stops rising at about the sixth decade. At the other extreme, some elderly people develop a tendency toward *postural (orthostatic) hypotension*—a sudden drop in blood pressure when they rise to standing.

Heart Rate and Rhythm.   In older adults, resting heart rate remains unchanged, but pacemaker cells decline in the sinoatrial node, as does maximal heart rate, affecting response to physiologic stress.[7]

Elderly people are more likely to have abnormal heart rhythms such as atrial or ventricular ectopy. Asymptomatic rhythm changes are generally benign. Like postural hypotension, however, they may cause *syncope,* or temporary loss of consciousness.

Respiratory Rate and Temperature.   Respiratory rate is unchanged, but changes in temperature regulation lead to susceptibility to *hypothermia.*

Skin, Nails, and Hair.
With age, the skin wrinkles, becomes lax, and loses turgor. The vascularity of the dermis decreases, causing lighter skin to look paler and more opaque. Skin on the backs of the hands and forearms appears thin, fragile, loose, and transparent. There may be purple patches or macules, termed *actinic purpura,* that fade over time. These spots and patches come from blood that has leaked through poorly supported capillaries and spread within the dermis.

Nails lose luster with age and may yellow and thicken, especially on the toes.

Hair undergoes a series of changes. Scalp hair loses its pigment, producing the well-known graying. Hair loss on the scalp is genetically determined. As early as age 20, a man's hairline may start to recede at the temples; hair loss at the vertex follows. In women, hair loss follows a similar, but less severe pattern. In both sexes, the number of scalp hairs decreases in a generalized pattern, and the diameter of each hair gets smaller. Less familiar, but probably more important clinically, is normal hair loss elsewhere on the body: the trunk, pubic areas, axillae, and limbs. As women reach age 55, coarse facial hairs appear on the chin and upper lip, but do not increase further thereafter.

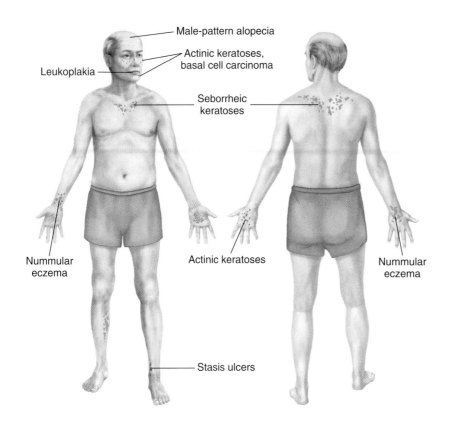

Male-pattern alopecia

Actinic keratoses, basal cell carcinoma

Leukoplakia

Seborrheic keratoses

Nummular eczema

Actinic keratoses

Nummular eczema

Stasis ulcers

Many of the changes described here pertain to lighter-skinned people and do not necessarily apply to those with darker skin tones. For example, Native American men have relatively little facial and body hair compared with lighter-skinned men and should be evaluated according to their own norms.

Head and Neck.　The eyes, ears, and mouth bear the brunt of old age. The fat that surrounds and cushions the eye within the bony orbit may atrophy, allowing the eyeball to recede somewhat. The skin of the eyelids becomes wrinkled, occasionally hanging in loose folds. Fat may push the fascia of the eyelids forward, creating soft bulges, especially in the lower lids and the inner third of the upper lids. Because their eyes produce fewer lacrimal secretions, aging patients may complain of dry eyes. The corneas lose some of their luster.

The pupils become smaller, which makes it more difficult to examine the ocular fundi. The pupils may also become slightly irregular but should continue to respond to light and near effort.

Visual acuity remains fairly constant between 20 and 50 years of age. It diminishes gradually until about age 70 and then more rapidly. Nevertheless, most elderly people retain good to adequate vision (20/20 to 20/70 as measured by standard charts). Near vision, however, begins to blur noticeably for virtually everyone. From childhood on, the lens gradually loses its elasticity, and the eye grows progressively less able to accommodate and focus on nearby objects. Ensuing *presbyopia* usually becomes noticeable during the fifth decade.

Aging affects the lenses and increases risk for *cataracts, glaucoma*, and *macular degeneration*. Thickening and yellowing of the lenses impair the passage of light to the retinas, requiring elderly people to need more light for reading and doing fine work. Cataracts affect 1 in 10 people in their 60s and 1 in 3 people in their 80s. Because the lens continues to grow over the years, it may push the iris forward, narrowing the angle between iris and cornea and increasing the risk of *narrow-angle glaucoma* (p. 215).

Acuity of hearing, like that of vision, usually diminishes with age. Early losses, which start in young adulthood, involve primarily the high-pitched sounds beyond the range of human speech and have relatively little functional significance. Gradually, loss extends to sounds in the middle and lower ranges. When a person fails to catch the upper tones of words while hearing the lower ones, words sound distorted and are difficult to understand, especially in noisy environments. Hearing loss associated with aging, known as *presbycusis*, becomes increasingly evident, usually after age 50.

Diminished salivary secretions and a decreased sense of taste accompany aging, but medications or various diseases probably contribute considerably to such changes. Teeth may wear down, become abraded, or be lost to dental caries or other conditions over time (pp. 235–236). Periodontal disease is the chief cause of tooth loss in most adults (p. 235). If a person has no teeth, the lower portion of the face looks small and sunken, with accentuated "purse-string" wrinkles radiating from the mouth. Overclosure of the mouth may lead to maceration of the skin at the corners, a condition known as *angular cheilitis* (p. 230). The bony ridges of the jaws that once surrounded the tooth sockets are gradually resorbed, especially in the lower jaw.

The frequency of palpable cervical nodes gradually diminishes with age and, according to one study, falls below 50% between 50 and 60 years of age. In contrast to the lymph nodes, the submandibular glands become easier to feel.

Thorax and Lungs.   As people age, their capacity for exercise decreases. The chest wall becomes stiffer and harder to move, respiratory muscles may weaken, and the lungs lose some of their elastic recoil. Lung mass declines, and residual volume increases. The speed of breathing out with maximal effort gradually diminishes, and cough becomes less effective.

Skeletal changes associated with aging may accentuate the dorsal curve of the thoracic spine, producing kyphosis and increasing the anteroposterior diameter of the chest. The resulting "barrel chest," however, has little effect on function.

Cardiovascular System.   Cardiovascular findings vary significantly with age. Review the effects of aging on blood pressure and heart rate described on p. 292. Aging also affects vascular sounds in the neck and adds to the significance of extra heart sounds like S_3 and S_4 and of selected systolic murmurs.

Neck Vessels. Lengthening and tortuosity of the aorta and its branches occasionally result in kinking or buckling of the carotid artery low in the neck, especially on the right. The resulting pulsatile mass, occurring chiefly in hypertensive women, may be mistaken for a carotid aneurysm—a true dilatation of the artery. A tortuous aorta occasionally raises the pressure in the jugular veins on the left side of the neck by impairing their drainage within the thorax.

In older adults, systolic bruits heard in the middle or upper portions of the carotid arteries suggest, but do not prove, partial arterial obstruction from atherosclerosis. In contrast, cervical bruits in younger people are usually innocent.

Extra Heart Sounds—S_3 and S_4. A physiologic *third heart sound,* commonly heard in children and young adults, may persist as late as age 40, especially in women. After age 40, however, an S_3 strongly suggests congestive heart failure from volume overload of the left ventricle, as in coronary artery disease or valvular heart disease (e.g., mitral regurgitation). In contrast, a *fourth heart sound* is seldom heard in young adults other than well-conditioned athletes. An S_4 can be heard in otherwise healthy older people, but often suggests decreased ventricular compliance and impaired ventricular filling. (See Table 8-7, Extra Heart Sounds in Diastole, p. 330.)

Cardiac Murmurs. Middle-aged and older adults commonly have a *systolic aortic murmur.* This murmur is detected in approximately one third of people close to age 60, and in well more than half of those reaching 85 years. Aging thickens the bases of the aortic cusps with fibrous tissue. Calcification follows, resulting in audible vibrations. Turbulence produced by blood flow into a dilated aorta may further augment this murmur. In most people, the process of fibrosis and calcification—known as *aortic sclerosis*—does not impede blood flow. In some, the aortic valve leaflets become calcified and immobile, resulting in *aortic stenosis* and outflow obstruction. A brisk carotid upstroke may help distinguish aortic sclerosis from aortic stenosis, with its delayed upstroke, but clinical differentiation between aortic sclerosis and aortic stenosis may be difficult. Both carry increased risk for cardiovascular morbidity and mortality.

Similar changes alter the mitral valve, usually approximately one decade later than aortic sclerosis. Calcification of the mitral valve annulus, or valve ring, impedes normal valve closure during systole, causing the systolic murmur of *mitral regurgitation.* This murmur may become pathologic as volume overload increases in the left ventricle.

Breasts and Axillae. The normal adult breast may be soft, but also granular, nodular, or lumpy. This uneven texture represents physiologic nodularity. It may be bilateral and palpable throughout the breast or only in parts of it. With aging, the female breasts tend to diminish as glandular tissue atrophies and is replaced by fat. Although the proportion of fat increases, its total amount may decrease. The breasts often become flaccid and more pendulous. The ducts surrounding the nipple may become more easily palpable as firm, stringy strands. Axillary hair diminishes.

Abdomen.   During the middle and later years, fat tends to accumulate in the lower abdomen and near the hips, even when total body weight is stable. This accumulation, together with weakening of the abdominal muscles, often produces a potbelly. Occasionally a person notes this change with alarm and interprets it as fluid or evidence of disease.

Aging may blunt the manifestations of acute abdominal disease. Pain may be less severe, fever is often less pronounced, and signs of peritoneal inflammation, such as muscular guarding and rebound tenderness (p. 377), may be diminished or even absent.

Male and Female Genitalia, Anus, Rectum, and Prostate.   As men age, sexual interest appears to remain intact, although frequency of intercourse declines. Several physiologic changes accompany decreasing testosterone levels. Erections become more dependent on tactile stimulation and less responsive to erotic cues. The penis decreases in size, and the testicles drop lower in the scrotum. Protracted illnesses, more than aging, lead to decreased testicular size. Pubic hair may decrease and become gray. Erectile dysfunction, or the inability to have an erection, affects approximately 50% of older men. It usually is caused by hypogastric-cavernous arterial insufficiency or venous leakage through the subtunical venules.[8]

In women, ovarian function usually starts to diminish during the fifth decade; on average, menstrual periods cease between 45 and 52 years of age. As estrogen stimulation falls, many women experience hot flashes, sometimes for up to 5 years. Symptoms range from flushing, sweating, and palpitations to chills and anxiety. Sleep disruption and mood changes are common. Women may report vaginal dryness, urge incontinence, or dyspareunia. Several vulvovaginal changes occur: pubic hair becomes sparse as well as gray; the labia and clitoris become smaller. The vagina narrows and shortens, and the vaginal mucosa becomes thin, pale, and dry, with loss of lubrication. The uterus and ovaries diminish in size. Within 10 years after menopause, the ovaries are usually no longer palpable. The suspensory ligaments of the adnexa, uterus, and bladder may also relax. Sexuality and sexual interest are often unchanged, particularly in the absence of partner issues, partner loss, or unusual work or life stress.[9]

In men, proliferation of prostate epithelial and stromal tissue, termed benign prostatic hyperplasia (BPH), begins in the third decade, "yet prostate enlargement results in only about half, and symptoms occur in only about half of men with enlargement."[10] Symptoms of urinary hesitancy, dribbling, and incomplete emptying can often be traced to causes other than BPH, such as coexisting disease, use of medication, and lower tract abnormalities. Hyperplasia continues to increase prostate volume until the seventh decade then appears to plateau. These changes are androgen dependent.

Peripheral Vascular System.   Aging itself conveys relatively few clinically important changes for the peripheral vascular system. Although arterial and venous disorders, especially atherosclerosis, do affect older people more frequently, they probably cannot be considered part of normal aging. Peripheral arteries tend to lengthen, become tortuous, and feel harder and less resilient. These changes do not necessarily indicate atherosclerosis, however, or pathologic changes in the coronary or cerebral vessels.

The common changes in skin, nails, and hair discussed earlier are not specific for arterial insufficiency, even though they are classically associated with it. Loss of arterial pulsations is not typical, however, and demands careful evaluation. Rarely, in those older than 50 years, the temporal arteries may become subject to giant cell, or temporal, arteritis, leading to loss of vision in 15% of those affected, and to complaints of headache and jaw claudication. Mean age of onset is 72 years. An important concern is possible aneurysm in the abdominal aorta in older adults with abdominal or back pain, especially those who are male, smoke, and have coronary disease.

Musculoskeletal System.   Musculoskeletal changes continue throughout the adult years. Soon after maturity, subtle losses in height begin; significant shortening is obvious by old age. Most loss of height occurs in the trunk as intervertebral discs become thinner and the vertebral bodies shorten or even collapse from osteoporosis. Flexion at the knees and hips may also contribute to shortened stature. Alterations in the discs and vertebrae also contribute to the kyphosis of aging and increase the anteroposterior diameter of the chest, especially in women. For these reasons, the limbs of an elderly person tend to look long in proportion to the trunk.

With aging, skeletal muscles decrease in bulk and power, and ligaments lose some of their tensile strength. Range of motion diminishes, partly because of osteoarthritis.

Nervous System.   Aging may affect all aspects of the nervous system, from mental status to motor and sensory function and reflexes. Age-related losses can exact a heavy toll. Older adults experience the death of loved ones and friends, retirement from valued employment, diminution in income, decreased physical capacities including impairments in vision and hearing, and often growing social isolation. Moreover, the aging brain experiences biologic changes. Brain volume and the number of cortical brain cells decrease, and both microanatomical and biochemical changes have been identified. Nevertheless, most adults adapt well to getting older. They maintain self-esteem, adapt to their changing capacities and circumstances, and eventually prepare themselves for death.

Most elderly people do well on the mental status examination, but selected impairments may become evident, especially at advanced ages. Many older people complain about their memories. "Benign forgetfulness" is the usual explanation and may occur at any age. This term refers to difficulty recalling the names of people or objects or certain details of specific events. Identifying this common phenomenon, when appropriate, may assuage worries about Alzheimer's disease. In addition to this circumscribed forgetfulness, elderly people retrieve and process data more slowly, and they take more time to learn new material. Their motor responses may slow, and their ability to perform complex tasks may become impaired.

Frequently, the clinician must try to distinguish these age-related changes in the nervous system from manifestations of specific mental disorders whose prevalence increases with aging, such as depression and dementia. Sorting out these ailments from medical complaints may be difficult, particularly because both mood disturbances and cognitive changes can alter the patient's ability to recognize or report symptoms. Older patients are also more susceptible to delirium, a temporary state of confusion that may be the first clue to infection or problems with medications. The clinician must learn to recognize these conditions promptly and to protect the patient from harm. (Review Chapter 16, The Nervous System: Mental Status and Behavior, pp. 573–593; Table 16-1, p. 590; and Table 20-1, p. 873.)

In assessing the nervous system of an older person, it is sometimes difficult to distinguish the changes of normal aging from those of age-related or other diseases. Some findings that would be abnormal in younger people, however, occur so often in the elderly that they can be attributed to aging alone, such as the changes in hearing, vision, extraocular movements, and pupillary size, shape, and reactivity described earlier.

Changes in the motor system are common. Older adults move and react with less speed and agility than younger ones, and skeletal muscles decrease in bulk. The hands of an aged person often look thin and bony as a result of atrophy of the interosseous muscles, causing muscle wasting in the backs of the hands that leaves concavities or grooves. As illustrated on page 617, this change may first appear between the thumb and the hand (1st and 2nd metacarpals) but may also be seen between the other metacarpals. Small muscle wasting may also flatten the thenar and hypothenar eminences of the palms. Arm and leg muscles can also show signs of atrophy, exaggerating the apparent size of adjacent joints. Muscle strength, though diminished, is relatively well maintained.

Occasionally, an older person develops a benign essential tremor in the head, jaw, lips, or hands that may be confused with parkinsonism (p. 653). Unlike parkinsonian tremors, however, benign tremors are slightly faster and disappear at rest, and there is no associated muscle rigidity.

Aging may also affect vibratory sense and reflexes. Older adults frequently lose some or all vibration sense in the feet and ankles (but not in the fingers or over the shins). Less commonly, position sense may diminish or disappear. The gag reflex may be diminished or absent. Abdominal reflexes may diminish or disappear. Ankle reflexes may be symmetrically decreased or absent, even when reinforced. Less commonly, knee reflexes are similarly affected. Partly because of musculoskeletal changes in the feet, the plantar responses become less obvious and more difficult to interpret. If other neurologic abnormalities accompany these changes, or if atrophy and reflex changes are asymmetric, you should search for an explanation other than age alone.

THE HEALTH HISTORY

■ APPROACH TO THE PATIENT

As you talk with older adults, begin to refine your usual techniques for obtaining the Health History. Your demeanor should convey respect, patience, and cultural awareness. Be sure to address patients by their last name.

Approach to the Older Adult Patient

- Adjusting the office environment
- Shaping the content and pace of the visit
- Eliciting symptoms
- Addressing the cultural dimensions of aging

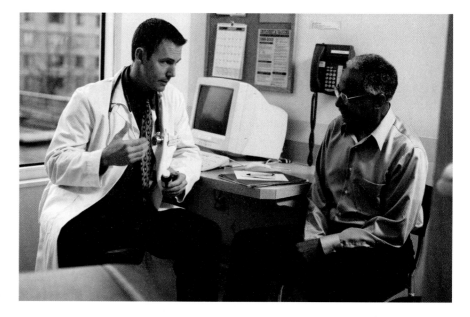

Adjusting the Office Environment. First, take the time to adapt the environment of the office, hospital, or nursing home to ensure the patient's ease in responding to your questions. Recall the physiologic changes in temperature regulation, and make sure the office is neither too cool nor too warm. Brighter lighting helps compensate for changes in lens proteins—a well-lit room allows the older adult to see your facial expressions and gestures. Face the patient directly, sitting at eye level.

More than 50% of older adults have hearing deficits, especially loss of high-tone discrimination, making a comfortable room, free of distractions or noise, conducive to accurate reactions and responses. In the hospital setting, ask about turning off the radio or television before starting your discussions. If appropriate, consider using a "pocket talker," a microphone that amplifies your voice and connects to an earpiece inserted by the patient. Try to adopt low speaking tones, and make sure the patient is appropriately using glasses, hearing aids, and dentures to assist with communication. Patients with quadriceps weakness benefit from chairs with higher seating and a wide stool with a handrail leading up to the examining table.[11]

Shaping the Content and Pace of the Visit. With older adults, you will often need to alter the traditional format of the initial or follow-up visit.

From middle age on, people begin to measure their lives in terms of years left rather than years lived. Older people often reminisce about the past and reflect on previous experiences. Listening to this process of life review provides important insights and helps you support patients as they work through painful feelings or recapture joys and accomplishments.

At the same time, it is important to balance the need to assess complex problems with the patient's endurance and possible fatigue. To provide enough time to fully listen to the patient but prevent him or her from becoming exhausted, make ample use of brief screening tools (see p. 858), information from home visits and the medical record, and reports from family members, caretakers, and allied health disciplines. Consider dividing the initial assessment into two visits. Two or more shorter visits may be less fatiguing and more productive because older patients frequently need more time to respond to questions, and their explanations may be slow and lengthy.

Eliciting Symptoms in the Older Adult. Eliciting the history from older adults calls for the clinician to be careful and astute: patients may accidentally or purposefully underreport symptoms; the presentation of acute illnesses may be different; common symptoms may mask a geriatric syndrome; patients may have cognitive impairment.

Older patients tend to overestimate healthiness even when increasing disease and disability are obvious.[11] It is best to start the visit with open-ended questions like "How can I help you today?" Older patients may be reluctant to report their symptoms. Some are afraid or embarrassed; others try to avoid medical expenses or the discomforts of diagnosis and treatment. Still others overlook their symptoms, thinking them to be merely part of aging, and simply forget about them. To reduce the risk for late recognition and delayed intervention, you may need to adopt more directed questions or health screening tools, as well as consult with family members and caretakers.

Acute illnesses present differently in older adults than in younger age groups. Older patients with infections are less likely to have fever. In those with myocardial infarction, reports of chest pain fall with increasing age, and complaints of shortness of breath, syncope, stroke, and acute confusion become more common.[12] Older patients with hyperthyroidism and hypothyroidism present with fewer symptoms and signs. In hyperthyroidism, fatigue, weight loss, and tachycardia comprise the most common symptom triad in patients older than 50 years. Older patients are more likely to have anorexia and atrial fibrillation; heat intolerance, increased sweating, and hyperreflexia are considerably rarer.[13] In hypothyroidism, older patients present with fewer symptoms and signs. Fatigue and weakness are common but notably nonspecific; the usual chilliness, paresthesias, weight gain, and cramps found in younger patients are uncommon.[14]

Managing an increasing number of chronic conditions calls for recognizing the symptom clusters typical of different *geriatric syndromes.* Geriatric syndromes are characterized by the interaction and probable synergism among multiple risk factors, for example, falls, dizziness, depression, urinary incontinence, and functional impairment.[15] Student clinicians need to learn about these syndromes because one symptom may relate to several others in a pattern of which the patient is unaware. Searching for the usual "unifying diagnosis" may pertain to fewer than 50% of older adults.[16]

Finally, the student must be knowledgeable about how cognitive impairment affects the patient's history. Evidence suggests that when older patients do report symptoms, their reports are reliable and contain more symptoms than reports from family or collateral sources.[17–20] When compared with unimpaired counterparts, even elders with mild cognitive impairment provide sufficient history to reveal concurrent disorders.[17] Use simple sentences with prompts about necessary information. For patients with more severe impairments, confirm key symptoms with family members or caretakers in the patient's presence and with his or her consent.

Learn to recognize and avoid stereotypes that keep you from viewing each patient as a unique person with a treasure of life experiences. When listening to them, discover how these patients see themselves and their situations, as well as their priorities, goals, and coping skills. Such knowledge strengthens your alliance with older patients as you collaborate on plans for care and treatment.

TIPS FOR COMMUNICATING EFFECTIVELY WITH OLDER ADULTS

- Provide a well-lit, moderately warm setting with minimal background noise and safe chairs and access to the examining table.
- Face the patient and speak in low tones; make sure the patient is using glasses, hearing devices, and dentures if needed.
- Adjust the pace and content of the interview to the stamina of the patient; consider two visits for initial evaluations when indicated.
- Allow time for open-ended questions and reminiscing; include family and caretakers when needed, especially if the patient has cognitive impairment.
- Make use of brief screening instruments, the medical record, and reports from allied disciplines.
- Carefully assess symptoms, especially fatigue, loss of appetite, dizziness, and pain, for clues to underlying disorders.
- Make sure written instructions are in large print and easy to read.

Addressing Cultural Dimensions of Aging. Clinicians must acquire new knowledge and awareness about the health beliefs and culture that shape the older adult's response to illness and the health care system. Between 1990 and 2000, Hispanics, African Americans, Native Americans, and other ethnic groups accounted for approximately 43% of the total growth of the population.[21] By 2050, the overall older adult population will increase by 230%, with the minority older adult population growing by 510%.[22] The broad categories used for federal reporting no longer capture the wide array of cultural differences that affect how older adults understand suffering, illness, and decisions about care, ranging from use of alternative therapies to timing of health care visits. Immigrant and refugee groups in the United States with particular health care needs include Vietnamese, Laotians, Haitians, Somalis, Russians and Eastern Europeans, Afghans, and Bosnians.

Cultural differences affect the epidemiology of illness and mental health, the process of acculturation, the specific concerns of the elderly, the potential for misdiagnosis, and disparities in health outcomes.[22–24] Take a few minutes to review the components of self-awareness needed for cultural competency discussed in Chapter 2 (pp. 55–56). Learn culturally specific ways to show respect to elders and use appropriate nonverbal communication styles. Direct eye contact or handshaking, for example, may not be culturally syntonic. Identify critical experiences that affect the patient's outlook and psyche arising from the country of origin or migration history. Ask about spiritual advisors and native healers.

Cultural values particularly affect decisions about the end of life. Elders, family, and even an extended community group may make these decisions with or for the older patient. Such group decision making is in contrast to the patient autonomy and informed consent that many contemporary health care providers value, expect, and automatically assume to be desired by all.[21] Being sensitive to the stresses of migration and acculturation, using translators effectively (see p. 45), enlisting "patient navigators" from the family and community, and accessing culturally validated assessment tools like the Geriatric Depression Scale are important for empathic care of older adults.[23]

◼ SPECIAL AREAS OF CONCERN WHEN ASSESSING COMMON OR CONCERNING SYMPTOMS

Common Concerns

- Activities of daily living
- Instrumental activities of daily living
- Medications
- Nutrition
- Acute and chronic pain
- Smoking and alcohol
- Advance directives and palliative care

As we have seen, symptoms in the older adult can have many meanings and interconnections, as in the geriatric syndromes. Explore the meaning of these symptoms as you would with all patients, and review the Common or Concerning Symptoms sections in previous chapters. For older adults, be sure to place these symptoms in the context of your overall functional assessment. Several areas warrant special attention as you gather the health history. Approach the following areas with extra thoroughness and sensitivity, always focusing on helping the older adult to maintain optimal well-being and level of function.

Activities of Daily Living. Learning how older adults, especially those with chronic illness, function in terms of daily activities is essential and provides an important baseline for the future. First, assess the patient's ability for self-care. Ask about his or her capacity to perform the *Activities of Daily Living (ADLs)*—these consist of basic self care abilities—then move on to inquiries about capacity for higher level functions of the *Instrumental Activities of Daily Living (IADLs)* listed below. Can the patient perform these activities independently, does he or she need some help, or is the patient entirely dependent on others?

You may wish to start with an open-ended request like "Tell me about your typical day" or "Tell me about your day yesterday." Then move to a greater level of detail . . . You got up at 8 AM? How is it getting out of bed? . . . "What did you do next?" Ask how things have changed, who is available for help, and what helpers actually do. Remember that assessing the patient's safety is one of your priorities.

ACTIVITIES OF DAILY LIVING AND INSTRUMENTAL ACTIVITIES OF DAILY LIVING

Physical Activities of Daily Living (ADLs)	*Instrumental Activities of Daily Living (IADLs)*
Bathing	Using the telephone
Dressing	Shopping
Toileting	Preparing food
Transferring	Housekeeping
Continence	Laundry
Feeding	Transportation
Managing money	Taking medicine

Medications. Statistics related to prescription drugs expose the dramatic rationale for obtaining a complete drug history.[3] Approximately 80% of older adults have at least one chronic disease and take at least one prescription drug each day. Adults older than 65 receive approximately 30% of all prescriptions. Roughly 30% take more than eight prescribed drugs each day! Older adults have more than 50% of all reported adverse drug reactions causing hospital admission, reflecting pharmacodynamic changes in the distribution, metabolism, and elimination of drugs that place them at increased risk.

Take a thorough medication history, including name, dose, frequency, and indication for each drug. Be sure to explore all components of polypharmacy, including suboptimal prescribing, concurrent use of multiple drugs, underuse, inappropriate use, and nonadherence. Ask about use of over-the-counter medications, vitamin and nutrition supplements, and mood-altering drugs such as narcotics, benzodiazepines, and recreational substances. Assess medications for drug interactions. Be particularly careful when treating insomnia, estimated to occur in approximately 40% of older adults. Increased exercise may be the best remedy. Recall that medications are the most common modifiable risk factor associated with falls. Review strategies for avoiding polypharmacy with your instructors. It is wise to keep the number of drugs prescribed to a minimum. Learn about drug–drug interactions and drugs contraindicated in older adults.[25,26]

Nutrition.   Taking a diet history and using the Rapid Screen for Dietary Intake and the Nutrition Screening Checklist (p. 115) are especially important in older adults. Prevalence of undernutrition increases with age, affecting 5% to 10% of elderly outpatients and 30% to 50% of hospitalized elders.[27] Those with chronic disease are particularly at risk, especially those with poor dentition, oral or gastrointestinal disorders, depression or other psychiatric illness, and drug regimens that affect appetite and oral secretions. For those underweight elders who give limited histories, the serum albumin is an independent risk factor for all-cause mortality.[28]

Acute and Chronic Pain.   Pain and associated complaints account for 80% of clinician visits. Prevalence of pain may reach 25% to 50% in community-dwelling adults and 40% to 80% in nursing home residents. Pain usually arises from musculoskeletal complaints like back and joint pain.[29] Headache, neuralgias from diabetes and herpes zoster, nighttime leg pain, and cancer pain are also common. Older patients are less likely to report pain, leading to undue suffering, depression, social isolation, physical disability, and loss of function.

■ Characteristics of Acute and Chronic Pain	
Acute Pain	**Chronic Pain**
Distinct onset	Lasts more than 3 months
Obvious pathology	Often associated with psychological or functional impairment
Short duration	Can fluctuate in character and intensity over time
Common causes: postsurgical, trauma, headache	Common causes: arthritis, cancer, claudication, leg cramps, neuropathy, radiculopathy

(Source: Reuben DB, Herr KA, Pacala JT, et al. Geriatrics at Your Fingertips: 2004, 6th ed. p. 119. Malden, MA: Blackwell Publishing, Inc., for the American Geriatrics Society, 2004.)

Inquire about pain, now considered "the fifth vital sign," each time you meet with the older patient. Ask specifically "Are you having any pain right now? How about during the past week?" Learn to distinguish acute pain from chronic pain and thoroughly investigate its cause. Many multidimensional and unidimensional pain scales are available. Unidimensional scales such as the Visual Analog Scale, graphic pictures, and the Verbal 0–10 Scale have all been validated and are easiest to use.[29] Study the many modalities of pain relief and which analgesics are most appropriate for older adults.

Smoking and Alcohol.   Smoking is harmful at all ages. At each visit, advise elderly smokers to quit. The commitment to stop smoking may take time, but quitting is an important step in reducing risk for heart disease, pulmonary disease, malignancy, and loss of daily function.

An estimated 5% to 10% of adults older than 65 years have alcohol-related problems.[30] Lifelong prevalence of alcohol abuse or dependency among community residents older than 65 years ranges from 4% to 8%.[31] Rates of alcoholism in older patients in hospital, emergency room, and clinic settings have been reported to reach 21%, 24%, and 36% respectively, and account for approximately 1% of hospital admissions for this age group.[31] The number of older people with problem drinking is expected to rise as the population ages over the coming decades. Despite the prevalence of alcohol problems among the elderly, rates of detection and treatment are low.

Use the CAGE questions to uncover problem drinking. Although symptoms and signs are subtler in older adults, making early detection more difficult, the four CAGE questions (see p. 50) remain sensitive and specific in this age group using the conventional cut-off score of 2 or more.[30,31]

Advance Directives and Palliative Care.   Many older patients are interested in expressing their wishes about end-of-life decisions and would like providers to initiate these discussions before any serious illness develops.[32] Advance care planning involves several tasks—providing information, invoking the patient's preferences, identifying proxy decision makers, and conveying empathy and support. Use clear and simple language. You can often begin the discussion by relating these decisions to a current illness or experiences with relatives or friends. Ask about preferences relating to written "Do Not Resuscitate" orders specifying life support measures "if the heart or lungs were to stop or give out." Second, encourage the patient to establish in writing a health care proxy or durable power of attorney for health care, "someone who can make decisions reflecting your wishes in case of confusion or emergency." These conversations, although difficult at first, convey your respect and concern for patients and help them and their families prepare openly and in advance for a peaceful death.[33] Plan to include these discussions in an office setting rather than in the uncertain and stressful environment of emergency or acute care.

For patients with advanced or terminal illnesses, include these discussions in an overall plan for palliative care. The goal of palliative care is "to relieve suffering and improve the quality of life for patients with advanced illnesses and their families through specific knowledge and skills, including communication with patients and family members; management of pain and other symptoms; psychosocial, spiritual, and bereavement support; and coordination of an array of medical and social services."[34] To ease patient and family distress, refining your communication skills is especially important: making good eye contact; asking open-ended questions; responding to anxiety, depression, or changes in the patient's affect; and showing empathy.

HEALTH PROMOTION AND COUNSELING

Important Topics for Health Promotion and Counseling in the Older Adult

- When to screen
- Vision and hearing
- Exercise
- Immunizations
- Household safety

- Cancer screening
- Depression
- Dementia
- Elder mistreatment

As the life span for older adults extends into the 80s, new issues for screening emerge. Given the heterogeneity of the aging population, guiding principles for deciding who might benefit from screening and when screening might be stopped are helpful, especially because evidence for making screening decisions is not always available. In general, base screening decisions on each older person's particular circumstances, rather than on his or her age alone. Three factors should be considered: life expectancy, time interval until benefit from screening accrues, and patient preference.[35] The American Geriatrics Society recommends that if life expectancy is short, give priority to treating conditions that will benefit the patient in the time that remains. Consider deferring screening if it places added burdens on the older adult with multiple medical problems, a shortened life expectancy, or dementia. Tests that help with prognosis and planning, however, are still warranted even if the patient would not pursue treatment.[36]

Screening for age-related changes in *vision* and *hearing* is important in helping older adults maintain optimal function, and is included in the 10-Minute Geriatric Screener (see p. 858).[37] Test *vision* objectively using an eye chart. Asking the patient about any *hearing* loss may be adequate, followed by the whisper test and more formal testing if indicated (see p. 190).

Recommend regular aerobic *exercise* to improve strength and aerobic capacity, increase physiologic reserve, improve energy levels for ADLs, and slow the onset of disability. Resistance training and Tai Chi may be especially helpful for improving balance, combating the negative effects of inactivity on cardiovascular disease and arthritis, and enhancing recovery from chronic diseases. Exercise programs can begin with brisk walking. Physical therapists can provide more tailored recommendations.

Immunizations should include the pneumococcal vaccine once after age 65 and annual influenza vaccinations after age 65. Unvaccinated older adults should have the primary series of three tetanus immunizations. Vaccinated older adults should receive the single booster dose of tetanus immunization every 10 years.

Survey older patients about *household safety.* Poor lighting, chairs at awkward heights, slippery or irregular surfaces, and environmental hazards can be readily corrected. Use of restraints should be avoided whenever possible.

Cancer screening for selected conditions can be controversial because of limited evidence supporting its use for adults older than age 70 to 80. The American Geriatrics Society recommends annual or biennial mammography for breast cancer screening up to age 75, then every 2 to 3 years if life expectancy remains more than 4 years. Although the prevalence of cervical cancer has declined in the United States, 40% to 50% of deaths from cervical cancer are in women older than 65 years. Provide Pap smears every 1 to 3 years until age 65 to 70 when there is no history of cervical pathology. Colonoscopy is recommended for colon cancer screening every 10 years beginning at age 50. This examination is difficult for many older patients, who may decline despite encouragement. Review the discussion about colonoscopy, fecal occult blood tests, and the pitfalls of the prostate-specific antigen test and the digital rectal examination on pages 462–463. Screening for lung cancer and ovarian cancer is not recommended. Check for skin cancer and oral cancers in high-risk patients.[38]

Depression commonly affects older adults but is both underdiagnosed and undertreated. A positive response to asking "Do you often feel sad or depressed?" is approximately 80% sensitive and specific and should prompt further investigation, possibly with the Geriatric Depression Scale. Depressed men older than 65 years are at increased risk for suicide; they require particularly careful evaluation.

Dementia, a "global impairment of cognitive function that interferes with normal activities," affects 16% of Americans older than 65 years.[39] Prominent features include short- and long-term memory deficits and impaired judgment. Thought processes are impoverished; speech may be hesitant as a result of difficulty in finding words. Loss or orientation to place may make navigating by foot or car problematic or even dangerous. Most dementias represent Alzheimer's disease (50% to 85%) or vascular multi-infarct dementia (10% to 20%). Watch for Alzheimer's disease in patients with a positive family history because their risk is three times higher than the risk in the general population.

Dementia often has a slow insidious onset and may escape detection by both families and clinicians, especially in the early stages of *mild cognitive impairment.* Look for problems with memory, then later for changes in cognitive function or ADLs. Watch for family complaints of new or unusual behaviors. Testing with the Mini-Mental State Examination may be helpful, although level of education and cultural variables such as language may affect scores. If you identify cognitive changes, investigate contributing factors such as medications, depression, metabolic abnormalities, or other medical and psychiatric conditions. In patients with dementia, counsel families about the potential for disruptive behavior, accidents, falls, and termination of driving privileges. Foster discussion of legal arrangements such as power of attorney and advance directives while the patient can still contribute to decision making. Useful tools for assessing memory loss and depression from the Practicing

Physician Education Project can be found at www.americangeriatrics.org/education/ppep_index.shtml.

Finally, consider screening all older patients for possible *elder mistreatment,* which includes abuse, neglect, exploitation, and abandonment. Depression, dementia, and malnutrition are all considered independent risk factors. Prevalence of elder mistreatment is approximately 1% to 5% of the older population; however, that statistic is based solely on self-reported cases of elder mistreatment, and many more cases may remain undetected. Although several screening instruments are available, no single instrument has emerged for rapid yet accurate assessment and diagnosis of this important problem.[40,41]

TECHNIQUES OF EXAMINATION

As you have gathered, assessment of the older adult does not follow the traditional format of the history and physical examination. It calls for enhanced techniques of interviewing, special emphasis on daily function and key topics related to elder health, and a focus on functional assessment during the physical examination. Because of its importance to the health of older adults and the order of your assessment, this section begins with Assessing Functional Status: The "Sixth Vital Sign." This segment includes how to evaluate risk for falls, one of the greatest threats to health and well-being in elders. Next follows features of the traditional "head-to-toe" examination tailored to the older adult.

▰ASSESSING FUNCTIONAL STATUS: THE "SIXTH VITAL SIGN"

During assessment of older adults, the clinician places a special premium on maintaining the patient's health and well-being. In a sense, all visits are opportunities for health promotion and counseling directed to sustaining the patient's independence and optimal level of function. Although the specific goals of care may vary, a primary focus is preserving the patient's functional status, the "sixth vital sign." Functional status specifically means the ability to perform tasks and fulfill social roles associated with daily living across a wide range of complexity.[42] As noted in the General Survey section on p. 861, your assessment of functional status begins when the patient enters the room. Several well-validated and time-efficient assessment tools can help maintain focus on these observations and assist with this approach.

Assessing Functional Ability.　Deficits in function are now recognized as better predictors of mortality and patient outcomes after hospitalization than admitting diagnoses.[43] Several performance-based assessment instruments are available. The screening tool on page 858 is brief, has high interrater agreement, and can be used easily by office staff. It also covers the three important domains of geriatric assessment: physical, cognitive, and psychosocial function. Note that it addresses vision and hearing, key sensory modalities, and includes questions about urinary incontinence, an often unreported problem that greatly affects social interactions and self-esteem in the elderly. One mnemonic that helps students assess causes of incontinence is DIAPERS: **D**elirium, **I**nfection, **A**trophic urethritis/vaginitis, **P**harmaceuticals, **E**xcess urine output (i.e., congestive heart failure, hyperglycemia), **R**estricted mobility, **S**tool impaction.[44]

■ *10-Minute Geriatric Screener*

Problem	Screening Measure	Positive Screen

Vision	2 Parts:
	    Ask: "Do you have difficulty driving, or watching television, or reading, or doing any of your daily activities because of your eyesight?"
	If yes, then:
	    Test each eye with Snellen chart while patient wears corrective lenses (if applicable).
		Yes to question and inability to read greater than 20/40 on Snellen chart

Hearing	Use audioscope set at 40 dB. Test hearing using 1,000 and 2,000 Hz.	Inability to hear 1,000 or 2,000 Hz in both ears or either of these frequencies in one ear
Leg mobility	Time the patient after asking: "Rise from the chair. Walk 20 feet briskly, turn, walk back to the chair and sit down."	Unable to complete task in 15 seconds

Urinary incontinence	2 Parts:
	    Ask: "In the last year, have you ever lost your urine and gotten wet?"
	If yes, then ask:
	    "Have you lost urine on at least 6 separate dates?"
		Yes to both questions

Nutrition/ weight loss	2 Parts: Ask: "Have you lost 10 lbs over the past 6 months without trying to do so?" Weigh the patient.	Yes to the question or weight <100 lbs
Memory	Three-item recall	Unable to remember all three items after 1 minute.
Depression	Ask: "Do you often feel sad or depressed?"	Yes to the question.

Physical disability	Six questions:
	    "Are you able to . . . :
	    "Do strenuous activities like fast walking or bicycling?"
	    "Do heavy work around the house like washing windows, walls, or floors?"
	    "Go shopping for groceries or clothes?"
	    "Get to places out of walking distance?"
	    "Bathe, either a sponge bath, tub bath, or shower?"
	    "Dress, like putting on a shirt, buttoning and zipping, or putting on shoes?"
		Yes to any of the questions.

(Source: Moore AA, Siu AL. Screening for common problems in ambulatory elderly: clinical confirmation of a screening instrument. Am J Med 100:438–440, 1996.)

Further Assessment of Falls.　There is a veritable avalanche of evidence linking falls to morbidity and mortality in the older population. Each year approximately 35% to 40% of healthy community-dwelling older adults experience falls. Incidence rates in nursing homes and hospitals are almost three times higher, with related injuries in approximately 25%. Loss of confidence from fear of falling and postfall anxiety syndrome further impair functional status even after recovery.[44,45]

The American Geriatrics Society recommends risk factor assessment for falls during routine primary care visits, with more intensive assessment in high-risk groups—those with first or recurrent falls, nursing home residents, and those prone to fall-related injuries. The Society has published an algorithm for assessing and managing falls. Fall-related assessments should include details about the how the fall occurred, especially from witnesses, and identification of risk factors, medical comorbidities, functional status, and environmental risks—coupled with interventions for prevention.[45] Effective single interventions include gait and balance training and exercise to strengthen muscles, reduction of home hazards, discontinuation of psychotropic medication, and multifactorial assessment with targeted interventions. Additional useful strategies include addressing change in postural blood pressure, attention to concurrent acute illness, reduction in medications to fewer than four, detection of sensory neuropathy and impairment of proprioception, investigation of any episodes of syncope, patient and family education, treatment of osteoporosis, and possible use of hip protectors.[46] Specific recommendations from the American Geriatrics Society about assessment and multifactorial interventions can be found in the diagram on Prevention of Falls in Older Adults on p. 860.

Review the easy-to-use tools for practicing clinicians on falls and urinary incontinence from the Practicing Physician Education Project at the Web site given on p. 872.

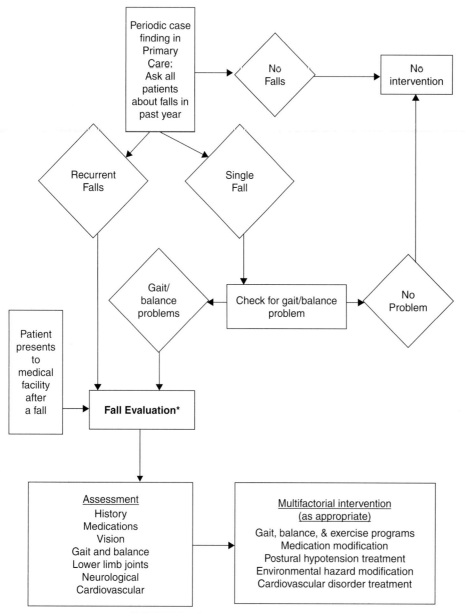

PREVENTION OF FALLS IN OLDER ADULTS

American Geriatric Society, British Geriatrics Society, American Academy of Orthopaedic Surgeons. Guideline for the prevention of falls in older persons. J Am Geriatr Soc. 49(5):664–672, 2001.

◼ PHYSICAL EXAMINATION OF THE OLDER ADULT

General Survey.   Deepen the observations about the patient that you have been compiling since the visit began. What is the patient's apparent state of health and degree of vitality? What about mood and affect? Note the patient's hygiene and how the patient is dressed. How does the patient walk into the room? Move onto the examining table? Are there changes in posture or involuntary movements?

Flat or impoverished affect may be seen in *depression, Parkinson's disease,* or *Alzheimer's disease.*

Undernutrition, slowed motor performance, loss of muscle mass, or weakness suggests frailty.

Kyphosis or abnormal gait can impair balance and increase risk for falling.

Vital Signs.   Measure blood pressure using recommended techniques, checking for increased systolic blood pressure (SBP) and widened pulse pressure (PP), defined as systolic blood pressure minus diastolic blood pressure. With aging, systolic blood pressure and peripheral vascular resistance increase, whereas diastolic blood pressure decreases.

Assess the patient for orthostatic hypotension, defined as a drop in systolic blood pressure of ≥ 20 mm Hg or diastolic blood pressure of ≥ 10 mm Hg within 3 minutes of standing.[51,52] Measure blood pressure and heart rate in two positions: supine after the patient rests for up to 10 minutes, then within 3 minutes.

Review the JNC 7 categories of prehypertension to help you with early detection and treatment of hypertension (p. 109).

Isolated systolic hypertension (SBP ≥140) after age 50 triples the risk for coronary heart disease in men. PP ≥60 is a risk factor for cardiovascular and renal disease and stroke.[47–50]

Orthostatic hypotension occurs in 10% to 20% of older adults and in up to 30% of frail nursing home residents, especially when they first arise in the morning. It can present with lightheadedness, weakness, unsteadiness, visual blurring, and, in 20% to 30% of patients, syncope.

Causes include medications, autonomic disorders, diabetes, prolonged bed rest, blood loss, and cardiovascular disorders.[47,53–55]

Measure heart rate, respiratory rate, and temperature. The apical heart rate may yield more information about arrhythmias in older patients. Use thermometers accurate for lower temperatures

Respiratory rate ≥ 25 breaths per minute indicates lower respiratory infection.

Hypothermia is more common in elderly patients.[11]

Weight and height are especially important in the elderly and needed for calculation of the body mass index. Weight should be measured at every visit.

Low weight is a key indicator of poor nutrition.

Undernutrition is seen with depression, alcoholism, cognitive impairment, malignancy, chronic organ failure (cardiac, renal, pulmonary), medication use, social isolation, and poverty.

Skin.   Note physiologic changes of aging, such as thinning, loss of elastic tissue and turgor, and wrinkling. Skin may be dry, flaky, rough, and often itchy *(asteatosis),* with a latticework of shallow fissures that creates a mosaic of small polygons, especially on the legs.

Observe any patchy changes in color. Check the extensor surface of the hands and forearms for white depigmented patches (*pseudoscars*) and for well-demarcated vividly purple macules or patches that may fade after several weeks (*actinic purpura*).

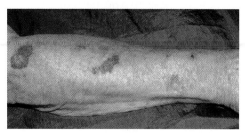

ACTINIC PURPURA

Look for changes from sun exposure. Areas of skin may appear weather beaten, thickened, yellowed, and deeply furrowed; there may be *actinic lentigines,* or "liver spots," and *actinic keratoses,* superficial flattened papules covered by a dry scale (p. 142).

Distinguish such lesions from a *basal cell carcinoma,* initially a translucent nodule that spreads and leaves a depressed center with a firm elevated border, and from a *squamous cell carcinoma,* a firm reddish-appearing lesion often emerging in a sun-exposed area (p. 142). A dark raised asymmetric lesion with irregular borders may be a *melanoma.*

Inspect for the benign lesions of aging, namely *comedones,* or blackheads, on the cheeks or around the eyes; *cherry angiomas* (p. 141), which often appear early in adulthood; and *seborrheic keratoses,* raised yellowish lesions that feel greasy and velvety or warty (p. 142).

Watch for any painful vesicular lesions in a dermatomal distribution.

Suspect *herpes zoster* from reactivation of latent varicella-zoster virus in the dorsal root ganglia. Risk increases with age and impaired cell-mediated immunity.[56]

In older bed-bound patients, especially when emaciated or neurologically impaired, inspect the skin thoroughly for damage or ulceration.

Pressure sores may develop from obliteration of arteriolar and capillary blood flow to the skin or from shear forces during movement across sheets or when lifted upright incorrectly. See Table 5-11, Pressure Ulcers.

HEENT.   Conduct a careful and thorough evaluation of the Head and Neck, as detailed in Chapter 6.

Inspect the eyelids, the bony orbit, and the eye. The eye may appear recessed from atrophy of fat in the surrounding tissues. Observe any *senile ptosis* arising from weakening of the levator palpebrae, relaxation of the skin, and increased weight of the upper eyelid. Check the lower lids for *ectropion* or *entropion* (p. 213). Note yellowing of the sclera, and *arcus senilis,* a benign whitish ring around the limbus (p. 216).

Test visual acuity, using a pocket Snellen chart or wall-mounted chart. Note any *presbyopia,* the loss of near vision arising from decreased elasticity of the lens related to aging.

More than 40 million Americans have refractive errors.

The pupils should respond to light and near effort. Except for possible impairment in upward gaze, extraocular movements should remain intact.

Using your ophthalmoscope, carefully examine the lenses and fundi.

Cataracts, glaucoma, and macular degeneration all increase with aging.[57]

Inspect each lens carefully for any opacities. Do not depend on the flashlight alone because the lens may look clear superficially.

Cataracts are the world's leading cause of blindness. Risk factors include cigarette smoking, exposure to UV-B light, high alcohol intake, diabetes, medications (including steroids), and trauma. See Table 6-8, p. 216.

In older adults, the fundi lose their youthful shine and light reflections, and the arteries look narrowed, paler, straighter, and less brilliant. Assess the cup-to-disc ratio, usually $\leq 1:2$.

An increased cup-to-disc ratio suggests open angle *glaucoma,* caused by irreversible optic neuropathy and leading to loss of peripheral and central vision and blindness. Prevalence is three to four times higher in African Americans than in the general population.

Inspect the fundi for colloid bodies causing alterations in pigmentation called *drusen*.

Macular degeneration causes poor central vision and blindness. Types include *dry atrophic* (more common but less severe) and *wet exudative,* or neovascular. Drusen may be hard and sharply defined, or soft and confluent with altered pigmentation, shown below and on p. 188.

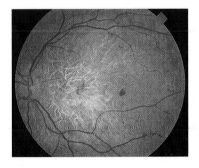

Test hearing by occluding one ear and using the techniques for whispered voice (see p. 190) or an audioscope.[58] Be sure to inspect the ear canals for cerumen.

Removing cerumen often quickly improves hearing.

Examine the oral cavity for odor, appearance of the gingival mucosa, any caries, mobility of the teeth, and quantity of saliva. Inspect closely for lesions on any of the mucosal surfaces. Ask the patient to remove dentures so you can check the gums for denture sores.

Malodor may occur with poor oral hygiene or periodontitis, caries. *Gingivitis* may arise from periodontal disease. Dental plaque and cavitation may cause caries. Increased tooth mobility from abscesses or advanced caries warrants removal to prevent aspiration. Decreased salivation may develop from medications, radiation, Sjögren's syndrome, or dehydration. Lesions may arise from *oral tumors,* usually on the lateral borders of the tongue and floor of the mouth.[59]

Continue your usual examination of the thyroid gland and lymph nodes.

Thorax and Lungs.   Complete the usual examination, making note of subtle signs of changes in pulmonary function.

Increased anteroposterior diameter, purse-lipped breathing, and dyspnea with talking or minimal exertion suggest *chronic obstructive pulmonary disease.*

Cardiovascular System.   Review your findings from measurement of the blood pressure and heart rate.

Isolated systolic hypertension and a widened pulse pressure are cardiac risk factors, prompting a search for *left ventricular hypertrophy (LVH).*

As with younger adults, begin by inspecting the JVP, palpating the carotid upstrokes, and listening for any overlying carotid bruits.

A *tortuous atherosclerotic aorta* can raise pressure in the left jugular veins by impairing their drainage into the right atrium. It may also cause kinking of the carotid artery low in the neck on the right, chiefly in women with hypertension, which can be mistaken for a carotid aneurysm.

Carotid bruits in the elderly warrant further investigation for possible carotid stenosis due to risk for ipsilateral stroke.

Assess the point of maximal impulse (PMI), then auscultate S_1 and S_2. Listen also for the extra sounds of S_3 and S_4.

Sustained PMI in LVH; diffuse PMI in congestive heart failure (see p. 311).

In older adults an S_3 suggests dilatation of the left ventricle from congestive heart failure or cardiomyopathy; an S_4 often accompanies hypertension.

Beginning in the second right interspace, listen for cardiac murmurs in all areas of auscultation (see p. 309). Describe the timing, shape, location of maximal intensity, radiation, intensity, pitch, and quality of each murmur you detect.

A systolic crescendo–decrescendo murmur in the second right interspace suggests aortic sclerosis or aortic stenosis, seen in approximately 30% and 2% of community-dwelling elders, respectively. Both carry increased risk for cardiovascular disease and death.[60]

For systolic murmurs over the clavicle, check for delay between the brachial and radial pulses.

Delay during simultaneous palpation (but not compression) of the brachial and radial pulses denotes aortic stenosis.[61]

A harsh holosystolic murmur at the apex suggests mitral regurgitation, also common in the elderly.

Breasts and Axillae. Palpate the breasts carefully for lumps or masses. Include palpation of the tail of Spence that extends into the axilla. Examine the axillae for lymphadenopathy.

Lumps or masses in older women, and rarely in older men, mandate further investigation for possible malignancy.

Abdomen. Continue your usual examination of the abdomen. Check for any bruits over the aorta, renal arteries, and femoral arteries. Inspect the upper abdomen; palpate to the left of the midline for any aortic pulsations. Try to assess the width of the aorta by pressing more deeply with one hand on each of its lateral margins (see pp. 384–385).

Bruits may be noted in atherosclerotic vascular disease.

Widened aorta and pulsatile mass may be found in *abdominal aortic aneurysm.*

Female Genitalia and Pelvic Examination.[62–64] Take special care to explain the steps of the examination and allow time for careful positioning. Ask an assistant to help the older woman move onto the examining table, then into the lithotomy position. Raising the head of the table may make her more comfortable. For the woman with arthritis or spinal deformities who cannot flex her hips or knees, an assistant can gently raise and support the legs, or help the woman into the left lateral position.

Inspect the vulva for changes related to menopause such as thinning of the skin, loss of pubic hair, and decreased distensibility of the introitus. Identify any labial masses. Note that bluish swellings may be varicosities. Bulging of the anterior vaginal wall below the urethra may indicate an urethrocele or urethral diverticulum.

Benign masses include condylomata, fibromas, leiomyomas, and sebaceous cysts. See Table 12-2, Bulges and Swellings of the Vulva, Vagina, and Urethra, p. 451.

Look for any vulvar erythema.

Erythema with satellite lesions results from infection with *Candida;* erythema with ulceration or necrotic center is associated with *carcinoma.* Multifocal reddened lesions with white scaling plaques are consistent with *Paget's disease.*

Inspect the urethra for *caruncles,* or prolapse of fleshy erythematous mucosal tissue at the urethral meatus. Note any enlargement of the clitoris.

Clitoral enlargement may accompany *androgen-producing tumors* or use of androgen creams.

Spread the labia, press downward on the introitus to relax the levator muscles, and gently insert the speculum after moistening it with warm water or a water-soluble lubricant. If you find severe vaginal atrophy, a gaping introitus, or an introital stricture from estrogen loss, you will need to vary the size of the speculum.

Inspect the vaginal walls, which may be atrophic, and the cervix. Note any thin cervical mucus or vaginal or cervical discharge.

Estrogen-stimulated cervical mucus with ferning is seen with use of hormone replacement therapy, *endometrial hyperplasia,* and *estrogen-producing tumors.*

Discharge may accompany vaginitis or cervicitis. See Table 12-6, Vaginal Discharge, p. 454.

Use a wooden spatula or endocervical brush to obtain endocervical cells for the Pap smear. A blind swab may be indicated if the atrophic vagina is too small.

See Table 12-7, Positions of the Uterus, p. 455, and Table 12-8, Abnormalities of the Uterus, p. 456.

After removing the speculum, ask the patient to bear down to detect uterine prolapse, cystocele, urethrocele, or rectocele.

Perform the bimanual examination. Check for motion of the cervix and for any uterine or adnexal masses.

Mobility of the cervix is restricted with inflammation, malignancy, or surgical adhesion. Enlarging uterine fibroids, or leiomyomas, are found in *malignant leiomyosarcoma.* The ovaries are palpable with *ovarian cancer.*

Perform the rectovaginal examination. Assess for uterine and adnexal irregularities through the anterior rectal wall, and for rectal masses. Change gloves first if blood from the bimanual examination is on the vaginal examining glove to obtain an accurate stool sample.

A uterus that is enlarged, fixed, or irregular may indicate adhesions or possible malignancy. Rectal masses are found in *colon cancer.*

Male Genitalia and Prostate. Examine the penis, retracting the foreskin if present. Examine the scrotum, testes, and epididymis.

Findings include smegma, penile cancer, and scrotal hydroceles.

Proceed with the rectal examination, paying special attention to any rectal masses and any nodularity or masses of the prostate. Note that the anterior and median lobes of the prostate are inaccessible to rectal palpation, limiting the utility of the digital rectal examination for detecting prostate enlargement or possible malignancy.

Rectal masses are found in *colon cancer. Prostate hyperplasia* may be linked with enlargement; *prostate cancer* is possible with nodules or masses.

Peripheral Vascular System. Auscultate the abdomen for aortic, renal, or femoral artery bruits.

Bruits over these vessels are found in *atherosclerotic disease.*

Assess the width of the abdominal aorta in the epigastric area and examine for a pulsatile mass.

Consider *abdominal aortic aneurysm* if aortic width is ≥ 3 cm or with a pulsatile mass, especially in older male smokers with coronary disease.

Palpate pulses carefully.

Diminished or absent pulses may indicate *arterial occlusion.* Consider confirmation with an office ankle–brachial index. Note that ≤33% of patients with peripheral vascular disease have symptoms of claudication.[65]

Musculoskeletal System. Begin your evaluation with the screening evaluation on p. 858. If you find joint deformity, deficits in mobility, or pain with movement, conduct a more thorough examination. Review the techniques for examining individual joints in Chapter 15, The Musculoskeletal System.

Degenerative joint changes in *osteoarthritis;* joint inflammation in *rheumatoid* or *gouty arthritis.*

See Tables 15-1 to 15-10.

Nervous System. As with the musculoskeletal examination, begin your evaluation of the nervous system with the 10-Minute Geriatric Screener on p. 858.

Pursue further examination if you note any deficits. Focus especially on memory and affect.

Learn to distinguish delirium from depression and dementia (see Table 20-1). Nonetheless, careful search for underlying causes is warranted.

Also pay close attention to gait and balance, particularly standing balance; timed 8-foot walk; stride characteristics like width, pace, and length of stride; and careful turning.

Abnormalities of gait and balance, especially widening of base, slowing and lengthening of stride, and difficulty turning, are correlated with risk for falls.[66–68]

Note that standard neuromuscular tests have not been shown to predict impairments in mobility.[69] Further, although neurologic abnormalities are common in the older population, their prevalence without identifiable disease increases with age, ranging from 30% to 50%.[70] Examples of age-related abnormalities include unequal pupil size, decreased arm swing and spontaneous movements, increased leg rigidity and abnormal gait, presence of the snout and grasp reflexes, and decreased toe vibratory sense.

Search for evidence of tremor, rigidity, bradykinesia, micrographia, shuffling gait, and difficulty turning in bed, opening jars, and rising from a chair.

These findings are seen in *Parkinson disease,* found in 1% of adults 65 years or older and 2% of those 85 years or older.[71] Tremor is of slow frequency and occurs at rest, with a "pill-rolling" quality. It is aggravated by stress and inhibited during sleep or movement. *Essential tremor* if bilateral and symmetric, with positive family history, and if diminished by alcohol.

Persistent blinking after glabellar tap and difficulty walking heel-to-toe in *Parkinson disease* are also more common.

RECORDING YOUR FINDINGS

Note that initially you may use sentences to describe your findings; later you will use phrases. The style below contains phrases appropriate for most write-ups. As you read through this physical examination, you will notice some atypical findings. Try to test yourself. See if you can interpret these findings in the context of all you have learned about the examination of the older adult.

Recording the Physical Examination—The Older Adult

Mr. J is an older adult who appears healthy but underweight, with good muscle bulk. He is alert and interactive, with good recall of his life history. He is accompanied by his son.

Vital Signs: Ht (without shoes) 160 cm (5′). Wt (dressed) 65 kg (143 lbs). BMI 28. BP 145/88 right arm, supine; 154/94 left arm supine. Heart rate (HR) 98 and regular. Respiratory rate (RR) 18. Temperature (oral) 98.6°F.

10-Minute Geriatric Screener   (see p. 858)

Vision: Patient reports difficulty reading. Visual acuity 20/60 on Snellen chart.

Needs further evaluation for glasses and possibly hearing aid.

Hearing: Cannot hear whispered voice in either ear. Cannot hear 1,000 or 2,000 Hz with audioscope in either ear.

Leg Mobility: Can walk 20 feet briskly, turn, walk back to chair, and sit down in 14 seconds.

Urinary Incontinence: Has lost urine and gotten wet on 20 separate days.

Needs further evaluation for incontinence, including "DIAPER" assessment (see p. 858), prostate examination, and postvoid residual, which is normally ≤ 50 ml (requires bladder catheterization).

Nutrition: Has lost 15 lbs over the past 6 months without trying.

Needs nutritional screen, p. 853.

Memory: Can remember three items after 1 minute.

Depression: Does not often feel sad or depressed.

Physical Disability: Can walk fast but cannot ride a bicycle. Can do moderate but not heavy work around the house. Can go shopping for groceries or clothes. Can get to places out of walking distance. Can bathe each day without difficulty. Can dress, including buttoning and zipping, and can put on shoes.   *(continued)*

Consider exercise regimen with strength training.

Physical Examination

Skin. Warm and moist. Nails without clubbing or cyanosis. Hair thinning at crown.

Head, Eyes, Ears, Nose, Throat (HEENT). Scalp without lesions. Skull NC/AT. Conjunctiva pink, sclera muddy. Pupils 2 mm constricting to 1 mm, round, regular, equally reactive to light and accommodation. Extraocular movements intact. Disc margins sharp, without hemorrhages or exudates. Mild arteriolar narrowing. TMs with good cone of light. Weber midline. AC ≥ BC. Nasal mucosa pink. No sinus tenderness. Oral mucosa pink. Dentition fair. Caries present. Tongue midline, slight beefy redness. Pharynx without exudates.

Neck. Supple. Trachea midline. Thyroid lobes slightly enlarged, no nodules.

Lymph Nodes. No cervical, axillary, epitrochlear, or inguinal lymph nodes.

Thorax and Lungs. Thorax symmetric. Kyphosis noted. Lungs resonant with good excursion. Breath sounds vesicular. Diaphragms descend 4 cm bilaterally.

Cardiovascular. JVP 6 cm above the left atrium. Carotid upstrokes brisk, without bruits. PMI tapping, in the 5th ICS, 9 cm lateral to the midsternal line. II/VI harsh holosystolic murmur at the apex, radiating to the axilla. No S_3, S_4, or other murmurs.

Abdomen. Scaphoid, with active bowel sounds. Soft, nontender. No masses or hepatosplenomegaly. Liver span 7 cm in right midclavicular line; edge smooth and palpable at the RCM. No CVAT.

Genitourinary. Circumcised male. No penile lesions. Testes descended bilaterally, smooth.

Rectal. Rectal vault without masses. Stool brown, negative for occult blood.

Extremities. Warm and without edema. Calves supple.

Peripheral Vascular. Pulses 2+ and symmetric.

Musculoskeletal. Mild degenerative changes at the knees, with quadriceps wasting. Good range of motion in all joints.

Neurological. Oriented to person, place, and time. Mini-Mental State: score 29. Cranial Nerves II–XII intact. Motor: Decreased quadriceps bulk. Tone intact. Strength 4/5 throughout. RAMs, finger-to-nose intact. Gait with widened base. Sensation intact to pinprick, light touch, position, and vibration. Romberg negative. Reflexes 2+ and symmetric, with plantar response downgoing.

Bibliography

CITATIONS

1. Federal Agency Forum on Aging Related Statistics. Older Americans 2000: Key Indicators of Well-Being. Hyattsville, MD: National Center for Health Statistics, 2000.
2. Fries JF. Measuring and monitoring success in compressing morbidity. Ann Intern Med Suppl 139(5):455, 2003.
3. Bodenheimer T, Wagner EH, Grumbach K. Improving primary care for patients with chronic illness. JAMA 288(14): 1775–1779, 2002.
4. Perls TT. Understanding the determinants of exceptional longevity. Ann Intern Med Suppl 139(5):445, 2003.
5. Perls TT, Kunkel LM, Puca AA. The genetics of exceptional human longevity. J Am Geriatr Soc 50:359–368, 2002.
6. Rowe JW, Kahn RL. Human aging: usual and successful. Science 237:143–149, 1987.

BIBLIOGRAPHY

7. Taffet GE. Physiology of aging. In Cassel CK, Leipzig RM, Cohen HJ, et al (eds). Geriatric Medicine, 4th ed, pp. 27–36. New York: Springer, 2003.

8. Mulligan T, Saddiqi W. Changes in male sexuality. In Cassel CK, Leipzig RM, Cohen HJ, et al (eds). Geriatric Medicine, 4th ed., pp. 719–726. New York: Springer, 2003.

9. Kaiser FE. Sexual function and the older woman. In Cassel CK, Leipzig RM, Cohen HJ, et al (eds). Geriatric Medicine, 4th ed., pp. 727–736. New York: Springer, 2003.

10. DuBeau CE. Benign prostatic hyperplasia. In Cassel CK, Leipzig RM, Cohen HJ, et al (eds). Geriatric Medicine, 4th ed., pp. 755–768. New York: Springer, 2003.

11. Tangarorang GL, Kerins GJ, Besdine RW. Clinical approach to the older patient: an overview. In Cassel CK, Leipzig RM, Cohen HJ, et al (eds). Geriatric Medicine, 4th ed., pp. 149–162. New York: Springer, 2003.

12. Bayer AJ, Chadna JS, Farag RR, et al. Changing presentation of myocardial infarction with increasing old age. J Am Geriatr Soc 34:263–266, 1986.

13. Trivalle C, Doucet J, Chassagrie P, et al. Differences in the signs and symptoms of hyperthyroidism in older and younger patients. J Am Geriatr Soc 44:50–53, 1996.

14. Doucet J, Trivalle C, Chassagrie P, et al. Does age play a role in clinical presentation of hypothyroidism? J Am Geriatr Soc 42:984–986, 1994.

15. Tinetti ME, Williams CS, Gill TM. Dizziness among older adults: a possible geriatric syndrome. Ann Intern Med 132(5): 337–344, 2000.

16. Fried LP, Sotrer DJ, King DE, et al. Diagnosis of illness presentation in the elderly. J Am Geriatr Soc 39:117–123, 1991.

17. Davis PB, Robins LN. History-taking in the elderly with and without cognitive impairment. J Am Geriatr Soc 37:249–255, 1989.

18. Ferraro KF, Su YP. Physician-evaluated and self-reported morbidity for predicting disability. Am J Public Health Jan; 90(1): 103–108, 2000.

19. Kuczmarski MF, Kuczmarski RJ, Najjar M. Effects of age on validity of self-reported height, weight and body mass index: findings from the third National Health and Nutrition Examination Survey, 1988–1994. J Am Diet Assoc 101(1):28–34, 2001.

20. Lagaay AM, van der Meij JC, Hijmans W. Validation of medical history taking as part of a population based survey in subjects aged 85 and over. BMJ 304:1091–1092, 1992.

21. Nunez GR. Culture, demographics, and critical care issues: an overview. Crit Care Clin 19:619–639, 2003.

22. Xakellis G, Brangman SA, Ladson H, et al. Curricular framework: core competencies in multicultural geriatric care. J Am Geriatr Soc 52:137–142, 2004.

23. Goldstein MZ, Griswold K. Practical geriatrics: cultural sensitivity and aging. Psychiatric Serv 49:769–771, 1998.

24. Evans CA, Cunningham BA. Caring for the ethnic elder. Geriatr Nurs 17(3):105–109, 1996.

25. Fick DM, Cooper JW, Wade WE, et al. Updating the Beers criteria for potentially inappropriate medication use in older adults: results of a US consensus panel of experts. Arch Intern Med 163:2716–2724, 2003.

26. Reuben DB, Herr KA, Pacala JT, et al. Geriatrics at Your Fingertips, 6th ed., pp. 9–12. Malden, MA: Blackwell Science, Inc., for the American Geriatrics Society, 2004.

27. Takahashi PY, Okhravi HR, Lim LS, et al. Preventive health care in the elderly population: a guide for practicing physicians. Mayo Clinic Proc 79:416–427, 2004.

28. Corti MC, Guralnik JM, Salive ME, et al. Serum albumin level and physical disability as predictors of mortality in older persons. JAMA 272(13):1036–1042, 1994.

29. Ferrell BA. Acute and chronic pain. In Cassel CK, Leipzig RM, Cohen HJ, et al (eds). Geriatric Medicine, 4th ed., pp. 323–342. New York: Springer, 2003.

30. Jones TV, Lindsey BA, Yount P, et al. Alcoholism screening questionnaires: are they valid in elderly medical outpatients? J Gen Intern Med 8(12):674–678, 1993.

31. Callahan CM, Tierney WM. Health services use and mortality among older primary care patients with alcoholism. J Am Geriatr Soc 43(12):1378–1383, 1995.

32. Tulsky JA. Doctor-patient communication issues. In Cassel CK, Leipzig RM, Cohen HJ, et al (eds). Geriatric Medicine, 4th ed., pp. 287–298. New York: Springer, 2003.

33. Callahan D. The value of achieving a peaceful death. In Cassel CK, Leipzig RM, Cohen HJ, et al (eds). Geriatric Medicine, 4th ed., pp. 351–360. New York: Springer, 2003.

34. Morrison RS, Meier DE. Palliative care. N Engl J Med 350: 2582–2590, 2004.

35. Beck LH. Periodic health examination and screening tests in adults. Hosp Pract 15:121–126, 1999.

36. American Geriatrics Society Ethics Committee. American Geriatric Society Position Paper: Health Screening Decisions for Older Adults, 2001. Available at: www.americangeriatrics.org. Accessed October 1, 2004.

37. Bogardus ST, Yueh B, Shekelle PG. Screening and management of adult hearing loss in primary care: clinical applications JAMA 289(15):1986–1990, 2003.

38. Oddone EZ, Heflin MT, Feussner JR. Screening for cancer. In Cassel CK, Leipzig RM, Cohen HJ, et al (eds). Geriatric Medicine, 4th ed., pp. 375–392. New York: Springer, 2003.

39. U.S. Preventive Services Task Force. Screening for dementia. In Guide to Clinical Preventive Services, pp. 531–541. Baltimore, Williams & Wilkins, 1996.

40. Fulmer T, Guadagno L, Dyer CB, et al. Progress in elder abuse screening and assessment instruments. J Am Geriatr Soc 52: 297–304, 2004.

41. Fulmer T, Hernandez M. Elder mistreatment. In Cassel CK, Leipzig RM, Cohen HJ, et al (eds). Geriatric Medicine, 4th ed., pp. 1057–1066. New York: Springer, 2003.

42. Koretz B, Reuben DB. Instruments to assess functional status. Reuben DB. Comprehensive geriatric assessment and systems approaches to geriatric care. In Cassel CK, Leipzig RM, Cohen HJ, et al (eds). Geriatric Medicine, 4th ed., pp. 185–194; pp. 195–204. New York: Springer, 2003.

43. Moore AA, Siu AL. Screening for common problems in ambulatory elderly: clinical confirmation of a screening instrument. Am J Med 100: 438–440, 1996.

44. Resnick NM. Urinary incontinence. In Cassel CK, Leipzig RM, Cohen HJ, et al (eds). Geriatric Medicine, 4th ed., pp. 931–956. New York: Springer, 2003.

45. American Geriatrics Society, British Geriatrics Society, American Academy of Orthopedic Surgeons. Guideline for prevention of falls in older persons. J Am Geriatr Soc 49:664–672, 2001.

46. Tinetti ME. Preventing falls in elderly persons. N Engl J Med 348(1):42–48, 2003.

47. Bobrie G, Genes N, Vaur L, et al. Is "isolated home" hypertension as opposed to "isolated office" hypertension a sign of greater cardiovascular risk? Arch Intern Med 161(18): 2205–2211, 2001.

48. Chaudhry SI, Krumholz HM, Foody JM. Systolic hypertension in older persons. JAMA 292(9):1074–1080, 2004.

49. Papademetriou V. Comparative prognostic value of systolic, diastolic, and pulse pressure. Am J Cardiol 91(4):433–435, 2003.

50. Vaccarino V, Berger AK, et al. Pulse pressure and risk of cardiovascular events in the systolic hypertension in the elderly program. Am J Cardiol 88(9):980–986, 2001.

51. Carlson JE. Assessment of orthostatic blood pressure: measurement technique and clinical applications. South Med J 92(2):167–173, 1999.

52. Consensus Committee of the American Autonomic Society and the American Academy of Neurology. Consensus statement on the definition of orthostatic hypotension, pure autonomic failure, and multiple system atrophy. Neurology 46:1470, 1996.

53. McGee S, Abernethy WB, Simel DL. Is this patient hypovolemic? JAMA 281(11):1022–1029, 1999.

54. Ooi WL, Barrett S, Hossain M, et al. Patterns of orthostatic blood pressure change and their clinical correlates in a frail elderly population. JAMA 277(16):1299–1304, 1997.

55. Raiha I, Luntonen S, Piha J, et al. Prevalence, predisposing factors and prognostic importance of postural hypotension. Arch Intern Med 155:930–935, 1995.

56. Gnann JW, Whitely RJ. Herpes zoster N Engl J Med 347(5): 340–346, 2002.

57. Congdon NG, Friedman DS, Lietman T. Important causes of visual impairment in the world today. JAMA 290(15): 2057–2060, 2003.

58. Swan IRC, Browning GG. The whispered voice as a screening test for hearing impairment. J Royal Col Gen Pract 35:197, 1985.

59. Gordon SR, Jahnigen DW. Oral assessment of the dentulous elderly patient. J Am Geriatr Soc 34:276–281, 1986.

60. Otto CM, Lind BK, Kitzman DW, et al. Association of aortic–valve sclerosis with cardiovascular mortality and morbidity in the elderly. JAMA 341(3):142–147, 1999.

61. Leach RM, McBrien DJ. Brachiocardial delay: a new clinical indicator of the severity of aortic stenosis. Lancet 335: 1199–1201, 1990.

62. Dumesic DA. Pelvic examination: what to focus on in menopausal women. Consultant 36:39–46, 1996.

63. American Geriatrics Society. Screening for cervical carcinoma in older women. J Am Geriatr Soc 49: 655–657, 2001.

64. Hoffman MS, Cardosi RD, Roberts WS, et al. Accuracy of pelvic examination in the assessment of patients with operable cervical cancer. Am J Obstet Gynecol 190:986–993, 2004.

65. McDermott MM, Greenland P, Liu K, et al. The ankle brachial index is associated with leg function and physical activity: the walking and leg circulation study. Ann Intern Med 136(12): 873–883, 2002.

66. Baloh RW, Ying SH, Jacobson KM. A longitudinal study of gait and balance dysfunction in normal older people. Arch Neurol 60:835–839, 2003.

67. Guralnik JM, Ferrucci L, Simonsek E, et al. Lower extremity function in persons over the age of 70 years as a predictor of subsequent disability. N Engl J Med 332(9):556–561, 1995.

68. Tinetti ME, Williams TF, Mayewski R. Fall risk index for elderly patients based on number of chronic disabilities. Am J Med 80(3):429–434, 1986.

69. Tinetti ME, Ginter SF. Identifying mobility dysfunctions in elderly patients. JAMA 259(8):1190–1193, 1988.

70. Odenheimer G, Funkenstein HH, Beckett L, et al. Comparison of neurologic changes in 'successfully aging' persons vs. the total aging population. Arch Neurol 51:573–580, 1994.

71. Rao G, Fisch L, Srinivasan S, et al. Does this patient have Parkinson disease? JAMA 289(3):347–353, 2003.

ADDITIONAL REFERENCES

American Geriatrics Society. Available at http://www.american geriatrics.org. Accessed July 7, 2005.

American Geriatrics Society. Ethnogeriatrics Steering Committee. Doorway Thoughts: Cross-cultural Health Care for Older Adults. Sudbury, MA: Jones and Bartlett, 2004.

Amin SH, Kuhle CL, Fitzpatrick LA. Comprehensive evaluation of the older woman. Mayo Clin Proc 78(9):1157–1185, 2003.

Cassel, CK. Geriatric Medicine: An Evidence-based Approach, 4th ed. New York, Springer, 2003.

Cassetta M, Gorevic PD. Crystal arthritis. Gout and pseudogout in the geriatric patient. Geriatrics 59(9):25–30, 2004.

Clark CM, Karlawish JHT. Alzheimer disease: Current concepts and emerging diagnostic and therapeutic strategies. Ann Intern Med 138(5):400–410, 2003.

Hazzard WR. Principles of Geriatric Medicine and Gerontology, 5th ed. New York, McGraw-Hill/Professional, 2003.

Kennedy-Malone L, Fletcher KR, Plank LR. Management Guidelines for Gerontological Nurse Practitioners. Philadelphia, FA Davis, 2000.

Karlawish JHT, Clark CM. Diagnostic evaluation of elderly patients with mild memory problems. Ann Intern Med 138(5):411–419, 2003.

Landefeld CS. Current Geriatric Diagnosis & Treatment. New York, Lange Medical Books/McGraw-Hill, 2004.

Meldon S, Ma OJ, Woolard R, American College of Emergency Physicians. Geriatric Emergency Medicine. New York, McGraw-Hill, Medical Pub Division, 2004.

Springhouse. Handbook of Geriatric Nursing Care, 2nd ed. Philadelphia, Lippincott Williams & Wilkins, 2002

TABLE 20-1   Delirium and Dementia

Delirium and dementia are common and very important disorders that affect multiple aspects of mental status. Both have many possible causes. Some clinical features of these two conditions and their effects on mental status are compared below. A delirium may be superimposed on dementia.

	Delirium	Dementia
Clinical Features		
Onset	Acute	Insidious
Course	Fluctuating, with lucid intervals; worse at night	Slowly progressive
Duration	Hours to weeks	Months to years
Sleep/Wake Cycle	Always disrupted	Sleep fragmented
General Medical Illness or Drug Toxicity	Either or both present	Often absent, especially in Alzheimer's disease
Mental Status		
Level of Consciousness	Disturbed. Person less clearly aware of the environment and less able to focus, sustain, or shift attention	Usually normal until late in the course of the illness
Behavior	Activity often abnormally decreased (somnolence) or increased (agitation, hypervigilance)	Normal to slow; may become inappropriate
Speech	May be hesitant, slow or rapid, incoherent	Difficulty in finding words, aphasia
Mood	Fluctuating, labile, from fearful or irritable to normal or depressed	Often flat, depressed
Thought Processes	Disorganized, may be incoherent	Impoverished. Speech gives little information.
Thought Content	Delusions common, often transient	Delusions may occur.
Perceptions	Illusions, hallucinations, most often visual	Hallucinations may occur.
Judgment	Impaired, often to a varying degree	Increasingly impaired over the course of the illness
Orientation	Usually disoriented, especially for time. A known place may seem unfamiliar.	Fairly well maintained, but becomes impaired in the later stages of illness
Attention	Fluctuates. Person easily distracted, unable to concentrate on selected tasks	Usually unaffected until late in the illness
Memory	Immediate and recent memory impaired	Recent memory and new learning especially impaired
Examples of Cause	Delirium tremens (due to withdrawal from alcohol) Uremia Acute hepatic failure Acute cerebral vasculitis Atropine poisoning	*Reversible:* Vitamin B_{12} deficiency, thyroid disorders *Irreversible:* Alzheimer's disease, vascular dementia (from multiple infarcts), dementia due to head trauma

Subject Index

NOTE: Page numbers followed by b indicate in-chapter boxed material; those followed by t indicate end-of-chapter tables.

of floor of mouth, 238t
of lip, 231t
pancreatic, skin in, 146t
of penis, 422t
squamous cell, 862
of skin, 124, 142t
of vulva, 450t
Cardiac arrhythmias, 111, 649t–650t
blood pressure measurement and, 110
in infants, 697–698, 718
Cardiac circulation, 281
Cardiac conduction system, 287–288
Cardiac cycle, 282–284
Cardiac disease, in infants, noncardiac findings
in, 716, 716b
Cardiac examination, 307–321
anatomic location of sounds in, 307
auscultation in, 313–319
heart murmurs and, 316–319, 318b
inspection and palpation in, 308–313
of aortic area, 313
of left ventricular area, 309–311
of pulmonic area, 313
of right ventricular area, 311–313
integrating, 319
percussion in, 313
recording findings of, 321, 321b
sequence of, 307b
special techniques in, 319–321
for identifying systolic murmurs, 319–320,
320b
for paradoxical pulse, 320–321
for pulsus alternans, 320
timing of impulses and sounds in, 308
Cardiac output, 288
Cardiac syncope, 608
Cardinal directions, 159
Cardiogenic shock, 306
Cardiomegaly, in infants, 716
Cardiomyopathy, 310
Cardiovascular system, 279–335. See also Cardiac entries; Heart
age-related changes in, 292–293
anatomy and physiology of, 279–293
in comprehensive physical examination, 13
disease of, prevention of, 296–298, 297b,
299b, 299–301, 300b
examination techniques for, 302–321
carotid pulse as, 305–307
for heart, 307b, 307–319
for identification of murmurs, 319–320,
320b
integrating, 319
jugular venous pressure as, 302–304, 303b
jugular venous pulsations as, 304–305
in older adults, 861–868
for paradoxical pulse, 320–321
for pulsus alternans, 320
in health history, 293b, 293–295
health promotion and counseling and, 295b,
295–301
in older adults, 843–844
during pregnancy, 818
recording findings for, 321
in review of systems, 10

Carotene, 122
Carotenemia, 127, 133t
Carotid arteries, 168
examination techniques for, 200
in older adults, 844
Carotid bruit, 762, 762b, 763
Carotid pulse, 305–307
jugular artery pulsations versus, 303b
Carpal bones, 508
Carpal tunnel, 509
Carpal tunnel syndrome, 510, 514, 554t
examination techniques for, 541–542
Cartilage, articular, 485
Cartilaginous joints, 485, 485b
Caruncles, urethral, 451t
in older adults, 866
Cataracts, 175, 188, 216t
in infants, 708
in older adults, 843, 863
Cat scratches, 140t
Cauda equina, 598
CBE (clinical breast examination), 344
Cellulitis, 479
acute, 492t–493t
periorbital, Haemophilus influenzae, 815t
Central cyanosis, 122, 126
Central nervous system. See also Brain; Spinal
cord
anatomy and physiology of, 596–598
disorders of, 660t–661t
Cephalohematoma, 802t
Cephalohematomas, 703
Cerebellar ataxia, 628, 664t
Cerebellar disease, 626, 627
Cerebellar system, 601b, 602, 603
Cerebellum, 597
lesions of, 661t
Cerebral cortex, lesions of, 661t
Cerebral palsy, 654t, 731
Cervical cancer, 443, 453t
Pap smear to detect, 430, 435–437
in older adults, 856
during pregnancy, 827, 832
Cervical erosion, 819
Cervical eversion, 819
Cervical lymph nodes, 196
Cervical mucous, in older adults, 866
Cervical os, shapes of, 453t
Cervical sprain, 547t
Cervical systolic murmur/bruit, 293
Cervicitis, mucopurulent, 443, 453t
Cervix, uterine, 430, 460
cancer of, 443, 453t
Pap smear to detect, 430, 435–437, 827,
856
fetal DES exposure and, 453t
inspection of, 442–443
palpation of, 445
during pregnancy, 819, 832
variations in surface of, 452t
Chadwick's sign, 818, 819
Chalazion, 214t
Chancre, syphilitic, 140t, 231t
in females, 450t
in males, 422t

Chart, reviewing before interview, 26
Cheilitis
actinic, 230t
angular, 230t
in older adults, 843
Cherry angiomas, 141t
in older adults, 862
Chest. See Heart; Lung(s); Thorax
Chest pain, 248–249, 268t–269t
exertional, 293
Chest wall
anatomy of, 241
auscultatory findings related to, 286
Cheyne-Stokes breathing, 120t
Chickenpox, 140t, 144t
skin in, 147t
Chief complaints, 5b, 6
Child abuse
asking questions about, 52
diagnostic facies in, 804t
Child development, 672–680
during adolescence, 678–680
during childhood, 675–677
health promotion and counseling and,
681–684, 682b
during infancy, 674
key principles in, 672b, 672–673
during middle childhood, 677–678
Childhood illnesses, 7
Children (age 1-10), 738–774
assessment of, 738b–740b, 738–745
in early childhood, 739–742
in middle childhood, 742–745
development of, 675–678
diagnostic facies in, 803t–804t
examination techniques for, 745–774
for abdomen, 763b, 763–765
for ears, 753–756, 754b
for eyes, 751–752, 752b
for female genitalia, 766–769
general survey and, 745–747
for head, 750
for heart, 762b, 762–763
for male genitalia, 765
for mouth and pharynx, 757b, 757–760,
759b, 760b
for musculoskeletal system, 769–771
for neck, 750–751
for nervous system, 771–774
for nose and paranasal sinuses, 756–757
for rectal examination, 769
for skin, 750
for thorax and lungs, 760–761
for vital signs, 747–749
hymen configuration is, 811t
preventive health care recommendations for,
797t
Chills, 95
Chlamydial infection, genital, 443, 444
Chloasma, 828
Choanal atresia, 709
Cholecystitis
acute, 394t–395t, 408t
assessment techniques for, 390
chronic, 394t–395t

Gonococcal urethritis, 417
Gonococcemia, skin in, 146t
Gout, 488
    tophaceous, chronic, in hands, 553t
Gouty arthritis
    of feet, 556t
    joint pain in, 548t–549t
    in older adults, 867
Gower maneuver/sign, 773, 814t
Graded responses, 37
Grandeur, delusions of, 583b
Grand mal seizures, 652t
Granulomas, umbilical, 723
Graphesthesia, 632
Graves' disease, 180, 200
Gray matter, 596
    subcortical, lesions of, 661t
Great arteries, transposition of, in infants, 810
Great vessels, 279–281
    of neck, 168
Greeting patients, 29–30
Grip strength, testing, 512, 620
Groin, anatomy of, 413
Grooming
    in general survey, 104–105
    in mental status examination, 579
Gross hematuria, 369
Growth, somatic
    of adolescents, 776
    of children, 745–747, 747b
    of infants, 695–696
Growth hormone deficiency, 746
Growths, penile, 414
Grunting, in infants, 712, 712b
Gums
    examination techniques for, 194
    findings in, 235t–236t
    recession of, 235t236t
Gynecomastia, 350, 778

H

Habituation
    in infants, 709
    in newborns, 692b
Haemophilus influenzae infection, 815t
Hair, 121, 122
    examination of, 128
        techniques for, 177
    in health history, 123, 123b
    lanugo, 700
    loss of, 149t
        with arterial peripheral vascular disease, 478
        during pregnancy, 828
    of newborns, 700, 701
    of older adults, 842
    during pregnancy, 828
    pubic, sexual maturity rating and
        in boys, 780, 781b
        in girls, 782, 783b
Hairy leukoplakia, 237t
Hairy tongue, 237t
Halitosis, in children, 760
Hallucinations, 584b
Hallux valgus, 556t

Hamman's sign, 275t
Hammer toe, 557t
Hamstring muscle, 531
Hand(s), 508–514
    arterial supply to, evaluating, 488–489
    arthritis in, 553t
    bony structures of, 508
    deformities of, 554t
    examination techniques for, 509–514
        inspection as, 509–510
        palpation as, 510–511
        range of motion and maneuvers as, 513–514
    of infants, 727
    joints of, 508
    muscle groups of, 509
    swellings of, 554t
Handedness, clinical position for examination and, 102
Handle, of malleus, 161
Harlequin dyschromia, 699
Harm, avoiding doing, 58
Hashimoto's thyroiditis, 200
Hay fever, 173
Head, 153–167. *See also specific organs*
    anatomy and physiology of, 153, 169–170
    circumference of
        of children, 746
        of infants, 696
    in comprehensive physical examination, 12
    examination techniques for, 177
        for adolescents, 777
        for children, 750
        for infants, 702–705, 705b
        in older adults, 862–864
        during pregnancy, 828
    in health history, 170b, 171–175
    health promotion and counseling and, 175b, 175–176
    of infant, abnormalities of, 802t
    of older adults, 842–843
    in review of systems, 9
Headache, 171, 206t–209t, 607
Health care proxy, 43, 53
Health history, 4–11, 93b, 93–95. *See also* Interviewing
    abdomen in, 362b, 362–370
        gastrointestinal tract and, 362–368
        urinary tract and, 368–370
    anus, rectum, and prostate in, 461, 461b
    breast in, 340b, 340–341
    cardiovascular system in, 293b, 293–295
    chief complaints in, 6
    comprehensive, 25
        adult, 5b, 6–11
        focused health history versus, 4–5
    family, 8
    fatigue in, 94
    female genitalia in, 432b, 432–435
    fever, chills and night sweats in, 95
    focused (problem-oriented), 26
        comprehensive health history versus, 4–5
    format for, 25
    head in, 170b, 171–175
    male genitalia in, 413b, 413–415

medications in, 7
mental health, obtaining, 49–50
mental status in, 575b, 575–576
musculoskeletal system in, 487b, 487–490
neck in, 170b, 174–175
neurologic assessment in, 607b, 607–609
with older adults, 848b, 848–855
    content and pace of visit for, 849
    cultural dimensions of aging and, 851
    eliciting symptoms and, 849–850, 850b
    office environment and, 848–849
    past, 7–8
    peripheral vascular system in, 478b, 478–479
    personal and social, 8
    pregnancy in, 822b, 822–823
    review of systems in, 8–11
    sexual, obtaining, 48–49
    skin, hair, and nails in, 123, 123b
    subjective versus objective data in, 5–6, 6b
    thorax and lungs in, 248b, 248–250
    weakness in, 95
    weight changes and, 93–94
Health Insurance Portability and Accountability Act (HIPPA), 43
Health promotion and counseling, 95b, 95–96
    abdomen in, 370b, 370–373
    blood pressure and, 96
    breasts and, 341b, 341–344, 342b
    cardiovascular system and, 295b, 295–301
    diet and, 96
    exercise and, 96
    female genitalia and, 435b, 435–438
        family planning and, 437
        menopause and, 437–438
        Pap smear and, 435–437
        sexually transmitted diseases and, 437
    head and neck and, 175b, 175–176
    male genitalia and, 415b, 415–416
    mental status and, 576b, 576–577
    musculoskeletal system and, 490b, 490–492
    for older adults, 855–857
    optimal weight and nutrition and, 95–96
    pediatric, 681–684, 682b
    for peripheral vascular disease, 479–480
    prostate cancer and, 462–463
    skin cancer and, 124b, 124–125
    smoking cessation and, 250–251
    transient ischemic attack/stroke prevention and, 609–610
Health status
    apparent, in general survey, 103
    first prenatal visit and, 822
Hearing
    aging and, 843
    assessment of, 612, 615
        in children, 756
        in older adults, 855
    pathways of, 161–162
Hearing loss, 172–173
    assessment of, 190–191
    in infants, 709
    interviewing and, 46
    patterns of, 229t

Hyperresonance, as percussion note, 256b, 257, 263
Hypertension
  in adolescents, 776
  blood pressure level and, 109, 109b
  in children, 749, 798t
  control of, 610
  diet for, 118t
  in infants, 697
  lifestyle modifications to prevent or manage, 299b, 299–301
  in office ("white coat"), 110
  in older adults, 841
  prevention of, 295–296, 296b
  pulmonary, 312, 313
    in infants, 719
  systemic, 313
  systolic, isolation, 109
  with unequal blood pressure in arms and legs, 111
Hypertensive retinopathy, 223t
Hyperthyroidism, 175, 177, 183–184
  apical impulse in, 311
  diagnostic facies in, 804t
  signs and symptoms of, 239t
  skin in, 127, 146t
Hypertrophic cardiomyopathy, 333t, 649t–650t
Hypertrophic osteoarthropathy, 490
Hypertrophy, 617
Hyperventilation, 120t, 249
  anxiety with, dyspnea in, 270t–271t
  hypercapnia due to, 649t–650t
Hypervolemia, jugular venous pressure and, 303
Hypesthesia, 631
Hypoalbuminemia, 294
Hypocapnia, 649t–650t
Hypoglossal nerve, 598, 599b
  of children, 772b
  examination of, 612, 616
Hypoglycemia, 649t–650t
Hypomanic episodes, 590t
Hypospadias, 417, 422t, 725, 813t
Hypotension
  blood pressure level and, 109b, 110
  postural (orthostatic), 110, 649t–650t
    in older adults, 841
Hypothalamus, 596
Hypothermia, 112
  actinic, 841
Hypothyroidism, 175, 177
  congenital, 699, 702, 710
    facies in, 803t
  signs and symptoms of, 239t
  skin in, 127
Hypotonia, in newborns, 731
Hypotonic muscles, 618
Hypovolemia, jugular venous pressure and, 303
Hysterectomy, Pap smear following, 436
Hysterical fainting, 649t–650t

I

IADLs (instrumental activities of daily living), older adults and, 852, 852b

Ichthyosis, 139t
  congenital, 700
Identifying data, 5b, 6
Ileus, paralytic, 376
Iliac arteries, anatomy and physiology of, 360
Iliac crest, 523
Iliac spine
  anterior superior, 523
  posterior superior, 523
Iliac tubercle, 523
Iliofemoral thrombosis, 487
Iliopectineal bursa, 524
Iliopsoas bursa, 524
Iliopsoas muscles, 524
Ilium, 523
Illusions, 584b
Immunizations, 8
  for older adults, 856
Imperforate hymen, 442
Impetigo, 138t, 139t
Incisional hernia, 404t
Incoherence, 582b
Incus, 160
Indigestion, 362
Induration, penile, 417
Infant(s) (first year)
  abdomen of, 723b, 723–724
  assessment of, 685–694
    of newborn, 686b, 686–692
    sequence of, 685
    testing for developmental milestones and, 694
  breasts of, 722
  cries of, 711, 711b
  development of, 674–675
  diagnostic facies in, 803t–804t
  ears of, 708–709, 709b
  eyes of, 706–708, 708b
  female genitalia of, 725–726
  heart murmurs in, 809t–810t
  heart of, 714–722
    auscultation of, 718–722, 719b, 722b
    inspection of, 715b, 715–716, 716b
    palpation of, 716–718
  male genitalia of, 725
  mouth and pharynx of, 710–711
  musculoskeletal system of, 727–730
  neck of, 705–706
  newborn. See Newborns
  nose and paranasal sinuses of, 709–710
  postterm, 700
  premature, 689, 699
  preventive health care recommendations for, 797t
  rashes in, 800t
  rectal examination of, 726
  reflexes in, 733, 734, 735b–736b
  techniques of examination for, 695–737
    for abdomen, 723b, 723–724
    for breasts, 722
    for ears, 708–709, 709b
    for eyes, 706–708, 708b
    for female genitalia, 725–726
    general survey as, 695–698
    for head, 702–705, 705b

  for heart, 714–722
  for male genitalia, 725
  for mouth and pharynx, 710–711
  for musculoskeletal system, 727–730
  for neck, 705–706
  for nervous system, 730–737, 732b, 735b–737b
  for nose and paranasal sinuses, 709–710
  for rectal examination, 726
  for skin, 699–702
  for thorax and lungs, 711–714, 712b, 714b
  thorax and lungs of, 711–714, 712b, 714b
Infantile automatisms, 734
Infection(s). *See also specific infections*
  of Bartholin's gland, 451t
  of bladder, 368, 386
  corneal, 215t
  diarrhea due to, 398t–399t
  from oral-penile transmission, 414
  thenar space, 555t
  of vas deferens, 418
Infectious diarrhea, 398t–399t
Inferior rectus muscle, right, 159
Inferior vena cava, 281
  obstruction of, 375
Inflammation
  meningeal, testing for, 641
  signs of, 494
Inflammatory bowel disease
  in children, 769
  diarrhea due to, 398t–399t
Inflammatory diarrhea, 398t–399t
Information, in mental status examination, 586
Informed consent, 58–59
Infraclavicular lymph nodes, 340
Infranuclear ophthalmoplegia, 183
Infrapatellar bursitis, 532
Infraspinatus muscles, 499, 505
Ingrown toenails, 557t
Inguinal canal, 413
Inguinal hernias, 526, 765
  female, 448
Inguinal ligament, 526
Inguinal lymph nodes
  horizontal, 477
  in males, 412
  superficial, 477, 483
  vertical, 477
Inguinal ring, external, 413
Innocent flow murmurs, 318
Insect bites, 137t, 138t
  in children, 801t
Insight, 584
  in mental status examination, 574b, 584
Inspection
  of abdomen, of infants, 723
  in abdominal examination, 374–376
  of ankle and foot, 539
  of axillae, 350–351
  of breasts, 345–346
    during pregnancy, 829
  in cardiac examination, 308–313
    of aortic area, 313
    of left ventricular area, 309–311

anatomy and physiology of, 165–167
in comprehensive physical examination, 12
examination techniques for, 193–195
  for children, 757b, 757–760, 759b, 760b
  for infants, 710–711
health promotion and counseling and, 176
of older adults, 843
during pregnancy, 828
Movements. *See also* Extraocular movements; Range of motion; *specific joints*
  facial, assessment of, 612, 614–615
  fetal, palpation for, 829
  involuntary, 609
    in motor assessment, 616
  of jaw, assessment of, 612, 613
  in newborns, 691
  point-to-point, assessing, 626–627
  rapid alternating, assessing, 626
Mucoid sputum, 250
Mucosal rings/webs, 396t
Mucous patch of syphilis, 238t
Mucous plug, 819
Multinodular goiter, 239t
Multiple sclerosis, 386
Multisystem conditions, 73
Murphy's sign, 390
Muscles. *See also specific muscles*
  atrophy of, assessing for, 617–618
  axiohumeral, 499
  axioscapular, 499
  of elbow, 506
  of hands, 509
  of hip, 524
  hypotonic, 618
  of knee, 531
  lesions of, 662t
  scapulohumeral, 499
  of shoulder, 499
  of spine, 517, 517b
  of temporomandibular joint, 495
  of wrist, 509
Muscle strength
  assessment of, in children, 772–773
  in motor assessment, 618–624, 619b
Muscle tone, 601b
  assessment of, in stuporous or comatose patients, 645–646
  disorders of, 659t
  in motor assessment, 618
Muscle weakness
  in chest, 259b
  in infants, 713
Muscular dystrophy, 773
Musculoskeletal system, 483–557. *See also specific structures*
  anatomy and physiology of, 493–494
  examination techniques for, 493b–494b, 493–494
    for adolescents, 784–785, 786b–788b
    for children, 769–771
    for infants, 727–730
    in older adults, 867
  fractures and. *See* Fractures
  health promotion and counseling and and, 490b, 490–492

joints and. *See* Joint(s); *specific joints*
  in lower extremities, in comprehensive physical examination, 13, 14
  muscles and. *See* Muscles; *specific muscles*
  of older adults, 850
  during pregnancy, 818
  in review of systems, 10
Myalgias, 488
Mycoplasma pneumonia, cough and hemoptysis in, 272t
Mycosis fungoides, 135t
Mydriasis, 181
Myocardial contractility, 288
Myocardial dysfunction, in infants, 717, 718
Myocardial infarction, 649t–650t
  chest pain with, 268t–269t
Myoclonus, 652t
Myomas, 446
  uterine, 456t
Myopathy, 623
Myopia, 171, 178
Myringitis, bullous, 227t
Myxedema, facies in, 211t

N

Nabothian cysts, 452t
Naegele's rule, 823
Nail(s), 121, 122, 123
  examination of, 128
  findings in or near, 150t–151t
  in health history, 123, 123b
  in older adults, 842
Nail plate, 122
Narrow-angle glaucoma, 181
  in older adults, 843
Nasal bone, 153
Nasal congestion, 173
Nasal flaring, in infants, 712, 712b
Nasal mucosa, examination techniques for, 192
Nasal obstruction, testing for, 192
Nasal septum, 162
  examination techniques for, 193
Nasolacrimal duct, 155
  obstruction of, 180
    examination techniques for, 201
  in infants, 708
Nausea, 362, 363
  during pregnancy, 821b
NAVEL mnemonic, 526
Near reaction, 158
Near response, 612
Near-sightedness, 171
Near syncope, 608
Neck
  abnormalities of, in children, 807t
  anatomy and physiology of, 168–170
  in comprehensive physical examination, 12
  examination techniques for, 196–200
    for adolescents, 777
    for children, 750–751
    for infants, 705–706
    during pregnancy, 828
  in health history, 170b, 174–175
  health promotion and counseling and, 175b, 175–176

inspection of, 253
movement of
  assessment of, 612, 615–616, 641
  in children, 750–751
  of older adults, 843
  in review of systems, 9
Neck pain, 488, 547t
Negative predictive value, 76b, 78b
Neglect, one-sided, 579
Neisseria gonorrhoeae cervicitis, 443
Neologisms, 582b
Neonates. *See* Newborns
Neovascularization, retinal, 222t
Nephrotic syndrome, facies in, 211t
Nervous system, 573–593, 595–667. *See also* Cranial nerves; Mental status examination; Motor system; Reflexes; Sensory system
  anatomy and physiology of, 595–605
    of central nervous system, 596–598
    of motor pathways, 601b, 601–603
    of peripheral nervous system, 598–600
    of sensory pathways, 603–605
    of spinal reflexes, 600–601
  in comprehensive physical examination, 14
  disorders of, constipation due to, 397t
  examination techniques for, 610b, 610–646
    for adolescents, 784–785, 786b–788b
    for children, 771–774
    for cranial nerves, 611–616
    for deep tendon reflexes, 632–639
    for infants, 730–737, 732b, 735b–737b
    for motor system, 616–629
    in older adults, 867–868
    for sensory system, 629–633
  in health history, 607–609, 697b
  health promotion and counseling and, 609–610
  in lower extremities, in comprehensive physical examination, 13, 14
  of older adults, 846–848
  recording findings for, 647, 647b
  in review of systems, 11
Neurocutaneous symptoms, pathologic, benign birthmarks versus, 799t
Neurodermatitis, 139t
Neurofibromatoses, 145t, 519, 799t
  in newborns, 700
  skin in, 146t
Neurologic evaluation, of stuporous or comatose patients, 644–646
Neuromuscular junction, lesions of, 662t
Neurons, of brain, 596
Neuropathic ulcers, 495t, 557t
Nevi
  benign, 143t
  elevated, 137t
  epidermal, 135t
  simplex, 701
Newborns
  ability for complex behavior, 692b
  Apgar score in, 687b–688b, 687–688
  assessment of, 686b, 686–692
    immediate, at birth, 687–689
    several hours after birth, 690–691

Temporal arteritis, headache and, 208t–209t
Temporal artery, superficial, 153
Temporal bone, 153
    mastoid portion of, 153
Temporal muscles, 495s, 496
    palpation of, 613
Temporomandibular joint, 495–496
Tenderness
    abdominal, 407t–408t
    in chest, 253
    of kidneys, 386
    musculoskeletal, 494
    of nonpalpable liver, 382
    rebound, 379
    spine and, 518
Tendinitis, 488
    bicipital, 551t
    calcific, of shoulder, 550t
    rotator cuff, 550t
Tenesmus, 367
Tenosynovitis, 488, 511, 512
    acute, 555t
    de Quervain's, 510, 511, 512
    gonococcal, 510
Tension headache, 171, 206t
Teres minor muscle, 499, 505
Terminal hair, 122
Terry's nails, 150t
Test(s), selection and use of, 75b, –76b
Testes, 418
    abnormalities of, 424t
    in boys, 781b
    pain in, 765
    painless nodules in, 418
    small, 424t
    torsion of, in children, 765
    tumors of, 424t
    undescended, 725, 813t
Testicular cancer, 418, 420
Testicular self-examination, 416, 420, 420b
Tetanus, 815t
Tetralogy of Fallot, in infants, 809t
Thalamus, 596, 604
Thelarche, premature, 722
Thenar atrophy, 554t
Thenar space infection, 555t
Therapeutic relationship, 35b, 35–41
    active listening for, 36
    building, 35
    empathic responses and, 38–39
    empowering patient and, 40–41, 41b
    guided questioning and, 36–38, 37b
    nonverbal communication and, 38
    partnering and, 40
    reassurance and, 39
    sexuality and, 57
    transitions and, 40
    validation and, 39
Thin patients, blood pressure measurement in,
    110
Third heart sound, in older adults, 844
Thoracic kyphosis, 519
Thoracoabdominal paradox, 713
Thoracohumeral muscle group, 505
Thorax. *See also* Chest *entries; specific organs*

anatomic terms for locations on, 246
anatomy and physiology of, 241–247
anterior, examination of, 261–264
    auscultation in, 264
    inspection in, 261
    palpation in, 261–262
    percussion in, 263–264
anterior, in comprehensive physical examina-
    tion, 13
anteroposterior diameter of, 253
deformities of, 273t
examination techniques for, 252–265
    for children, 760–761
    for infants, 711–714, 712b, 714b
    in older adults, 864
    during pregnancy, 828
expansion of, testing, 254, 261
in health history, 248b, 248–250
initial survey of, 252–253
locating findings on, 242–244
in older adults, 843
posterior, in comprehensive physical exami-
    nation, 12
posterior, examination of, 253–261
    auscultation in, 258–261
    inspection in, 253
    palpation in, 253–255
    percussion in, 255–258
recording findings for, 266, 266b
retraction of, in infants, 713
Thought content, in mental status examina-
    tion, 574b
Thought processes
    content of, in mental status examination,
        582–583, 583b
    in mental status examination, 574b,
        581–582, 582b
Thrills, 306
    in infants, 717
Throat. *See also* Pharynx
    in comprehensive physical examination, 12
    examination techniques for
        for adolescents, 777
        in older adults, 862–864
    in review of systems, 9
    strep (streptococcal pharyngitis), 174
        in children, 760, 807t
Thromboangiitis obliterans, 488, 492t–493t
Thrombocytopenic purpura, skin in, 147t
Thrombophlebitis, superficial, 479, 487,
    492t–493t
Thrombosis, iliofemoral, 487
Thrush, 711
    in children, 806t
    palatal, 233t
Thumbs
    abduction of, carpal tunnel syndrome and, 541
    opposition of, testing, 621
    range of motion and maneuvers for,
        513–514
Thyroglossal duct cysts, 706, 710
Thyroid
    enlargement of, 239t
    signs and symptoms of dysfunction of, 239t
    single nodules of, 239t

Thyroid cartilage, 169
Thyroid gland, 169
    examination techniques for, 198–200
    during pregnancy, 817, 828
Thyroid isthmus, 199
TIAs (transient ischemic attacks), prevention
    of, 609–610
Tibia, 538
    torsion of, in infants, 729
Tibial artery, posterior, 474
Tibial plateau, lateral, 533
Tibial pulse, posterior, 485
Tibial torsion, in children, 770
Tibial tuberosity, 530
Tibia vara, 770
Tibiofemoral joints, 530
Tibiotalar joint, 538, 540
Tics, 654t
Time, orientation to, 585
Timing, clustering clinical data by, 73
Tinea capitis, 149t
    in children, 801t
Tinea corporis, 135t
    in children, 801t
Tinea faciale, 135t
Tinea versicolor, 132t, 134t
Tinel's sign, carpal tunnel syndrome and, 541
Tinnitus, 173
Titles, addressing patients using, 29
TMJ syndrome, 496
Tobacco use
    in health history, 7
    smoking cessation and, 250–251
    teeth and, 176
Toe(s), abnormalities of, 557t
Toenails, ingrown, 557t
Tongue, 166
    cancer of, 194–195
    of children, 759
    examination techniques for, 194
    findings in or under, 237t–238t
    sore, 174
    symmetry and position of, assessment of,
        612, 616
Tongue tie, 710
Tonic-clonic seizures, 652t
Tonic neck reflex, asymmetric, 735b
Tonic pupil, 182, 217t
Tonsil(s)
    of children, 760
    normal, large, 232t
Tonsillar fossa, 167
Tonsillar lymph nodes, 196
Tonsillar nodes, pulsating, 196
Tonsillitis, exudative, 232t
Tophi, 226t
Tori mandibulares, 238t
Torticollis, 518, 520, 704
    congenital, 706
Torus palatinus, 194, 233t
Total-body skin examination, 124
Touch sensation, 603–604
Tourette's syndrome, 654t
Toxic liver damage, 368
Toxoplasmosis, congenital, retinal changes in, 708

Trachea
    anatomy and physiology of, 246
    examination techniques for, 198
Tracheal breath sounds, 259b
Tracheal rings, 169
Tracheitis, bacterial, in infants, 712
Tracheobronchitis
    chest pain with, 268t–269t
    cough and hemoptysis in, 272t
Tragus, 160
Transformation zone, 430, 431
Transient ischemic attacks (TIAs), prevention
    of, 609–610
Transitions, in interview, 40
Transposition of the great arteries, in infants,
    810
Transverse lie, 833
Trapezius muscles, 517
Traube's space, 382
Treatment plans, negotiating, 34
Tremors, 653t–654t
    intention, 626
    in newborns, 691
    in older adults, 847, 868
Trendelenburg's sign, 770
Trendelenburg test, 490–491
Triceps muscle, 499, 506
Triceps reflex, 601, 635
Trichomonal vaginitis, 454t
Trichotillomania, 149t
Tricuspid regurgitation, 331t
Tricuspid stenosis, 304
Tricuspid valve, 281
    auscultation of sounds from, 286, 314
Trigeminal nerve, 495, 598, 599b
    of children, 772b
    examination of, 612, 613–614
    of infants, 732t
Trigeminal neuralgia, headache and, 208t–209t
Trigger finger, 513, 554t
Tripod position, 751
Trochanter, greater, 523, 524
Trochanteric bursa, 524, 526
Trochanteric bursitis, 488, 526
Trochlear groove, 530
Trochlear nerve, 598, 599b
    of children, 772b
    examination of, 611, 612
    in infants, 732b
    paralysis of, 218t
Truncus arteriosus, 717
Trunk, muscle strength of, testing, 622
Trunk incurvation reflex, 736b
Tubal pregnancy, ruptured, 457t
Tuberculosis, cough and hemoptysis in, 272t
Tuberous sclerosis, 799t
    skin in, 147t
Tug test, 189
Tumors. See also Cancer; specific tumors
    abdominal, 405t
    adrenal, in children, 765
    of brain, headache and, 208t–209t
    headache due to, 171
    oral, in older adults, 864
    pituitary, in children, 765

of skin, 142t
    testicular, 424t
Tunica vaginalis, 411, 412
Turbinates, 163
Turgor, of skin, in newborns, 702
Turner's syndrome, 701
T wave, 287
Two-point discrimination, 632
Tympanic membrane, 160, 161
    examination techniques for, 189–190
    temperature of, measuring, 113
Tympanosclerosis, 227t
Tympany, as percussion note, 256b

U
Ulcer(s)
    aphthous, 174, 194, 238t
    in arterial insufficiency, 495t
    nasal, 193
    neuropathic, 495t, 557t
    peptic, 394t–395t
    pressure, 128, 148t
        in older adults, 862
    of skin, 140t, 144t
    in venous insufficiency, 495t
    venous stasis, 479
Ulcerative colitis, 490
    diarrhea due to, 398t–399t
    skin in, 147t
Ulcerative gingivitis, acute necrotizing, 235t
Ulnar artery, 473
Ulnar nerve, 506
    compression of, 510
    disorders of, 554t
Ulnar pulse, 488
Umbilical artery, single, 723
Umbilical cord, 723
Umbilical granulomas, 723
Umbilical hernias, 404t, 723
Umbilicus amnioticus, 723
Umbilicus cutis, 723
Unreality, feelings of, 583b
Upper motor neurons, 603
Ureteral colic, 370
Urethral caruncles, 441, 451t
Urethral meatus, 411, 412, 429
Urethral mucosa, 441
    prolapse of, 451t
Urethral obstruction, 724
Urethral strictures, 386, 417
Urethritis
    gonococcal, 417
    nongonococcal, 417
Urge incontinence, 369, 402t–403t
Urinary frequency, 368–369, 401t
    during pregnancy, 821b
Urinary incontinence, 402t–403t
    functional, 369, 402t–403t
    overflow, 369, 402t–403t
    secondary to medications, 402t–403t
    stress, 368, 402t–403t
    urge, 369, 402t–403t
Urinary system
    in health history, 368–370
    in review of systems, 10

Urinary urgency, 368–369
Urine, color of, 367
Urticaria, 137t, 145t
    in children, 801t
Uterus, 430. See also Cervix, uterine
    abnormalities of, 456t
    anatomy and physiology of, 361
    bicornuate, 832–833
    contractions of, during pregnancy, 830
    palpation of, 445
    positions of, 455t
        during pregnancy, 818–819
    prolapse of, 456t
    retroflexion of, 446, 455t
    retroversion of, 446, 455t
Uvula, 167
    of children, 760

V
Vaccines, diseases preventable by, 815t
Vagina, 430
    inspection of, 445
        during pregnancy, 818, 832
Vaginal bleeding
    in children, 767
    intermenstrual, 433
    postcoital, 433
    postmenopausal, 432, 433
Vaginal discharge, 434, 454t
    in adolescents, 782
    in children, 767
Vaginismus, 434
Vaginitis
    candidal, 454t
    trichomonal, 454t
Vaginosis, bacterial, 454t
Vagus nerve, 598, 599b
    of children, 772b
    examination of, 612, 615
    of infants, 732t
Valgus stress test, 536b
Validation, in interview, 39
Validity, of tests, 75b
Valsalva maneuver
    to identify systolic murmurs, 320
    inguinal hernias and, 765
Values, 55
Valves
    cardiac. See Heart valves
    venous, evaluating competency of, 490–491
Valves of Houston, 460
Varicella, 815t
    skin in, 147t
Varicocele, 425t
Varicose veins, 487
    mapping, 490
        during pregnancy, 833
    of tongue, 238t
Varus stress test, 536b–537b
Vascular lesions, of skin, 141t
Vascular markings, in newborns, 701
Vascular rings, in infants, 712
Vas deferens, 411, 412
    infection of, 418
Vasodepressor syncope, 608, 649t–650t